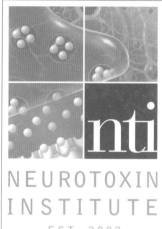

SCIENTIFIC AND THERAPEUTIC ASPECTS OF BOTULINUM TOXIN

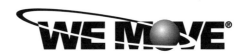

WE MOVE
204 W. 84th St.
New York, NY 10024
www.wemove.org

SCIENTIFIC AND THERAPEUTIC ASPECTS OF BOTULINUM TOXIN

Editors

Mitchell F. Brin, M.D., Mark Hallett, M.D.,
Joseph Jankovic, M.D.

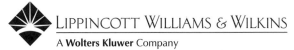

LIPPINCOTT WILLIAMS & WILKINS
A **Wolters Kluwer** Company
Philadelphia · Baltimore · New York · London
Buenos Aires · Hong Kong · Sydney · Tokyo

Editor: Charley Mitchell
Managing Editor: Jennifer Kullgren
Marketing Manager: Kate Rubin
Production Editor: Richard Adin
Purchasing Manager, Clinical and Healthcare: Jennifer Jett
Compositor: Maryland Composition
Printer: Edwards Brothers

On the cover: The three-dimensional x-ray crystallographic structure of botulinum toxin, the symbol of Toxins '99. Courtesy of Ray Stevens, Ph.D.

Library of Congress Cataloging-in-Publication Data

Scientific and therapeutic aspects of botulinum toxic / editors, Mitchell F. Brin, Joseph Jankovic, Mark Hallett.
    p. ; cm.
    Includes bibliographical references and index.
    ISBN 0-7817-3267-0 (alk. paper)
    1. Botulinum toxin. 2. Botulinum toxin—Therapeutic use. I. Brin, Mitchell F. II. Jankovic, Joseph. III. Hallett, Mark.
    [DNLM: 1. Botulinum Toxins—therapeutic use. 2. Tetanus Toxin—therapeutic use. 3. Botulinum Toxins—pharmacology. 4. Tetanus Toxin—pharmacology. QW 630.5.N4 S416 2002]
QP632.B66 S256 2002
615′.329364—dc21   2002141563

10 9 8 7 6 5 4 3 2 1

Preface

In November 1999, over 600 basic scientists and clinicians from throughout the world gathered in Orlando, Florida, to discuss the scientific and clinical aspects of botulinum and tetanus toxins. This conference was planned and produced by WE MOVE (Worldwide Education and Awareness for Movement Disorders), as an outgrowth of previous meetings devoted to either the basic science of neurotoxins (Madison, Wisconsin, 1992; Oxford, England, 1997), or to their use in clinical practice (Munich 1995). Our goal for this meeting was to provide an opportunity to share scientific and clinical experiences and to provoke further interest in fundamental neurotoxin research. The present volume is both a summary and an extension of that landmark event.

Botulinum toxin, produced by the bacterium *Clostridium botulinum,* has been under clinical investigation since the late 1970s. Beginning with the pioneering work of Dr. Alan Scott in the treatment of strabismus, the range of clinical applications has grown to encompass dystonia, spasticity, hyperhidrosis, gastrointestinal and genitourinary disorders, pain, headache, cosmetic conditions, and a host of additional novel applications associated either with excessive muscle contraction or pain. Over the years, the number of primary clinical publications has grown exponentially, and continues to increase every year. At the same time, basic scientific work on toxin structure and function has illuminated the fundamental mechanisms of action of these unique molecules, shedding light not only on the pharmacologic effects, but also the basic cell biology of synaptic vesicle release and recycling.

This unique therapy has also had an impact on our clinical practices. It has provided a new and powerful tool for therapeutic and medical management. It has raised both scientific and public awareness about dystonia, and other muscle-contraction or painful disorders. It has resulted in additional patients for clinical research. It has also brought together multiple disciplines to address and rethink human neurophysiology, and stretched our basic thinking about the pathophysiology of disease. These developments have highlighted the critical importance of understanding and supporting the basic science and clinical research of neurotoxins.

Toxin therapy provides a key example of the value of translational research, which relies on the iterative interplay between clinical observation and laboratory discovery. There are clinical applications of botulinum toxin therapy for which we do not fully understand why the therapy is efficacious. Basic scientific investigation has the potential to illuminate these mysteries, which, in turn, will allow us to address therapeutic issues more precisely.

The future of toxin therapy is predicated on the quality of the interaction of basic science and clinical science. It is our hope that this publication will further that interaction and lead to greater understanding and appreciation of these unique molecules and remarkable therapies.

We recognize that each botulinum neurotoxin product is distinct, and it is with great enthusiasm that we welcome novel serotypes and formulations into the therapeutic arena. The unique properties of each preparation may lead to treatment opportunities heretofore unexplored. Research is proceeding apace to further characterize the distinctive basic and clinical attributes of these fascinating proteins.

Neither a meeting of this scope nor a book of this depth would be possible without the generous efforts of many different people. We are grateful to the members of the Organizing Committee who worked diligently to bring the conference to fruition, and also to the corporate sponsors who supported this landmark meeting. Working in conjunction with WE MOVE staff, Dr. Linda Lyle, and Richard Robinson provided the editorial and organizational skills to produce this book. Finally, we are deeply grateful to Judith Blazer, Executive Director of WE MOVE, whose dedication and unstinting hard work made it all possible.

Mitchell F. Brin, MD
Mark Hallett, MD
Joseph Jankovic, MD

International Conference 1999 Basic and Therapeutic Aspects of Botulinum and Tetanus Toxins Orlando, Florida, November 16–18, 1999

Chairman

Mitchell F. Brin

Basic Science Committee

Michael Adler	Shunji Kozaki
Oliver Dolly	Elaine Neale
Keith Foster	Cesare Montecucco
Jane Halpern	Heiner Neimann
Eric Johnson	Lance Simpson

Clinical Science Committee

Alberto Albanese	Joseph Jankovic
Stephen Arnon	Ryuji Kaji
Michael Barnes	Andrew Lees
Reiner Benecke	Ivan Lorentz
Andrew Blitzer	Werner Poewe
Cynthia Comella	Eduardo Tolosa
Mark Hallett	

Sponsor

WE MOVE

Funded in part by unrestricted educational grants from:

Allergan, Inc.
Elan Phamaceuticals, Inc.
Ipsen, Ltd.

Contents

I. Basic Sciences: Mechanism of Action

1. The Metalloprotease Activity of Tetanus and Botulinum Neurotoxins 3
   Ornella Rossetto, Paola Caccin, Michela Rigoni, Michela Seveso,
   Fiorella Tonello, Cesare Montecucco

2. Structural View of Botulinum Neurotoxin in Numerous Functional States 11
   Michael A. Hanson, Raymond C. Stevens

3. Crystal Structure of *Clostridium botulinum* Neurotoxin Serotype B 29
   Subramanyam Swaminathan, Subramaniam Eswaramoorthy

4. The Receptor Binding Domains of Clostridial Neurotoxins 41
   J. Mark Sutton, Lindsey Spaven, Nigel J. Silman, Bassam Hallis,
   Oliver Chow-Worn, Clifford C. Shone

5. Neurospecific Binding and Trafficking of Tetanus Toxin 49
   Giovanna Lalli, Judit Herreros, Giampietro Schiavo

6. Botulinum Neurotoxin A and Synaptic Vesicle Trafficking 61
   Elaine A. Neale

7. Molecular Basis of the Unique Endopeptidase Activity of Botulinum
   Neurotoxin 75
   Bal Ram Singh

II. Pharmacology of Botulinum Neurotoxins

8. Insights into the Extended Duration of Neuroparalysis by Botulinum
   Neurotoxin A Relative to the Other Shorter-Acting Serotypes: Differences
   Between Motor Nerve Terminals and Cultured Neurons 91
   J. Oliver Dolly, Godfrey Lisk, Patrick G. Foran, Frederic Meunier,
   Nadiem Mohammed, G. O'Sullivan, Anton de Paiva

9. Immunologic and Other Properties of Therapeutic Botulinum Toxin
   Serotypes 103
   K. Roger Aoki

10. Production, Quality, and Stability of Botulinum Toxin Type B
    (MYOBLOC℠) for Clinical Use 115
    James E. Callaway, Andrew J. Grethlein

11. Spread of Paralysis to Nearby and Distant Noninjected Muscles in a
    Monkey Hand Model: Comparison of BoNT-B and BoNT-A 123
    Joseph C. Arezzo, Mona S. Litwak, Florence A. Caputo, Kathleen E. Meyer,
    George M. Shopp

12. The Glycogen Depletion Assay and the Measurement of Botulinum Toxin
Injections 135
Asif Amirali, Ira Sanders

III. Clinical Diseases

13. Clinical Botulism 145
Stephen S. Arnon

14. Clinical Aspects of Tetanus 151
John C. Morgan, Thomas P. Bleck

IV. Neurophysiology

15. Effects of Botulinum Toxin at the Neuromuscular Junction 167
Mark Hallett

16. Effects of Botulinum Toxin Type A on Central Nervous System Function ... 171
Alfredo Berardelli, Francesca Gilio, Antonio Currà

17. Impact of Botulinum Toxin on Laryngeal Physiology 179
Christy L. Ludlow

V. Clinical Therapeutics

18. The Role of Botulinum Toxin Type A in the Management of Strabismus 189
Alan Scott

19. The Role of Botulinum Toxin Type A (BOTOX®) in the Management of
Blepharospasm and Hemifacial Spasm 197
Joseph A. Mauriello, Jr.

20. Botulinum Toxin Type A Injections for the Management of the
Hyperfunctional Larynx 207
Andrew Blitzer, Craig Zalvan, Omar Gonzalez-Yanez, Mitchell F. Brin

21. The Use of Botulinum Toxin in Juvenile Cerebral Palsy 217
Mauricio R. Delgado

22. Botulinum Toxin Type A in the Treatment of Spasticity 223
A.P. Moore

23. Botulinum Toxin Type A BOTOX® for Pain and Headache 233
*Mitchell F. Brin, William Binder, Andrew Blitzer, Lawrence Schenrock,
Janice M. Pogoda*

24. The Role of Botulinum Toxin Type A in the Management of Occupational
Dystonia and Writer's Cramp 251
Barbara Illowsky Karp

25. Botulinum Toxin A Therapy for Temporomandibular Disorders 259
Marvin Schwartz, Brian Freund

26. The Role of Botulinum Toxin in Gastrointestinal Disorders 269
   Giuseppe Brisinda, Giorgio Maria, Anna Rita Bentivoglio, Alberto Albanese

27. Botulinum Toxin Type A in the Treatment of Hyperfunctional Facial Lines
   and Cosmetic Disorders 287
   Alastair Carruthers, Jean Carruthers

28. Botulinum Toxin for Achalasia and Related Disorders 295
   Willemijntje A. Hoogerwerf, Dennis D. Dykstra, Pankaj J. Pasricha

29. Treatment of Focal Hyperhidrosis with Botulinum Toxin A 303
   Markus Naumann

30. The Use of Botulinum Toxins in the Management of Myofascial Pain and
   Other Conditions Associated with Painful Muscle Spasm 309
   Mike A. Royal

31. Botulinum Toxin Treatment in Tremors 323
   Jyh-Gong Hou, Joseph Jankovic

32. Botulinum Toxin in the Treatment of Tics 337
   Carolyn H. Kwak, Joseph Jankovic

33. Botulinum Toxin Type A in the Management of Oromandibular Dystonia
   and Bruxism 343
   Ron Tintner, Joseph Jankovic

34. Use of Botulinum Toxin in Urologic Disorders 351
   Dennis D. Dykstra

VI. Clinical Trials

35. Cervical Dystonia: Treatment with Botulinum Toxin Serotype A as
   BOTOX® or Dysport® 359
   Cynthia L. Comella

36. Studies with Dysport® in Cervical Dystonia 365
   Werner Poewe, Tanja Entner

37. Review of Clinical Efficacy Studies with Botulinum Toxin Type B
   (MYOBLOC™) for Cervical Dystonia 371
   Stewart A. Factor

VII. Immunology of Botulinum Toxin

38. Immune Recognition and Cross-Reactivity of Botulinum Neurotoxins 385
   M. Zouhair Atassi

39. Botulinum Toxin: Clinical Implications of Antigenicity and
   Immunoresistance 409
   Joseph Jankovic

40. Managing Patients with Botulinum Toxin Antibodies 417
   Dirk Dressler

41. Vaccines for Preventing Botulism 427
   Leonard A. Smith, Michael P. Byrne

VIII. Other Serotypes and Chemodenervating Agents

42. Botulinum Neurotoxin Serotypes C and E: Clinical Trials 441
   Roberto Eleopra, Valeria Tugnoli, Rocco Quatrale, Ornella Rossetto,
   Cesare Montecucco, Domenico De Grandis

43. Long-Term Use of Botulinum Toxin Type F to Treat Patients Resistant to
   Botulinum Toxin Type A 451
   Paul E. Greene

44. Muscle Afferent Block for Dystonia: Implications for the Physiological
   Mechanism of Action of Botulinum Toxin 455
   Ryuji Kaji

45. Electromyography-Guided Chemodenervation with Phenol in Cervical
   Dystonia (Spasmodic Torticollis) 459
   Janice M. Massey

46. Immunotoxin 463
   Mark Hallett

IX. Novel Toxin Constructs

47. Hybrid and Chimeric Botulinum Toxin Molecules 469
   Eric A. Johnson, Michael C. Goodnough, Carl M. Malizio,
   William H. Tepp, Sean S. Dineen, Marite Bradshaw

48. Novel Toxin Developments: Delivery of Endopeptidase Activity of
   Botulinum Neurotoxin to New Target Cells 477
   Keith A. Foster

49. Neuronal Delivery Vectors Derived from Tetanus Toxin 485
   Paul S. Fishman

Index 495

Contributors

Alberto Albanese, M.D.
Istituto Nazionale Neurologico Carlo Besta
Università Cattolica del Sacro Cuore
Milano, Italy

Asif Amirali, M.D.
Department of Otolaryngology
Mount Sinai School of Medicine
New York, New York USA

K. Roger Aoki, Ph.D.
Biological Sciences
Allergan, Inc.
Irvine, California USA

Joseph C. Arezzo, Ph.D.
Departments of Neuroscience and Neurology
Albert Einstein College of Medicine
Bronx, New York USA

Stephen S. Arnon, M.D.
Founder and Chief
Infant Botulism Treatment and Prevention
*   Program*
California Department of Health Services
Berkeley, California USA

M. Zouhair Atassi, Ph.D., D.Sc.
Department of Biochemistry and Molecular
*   Biology*
Department of Immunology
Baylor College of Medicine
Houston, Texas USA

Anna Rita Bentivoglio, M.D., Ph.D.
Istituto di Neurologia
Università Cattolica del Sacro Cuore
Roma, Italy

Alfredo Berardelli
Dipartimento di Scienze Neurologiche
Università di Roma ''La Sapienza''
Roma and Istituto Neurologico Mediterraneo
*   ''Neuromed'', IRCCS*
Pozzilli, Italia

William Binder, M.D.
Associate Clinical Professor, UCLA School of
*   Medicine*
Attending Surgeon, Cedars Sinai Medical Center
Beverly Hills, California USA

Thomas P. Bleck, M.D., FCCM
Professor of Neurology, Neurological Surgery, and
*   Medicine*
The Louise Nerancy Eminent Scholar in Neurology
Director, Division of Critical Care
Department of Neurology
University of Virginia
Charlottesville, Virginia USA

Andrew Blitzer, M.D., D.D.S.
Professor of Clinical Otolaryngology
Columbia University
Director, New York Center for Voice and
*   Swallowing Disorders*
St. Luke's/Roosevelt Hospital Center
New York, New York USA

Marite Bradshaw, Ph.D.
Department of Food Microbiology and Toxicology
Food Research Institute
University of Wisconsin
Madison, Wisconsin USA

Mitchell F. Brin, M.D.
Vice President Development, and Therapeutic Area
*   Head*
BOTOX/Neurology
Allergan, Inc.
Irvine, California USA
*   and*
Bachmann-Strauss Professor of Neurology
The Mount Sinai School of Medicine
New York, New York USA

Giuseppe Brisinda, M.D.
Istituto di Clinica Chirurgica
Università Cattolica del Sacro Cuore
Roma, Italy

Michael P. Byrne, Ph.D.
Human Genome Sciences, Inc.
Rockville, Maryland USA

Paola Caccin
Centro CNR Biomembrane and Dipartimento di Scienze Biomediche
Università di Padova
Padova, Italy

James E. Callaway, Ph.D.
Elan Pharmaceuticals
San Diego, California USA

Florence A. Caputo, Ph.D.
Sierra BioMedical, Inc.
Sparks, Nevada USA

Alastair Carruthers, M.D.
Division of Dermatology
University of British Columbia
Vancouver, British Columbia Canada

Jean Carruthers, M.D.
Department of Ophthalmology
University of British Columbia
Vancouver, British Columbia Canada

Oliver Chow-Worn
Centre for Applied Microbiology and Research (CAMR),
Porton Down,
Salisbury, Wiltshire UK

Cynthia L. Comella, M.D.
Department of Neurological Sciences
Rush-Presbyterian-St. Luke's Medical Center
Chicago, Illinois USA

Antonio Currà
Dipartimento di Scienze Neurologiche
Università di Roma "La Sapienza"
Roma and Istituto Neurologico Mediterraneo "Neuromed", IRCCS
Pozzilli, Italia

Domenico De Grandis, M.D.
Department of Clinical Neuroscience, Neurology Section
Hospital of Rovigo
Rovigo, Italy

Mauricio R. Delgado, M.D., F.R.C.P.(C)
Professor of Neurology
University of Texas Southwestern Medical School
Director of Pediatric Neurology
Texas Scottish Rite Hospital for Children
Dallas, Texas USA

Anton de Paiva, B.Sc., Ph.D.
Centre for Neurobiochemistry
Dept. Biological Sciences
Imperial College of Science, Technology & Medicine
London, UK

Sean S. Dineen, B.S.
Department of Food Microbiology and Toxicology
Food Research Institute
University of Wisconsin
Madison, Wisconsin USA

J. Oliver Dolly, B.Sc. (Hons.), M.Sc., Ph.D.
Centre for Neurobiochemistry
Dept. Biological Sciences
Imperial College of Science, Technology & Medicine
London, UK

Dirk Dressler, M.D.
Department of Neurology
Rostock University
Rostock, Germany

Dennis D. Dykstra, M.D., Ph.D., M.H.A.
Department of Physical Medicine and Rehabilitation
University of Minnesota
Minneapolis, Minnesota USA

Roberto Eleopra, M.D.
Neurologist and Clinical Neurophysiologist
Department of Clinical Neuroscience, Neurology Section
University Hospital S. Anna
Ferrara, Italy

Tanja Entner, M.D.
Department of Neurology
University Hospital Innsbruck
Innsbruck, Austria

Subramaniam Eswaramoorthy, Ph.D.
Biology Department
Brookhaven National Laboratory
Upton, New York USA

Stewart A. Factor, D.O.
Professor of Neurology
Riley Family Chair in Parkinson's Disease
Parkinson's Disease and Movement Disorder Center of Albany Medical Center
Albany, New York USA

Paul S. Fishman, M.D., Ph.D.
Department of Neurology
University of Maryland, School of Medicine
Baltimore VA Medical Center
Baltimore, Maryland USA

Patrick G. Foran, B.Sc., Ph.D.
Centre for Neurobiochemistry
Dept. Biological Sciences
Imperial College of Science, Technology &
*   Medicine*
London, UK

Keith A. Foster, M.A., Ph.D.
Centre for Applied Microbiology and Research
*   (CAMR)*
Porton Down, Salisbury
Wiltshire, UK

Brian Freund, B.Sc., D.D.S., M.D.,
**   F.R.C.P.C.**
The Crown Institute
Toronto, Ontario Canada

Francesca Gilio
Dipartimento di Scienze Neurologiche
Università di Roma ''La Sapienza''
Roma and Istituto Neurologico Mediterraneo
*   ''Neuromed,'' IRCCS*
Pozzilli, Italy

Omar Gonzalez-Yanez, M.D.
New York Center for Voice and Swallowing
*   Disorders at*
St. Luke's/Roosevelt Hospital Center
Columbia University
New York, New York USA

Michael C. Goodnough, Ph.D.
Department of Food Microbiology and Toxicology
Food Research Institute
University of Wisconsin
Madison, Wisconsin USA

Paul E. Greene, M.D.
Columbia-Presbyterian Medical Center
New York, New York USA

Andrew J. Grethlein, Ph.D.
Elan Pharmaceuticals
South San Francisco, California USA

Mark Hallett, M.D.
Chief, Human Motor Control Section, NINDS
National Institutes of Health
Bethesda, Maryland USA

Bassam Hallis, Ph.D.
Centre for Applied Microbiology and Research
*   (CAMR)*
Porton Down
Salisbury, Wiltshire UK

Michael A. Hanson
Department of Chemistry
The Scripps Research Institute
La Jolla, California USA

Judit Herreros, Ph.D.
Molecular NeuroPathobiology Laboratory
Imperial Cancer Research Fund
London, UK

Willemijntje A. Hoogerwerf, M.D.
Division of Gastroenterology
University of Texas Medical Branch
Galveston, Texas USA

Jyh-Gong Hou, M.D., Ph.D.
Parkinson's Disease Center and Movement
*   Disorders Clinic*
Department of Neurology
Baylor College of Medicine
Houston, Texas USA

Joseph Jankovic, M.D.
Parkinson's Disease Center and Movement
*   Disorders Clinic*
Department of Neurology
Baylor College of Medicine
Houston, Texas USA

Eric A. Johnson, Sc.D.
Department of Food Microbiology and Toxicology
Food Research Institute
University of Wisconsin
Madison, Wisconsin USA

Ryuji Kaji, M.D., Ph.D.
Professor and Chairman
Department of Clinical Neuroscience
Hospital of the University of Tokushima
Tokushima City, Tokushima Japan

Barbara Illowsky Karp, M.D.
Office of the Clinical Director
National Institute of Neurological Disorders and
*   Stroke*
National Institutes of Health
Bethesda, Maryland USA

Carolyn H. Kwak, M.S., PA-C
*Parkinson's Disease Center and Movement
    Disorders Clinic*
Department of Neurology
Baylor College of Medicine
Houston, Texas USA

Giovanna Lalli, Ph.D.
Molecular NeuroPathobiology Laboratory
Imperial Cancer Research Fund
London, UK

Godfrey Lisk, B.Sc. (Hons.)
Centre for Neurobiochemistry
Dept. Biological Sciences
*Imperial College of Science, Technology &
    Medicine*
London, UK

Mona S. Litwak
Departments of Neuroscience and Neurology
Albert Einstein College of Medicine
Bronx, New York USA

Christy L. Ludlow, Ph.D.
Chief, Laryngeal and Speech Section
Medical Neurology Branch
*National Institute of Neurological Disorders and
    Stroke*
Bethesda, Maryland USA

Carl M. Malizio, B.S.
Department of Food Microbiology and Toxicology
Food Research Institute
University of Wisconsin
Madison, Wisconsin USA

Giorgio Maria, M.D.
Istituto di Clinica Chirurgica
Università Cattolica del Sacro Cuore
Roma, Italy

Janice M. Massey, M.D.
Professor of Neurology
Duke University Medical Center
Durham, North Carolina USA

Joseph A. Mauriello, Jr., M.D.
Clinical Associate Professor of Ophthalmology
Department of Ophthalmology
UMD-New Jersey Medical School
Summit, New Jersey USA

Frederic Meunier, B.Sc., Ph.D.
Centre for Neurobiochemistry
Dept. Biological Sciences
*Imperial College of Science, Technology &
    Medicine*
London, UK

Kathleen E. Meyer, Ph.D.
Elan Pharmaceuticals
South San Francisco, California USA

Nadiem Mohammed, B.Sc., Ph.D.
Centre for Neurobiochemistry
Dept. Biological Sciences
*Imperial College of Science, Technology &
    Medicine*
London, UK

Cesare Montecucco, Ph.D.
*Centro CNR Biomembrane and Dipartimento di
    Scienze Biomediche*
Università di Padova
Padova, Italy

**A.P. Moore, M.B., Ch.B., F.R.C.P.(UK),
M.D.**
Senior Lecturer in Neurology
Department of Neuroscience, Liverpool University
*The Walton Centre for Neurology and
    Neurosurgery*
Liverpool, UK

John C. Morgan, M.D., Ph.D.
Department of Neurology
University of Virginia
Charlottesville, Virginia USA

Markus Naumann, M.D.
Assistant Professor of Neurology
Department of Neurology
University of Würzburg
Germany

Elaine A. Neale, Ph.D.
Laboratory of Developmental Neurobiology
*National Institute of Child Health and Human
    Development*
National Institutes of Health
Bethesda, Maryland USA

G. O'Sullivan, B.Sc., Ph.D.
Centre for Neurobiochemistry
Dept. Biological Sciences
*Imperial College of Science, Technology &
    Medicine*
London, UK

Pankaj J. Pasricha, M.D.
*Enteric Neuromuscular Disorders and Pain
  Laboratory
Division of Gastroenterology and Hepatology
University of Texas Medical Branch
Galveston, Texas USA*

Werner Poewe, M.D.
*Department of Neurology
University Hospital Innsbruck
Innsbruck, Austria*

Janice M. Pogoda, Ph.D.
*Statology
Rocklin, California USA*

Rocco Quatrale, M.D.
*Department of Clinical Neuroscience, Neurology
  Section
University Hospital S. Anna
Ferrara, Italy*

Michela Rigoni
*Centro CNR Biomembrane and Dipartimento di
  Scienze Biomediche
Università di Padova
Padova, Italy*

Ornella Rossetto, Ph.D.
*Centro CNR Biomembrane and Dipartimento di
  Scienze Biomediche
Università di Padova
Padova, Italy*

Mike A. Royal, M.D.
*Elan Biopharmaceuticals
San Diego, California USA*

Ira Sanders, M.D.
*Department of Otolaryngology
Mount Sinai School of Medicine
New York, New York USA*

Lawrence Schenrock, M.D.
Deceased

Giampietro Schiavo, Ph.D.
*Molecular NeuroPathobiology Laboratory
Imperial Cancer Research Fund
London, UK*

Marvin Schwartz, B.Sc., D.D.S., M.Sc.
*The Crown Institute
Toronto, Ontario Canada*

Alan B. Scott, M.D.
*Smith–Kettlewell Eye Research Institute
San Francisco, California USA*

Michela Seveso, Ph.D.
*Centro CNR Biomembrane and Dipartimento di
  Scienze Biomediche
Università di Padova
Padova, Italy*

Clifford C. Shone, Ph.D.
*Centre for Applied Microbiology and Research
  (CAMR)
Porton Down
Salisbury, Wiltshire UK*

George M. Shopp, Ph.D.
*Elan Pharmaceuticals
South San Francisco, California USA*

Nigel J. Silman, Ph.D.
*Centre for Applied Microbiology and Research
  (CAMR)
Porton Down
Salisbury, Wiltshire UK*

Bal Ram Singh, Ph.D.
*Department of Chemistry and Biochemistry
School of Marine Science and Technology
University of Massachusetts Dartmouth
Dartmouth, Massachusetts USA*

Leonard A. Smith, Ph.D.
*Chief, Department of Immunology and Molecular
  Biology
Division of Toxinology and Aerobiology
United States Army Medical Research Institute of
  Infectious Diseases
Fort Detrick, Maryland USA*

Lindsey Spaven
*Centre for Applied Microbiology and Research
  (CAMR)
Porton Down
Salisbury, Wiltshire UK*

Raymond C. Stevens, Ph.D.
*Departments of Chemistry and Molecular Biology
The Scripps Research Institute
La Jolla, California USA*

J. Mark Sutton, Ph.D.
*Centre for Applied Microbiology and Research
  (CAMR)
Porton Down
Salisbury, Wiltshire UK*

Subramanyam Swaminathan, Ph.D.
Biology Department
Brookhaven National Laboratory
Upton, New York USA

William H. Tepp, B.S.
Department of Food Microbiology and Toxicology
Food Research Institute
University of Wisconsin
Madison, Wisconsin USA

Ron Tintner, M.D.
Parkinson's Disease Center and Movement
Disorders Clinic
Department of Neurology
Baylor College of Medicine
Houston, Texas USA

Fiorella Tonello, Ph.D.
C.R.I.B.I.
Università di Padova
Padova, Italy

Valeria Tugnoli, M.D.
Department of Clinical Neuroscience, Neurology
Section
University Hospital S. Anna
Ferrara, Italy

Craig Zalvan, M.D.
New York Center for Voice and Swallowing
Disorders
St. Luke's/Roosevelt Hospital Center
Columbia University
New York, New York USA

BASIC SCIENCES: MECHANISM OF ACTION

Scientific and Therapeutic Aspects of Botulinum Toxin
edited by M.F. Brin, J. Jankovic, and M. Hallett
Lippincott Williams & Wilkins, Philadelphia, © 2002.

1

The Metalloprotease Activity of Tetanus and Botulinum Neurotoxins

Ornella Rossetto, Paola Caccin, Michela Rigoni, Michela Seveso,
Fiorella Tonello, and Cesare Montecucco

Metalloproteases are hydrolytic enzymes that catalyze a metal-dependent cleavage of peptide bonds. The active site metal atom is usually zinc. They include aminopeptidases, carboxypeptidases, and endopeptidases depending on whether they remove an N- or a C-terminal residue or cleave internal peptide bonds of the protein substrate. The signature of zinc-dependent endopeptidases is an active site zinc-binding motif consisting of His-Glu-X-X-His (1). Perhaps thousands of different metalloproteases are produced by microorganisms; most of them are still to be characterized. They can nowadays be identified by genomic searches using the metalloprotease signature. They are involved in metabolic activities or are released extracellularly to cleave substrates not elaborated by the microorganism itself.

The recent determination of the primary sequence of clostridial neurotoxins, which are responsible for tetanus and botulism, has led to the discovery of their metalloproteolytic activity. The protease domain of these toxins enters into the cytosol where it displays a zinc-dependent endopeptidase activity of remarkable specificity. Tetanus and botulinum toxins cleave three protein components of the neuroexocytosis machinery leading to the blockade of neurotransmitter release and consequent paralysis. Botulinum neurotoxins (BoNTs) are increasingly used in medicine for the treatment of human diseases characterized by hyperfunction of cholinergic terminals, while tetanus neurotoxin (TeNT) still awaits the exploitation of its therapeutic potentials.

TeNT and BoNT were identified as the sole cause of tetanus and botulism, respectively, a little over a century ago, after the discovery of the anaerobic and spore-forming bacteria of the genus *Clostridium* (2–4). Seven types of BoNT (indicated with letters from A to G) differing in antigenicity and biochemical activity are known (5,6). BoNTs bind to and enter peripheral cholinergic terminals, causing a sustained block of acetylcholine (ACh) release, with ensuing flaccid paralysis and autonomic symptoms. Tetanus neurotoxin blocks neurotransmitter release at the inhibitory interneurons of the spinal cord, resulting in a frequently lethal spastic paralysis. Hence, despite the opposite clinical symptoms of tetanus and botulism, clostridial neurotoxins affect the same neuronal function: neuroexocytosis (7,8).

GENETICS AND STRUCTURE

Clostridial neurotoxins are always encoded by genes located on mobile genetic elements, which explains why nontoxigenic and toxigenic strains of *Clostridium tetani* and *Clostridium botulinum* are known and why they can be interconverted. TeNT and BoNT/G encoding genes are contained within large plasmids. In *C. botulinum,* the neurotoxin genes for A, B, E, and F have a chromosomal localization, whereas the C and D toxin encoding genes are present within bacteriophages. Usually one bacterium harbors one toxin gene, but several cases of multiple toxin genes have been reported (9). The clostridial neurotoxins are made in the bacterial cytosol and are released by bacterial autolysis as single polypeptide chains of 150 kDa, which are later activated by a specific proteolytic cleavage within a loop subtended by a highly conserved disulfide bridge (10). The heavy chain (H, 100 kDa) and the light chain (L, 50 kDa) remain associated via noncovalent interactions and by the conserved interchain S-S bond. The integrity of this disulfide bond is essential for neurotoxicity, but it has to be reduced to free the metalloproteolytic activity of the L chain in the cytosol (11) (Fig. 1.1).

The crystallographic structures of BoNT/A and BoNT/B and of the C-terminal part of the heavy chain of TeNT revealed that the 50-kDa receptor-binding domain, termed H_c, consists of two subdomains (12–14). The N-terminal part of H_c (H_cN) consists of 16 β-strands and 4 α-helices arranged in a jelly roll motif, closely similar to that of carbohydrate-binding proteins of the legume lectin family (14,15). The amino acid sequence of this subdomain is highly conserved among BoNTs and TeNT, suggesting a closely similar three-dimensional structure. At variance, the sequence of the C-terminal part of H_c (H_cC) is poorly conserved, but folds similarly to proteins of the trypsin inhibitor family. On the basis of experiments performed with TeNT, it was suggested that H_cC plays a major role in neurospecific binding (16).

The N-terminal part of the heavy chain (H_N) features two ~100-Å-long antiparallel α-helices, similar to those of the membrane interacting proteins, colicins and influenza hemagglutinin (14,15). The H_N domains of the clostridial neurotoxins (CNTs) are highly homologous and their predicted secondary structures are also highly similar, in agreement with their proposed role in transmembrane translocation of the L chain (15,17). The N-terminal domain is the L chain of clostridial neurotoxins and it is the metalloprotease which exerts its action in the cytosol of nerve terminals.

The structural organization of the CNTs is tailored to perform their mode of neuron intoxication, which consists of four steps (17,18): (a) binding; (b) internalization; (c) membrane translocation; and (d) proteolytic cleavage of their substrates (Fig. 1.2).

NEURONAL INTOXICATION

From the site of production or adsorption (intestine or wounds), BoNTs and TeNT diffuse in the body fluids, up to the presynaptic membrane of cholinergic terminals where they bind very specifically. The H_c domain plays a major role in neurospecific binding (19), but additional regions may be involved in determining the remarkable specificity for cholinergic terminals of CNTs.

Several investigators have attempted to identify the presynaptic receptor(s) of CNTs. Polysialogangliosides are certainly involved (20–22) together with as yet unidentified proteins of the presynaptic membrane (23). The presence of both lectin-like and protein binding subdomains in the H_c domain supports the suggestion that CNTs bind strongly and specifically to the presynaptic membrane because they display multiple interactions with sugar- and protein-binding sites (14,15). Identification of the receptors for the various CNTs will constitute a major advance in the understanding of the mechanism of neuron intoxication and will help to improve current therapeutic protocols employing BoNT to treat human syndromes of hyperfunction of cholinergic terminals and excessive muscle contraction.

As depicted in Fig. 1.2, the L chains of CNTs block neuroexocytosis by acting in the cytosol and they reach this cell compartment following endocytosis and membrane translocation. They are internalized inside acidic cellular compartments via endocytosis (24). Nerve stimulation facilitates intoxication by CNTs (25) and a close link exists between stimulus-contraction coupling and endocytosis at nerve terminals (26). Endocytosis and other factors such as nerve stimulation-dependent proteolytic activity in the cytosol (27) may partly account for this effect, which is potentially very relevant for the development of novel protocols of therapy employing BoNT. The protein receptor of TeNT is responsible for its entry inside vesicles moving retrogradely inside the axon, whereas BoNTs protein receptors guide them inside vesicles that acidify within the neuromuscular junction (NMJ). The TeNT-containing vesicles carry the toxin up

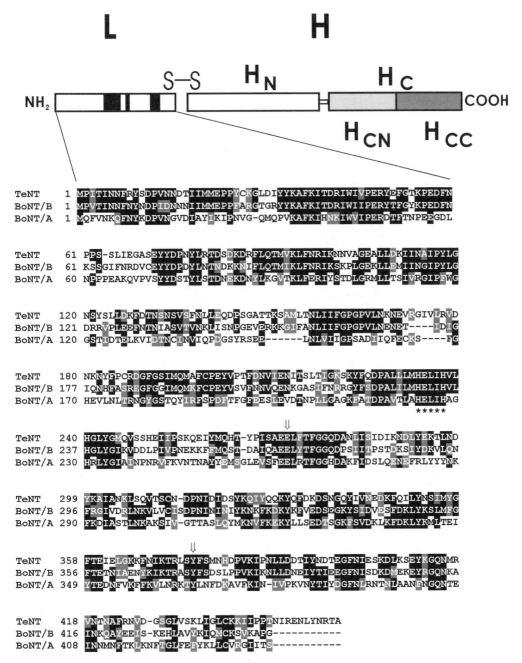

FIG. 1.1. The three-functional domain structure of clostridial neurotoxins (CNTs). Schematic structure of activated di-chain CNTs and aminoacidic sequence of TeNT, BoNT/B and BoNT/A L-chains. The neurotoxins are composed of two polypeptide-chain held together by a single disulfide bridge. The C-terminal portion of the heavy chain (H, 100 kDa) is responsible for neurospecific binding (domain H_C) while the N-terminus (H_N) is implicated in the translocation of the light chain in cytosol and pore formation. Structurally H_C can be further subdivided into two portions of 25 kDa: H_CN and H_CC. The light chain (L, 50 kDa) is a zinc-endopeptidase responsible for the intracellular activity of CNTs. The zinc-binding motif in the central part of the L chain is indicated by an asterisk. Amino acids E262 and Y366 that we mutated in BoNT/A are indicated by an arrow.

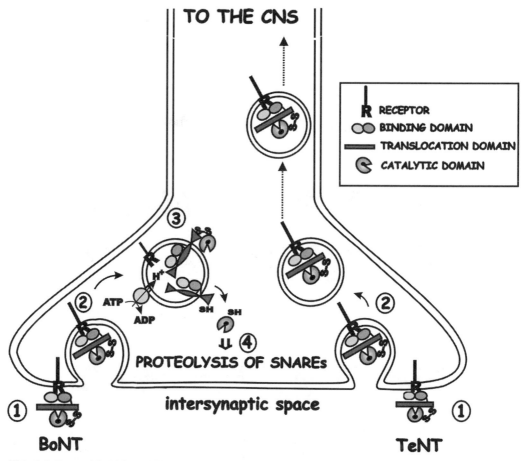

FIG. 1.2. Entry of BoNTs and TeNT inside nerve terminals. (1) BoNTs and TeNT bind to the presynaptic membrane at as-yet unidentified receptors of peripheral nerve terminals. (2) The protein receptor of TeNT is responsible for its inclusion in an endocytic vesicle that moves in a retrograde direction along the axon to the inhibitory interneurons of the spinal cord (CNS), whereas BoNT protein receptors guide them inside vesicles that acidify within the neuromuscular junction (NMJ). (3) At low pH, BoNTs and TeNT change conformation, insert into the lipid bilayer of the vesicle membrane and translocate the L chain into the cytosol of peripheral and central neurons respectively. (4) Inside the cytosol, the L chain catalyzes the proteolysis of one of the three SNARE proteins.

dendritic terminals and release it in the intersynaptic space. TeNT then enters the inhibitory interneurons of the spinal cord via synaptic vesicle endocytosis.

To reach the cytosol the L chain has to translocate across the vesicle membrane (Fig. 1.2) and the acidity of the lumen is essential for such a movement. Clostridial neurotoxins have to be acidified for nerve intoxication to occur (28) because the acidic environment causes a conformational change from a water-soluble "neutral" structure to an "acid" structure characterized by

the surface exposure of hydrophobic patches, which lead the H and L chains in the hydrocarbon core of the lipid bilayer (29). Following the low-pH-induced membrane insertion, BoNTs and TeNT form transmembrane ion channels in planar lipid bilayers of low conductance (30,31). There is a general consensus that the toxin channels participate in the process of transmembrane translocation of the L domain, from the vesicle membrane to the nerve terminal cytosol, but there is no agreement on how this process may take place. One hypothesis envisages that the L chain translocates across the vesicle membrane within a channel opened laterally to lipids, whereas the alternative model proposes that the L chains move inside a proteinaceous pore (18).

METALLOPROTEASE ACTIVITY OF CLOSTRIDIAL NEUROTOXINS

Once in the cytosol, the L chain of clostridial neurotoxins displays its metalloproteolytic activity. These enzymes are characterized by a long, cleft-shaped, active site containing the zinc atom coordinated via the two histidines and the glutamic acid of the zinc-binding motif, and by Glu262 in BoNT/A and Glu268 in BoNT/B, a residue conserved among clostridial neurotoxins which corresponds to Glu271 of TeNT (Fig. 1.1). The Glu residue of the motif (Glu224 in BoNT/A, Glu231 in BoNT/B and Glu234 in TeNT) plays the fundamental role of coordinating the water molecule which performs the hydrolytic reaction of proteolysis. Its mutation leads to complete inactivation of these neurotoxins (32,33). The critical role of Glu271 of TeNT and Glu262 in BoNT/A is that of providing a negatively charged carboxylate moiety (34 and below). This active site architecture is similar to that of thermolysin and identifies a primary sphere of residues essential to the catalytic function, which coincides with the zinc coordinating residues. In addition, it appears that a secondary layer of residues, less close to the zinc center, is present at the active site of clostridial neurotoxins. Among these residues, Arg363 and Tyr366 in BoNT/A could play a role in the catalytic activity of this family of metalloproteases. In particular, the phenolic ring of Tyr366 in BoNT/A (corresponding to Tyr373 in BoNT/B and to Tyr375 in TeNT) points inside the cleft-shaped active site of the toxin (14,15). The Ala substitution of Tyr375 inactivates the TeNT L chain, clearly indicating that this residue plays a critical role in the hydrolysis of the substrate (34). It has been proposed that Tyr373 of BoNT/B assists the hydrolysis reaction by donating a proton to the amide nitrogen of vesicle-associated membrane protein (VAMP) Phe77 which, together with bound water molecules, stabilizes the leaving group (35).

The active site of the L chain faces the H chain in the unreduced toxin and becomes accessible to the substrate upon reduction of the interchain S-S bond. Their proteolytic activity is zinc-dependent and heavy metal chelators such as orthophenanthroline, which remove bound zinc, generating inactive apo-neurotoxins, but the active site metal atom can be reacquired upon incubation of apo-toxin in zinc-containing buffers (11).

BoNTs and TeNT are remarkably specific proteases that recognize and cleave only three proteins, the so-called SNARE [soluble NSF (N-ethylmaleimide-sensitive factor) attachment receptor] proteins, which form the core of the neuroexocytosis machinery (17,23). TeNT, BoNT/B, /D, /F and /G cleave VAMP, at different single peptide bonds (17,36); BoNT/A and /E cleave synaptosomal-associated protein of 25 kDa (SNAP-25) at different sites within the COOH-terminus whereas BoNT/C cleaves both syntaxin and SNAP-25 (37–39). Strikingly, TeNT and BoNT/B cleave VAMP at the same peptide bond (Gln76-Phe77), but they cause the opposite symptoms of tetanus and botulism, respectively (36), conclusively demonstrating that the different symptoms of the two diseases derive from different sites of intoxication rather than from a different molecular mechanism of action.

VAMP, SNAP-25, and syntaxin form a heterotrimeric coil-coiled complex, termed the SNARE complex, which induces the juxtaposition of vesicle to the target membrane complex (40) and is involved in their fusion (41). VAMP is a family of vesicular SNAREs with a short C-terminal tail facing the vesicle lumen, a single transmembrane domain and the remaining N-terminal part exposed to the cytosol. VAMP-1 and -2 are the isoforms mainly involved in the binding and fusion of neurotransmitter-containing synaptic vesicles with the presynaptic membrane (neuroexocytosis). Syntaxin is anchored to target membranes via a C-terminal hydrophobic tail. Of the many syntaxin isoforms presently known, syntaxins 1A, 1B, and 2 are the isoforms mainly involved in neuroexocytosis. SNAP-25 (of which there are several isoforms) are 25-kDa SNARE proteins bound to the target membrane via fatty acids covalently linked to cysteine residues present in the middle of the polypeptide chain. The proteolysis of one SNARE protein prevents the formation of the complex and, consequently, the release of the neurotransmitter.

The molecular basis of the specificity of the metalloprotease activity of the clostridial neurotoxins for the three SNAREs is only partially known. Experimental evidence implicates a nine-residue-long motif (termed SNARE motif), characterized by three carboxylate residues alternated with hydrophobic and hydrophilic residues (42–44). The motif is present in two copies in VAMP and syntaxin, and in four copies in SNAP-25. The various clostridial neurotoxins differ with respect to the specific interaction with the SNARE motif (23). The findings that only protein segments including at least one SNARE motif are cleaved by the toxins and that the motif is exposed at the protein surface (42,43,45) clearly indicate the involvement of the SNARE motif in the specificity of action of botulinum neurotoxins. Moreover, different SNARE isoforms coexist within the same cell (46), but only some of them are susceptible to proteolysis by the CNTs and it has been shown that resistance is associated with mutations in SNARE motifs at the cleavage site (17).

MUTAGENESIS OF THE ACTIVE SITE OF BONT/A L CHAIN

The crystallographic structures of BoNT/A (13) and of BoNT/B (14) provide a firm structural basis for the design of mutants addressing in a rational way the problem of the relation between structure and function in these molecules. The analysis of the available structures reveals that, in addition to the three residues of the zinc-binding motif, another glutamic acid (Glu262 in BoNT/A and Glu268 in BoNT/B) is involved as a fourth ligand. Structural and spectroscopic studies suggested the possibility that Tyr366 in BoNT/A plays a fundamental role in catalysis. To determine the specific contribution of Glu262 and of Tyr366 in zinc binding and in the proteolytic activity of BoNT/A, they were substituted with Ala (Fig. 1.1). The mutants were generated by PCR and expressed in *Escherichia coli* as fusion proteins with GST. After

affinity purification, the native and mutant recombinant BoNT/A L chains were released by thrombin cleavage and further passed through a HPLC gel filtration column. The mutants were characterized by spectroscopic analysis and compared with the corresponding wild-type chain. Circular dichroism and fluorescence spectra of the all mutants were essentially indistinguishable from that of the wild-type protein. Both far and near ultraviolet (UV) spectra of the mutants indicate they achieved a folding status closely similar, if not identical, to that of the native molecules (not shown).

The zinc-dependent endopeptidase activity of TeNT and BoNTs can be assayed conveniently by following the formation of the proteolytic fragments of their substrate by quantitative sodium dodecyl sulfate-polyacrylamide gel electrophoresis (SDS-PAGE) (11). Figure 1.3 shows that mutation of Glu to Ala in position 262 of BoNT/A LC dramatically impairs the endopeptidase activity of the toxin, indicating that the critical role of Glu262 is to provide a negatively charged carboxylate moiety, and that the distance of the carboxylate from the zinc atom is not a strong determinant for activity. The Y366A mutant of BoNT/A has a strongly reduced activity. The exact catalytic function of Tyr366 of

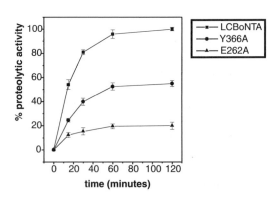

FIG. 1.3. Proteolytic activity of recombinant L chain of BoNT/A and of its mutants. Time course of the proteolytic activity of the recombinant L chain of BoNT/A and of its mutants at the 262 position and at the 366 position was measured on the GST-SNAP25 substrate at 37°C (98.6°F). Values are expressed as percentage of maximal cleavage. Bars are the ±SD of three different experiments.

BoNT/A L chain is not apparent from this particular experiment because we cannot distinguish between an effect on the binding and positioning of the substrate and a direct role in the hydrolysis reaction. The latter possibility is favored by the result of the competition experiment in which the activity of wild-type tetanus toxin is determined in the presence of the two inactive TeNT L-chain Ala mutants (E271A and Y375A) to compare their efficiency in substrate binding (34). It was suggested that in the L chain of BoNT/B, Tyr373 donates a proton to the amide nitrogen of VAMP Phe77 and stabilizes the leaving group through hydrogen bonding interaction with its amine (14). The present findings support this proposal and extend it to BoNT/A.

ACKNOWLEDGMENTS

Work performed in the authors' laboratory is supported by Telethon-Italia grant 1068 and MURST -grant 990698133.

REFERENCES

1. Rawlings ND, Barrett AJ. Evolutionary families of metallopeptidases. *Methods Enzymol* 1995;248: 183–228.
2. Emergem EV. Ueber einen neuen anaeroben Bacillus und seine Beziehungen zum Botulism. *Z. Hyg Infekt* 1897;26:1–56.
3. Faber K. Die Pathogenie des Tetanus. *Berl Klin Wochenschr* 1890;27:717–720.
4. Tizzoni G, Cattani G. Uber das Tetanusgift. *Zentralbl Bakt* 1890;8:69–73.
5. Smith LD, Sugiyama H. *Botulism: the organism, its toxins, the disease.* Springfield, IL: C.C. Thomas Publisher, 1988.
6. Hatheway CL. Botulism: the present status of the disease. *Curr Top Microbiol Immunol* 1995;195:55–75.
7. Burgen ASV, Dickens F, Zatman LJ. The action of botulinum toxin on the neuro-muscular junction. *J Physiol* 1949;109:10–24.
8. Brooks VB, Curtis DR, Eccles JC. Mode of action of tetanus toxin. *Nature* 1955;175:120–121.
9. Popoff MR, Marvaud JC. Structural and genomic features of clostridial neurotoxins. In: Alouf JE, Freer JH, eds. *The comprehensive sourcebook of bacterial protein toxins, 2nd ed.* London: Academic Press, 1999: 174–201.
10. Das Gupta BR. Structures of botulinum neurotoxin, its functional domains, and perspectives on the crystalline type A toxin. In: Jankovic J, Hallett M, eds. *Therapy with botulinum toxin.* New York: Marcel Dekker, 1994: 15–39.
11. Schiavo G, Montecucco C. Tetanus and botulism neurotoxins: isolation and assay. *Methods Enzymol* 1995;248: 643–652.
12. Umland TC, Wingert LM, Swaminathan S, et al. Structure of the receptor binding fragment HC of tetanus neurotoxin. *Nat Struct Biol* 1997;4:788–792.
13. Lacy DB, Tepp W, Cohen AC, DasGupta BR, Stevens RC. Crystal structure of botulinum neurotoxin type A and implications for toxicity. *Nat Struct Biol* 1998;5: 898–902.
14. Swaminathan S, Eswaramoorthy S. Structural analysis of the catalytic and binding sites of *Clostridium botulinum* neurotoxin B. *Nat Struct Biol* 2000;7:693–699.
15. Lacy DB, Stevens RC. Sequence homology and structural analysis of the clostridial neurotoxins. *J Mol Biol* 1999;291:1091–1104.
16. Halpern JL, Loftus A. Characterization of the receptor-binding domain of tetanus toxin. *J Biol Chem* 1993;268: 11188–11192.
17. Schiavo G, Matteoli M, Montecucco C. Neurotoxins affecting neuroexocytosis. *Physiol Rev* 2000;80:717–766.
18. Montecucco C, Papini E, Schiavo G. Bacterial protein toxins penetrate cells via a four-step mechanism. *FEBS Lett* 1994;346:92–98.
19. Lalli G, Herreros J, Osborne SL, et al. Functional characterisation of tetanus and botulinum neurotoxins binding domains. J Cell Sci 1999;112:2715–2724.
20. Halpern JL, Neale EA. Neurospecific binding, internalization, and retrograde axonal transport. *Curr Top Microbiol Immunol* 1995;195:221–241.
21. Nishiki T, Tokuyama Y, Kamata Y, et al. The high-affinity binding of *Clostridium botulinum* type B neurotoxin to synaptotagmin II associated with gangliosides GT1b/GD1a. *FEBS Lett* 1996;378:253–257.
22. Kitamura M, Takamiya K, Aizawa S, et al. Gangliosides are the binding substances in neural cells for tetanus and botulinum toxins in mice. *Biochim Biophys Acta* 1999; 1441:1–3.
23. Rossetto O, Seveso M, Caccin P, et al. Tetanus and botulinum neurotoxins: turning bad guys into good by research. *Toxicon* 2001b;39:27–41.
24. Dolly JO, Black J, Williams RS, et al. Acceptors for botulinum neurotoxin reside on motor nerve terminals and mediate its internalization. *Nature* 1984;307: 457–460.
25. Hughes R, Whaler BC. Influence of nerve-endings activity and of drugs on the rate of paralysis of rat diaphragm preparations by Clostridium botulinum type A toxin. *J Physiol* 1962;160:221–233.
26. Cremona O, De Camilli P. Synaptic vesicle endocytosis. *Curr Opin Neurobiol* 1997;7:323–330.
27. Hua SY, Charlton MP. Activity-dependent changes in partial VAMP complexes during neurotransmitter release. *Nat Neurosci* 1999;2:1078–1083.
28. Simpson LL, Coffield JA, Bakry N. Inhibition of vacuolar adenosine triphosphatase antagonizes the effects of clostridial neurotoxins but not phospholipase A2 neurotoxins. *J Pharmacol Exp Ther* 1994;269:256–262.
29. Montecucco C, Schiavo G, Dasgupta BR. Effect of pH on the interaction of botulinum neurotoxins A, B, and E with liposomes. *Biochem J* 1989;259:47–53.
30. Hoch DH, Romero Mira M, Ehrlich BE, et al. Channels formed by botulinum, tetanus, and diphtheria toxins in planar lipid bilayers: relevance to translocation of proteins across membranes. *Proc Natl Acad Sci U S A* 1985; 82:1692–1696.

31. Boquet P, Duflot E. Tetanus toxin fragment forms channels in lipid vesicles at low pH. *Proc Natl Acad Sci U S A* 1982;79:7614–7618.

32. Li Y, Foran P, Fairweather NF, de Paiva A, et al. A single mutation in the recombinant light chain of tetanus toxin abolishes its proteolytic activity and removes the toxicity seen after reconstitution with native heavy chain. *Biochemistry* 1994;33:7014–7020.

33. Li L, Binz T, Niemann H, et al. Probing the mechanistic role of glutamate residue in the zinc-binding motif of type A botulinum neurotoxin light chain. *Biochemistry* 2000;39:2399–2405.

34. Rossetto O, Caccin P, Rigoni M, et al. Active-site mutagenesis of tetanus neurotoxin implicates TYR-375 and GLU-271 in metalloproteolytic activity. *Toxicon* 2001; 39:1151–1159.

35. Hanson, MA, Stevens RC. Cocrystal structure of synaptobrevin-II bound to botulinum neurotoxin type B at 2.0 Å resolution. *Nat Struct Biol* 2000;7:687–692.

36. Schiavo G, Benfenati F, Poulain B, et al. Tetanus and botulinum-B neurotoxins block neurotransmitter release by proteolytic cleavage of synaptobrevin. *Nature* 1992; 359:832–835.

37. Blasi J, Chapman ER, Link E, et al. Botulinum neurotoxin A selectively cleaves the synaptic protein SNAP-25. *Nature* 1993;365:160–163.

38. Blasi J, Chapman ER, Yamasaki S, et al. Botulinum neurotoxin C1 blocks neurotransmitter release by means of cleaving HPC-1/syntaxin. *Embo J* 1993;12: 4821–4828.

39. Schiavo G, Santucci A, Dasgupta BR, et al. Botulinum neurotoxins serotypes A and E cleave SNAP-25 at distinct COOH-terminal peptide bonds. *FEBS Lett* 1993; 335:99–103.

40. Sutton RB, Fasshauer D, Jahn R, Brunger AT. Crystal structure of a SNARE complex involved in synaptic exocytosis at 2.4 Å resolution. *Nature* 1998;395: 347–353.

41. Chen YA, Scales SJ, Patel SM, et al. SNARE complex formation is triggered by Ca^{2+} and drives membrane fusion. *Cell* 1999;97:165–174.

42. Rossetto O, Schiavo G, Montecucco C, et al. SNARE motif and neurotoxins. *Nature* 1994;372:415–416.

43. Pellizzari R, Rossetto O, Lozzi L, et al. Structural determinants of the specificity for synaptic vesicle-associated membrane protein/synaptobrevin of tetanus and botulinum type B and G neurotoxins. *J Biol Chem* 1996;271: 20353–20358.

44. Vaidyanathan VV, Yoshino K, Jahnz M, et al. Proteolysis of SNAP-25 isoforms by botulinum neurotoxin types A, C, and E: domains and amino acid residues controlling the formation of enzyme-substrate complexes and cleavage. *J Neurochem* 1999;72:327–337.

45. Washbourne P, Pellizzari R, Baldini G, et al. Botulinum neurotoxin type-A and type-E require the SNARE motif in SNAP-25 for proteolysis. *FEBS Lett* 1997;418:1–5.

46. Bock JB, Scheller RH. SNARE proteins mediate lipid bilayer fusion. *Proc Natl Acad Sci U S A* 1999;96: 12227–12229.

Scientific and Therapeutic Aspects of Botulinum Toxin
edited by M.F. Brin, J. Jankovic, and M. Hallett
Lippincott Williams & Wilkins, Philadelphia, © 2002.

2

Structural View of Botulinum Neurotoxin in Numerous Functional States

Michael A. Hanson and Raymond C. Stevens

Different strains of *Clostridium botulinum* produce seven immunologically distinct forms of botulinum neurotoxin (BoNT) designated A-G (1). The toxin is synthesized as an inactive ~150-kDa single-chain protein, and secreted as a large complex with nontoxic proteins that protect it during passage through the gastrointestinal tract (Fig. 2.1). The toxin is posttranslationally proteolyzed to form the active di-chain molecule in which the ~50-kDa light chain and the ~100-kDa heavy chain remain linked by a disulfide bond. The active di-chain molecule is composed of three ~50-kDa functional domains: binding, translocation, and catalytic (2). The binding domain comprises the C-terminal half of the heavy chain, while the translocation domain is located in its N-terminal half. The catalytic domain, a zinc-endopeptidase, is confined to the N-terminal 50-kDa light chain (Fig. 2.2).

Each BoNT domain is associated with one step of a three-step model for toxicity (3). In the first step, the binding domain mediates interaction between the toxin and the presynaptic nerve terminal membrane (4). This interaction is thought to occur with both a ganglioside and protein receptor (5). Following binding, the protein is internalized by receptor-mediated endocytosis (6,7). The acidity of the endosome is thought to cause a structural change in the translocation domain, which then forms a pore in the endosomal membrane. This pore provides passage for the catalytic domain into the cytosol of the presynaptic neuron. The third step involves proteolysis of a SNARE [soluble NSF (*N*-ethyl-

maleimide–sensitive factor) attachment receptor] protein, which is a crucial component in synaptic vesicle membrane fusion (Fig. 2.3). Each toxin serotype (A-G) specifically cleaves a different peptide bond on one SNARE protein, effectively disabling neurotransmitter vesicle exocytosis and resulting in paralysis of the infected host (Fig. 2.4).

TOXIN COMPLEX STRUCTURE AND STABILITY

The most common method of intoxication by botulinum neurotoxins is oral ingestion of toxin complex found in contaminated foods. This route of intoxication exposes the toxin complex to extremes in pH and a wide variety of proteolytic enzymes. These conditions are, of course, designed to degrade ingested protein, so it is somewhat surprising that the toxin complex is able to withstand these harsh conditions and still function as a highly potent neurotoxin. It has been demonstrated that the neurotoxin-associated proteins protect the 150-kDa holotoxin in the gastrointestinal tract (8).

For most serotypes, the bacterial secreted neurotoxin complex is produced in clostridia with nontoxic neurotoxin-associated proteins (NAPs) in complex with the neurotoxin itself. For example, serotype A is secreted as one of three sizes—300 kDa, 500 kDa, or 900 kDa—whereas tetanus neurotoxin is not known to be secreted with neurotoxin associated proteins (9). The 900-kDa species represents a complex containing the full contingency of NAPs, and its three-dimensional structure has been characterized by two-dimensional electron diffraction

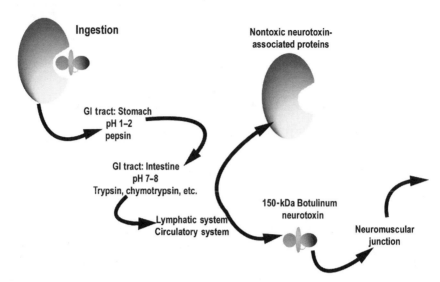

FIG. 2.1. Route of invasion in oral botulism intoxication.

(10). Complex stability and equilibrium of association between holotoxin and NAPs has been studied at the molecular level through a variety of biophysical experiments on botulinum neurotoxin, toxin complex, and the isolated neurotoxin-associated proteins (11,12).

A two-dimensional representation of the 900-kDa complex of botulinum neurotoxin type A (BoNT/A) was determined at low resolution from projection density maps calculated from the electron diffraction of two-dimensional toxin complex crystals (10) (Fig. 2.5). These maps show the toxin complex as a triangular species composed of six density "blobs." This central triangle is surrounded by two less-dense triangular structures. This information can be related

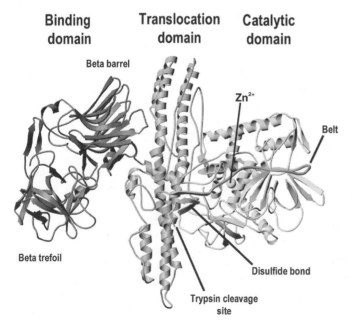

FIG. 2.2. The three-dimensional structure of the 150-kDa botulinum neurotoxin type A (14). The toxin is produced as a single-chain, three-domain protein. The toxin is picked by the protease trypsin to produce the di-chain species with the catalytic domain fastened to the translocation domain by a disulfide bond. One unusual feature of the holotoxin is the 54-residue translocation domain belt that wraps around the catalytic domain. It is thought the belt serves to protect the catalytic domain active site cleft.

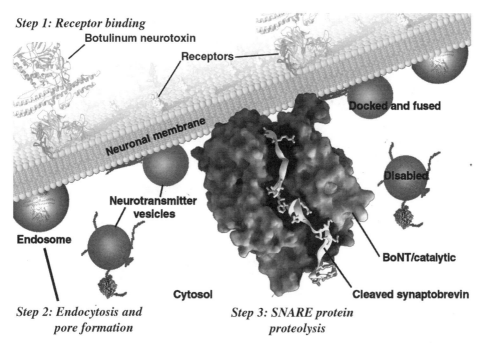

FIG. 2.3. Diagram of the three-step model for botulinum neurotoxin toxicity (3). Step 1 involves binding of the toxin to ganglioside and protein receptors on the surface of the presynaptic neuron. Step 2 involves receptor-mediated endocytosis and acid-induced pore formation enacted by the translocation domain. Step 3 involves selective proteolysis of the toxin's SNARE (soluble *N*-ethylmaleimide–sensitive factor attachment receptor) substrate. The exact identity of the substrate is serotype specific (BoNT/B and it's substrate synaptobrevin are shown here), but the end result is generally neurotransmitter vesicles that are disabled and can neither fuse to the neuronal membrane nor release neurotransmitter into the synapse. The result is flaccid paralysis.

to relevant biochemical data to draw important conclusions about the dimensions and shape of the toxin complex.

Both analytical ultracentrifugation (11a) and dynamic light scattering (12) have been used to determine the molecular weight of the BoNT/A complex. The ultracentrifugation data suggests that the complex is a prolate ellipsoid with a molecular weight of 900 kDa. Dynamic light scattering data, assuming a spherical molecule, indicates that the hydrodynamic radius of the complex is 110 Å, giving a calculated molecular weight of 1,200 kDa. The discrepancy between these two results suggests that the complex is elliptical with an axis of 220 Å. Indeed, the projection maps of the toxin complex agree with this data only if the six major blobs in the density projection map are assumed to be elliptical with a height of approximately 100 Å. In summary,

it is most likely that the 900 kDa complex is composed of six cylinders 40 × 100 Å, arranged in an equilateral triangle 130 Å on each side and hollow in the middle. In addition, six smaller structures project 110 Å from the center of the triangle, yielding a complex with overall dimensions of 100 × 220 Å (10).

To gain a more detailed view of the toxin complex and to determine how the holotoxin- and neurotoxin-associated proteins protect each other, a three-dimensional reconstruction of the toxin was created by tilting the two-dimensional crystals through angles from −60 degrees to 60 degrees. From this reconstruction, it was possible to locate the density associated with the 150-kDa holotoxin and determine which regions interact with the neurotoxin-associated proteins (13) (Fig. 2.6).

Chen et al. performed antibody mapping stud-

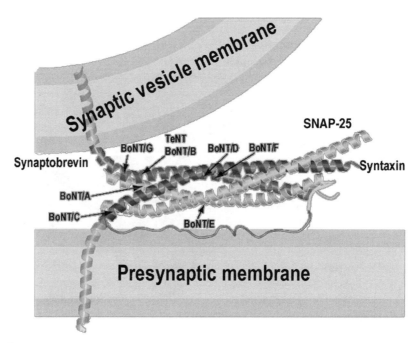

FIG. 2.4. Synaptic vesicle membrane fusion is mediated by the formation of the SNARE complex. SNARE complex formation involves the interaction of the three neuronal SNARE proteins (SNAP-25, syntaxin, and synaptobrevin) to form a four-helix bundle. Each botulinum neurotoxin serotype has a specific proteolytic site on one of the three neuronal SNARE proteins. (From Sutton RB, Fasshauer D, Jahn R, Brunger AT. Crystal structure of a SNARE complex involved in synaptic exocytosis at 2.4-Å resolution. *Nature* 1998;395:347–353, with permission.)

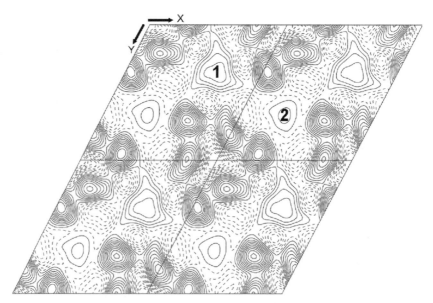

FIG. 2.5. A projection density map from electron diffraction studies of the 900-kDa toxin complex type A (10). The toxin complex is represented by the central triangle composed of six "blobs" and the two less-dense blobs surrounding the triangle labeled *1* and *2*.

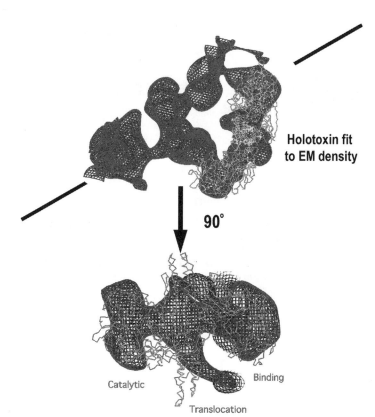

Holotoxin fit to EM density

90°

Catalytic

Binding

Translocation

FIG. 2.6. The structure of botulinum neurotoxin A fit into the three-dimensional reconstruction of the two-dimensional electron diffraction images (13). The two views putatively show how the 150-kDa toxin species interacts with the nontoxic neurotoxin-associated proteins in the toxin complex.

ies in order to gain a greater understanding of the domain organization of the toxin and how it interacts with the NAPs in forming the toxin complex of serotype A (11). In this study, 44 monoclonal single-chain variable antibody fragments that bind to specific regions on each domain of the holotoxin were used to determine which domain regions were involved in packing interactions with other domains and with the NAPs in the toxin complex (11). The results of this study are shown schematically in Fig. 2.7. Briefly, the 15 antibody-binding sites (Ab sites) were identified on the separated catalytic domain, 5 Ab sites were identified on the translocation domain, and 26 Ab sites were identified on the binding domain. When the same analysis was done on the intact holotoxin, the translocation domain lost two Ab sites, the binding domain lost six Ab sites and the catalytic domain didn't lose any. When the Ab site analysis was performed on the toxin complex, neither the translocation domain nor the catalytic domain

lost any additional Ab sites; however, the binding domain lost all but two. This seems to indicate that the holotoxin interacts with the NAPs primarily through interactions with the binding domain.

Dynamic light scattering is a biophysical technique that measures the diffusion coefficient of a particle in solution. From this information the dynamic hydrated radius and an estimate of the molecular weight of the particle can be calculated. The distribution of particle sizes is indicated by the polydispersity value, which is represented by error bars in Fig. 2.8. A larger polydispersity value indicates a larger distribution of particle sizes in solution. The three toxin species mentioned previously were examined by dynamic light scattering over a pH range from 1 to 10 (12).

The molecular mass of the serotype A holotoxin species was determined to be approximately 150 kDa between pH 10 and 4. However, as the pH dropped below 4, the estimated molec-

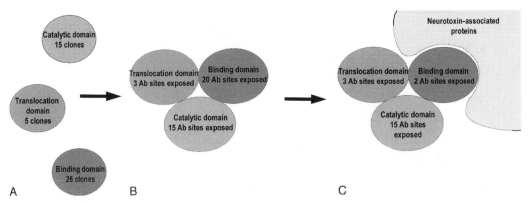

FIG. 2.7. Diagram of the antibody mapping studies of BoNT/A (11). **A:** Starting with each domain of the toxin separately, a baseline is established for the number of antibody binding sites. **B:** When the toxin is in the single-chain holotoxin form, some of the antibody-binding sites are occluded, presumably because of packing interaction with adjacent domains. **C:** In the toxin complex form, all but two antibody-binding sites on the binding domain of the toxin are occluded. Therefore, most of the interactions between the holotoxin and the neurotoxin-associated proteins occur through the binding domain.

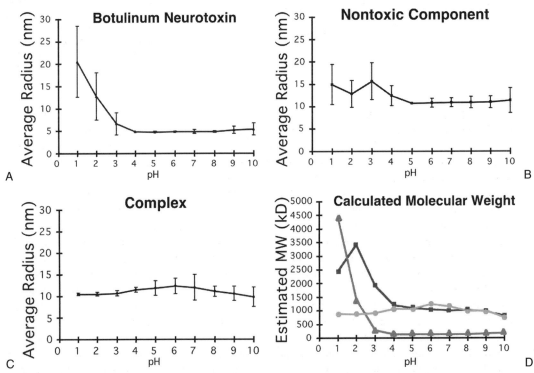

FIG. 2.8. Results from light-scattering studies involving different species of botulinum neurotoxin serotype A over a range of physiologically relevant pH (12). **A:** The calculated hydrodynamic radius of the 150-kDa holotoxin as a function of pH. **B:** The hydrodynamic radius of the nontoxic neurotoxin-associated proteins without toxin as a function of pH. **C:** The hydrodynamic radius of the intact toxin complex as a function of pH. **D:** The calculated molecular weight of all three species as a function of pH.

ular weight and polydispersity of the holotoxin began to increase (Fig. 2.8A and D). This increase in polydispersity was likely a result of general denaturation and degradation of the holotoxin at acidic pH associated with the conditions in the stomach.

The isolated neurotoxin-associated proteins associated with serotype A, had an apparent molecular weight of 962 kDa between pH 10 and 5, indicating that it did not aggregate or disassemble under these conditions. Surprisingly, as the pH dropped below 5, the neurotoxin-associated proteins began to aggregate, disassemble or denature as indicated by a sharp jump in polydispersity (Fig. 2.8B and D). These results indicate that the neurotoxin-associated proteins are not exceptionally stable in the acidic conditions of the stomach either. However, when a similar test was performed on the intact toxin complex (comprising the holotoxin type A and its neurotoxin-associated proteins) it was found that it was most stable at acidic pH. Interestingly basic pH conditions associated with the small intestine seemed to destabilize the complex (Fig. 2.8C and D). Together, these results indicate that the type A holotoxin and its neurotoxin-associated proteins protect each other in the complex form, while in the acidic conditions of the stomach. However, as the complex moves into basic conditions of the small intestine, the equilibrium between the toxin complex and its two components shifts and the complex starts to disassociate (12).

A similar effect was seen upon exposure of these three species of type A to a variety of proteases. Both the holotoxin and the neurotoxin-associated proteins were susceptible to proteolytic degradation. However, the toxin complex was found to be remarkably resistant to proteolysis under both acidic and basic conditions (12).

It appears as if the main function of the neurotoxin-associated proteins is to protect the toxin from the gastrointestinal tract defenses and deliver intact toxin to the small intestine. Once in the small intestine, the basic pH may cause a shift in equilibrium to favor a release of the toxin from its associated proteins. The free toxin would then be absorbed into the blood stream, where it makes its way to the neuromuscular junction.

HOLOTOXIN STRUCTURE

To date, two structures of the intact botulinum neurotoxin (holotoxin) structure have been solved. The structure of BoNT/A (PDB accession code 3BTA) was solved at 3.3-Å resolution (14) and the structure of BoNT/B (PDB accession code 1EPW) was solved at 1.8-Å resolution (15). Overall, the two structures are very similar, the major differences being in the binding and catalytic domains where the amino acid sequences are also less homologous. These two structures show that the BoNT binding domain is structurally similar to the tetanus neurotoxin (TeNT) binding domain (16), and can be divided into two subdomains, an N-terminal β-barrel and a C-terminal β-trefoil fold.

The BoNT/TeNT translocation domain fold is markedly different from the folds observed in other toxins that undergo pore formation and translocation (17). Most notable are a kinked pair of α-helices, 105 Å in length, and a 54 residue "belt" that wraps around the perimeter of the catalytic domain. The translocation domain, in the holotoxin, occludes access to a large negatively charged cleft leading into the active site zinc of the catalytic domain. The zinc appears to be directly coordinated by His222, His226, and Glu261, with a water-mediated coordination through Glu223.

NEURONAL RECOGNITION

Two structures of the TeNT binding domain have been solved, one at 2.7 Å (PDB accession code 1AF9) (16) and one at 1.5 Å (PDB accession code 1A8D) (18). The main peptide chains of the two structures differ only in the orientation of two surface loops, located in crystal packing interfaces. As both structures were obtained in the same space group, these packing interface differences, along with temperature and X-ray source differences, are likely to account for the differences in resolution.

The structure of BoNT/A reveals the orientation of the binding domain with respect to the entire toxin and the accessibility of the surface loops in the presence of the translocation domain. The binding domain tilts away from the plane of the catalytic and translocation domains by ~60 degrees and projects away from the long axis of the translocation domain by ~40 degrees. The projection away from the long axis can vary at least 5 degrees (unpublished data). This observation is not surprising given the relatively small interface between the binding and translocation domains. (The binding domain buries ~400 Å^2 of the translocation domain while the translocation domain buries ~480 Å^2 of the binding domain.) In the absence of crystallographic packing interactions, in solution, the relative orientation of this domain could vary even more substantially (Fig. 2.9). The two sub-domains of the binding domain are linked by an α-helix and create a cleft at the subdomain interface (Fig. 2.9). The C-terminal subdomain buries ~500 Å^2 of the N-terminal subdomain, while the N-terminal subdomain buries ~540 Å^2 of the C-terminal domain. The contacts between the two subdomains are made through loops such that this interface could also be flexible, although the subdomain   -strands align almost identically in the three toxin-binding domain structures.

While the identification of a protein receptor-binding site is still under investigation, the ganglioside-binding site is fairly well characterized.

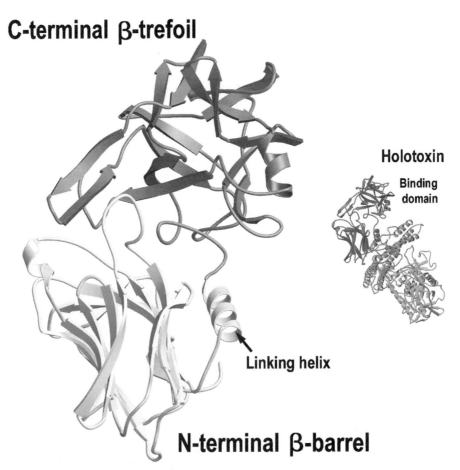

FIG. 2.9. The binding domain of botulinum neurotoxin type A (14). **Left:** An enlarged view of the binding domain showing the architecture of the two subdomains: the N-terminal β-barrel and C-terminal β-trefoil fold. Also shown is the helix that links the two subdomains. **Right:** A view of the entire holotoxin structure with the binding domain in the same orientation as shown on the left. Note the angle of the binding domain relative to the rest of the toxin.

A BoNT/A binding study using trypsin digests indicates that the 30 C-terminal residues of the C-terminal subdomain are involved in binding the GT1b ganglioside (19). A photo-affinity labeling study using a novel ganglioside probe implicates this same region in TeNT, showing labeling of H1295 (20). The functional significance of this region has also been identified in BoNT/E (21). A monoclonal antibody capable of neutralizing BoNT/E in mice also bound the peptide YLTHMRD. Comparison of this sequence location in BoNT/E aligns to residues 1292–1298 of TeNT and residues 1266–1272 of BoNT/A. In addition, a BoNT/A binding assay that monitored tryptophan fluorescence showed fluorescence quenching upon binding the ganglioside (22). However, with three tryptophans located within the 30 C-terminal residues, it was impossible to narrow the location of the binding site further. The BoNT/A structure shows that of the three tryptophans, only one (W1265) is solvent accessible. This highly hydrophobic residue is fully exposed to solvent and

makes contact with Q1269, the residue in BoNT/A that aligns to H1295 of TeNT, implicated in the photo-affinity labeling study. These two residues are both located on helix 22, beneath a loop whose orientation varies dramatically between BoNT/A and TeNT. In BoNT/A this loop points outward, creating a deep positively charged cleft between subdomains, while in TeNT the loop folds inward, creating a shallow, more neutral cleft.

More recently, four crystal structures of the TeNT binding domain in complex with four different carbohydrate moieties: N-acetylgalactosamine, sialic acid, lactose and galactose (PDB accession codes 1DOH, 1DFQ, 1DLL and 1DIW, respectively) have been reported (23) (Fig. 2.10). These four structures indicate that there are four different carbohydrate-binding pockets on the TeNT binding domain. N-Acetylgalactosamine (NGA) has two different binding sites, one of which is in common with sialic acid. Lactose and galactose each have one binding site. The lactose-binding site is equivalent to the

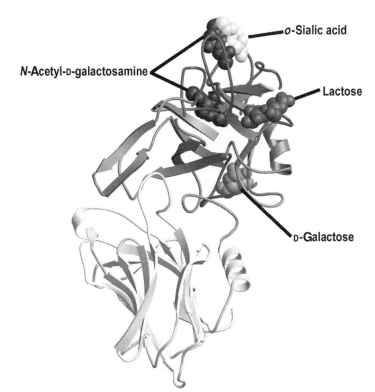

o-Sialic acid

N-Acetyl-D-galactosamine

Lactose

D-Galactose

FIG. 2.10. The structure of tetanus neurotoxin binding domain with the location of the ganglioside binding sites (23). The ganglioside moieties are rendered as space-filling models in their crystallographically determined binding sites. The lactose binding site has been verified by biochemical methods.

site identified by fluorescence quenching and neutralizing antibody studies described above. This lactose-binding site shares high sequence and structural homology with the other toxin serotypes, whereas the NGA- and galactose-binding sites have less homology because of differences in lengths and positions of the loops between the different serotypes. These data suggest that the toxin-binding domain exhibits multivalency, possessing primary and secondary carbohydrate-binding sites. Variation in the specificity of the primary or secondary binding sites among the toxin serotypes could explain the neuronal binding variability of the clostridial toxin family.

TOXIN TRANSLOCATION

The clostridial neurotoxin translocation domain is able to form channels in artificial bilayers (24–26) and in cell membranes (27). Visualization of these channels using electron cryomicroscopy suggests that the channels may be formed by the oligomerization of BoNT to form a tetramer (28). Efforts to identify the pore-forming segment(s) of the clostridial neurotoxins have focused on identifying amphipathic sequences capable of spanning the membrane (29,30). Three such sequences were identified using the MOMENT algorithm for determining hydrophobic moments (595–614, 625–647, and 648–691) (29). A peptide representing part of one of these sequences, 659–681 (Fig. 2.11), was shown to form channels in planar lipid bilayers (31). This sequence could possibly oligomerize to form a four-helix-bundle in the membrane. The structure of BoNT/A, solved at pH 7, does not refute or support this hypothesis. The previously identified amphipathic sequences do not correspond to the long pairs of kinked α-helices observed in the BoNT/A translocation domain. Instead, the sequences precede these helices and adopt primarily extended loop conformations (Fig. 2.11). Interestingly the structure of BoNT/B, solved at pH 6, indicates that part of the amphipathic sequence corresponds to a short helical segment as opposed to the extended loop structure found in BoNT/A solved

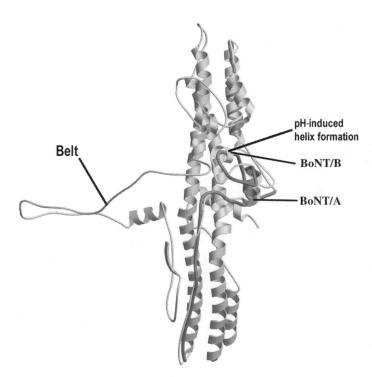

FIG. 2.11. The structure of the translocation domain of botulinum neurotoxin type A (14) with the amphipathic pore-forming sequence of botulinum neurotoxin type B overlaid (15). Note the two long helices 105 Å in length. Also note the putative pH induced helix formation.

at pH 7.0. It is possible that this structural difference is a manifestation of the pH-induced structural changes that induce pore formation.

The critical follow-up question after identifying the pore-forming segment is to identify the molecular mechanism by which pH triggers this sequence to change structure and form a membrane-spanning channel. The calculated pI for the BoNT/A translocation domain is 4.66 (as compared to 9.1 for the binding domain and 6.0 for the entire toxin). This low pI value is attributable to the first half of the domain containing the amphipathic loops (pI = 4.6) and the second half containing the kinked pair of α-helices (pI = 8.5). The low pI and charge distribution could predispose the translocation domain to respond structurally to acidic conditions. The three-dimensional charge distribution indicates several clusters of glutamate and aspartate residues on both sides of the translocation domain. The clustering of the negative charge is expected to raise the pKa of these residues, making them titratable at endosomal pH (4.5 to 5.5). We therefore propose that these residues and possibly any histidines present in this region of the structure will effect the structural changes required for pore formation.

The translocation domain only contains two histidines (H551 and H560) located immediately after the translocation domain belt (residues 492–545) and precedes a disordered loop in the structure. While H560 is solvent accessible, H551 is buried at the interface of the catalytic and translocation domains within 7 Å of their connecting disulfide. The idea that H551 protonation could disrupt this interface is supported by the fact that the residues following position 551 are likely to be very flexible. The role that the "belt" might play in translocation is unknown, although with movement in this loop region, it is not implausible to consider that the "belt" could move as well. In fact, evidence for this pH-induced belt movement exists in a comparison of the structure of BoNT/B and BoNT/A holotoxins. The belt in BoNT/B is in a significantly altered position when compared to that of BoNT/A. The belt in BoNT/B is located to the side of the catalytic domain cleft, leaving the active site

unobstructed (Fig. 2.12). It is reasonable to assume that the altered position of the belt in BoNT/B is a result of the lower pH employed in the crystallization conditions.

SUBSTRATE SPECIFICITY AND BINDING

The proteolytic activity of the clostridial neurotoxins is enhanced by the reduction of the disulfide bond and presumably the dissociation of the catalytic domain from the translocation domain. This is consistent with the active site of the catalytic domain being occluded by both the translocation domain belt and the main body of the translocation domain (14). Moreover, the separation of the catalytic domain results in a number of structural changes that appear to activate the domain for subsequent binding and catalysis. These structural changes and the mechanism of maintaining substrate specificity have been examined with two structures of the recombinant separated catalytic domain of botulinum neurotoxin type B (BoNT/B-LC) (32).

By comparing the structure of the separated BoNT/B-LC (apo-BoNT/B-LC; PDB accession code 1F82) with BoNT/B-LC in the holotoxin form (holo-BoNT/B-LC), the structural changes that occur upon separation can be visualized (Fig. 2.13). These structural changes are generally localized to four loops surrounding the active site cleft. Of these four loops, two become disordered (loops 50 and 200) and two have altered positions with respect to the active site (loop 250 and the catalytic loop) (Fig. 2.13). Loop 250 moves 18 Å relative to its position in holo-BoNT/B-LC, burying hydrophobic residues that were exposed after separation from the translocation domain. The movement of loop 250 forces the catalytic loop to move 4 Å further into the active site. The movement of loop 250 and disordering of loops 50 and 200 likely enable substrate binding by further exposing the substrate binding surface on the catalytic domain.

The structure of separate BoNT/B-LC soaked in synaptobrevin-II substrate (Sb2-BoNT/B-LC; PDB accession code 1F83) was solved to 2.0 Å

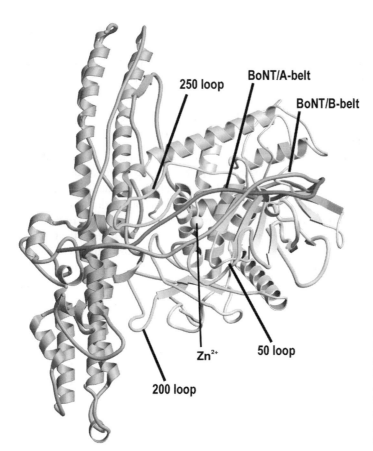

FIG. 2.12. The structure of BoNT/B translocation and catalytic domains (15). The translocation domain belt for BoNT/A (14) is overlaid to illustrate the structural differences that are putatively caused by the lowered pH of BoNT/B in the structure solution.

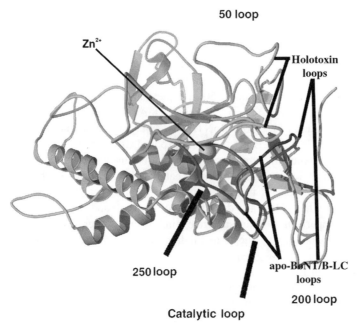

FIG. 2.13. The catalytic domain of BoNT/B solved to 2.2-Å resolution (apo-BoNT/B-LC) (32) with the catalytically important loops of the holotoxin overlaid to illustrate the structural differences. Loops 50 and 200 become disordered upon separation from the holotoxin and are not shown. Loop 250 moves approximately 18 Å to pack against the base of the active site cleft. This movement is thought to force the catalytic loop 4 Å further into the active site.

(32). The electron density for the synaptobrevin substrate was modeled as the cleaved peptide chain products. In the product-bound Sb2-BoNT/B-LC structure the loops 50 and 200 become ordered and participate in a number of interactions with the bound synaptobrevin product (Fig. 2.14). Loop 50 in Sb2-BoNT/B-LC is located 21 Å from its former position in holo-BoNT/B-LC, and participates in a number of interactions with the synaptobrevin peptide (Fig. 2.14). Loop 200 moves 13 Å closer to the active site relative to its position in holo-BoNT/B-LC and stabilizes the position of loop 250 through a number of hydrogen bonding interactions. Loops 50 and 200 appear to be stabilized through interactions with a short segment of synaptobrevin N-terminal to the cleaved bond.

The synaptobrevin peptide binds in a random coil conformation in the Sb2-BoNT/B-LC complex, consistent with NMR solution studies (33). The C-terminal region found to be slightly helical in solution, binds to the toxin in extended conformation, occupying the cleft vacated by the translocation domain belt of the BoNT/A. In the Sb2-BoNT/B-LC complex, the N-terminal synaptobrevin region is bound between loops 50 and 200. Eighteen hydrogen bonds and one aromatic T-stacking interaction hold the two proteins tightly together. The modeled conforma-

tion of the substrate peptide was recently verified by computational work, which indicates that the conformation of the peptide is energetically favorable (Dr. Mark Olson, personal communication). These calculations also support the existence of a cooperative binding site that involves the N-terminal portion of the substrate peptide. Therefore despite the low occupancy of the bound peptide and resulting weak electron density maps, as well as criticism of the peptide bound structure (34), we remain confident in the placement of the synaptobrevin peptide and the conclusions drawn from it.

Previous sequence alignments indicate that the clostridial neurotoxin catalytic domains have high sequence identity, up to 51.6% in the case of BoNT/B and TeNT (35). Despite the high sequence and presumably structural similarities, each serotype possesses an altered substrate profile, cleaving a different peptide bond on either synaptobrevin, syntaxin or SNAP-25 (the proteins involved in SNARE complex formation). This variation in specificity between serotypes may be because each catalytic domain has two substrate recognition sites. Binding of substrate to both of these sites is required for proteolysis to occur (36). This helps explain the requirement each serotype has for a very long minimum substrate length, and the fact that each botulinum

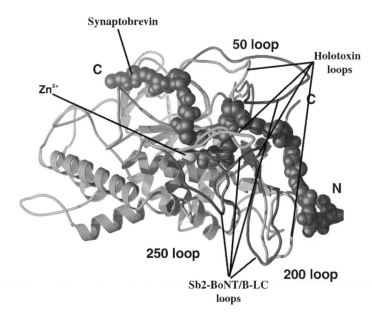

FIG. 2.14. The catalytic domain of BoNT/B with synaptobrevin proteolyzed products bound. This structure was solved to 2.0-Å resolution (32). Loops 50 and 200 become ordered upon binding of the N-terminal portion of the synaptobrevin substrate. Loop 50 moves 21 Å away from its former position in the holotoxin complex. Loop 200 moves 13 Å closer to the active site and makes stabilizing contacts with loop 250.

neurotoxin has a different substrate length requirement (2). Clostridial neurotoxin substrate specificity is therefore most likely a result of the spatial relationship between the substrate recognition sites in the three different synaptic vesicle fusion proteins (36).

The molecular requirement for two different binding sites can be explained by the assertion that binding of the substrate recognition site distal to the cleaved bond either induces a favorable conformation in the peptide substrate, or causes a favorable structural change in the enzyme (cooperative or allosteric effects). In the case of tetanus toxin, activity assays with different portions of the peptide substrate effectively ruled out the former possibility (37). Indeed, structural evidence for a cooperative mechanism exists in a comparison of the three BoNT/B catalytic domain structures introduced previously (holo-BoNT/B-LC, apo-BoNT/B-LC and Sb2-BoNT/B-LC).

The observed positions of loop 250 and the catalytic loop in apo-BoNT/B-LC are likely stabilized by crystal packing interactions. It would be reasonable to assume that in solution loop 250 is disordered after separation from the translocation domain, and the catalytic loop is in the same position as holo-BoNT/B-LC (Fig. 2.15A).

These assumptions have been reinforced by recent structural work by the author (unpublished results). The ordering of the 50 and 200 loops upon binding of synaptobrevin in solution would stabilize the previously observed position of loop 250 in the crystal lattice. The interactions between the synaptobrevin-stabilized position of loop 250 and the catalytic loop would force the catalytic loop further into the active site (Fig. 2.15B). This catalytic loop movement appears to contribute to toxin activation by reducing the distance between the conserved BoNT/B residues Arg369 and Tyr372 and the scissile bond of the substrate. Efficient proteolysis of the substrate could therefore be dependent on the loop changes caused by binding of the N-terminus of synaptobrevin, explaining structurally the kinetic results obtained (32,37).

THE PROTEOLYTIC MECHANISM OF BOTULINUM NEUROTOXINS

The positioning of Arg369 and Tyr372 on the catalytic loop is important for catalysis, given the proposed mechanism described below (Fig. 2.16). This catalytic mechanism is based on the proposed mechanism for thermolysin (38), which is thought to be similar to the clostridial

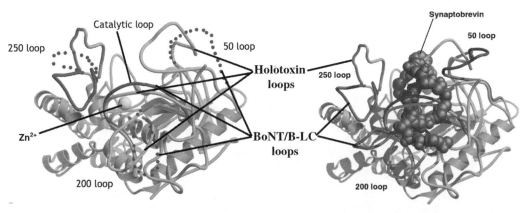

FIG. 2.15. Alternative view of toxin separation and substrate binding. **A:** When the catalytic domain separates from the holotoxin all of the loops become disordered. Loop 250 establishes equilibrium between the holotoxin position and the apo-BoNT/B-LC position. This equilibrium can be shifted by crystal lattice contacts or by substrate binding as shown in *B.* **B:** Synaptobrevin binds to BoNT/B-LC causing an ordering of loop 200, which stabilizes the position of loop 250. Loop 250 forces the catalytic loop 4 Å further into the active site, positioning two catalytically important residues. Substrate binding therefore enables catalysis through a cooperative mechanism (unpublished data).

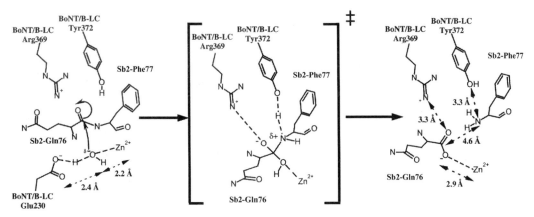

FIG. 2.16. The proposed reaction mechanism for synaptobrevin proteolysis by botulinum neurotoxin. Dotted lines represent noncovalent and hydrogen bonding interactions. Relevant interatomic distances are labeled in the reactants and products. Note the function of Arg369 and Tyr372, both of which are located on the catalytic loop (32).

catalytic domain and the Sb2-BoNT/B-LC structure described above.

The active site found in all clostridial neurotoxins is centered around a catalytic and structural zinc cation coordinated by a strictly conserved HEXXH + E motif. In the case of BoNT/B-LC, zinc coordinates His229, Glu230, and His233, all of which are located on a single helix. The fourth ligand, Glu267, is located in an adjacent helix. The side chains from His229, His233, and Glu267 form 2.1-Å coordinating bonds with the zinc ion. Glu230 indirectly coordinates the zinc ion through a bridging water molecule, with a side chain-to-water distance of 2.4 Å and a water-to-zinc bond distance of 2.2 Å. The bridging water molecule is thought to function as an activated nucleophile for attack on the carbonyl carbon of the synaptobrevin scissile bond. The negative charge that develops on the substrate carbonyl oxygen atom of Sb2-Gln76 in the transition state is stabilized by the zinc ion, in combination with the conserved Arg369 residue. The conserved active site residue Tyr372 likely donates a proton to the amide nitrogen of the scissile bond in the transition state. This allows conversion of the amine to a more favorable protonated leaving group, assisting in the hydrolysis reaction to yield the cleaved synaptobrevin products. Tyr372, together with bound water molecules, likely stabilizes the

leaving group through hydrogen bonding interactions with the synaptobrevin amine. The synaptobrevin cleaved fragments are observed in the Sb2-BoNT/B-LC structure, where the electrophilic carbonyl carbon atom of Sb2-Gln76 is situated more than 4 Å away from the amine of the cleaved Sb2-Phe77 residue.

CONCLUSIONS

The Clostridial neurotoxins represent a fascinating family of enzymes. Their ability to survive under extremely harsh conditions and to maintain a potency that is second to none among protein toxins is truly remarkable. The mechanisms by which these enzymes locate and disable their intended targets with such high specificity has intrigued scientists for almost a century. Some common themes that arise in the toxins' mode of action include their use of multiple recognition sites, both in the recognition of their neuronal targets and in the eventual proteolysis of their SNARE substrates. Another theme is the toxins' strategy of using protein mass to protect the toxic machinery under adverse conditions, starting with the complex-forming neurotoxin-associated proteins that protect the toxin from harsh extremes of pH and exposure to proteolytic enzymes. The complex may serve an additional function in the bloodstream by protecting the binding domain's multiple antigenic sites from recognition by the body's immune defenses. The translocation domain belt occluding the catalytic domain active site cleft ensures that peptide-like inhibitors cannot gain access to the proteolytic machinery. Finally the proposed cooperative mechanism of the catalytic domain enhances the substrate specificity of the toxin, ensuring that the enzyme doesn't attack multiple targets. These factors combine to deliver a highly potent neurotoxin to the areas were it can be the most effective.

REFERENCES

1. Simpson LL. *Botulinum neurotoxin and tetanus toxin.* San Diego: Academic Press, 1989.
2. Montecucco C, Schiavo G. Structure and function of tetanus and botulinum neurotoxins. *Q Rev Biophys* 1995;28:423–472.
3. Simpson LL. Kinetic studies on the interaction between botulinum toxin type A and the cholinergic neuromuscular junction. *J Pharmacol Exp Ther* 1980;212:16–21.
4. Dolly JO, Black J, Williams RS, et al. Acceptors for botulinum neurotoxin reside on motor nerve terminals and mediate its internalization. *Nature* 1984;307: 457–460.
5. Montecucco C. How do tetanus and botulinum toxins bind to neuronal membranes? *Trends Biochem Sci* 1986; 11:315–317.
6. Black JD, Dolly JO. Interaction of[125]I-labeled botulinum neurotoxins with nerve terminals. I. Ultrastructural autoradiographic localization and quantitation of distinct membrane acceptors for types A and B on motor nerves. *J Cell Biol* 1986;103:521–534.
7. Black JD, Dolly JO. Interaction of[125]I-labeled botulinum neurotoxins with nerve terminals. II. Autoradiographic evidence for its uptake into motor nerves by acceptor-mediated endocytosis. *J Cell Biol* 1986;103: 535–544.
8. Ohishi I, Sugii S, Sakaguchi G. Oral toxicities of *Clostridium botulinum* in response to molecular size. *Infect Immun* 1997;16:107–109.
9. Johnson EA, Bradshaw M. Clostridium botulinum and its neurotoxins: a metabolic and cellular perspective. *Toxicon* 2001;39:1703–1722.
10. Burkard F, Chen F, Kuziemko GM, et al. Electron density projection map of the botulinum neurotoxin 900-kilodalton complex by electron crystallography. *J Struct Biol* 1997;120:78–84.
11. Chen F, Kuziemko GM, Amersdorfer P, et al. Antibody mapping to domains of botulinum neurotoxin serotype A in the complexed and uncomplexed forms. *Infect Immun* 1997;65:1626–1630.
11a.Putnam FW, Lamanna C, Sharp DG. Physicochemical properties of crystalline *Clostridium botulinum* type A toxin. *J Biol Chem* 1948;176:401–412.
12. Chen F, Kuziemko G, Stevens RC. Biophysical characterization of the stability of the 150-kilodalton botulinum toxin, the nontoxic component, and the 900-kilo-

13. dalton botulinum toxin complex species. *Infect Immun* 1998;66:2420–2425.
13. Chen F. Botulinum neurotoxin complex: a structural and biophysical characterization. Dissertation. Berkeley: University of California at Berkeley, 1998.
14. Lacy DB, Tepp W, Cohen AC, et al. Crystal structure of botulinum neurotoxin type A and implications for toxicity. *Nat Struct Biol* 1998;5:898–902.
15. Swaminathan S, Eswaramoorthy S. Structural analysis of the catalytic and binding sites of *Clostridium botulinum* neurotoxin B. *Nat Struct Biol* 2000;7:693–699.
16. Umland TC, Wingert LM, Swaminathan S, et al. Structure of the receptor binding fragment HC of tetanus neurotoxin. *Nat Struct Biol* 1997;4:788–792.
17. Lacy DB, Stevens RC. Unraveling the structures and modes of action of bacterial toxins. *Curr Opin Struct Biol* 1998;8:778–784.
18. Knapp M, Segelke B, Rupp B. The 1.61 Angstrom structure of the tetanus toxin ganglioside binding region: Solved by MAD and MIR phase combination. *Am Cryst Assoc Papers* 1998;25:90.
19. Shone CC, Hambleton P, Melling J. Inactivation of *Clostridium botulinum* type A neurotoxin by trypsin and purification of two tryptic fragments. Proteolytic action near the COOH- terminus of the heavy subunit destroys toxin-binding activity. *Eur J Biochem* 1985;151:75–82.
20. Shapiro RE, Specht CD, Collins BE, Woods AS, Cotter RJ, Schnaar RL. Identification of a ganglioside recognition domain of tetanus toxin using a novel ganglioside photo-affinity ligand. *J Biol Chem* 1998;272: 30380–30386.
21. Kubota T, Watanabe T, Yokosawa N, et al. Epitope regions in the heavy chain of *Clostridium botulinum* type E neurotoxin recognized by monoclonal antibodies. *Appl Environ Microbiol* 1997;63:1214–1218.
22. Kamata Y, Yoshimoto M, Kozaki S. Interaction between botulinum neurotoxin type A and ganglioside: ganglioside inactivates the neurotoxin and quenches its tryptophan fluorescence. *Toxicon* 1997;35:1337–1440.
23. Emsley P, Fotinou C, Black I, et al. The structure of the H(C) fragment of tetanus toxin with carbohydrate subunit complexes provide insight into ganglioside binding. *J Biol Chem* 2000;275:8889–8894.
24. Blaustein RO, Germann WJ, Finkelstein A, et al. The N-terminal half of the heavy chain of botulinum type A neurotoxin forms channels in planar phospholipid bilayers. *FEBS Lett* 1997;226:115–120.
25. Donovan JJ, Middlebrook JL. Ion-conducting channels produced by botulinum toxin in planar lipid membranes. *Biochemistry* 1996;25:2872–2876.
26. Hoch DH, Romero-Mira M, Ehrlich BE, et al. Channels formed by botulinum, tetanus, and diphtheria toxins in planar lipid bilayers: relevance to translocation of proteins across membranes. *Proc Natl Acad Sci U S A* 1985: 82:1692–1696.
27. Sheridan RE. Gating and permeability of ion channels produced by botulinum toxin types A and E in PC12 cell membranes. *Toxicon* 1998:36:703–717.
28. Schmid MF, Robinson JP, DasGupta BR. Direct visualization of botulinum neurotoxin-induced channels in phospholipid vesicles. *Nature* 1993;364:827–830.
29. Lebeda FJ, Olson MA. Structural predictions of the channel-forming region of botulinum neurotoxin heavy chain. *Toxicon* 1995;33:559–567.
30. Montal MS, Blewitt R, Tomich JM, et al. Identification

of an ion channel-forming motif in the primary structure of tetanus and botulinum neurotoxins. *FEBS Lett* 1992; 313:12–18.

31. Oblatt-Montal M, Yamazaki M, Nelson R, Montal M. Formation of ion channels in lipid bilayers by a peptide with the predicted transmembrane sequence of botulinum neurotoxin A. *Protein Sci* 1994;4:1490–1497.

32. Hanson MA, Stevens RC. Cocrystal structure of synaptobrevin-II bound to botulinum neurotoxin type B at 2.0-Å resolution. *Nat Struct Biol* 1997;7:687–690.

33. Hazzard J, Sudhof TC, Rizo J. NMR analysis of the structure of synaptobrevin and of its interaction with syntaxin. *J Biomol NMR* 1999;14:203–207.

34. Rupp B, Segelke B. Questions about the structure of the botulinum neurotoxin B light chain in complex with a target peptide. *Nat Struct Biol* 2001;8:663–664.

35. Kurazono H, Mochida S, Binz T, et al. Minimal essential domains specifying toxicity of the light chains of tetanus toxin and botulinum neurotoxin type A. *J Biol Chem* 1992;267:14721–14729.

36. Pellizzari R, Rossetto O, Lozzi, L, et al. Structural determinants of the specificity for synaptic vesicle-associated membrane protein/synaptobrevin of tetanus and botulinum type B and G neurotoxins. *J Biol Chem* 1996;271: 20353–20358.

37. Cornille F, Martin L, Lenoir C, et al. Cooperative exosite-dependent cleavage of synaptobrevin by tetanus toxin light chain. *J Biol Chem* 1997;272:3459–3464.

38. Matthews BW. Structural basis of the action of thermolysin and related zinc peptidases. *Acc Chem Res* 1998;21:333–340.

39. Sutton RB, Fasshauer D, Jahn R, et al. Crystal structure of a SNARE complex involved in synaptic exocytosis at 2.4-Å resolution. *Nature* 1998;395:347–353.

Scientific and Therapeutic Aspects of Botulinum Toxin
edited by M.F. Brin, J. Jankovic, and M. Hallett
Lippincott Williams & Wilkins, Philadelphia, © 2002.

3

Crystal Structure of *Clostridium botulinum* Neurotoxin Serotype B

Subramanyam Swaminathan and Subramaniam Eswaramoorthy

The toxigenic strains of *Clostridium botulinum* produce seven serologically distinct types of neurotoxins labeled A to G (EC 3.4.24.69), while *Clostridium tetani* produces tetanus neurotoxin (EC 3.4.24.68). Botulinum and tetanus neurotoxins (BoNTs and TeNT) are produced as single inactive chains of molecular mass of approximately 150 kDa. Most of these neurotoxins are released after being cleaved into two chains, a heavy chain (H) of 100 kDa and a light chain (L) of 50 kDa held together by an interchain disulfide bond, by tissue proteinases. BoNT/E is released as a single chain but cleaved by host proteinases (1). *Clostridium botulinum* neurotoxins are extremely poisonous proteins with their LD_{50} for humans in the range of 0.1 to 1 ng kg^{-1} (2). Botulinum neurotoxins are responsible for neuroparalytic syndromes of botulism characterized by serious neurological disorders and flaccid paralysis. BoNTs block the release of acetylcholine at the neuromuscular junction causing flaccid paralysis while TeNT blocks the release of neurotransmitters like glycine and γ-aminobutyric acid (GABA) in the inhibitory interneurons of the spinal cord resulting in spastic paralysis. In spite of different clinical symptoms, their etiological agents intoxicate neuronal cells in the same way and these toxins have similar structural organization (3).

Both BoNTs and TeNT are classified as AB (activating–binding) proteins because they are characterized by similar functional and domain structures. In the case of neurotoxins, the heavy chain forms the B (binding) domain, whereas

the L chain serves as the A (activating) domain (4). The H chain can be cleaved into two chains by papain digestion; the C-terminal chain, H_C, is the binding domain and the N-terminal domain, H_N, the translocation domain. This three-domain organization is similar to that of diphtheria toxin (DT) and *Pseudomonas aeruginosa* exotoxin A (ETA) (5,6). However, the effect of these toxins on target cells is different. While in most cases toxins cause cell death, only the exocytosis is blocked by neurotoxins (7). The structural motif of these toxins is different from other AB proteins, such as Cholera toxin, where the B domain comprises an oligomer (8,9). Even though the general intoxication may be similar the details are different, with each class having a specific mode. The intoxication by neurotoxins is proposed to be a four-step process (7,10–12): (a) cell binding; (b) internalization; (c) translocation into cytosol; and (d) enzymatic modification of a cytosolic target.

These neurotoxins have been classified as zinc-endopeptidases because of the presence of a conserved zinc binding motif, HExxH, approximately in the middle of the light chain (13,14). The inhibition of exocytosis by neurotoxins in cytosol has been identified as a zinc-dependent specific proteolysis of components in the neuroexocytosis apparatus. They act specifically on protein components of the same neuroexocytosis apparatus present in cytosol. Each neurotoxin attacks a specific target component: BoNT-B, D, F, and G specifically cleave the vesicle-associated membrane protein (VAMP, also called synaptobrevin); BoNT-A and E cleave a synaptosomal-associated protein of 25 kDa (SNAP-25) by specific hydrolysis; and BoNT-C cleaves

---

Color images for this chapter are available at www.wemove.org/toxinsbook/

syntaxin (15–20). Söllner et al. showed that these proteins together form part of a complex responsible for mediating vesicle docking and fusion (21). The importance of Zn in the catalysis has been established by the fact that chelation of Zn or use of zinc inhibitors blocks this intoxication process. BoNT-A is being used and approved by the Food and Drug Administration to treat various neuromuscular disorders such as strabismus, torticollis, and blepharospasm because of its specificity in inhibiting neurotransmitter release at neuromuscular junctions (22). However, for therapeutics, botulinum neurotoxin in complex with their associated proteins (NAPs) is being used. Recently, the use of BoNT-B for similar purposes was also approved.

In spite of the availability of a large body of chemical, biologic, and pathogenic information for these neurotoxins, the most vital information—three-dimensional structures—has started to appear only recently. The three-dimensional structures of BoNT-A (23), BoNT-B (24), BoNT-B light chain (25), and the C fragment of TeNT (26) have helped us understand the structure–function relationships in clostridial neurotoxins. Here we present the crystal structure of *C. botulinum* neurotoxin serotype B. Because

these neurotoxins bind first to the large negatively charged surface of the presynaptic membrane, which consists of polysialogangliosides and other acidic lipids (10), the crystal structure of BoNT-B in complex with sialyl lactose, which partly mimics the sugar group of a ganglioside, is also presented. These structures have helped us to map the active site and binding site.

DESCRIPTION OF THE STRUCTURE

The BoNT-B molecule has three distinct structural domains, each one corresponding to one of the three steps of the mechanism of toxification; namely, binding, translocation, and catalytic activity. They are arranged sequentially in a linear fashion with the translocation domain in the middle. Accordingly, there are no interactions between the binding and catalytic domains. The catalytic domain has a compact globular structure and belongs to the α/β classification. The translocation domain is mainly α-helical. The binding domain is made up of two subdomains (Fig. 3.1). The sequence of BoNT-B along with its secondary structural elements is presented in Table 3.1. Even though the primary sequence starts with the catalytic domain, the domain structures are discussed below starting from the

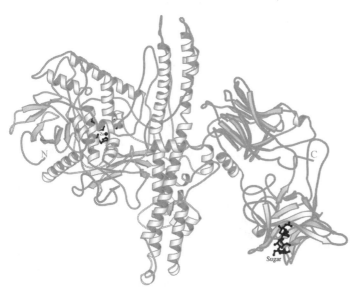

CATALYTIC   TRANSLOCATION   BINDING

FIG. 3.1. Ribbon representation of BoNT-B molecule. The three functional domains are marked as binding, translocation, and catalytic. The active site and its ligands are shown as ball-and-stick model in the catalytic domain and lie below the plane of the paper. The sialyl lactose molecule is also shown and is above the plane of the paper. This figure was generated by MOLSCRIPT (44).

TABLE 3.1. *The sequence of BoNT/B with the secondary structural elements marked below the sequence. E and H represent β strands and α helices as denoted in the line below the secondary structures. G and T represent 3/10 helices and turns, respectively.*

```
  1    PVTINNFNYN DPIDNNNIIM MEPPFARGTG RYYKAFKITD RIWIIPERYT
            TT              EEE EE GGGTT    EEEEEETT TEEEE
                           β1                 β2      β3
 51    FGYKPEDFNK SSGIFNRDVC EYYDPDYLNT NDKKNIFLQT MIKLFNRIKS
       TT  GGGG          TT     EE TTTT  HHHHHHHHHH HHHHHHHHTT
                           β4         EE          α1
101    KPLGEKLLEM IINGIPYLGD RRVPLEEFNT NIASVTVNKL ISNPGEVERK
       HHHHHHHHHH HHH          TT  TTEE  TTTEEEEE EEEEE    E
           α2                      β5        β6
151    KGIFANLIIF GPGPVLNENE TIDIGIQNHF ASREGFGGIM QMKFCPEYVS
       EEEE  EEEE        TT  E EE  EETTEE GGGTT    E EEE   EEE
       β7   β8              β9 β10 β11               β12
201    VFNAAAAAAA AAAFNRRGYF SDPALILMHE LIHVLHGLYG IKVDDLPIVP
       EE  TT   T T      EE   HHHHHHHH HHHHHHHHTT
       β13           β14        α3
251    NEKKFFMQST DAIQAEELYT FGGQDPSIIT PSTDKSIYDK VLQNFRGIVD
           TT      HHHHHH H TTGGGG    HHHHHHHHHH HHHHHHHHHH
                    α4                  α5
301    RLNKVLVCIS DPNININIYK NKFKDKYKFV EDSEGKYSID VESFDKLYKS
       HHHH  EE     TT  HHHHH HHHHHHTT E E TT  EE  HHHHHHHHHH
           β15            α6        β16    β17        α7
351    LMFGFTETNI AENYKIKTRA SYFSDSLPPV KIKNLLDNEI YTIEEGFNIS
       HHHT  HHHH HHHHT       EEEE EE  TT TTT   TTT T  G
           α8                β18
401    NKDMEKEYRG QNKAINKQAY EEISKEHLAV YKIQMCKSV- --GICIDVDN
       GGT  GGGGG G TTT GGG EE  GGG EE  EEEEE      EEEEEG
                          β19      β20 β21           β22
451    EDLFFIADKN SFSDDLSKNE RIEYNTQSNY IENDFPINEL ILDTDLISKI
       GG    GG G   GGG  E E          HHHH H
                 β23              α9
501    ELPSENTESL TDFNVDVPVY EKQPAIKKIF TDENTIFQYL YSQTFPLDIR
          EE            EEEEEEEE   HHHHH HTT    TT
          β24            β25         α10
551    DISLTSSFDD ALLFSNKVYS FFSMDYIKTA NKVVEAGLFA GWVKQIVNDF
          EEE  HHH HHH TTEEE  HHHHHHH T   HHHHH HHHHHHHHHH
          β26  α11    β27     α12         α13
601    VIEANKSNTM DKIADISLIV PYIGLALNVG NETAKGNFEN AFEIAGASIL
       HHHHHGGG     GGGT    TTHHHHH  T TTTT   HHH HHHHHGGGGG
                            α14                    α15
651    LEFIPELLIP VVGAFLLESY INNKNKIIKT IDNALTKRNE KWSDMYGLIV
                        EE      TT      HH HHHHHHHHHH HHHHHHHHH
                    β28                     α16
701    AQWLSTVNTQ FYTIKEGMYK ALNYQAQALE EIIKYRYNIY SEKEKSNINI
       HHHHHH HHH HHHHHHHHHH HHHHHHHHHH HHHHHHHHT   HHHHHT
```

(continued)

TABLE 3.1. *(continued)*

```
                  α17                                        α18
751   DFNDINSKLN EGINQAIDNI NNFINGCSVS YLMKKMIPLA VEKLLDFDNT
      HHHHHHHHH  HHHHHHHHHH HHHHHHHHHH HHHHH HHHH HHHHHHHHHH
                  α19                                        α20
801   LKKNLLNYID ENKLYLIGSA EYEKSKVNKA LKTIMPFDLS IYTNDTILIE
      HHHHHHHHHH H HHHH TTT TTTHHHHHHH TT      GG GT   HHHHH
                  α21                         α22
851   MFNKYNSEIL NNIILNLRYK DNNLIDLSGY GAKVEVYDGV ELNDKNQFKL
      HHHHHHT GG GG   EEEEE        EEE      EEEE TT EE TT EEEE
                    β29        β30          β31    β32    β33
901   TSSANSKIRV TQNQNIIFNS VFLDFSVSFW IRIPKYKNDG IQNYIHNEYT
        TT   EEE E   TT         EEEEEE EE     GGG HHHHH EEE
          β34                    β35                α23
951   IINCMKNNSG WKISIRGNRI IWTLIDINGK TKSVFFEYNI REDISEYINR
      EEEEEEETTEE EEEEEETTEE EEEEE TT  EEEEEEE             TT
        β36        β37        β38             β39
1001  WFFVTITNNL NNAKIYINGK LESNTDIKDI REVIANGEII FKLDGDIDRT
      EEEEEEE    EEEEEETTE  EEEEEE     EEE EEEEE       TT
        β40        β41        β42             β43
1051  QFIWMKYFSI FNTELSQSNI EERYKIQSYS EYLKDFWGNP LMYNKEYYMF
      EEEEEEEE E        HHHH HHHHHHHHH     TT      EE   EEEEE
        β44            α24                     β45   β46
1101  NAGNKNSYIK LKKDSPVGEI LTRSKYNQNS KYINYRDLYI GEKFIIRRKS
      ETT TTEEEE E TT   EEE EE                      EEEEE
        β47        β48                              β49
1151  NSASIADDIV RKEDYIYLDF FNLNQEWRVY TYKYFKKEEE KLFLAPISDS
        EE     TT EEEEEE  EETTEEEEEE  EETT     EE E EEEE
          β50        β51        β52          β53    β54
1201  DEFYNTIQIK EYDEQPTYSC QLLFKKDEES TDEIGLIGIH RFYESGIVFE
      TTEE   EEEE         E EEEEE      EEEEEEEE EEEEE       E
        β55    β56              β57          β58
1251  EYKDYFCISK WYLKEVKRKP YNLKLGCNWQ FIPKDEGWTE
      EEEEEEEEET THHHHTT    TT TT EE EE    TT
        β59        α25                    β60
```

C-terminal end in the sequential mode of action of the toxin.

Binding domain: The binding domain comprises two distinct domains corresponding to the N- and C-terminal halves (B_N and B_C). B_N contains two seven-stranded antiparallel β-sheets sandwiched together and resembles a jelly roll motif. This domain is very similar to the fold observed in legume lectins. Helix α24 runs almost parallel to the length of this β sandwich and connects B_N to B_C, and α22 is almost perpendicular to the sandwich and connects the binding domain to the translocation domain. One of the β-sheets has a concave surface and is exposed to the solvent region while the other

with a convex surface is packed against the translocation domain. In addition to a six-stranded β-barrel, the second subdomain (B_C) contains a β-trefoil motif formed by β strands β47, β48, β52, β55, β58 and β59. The β-trefoil is at the bottom of the molecule and is exposed to the solvent while the six-stranded β-barrel is closer to the β-sandwich of the B_N domain. The side chains from the hairpin bends at the bottom of the β-sandwich make van der Waals and hydrogen bond contacts with the B_C domain. The whole binding domain is tilted away from the central translocation domain and has minimal interaction with it. The structure of the binding domain is very similar to the C-fragment of tetanus toxin (TeNT-C) and the binding domain of BoNT-A (23,26), except for the conformation of long loops connecting β strands. Also, the interaction between the subdomains in BoNT-B is weaker than in BoNT-A or TeNT-C. Even though the overall sequence homology is poor for all clostridial neurotoxins in the C-terminal half of the binding domain, it was suggested that they would all adopt the same fold with the differences in sequences accounted for by the extended loop regions (26). The interface between B_N and B_C domains is filled with aromatic side chains.

Translocation domain: After toxins are bound to the membranes, a temperature- and energy-dependent process internalizes them. Neurotoxins have to cross the hydrophobic barrier of the vesicle membrane to attack their targets, the components of the neuroexocytosis apparatus, residing in the cytosol. This is common to all bacterial toxins with intracellular targets and is the least-understood step in the process. It has been proposed that the acidification of the vesicle lumen by a proton-pumping ATPase leads to conformational changes in the toxin. The acidic conformation then exposes a hydrophobic area of the toxin molecule, creates an ion channel in the membrane and inserts the L chain into cytosol (2,4,10). However, it is still not clear whether the L chain first unfolds to enter the ion channel or pore and then refolds within the cytosol.

The translocation domain consists of two, long, α-helical regions, each about 105 Å in length forming coiled-coil helices. Because of this coiled-coil nature, the helices have kinks or breaks in the helical structure and hence the two long helices are split into four helices, each approximately 50 Å in length. The core of the translocation domain consists of a four-helical bundle (α12, α13, α17, and α19) on one end and a three-helical bundle (α16, α20, and α21) on the other (Fig. 3.1). The three-helical bundle resembles the translocation region in other toxins like Colicin Ia (27). The putative translocation membrane region as predicted by the TMAP program lies in the region 639–667 (28). This region adopts an extended conformation and spans the molecule from the top to the middle of the molecule. The only α helix in this region is from 638–645 which is in the middle part of the molecule. Channel-forming regions in the heavy chain have also been predicted on the basis of hydrophobic moments (29). This region and the region immediately preceding it have about ten charged residues, most of which form strong hydrogen bonds through their side chains to adjacent residues either in the binding domain or in the translocation domain. It is apparent from this structure that this region is flexible and can change its conformation under favorable conditions. At low acidic pH, these side chains are expected to be protonated, thereby disturbing hydrogen bonding interactions which would further allow changes in conformation. Furthermore, if sequence upstream from 600 is considered (toward N-terminus), there are five more negatively charged residues that will also be affected by a change in pH. The structure of the region from 550 to 672 has both flexible regions and helices. The flexible regions should help in accommodating any change in the conformation.

In both BoNT-B and BoNT-A determined at pH 6.0 and 7.0, respectively, this region has a very flexible conformation—neither an extended nor a helical conformation. At this stage, it is difficult to speculate whether a further conformational change will take place at lower pH, because structures at lower pH are not known. There is a long loop formed by residues 481–532 that wraps around the catalytic domain and is aptly called the belt. Even though in the primary sequence this loop region is part of the translocation domain, in three dimensions it forms part of the catalytic domain. The conformation and position of the loop seem to play an important role in the catalytic action of the toxin.

Catalytic domain: In all BoNTs and TeNT, the L chain, responsible for the catalytic activity, contains a zinc-binding HExxH motif in the middle of the chain. Accordingly, the L chain has been identified as a zinc-endopeptidase. The L chain is released into the cytosol and attacks a specific target. Physicochemical measurements have shown that clostridial neurotoxins contain one zinc atom per molecule of toxin [except for BoNT-C which contains two zinc atoms (30)], bound to the L chain. As suggested by chemical modification and mutagenetic studies, two histidines and one glutamic acid provide ligands to zinc, similar to that in thermolysin (13,31). The fourth coordination is provided by a water molecule and is responsible for the hydrolysis of a peptide bond of the substrates.

The catalytic domain comprises a mixture of α helices and β sheets and strands (Fig. 3.1). This forms a compact globular-like protein structure. The active site zinc is found deep inside a large open cavity, which has a high negative electrostatic potential. This zinc is coordinated by two histidine residues (229 and 233) and a glutamate residue (267). In this structure the fourth coordination is supplied by an oxygen atom of a sulfate ion which is present in this structure. The protein was supplied as a precipitate in 60% ammonium sulfate which was removed by dialysis before the crystallization trials. It is proposed that the water molecule bound to the zinc ion was displaced by the sulfate ion when the protein was precipitated and remains tightly bound even after dialysis. However, because phosphate buffer was used throughout the protein purification, we cannot completely rule out the possibility of a phosphate ion in this position from crystallographic

studies alone. The presence of a sulfate or phosphate ion at the catalytic site has also been reported in the crystal structures of diphtheria repressor, carbonic anhydrase IV, and *Streptomyces griseus* aminopeptidase (32–34). The presence of a sulfate or phosphate ion also raises an interesting possibility: Could they be used to inhibit the toxin? We have also determined the crystal structure of BoNT-B where the sulfate ion was completely removed before crystallization. In this structure, the fourth coordination for the zinc ion is through a water molecule which is believed to be nucleophilic.

Figure 3.2 shows the zinc coordination in BoNT-B. Zinc is coordinated by protein atoms Nε2 of His229, Nε2 of His233, and Oε1 of Glu267. The fourth coordination is O of the nucleophilic water molecule. The coordination distances are 2.25, 2.20, 2.28, and 2.62 Å, respectively. This arrangement is very similar to that in thermolysin (31), where the HExxH motif is formed by residues 142 to 146. However, the distance between the nucleophilic water and the catalytic zinc ion in BoNT-B is much larger than in thermolysin (1.88 Å). Also, in thermolysin the nucleophilic water has two hydrogen bonds

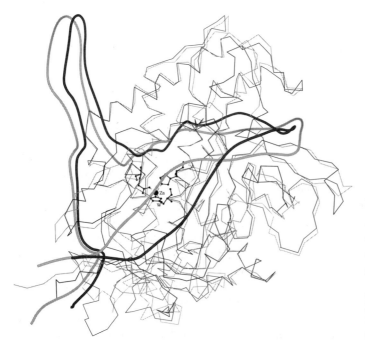

FIG. 3.2. The C-alpha trace of the light chains of BoNT-A and BoNT-B are superposed with the belt region shown in worm drawing. Light and dark shades correspond to BoNT-A and BoNT-B, respectively. In BoNT-A the zinc site is partially covered by the belt region. Zinc and its ligands of BoNT-B are shown in ball-and-stick model.

to Oϵ1 and Oϵ2 of residue Glu143 (corresponding to Glu230 in BoNT-B). It is argued that the nucleophilicity of this water is enhanced because of these hydrogen bonds in addition to the oxygen being coordinated to the zinc ion. A similar mechanism is also proposed for BoNT-A (35). In BoNT-B the situation is different, at least in the native structure. The coordination distance of the nucleophilic water to the zinc ion is 2.62 Å, much larger than in thermolysin. Also, the distance between the nucleophilic water and Oϵ1 or Oϵ2 of Glu230 is more than 3.6 Å, outside the hydrogen bonding distance. Under these circumstances, it is not clear how the water could be in an activated state. However, these distances are reported to be 2.2 and 2.4 Å, respectively, in BoNT-B-LC (25). The difference between BoNT-B and BoNT-B-LC could be a result of the differing pH. The mode of catalytic acta may be different in BoNT-B than in thermolysin. There is also very little similarity between the secondary structures of the two proteins in this site. The active site cavity is 15 $\times$ 24 $\times$ 25 Å in dimension, with a very wide mouth and an opening on the other side, which is partly shielded by Phe271. Modeling studies and inhibitor studies show that this cavity is big enough to accommodate medium-sized organic molecules. Our recent results (unpublished) with inhibitor-binding studies support this hypothesis. Modeling studies based on our polyalanine model of the catalytic domain with 7-*N*-phenyl-carbamoylamino-4-chloro-3-propyloxyisocoumarin show that the cavity is big enough to accommodate this molecule (M. Adler, Meeting of the Interagency Botulism Research Coordinating Committee, Orlando, 1999).

COMPARISON OF BONT-A AND -B

Overall, the three-dimensional structures of BoNT-A and -B are similar. Individual domains fold similarly and the C-alpha chains superpose with a root mean square deviation (rmsd) of less than 2.0 Å. The rmsd's between the binding, translocation, and the catalytic domains of BoNT-A and -B are 1.43, 1.56, and 1.43 Å, respectively for about 80% to 85% matched residues. However, when the molecules are considered as a whole, only 49% of the residues match with a rmsd of 2.06 Å, which indicates that the association of the three domains may be slightly different in the two molecules. In particular, the orientation of the binding domain with respect to the translocation domain is different. In BoNT-B the binding domain makes a smaller tilt to the translocation domain than in BoNT-A. Also the orientation of the belt region and its position with respect to the zinc site is different. Although the catalytic and translocation domains (except for the belt region) superpose fairly well, the binding domains, especially the C-terminal halves, do not. These differences may be because the pH of crystallization was different.

In BoNT-A there is a disulfide bridge between Cys1234 and Cys1279 in the C-terminal domain (B$_C$). This disulfide bond is absent in BoNT-B, even though sequence alignment shows cysteines aligned at these positions (36). The distance between the two Sγ's is about 10 Å. Of the ten cysteine residues present in the molecule, only Cys436 and Cys445 form a disulfide bond. All others, except Cys70, have an accessible surface area of zero, which suggests that they are all buried. Cys70 has a nonzero value and it is exposed to the solvent as predicted from biochemical studies (37).

THE ROLE OF THE BELT REGION

The loop region 481–532 of the translocation domain that wraps around the catalytic domain seems to play a significant role in botulinum neurotoxins. The substrates for all neurotoxins are long polypeptides with separate binding and cleavage sites. The separation between these two sites is speculated to play a role in the specificity of the targets. We speculate that either the substrates take the position of the belt in the separated light chain or perhaps the belt region helps in forming interactions with the substrates, if the L chain is not separated. Once they are bound to the toxin, the cleavage site may protrude inside the active site cavity. In BoNT-A the active site is shielded from the environment by the belt region (23). But it has a different disposition in BoNT-B than in BoNT-A (Fig. 3.2). In BoNT-A, the cavity is partially covered by the belt on looking down the cavity. This enables the zinc ion to be shielded from the environment. In BoNT-B, the belt region does not shield the zinc ion, thus making it completely accessible to inhibitor or substrate molecules. This difference in orientation of the belt region may be either a result of the shorter length of the belt region in BoNT-A than in B and E, or because of the different pH values at which BoNT-A and -B were crystallized. In any case, this fact presents interesting possibilities in the design of inhibitor molecules for various botulinum neurotoxins. It also suggests that the belt region in type E may be more similar to type B than to type A. Interestingly, all residues within a radius of 8 Å from zinc are identical in BoNT-A and -B, except for five. However, as the radius increases, differences set in and the belt region gets involved at about 15 Å. This similarity suggests that the difference in substrate specificity between the two molecules may not be a consequence of the residues in the immediate vicinity of zinc site, but may be a long-range effect especially near the mouth of the cavity.

TYROSINE PHOSPHORYLATION AND ENHANCED CATALYTIC ACTIVITY

It has been reported that nonreceptor tyrosine kinase Src phosphorylates botulinum neurotoxins A, B, and E, and tetanus neurotoxin. Tyrosine phosphorylation of serotypes A and E of *C. botulinum* neurotoxin increases their catalytic activity in addition to increasing their thermal stability. The effect is also reversed when the toxins are dephosphorylated. This led to the postulation that the toxin may exist in phosphorylated form inside the neuron (38). Tyr372, which is in the vicinity of the active site, is believed to be a proton donor to stabilize the leaving group after the scissile bond is cleaved (25,35,39). However, in the case of BoNT-B, the distance between the zinc and the OH of Tyr372 is more than 6.6 Å and the orientation seems not to be conducive for a proton donation. If Tyr372 is phosphorylated, in addition to its pKα value changing from phenolic to phosphoric value, the required OH for donating a proton comes much closer to zinc. A hypotheti-

cal model with Tyr372 phosphorylated brings the OH group of the phosphate group within 4.5 Å (figure not shown). The enhancement of the catalytic activity may be a result of this shorter distance.

REDUCED FORM OF BONT-B

Reduction of the interchain disulfide is a prerequisite for toxic activity and the rate-limiting step in toxicity (40). The absence of the toxic activity in the unreduced state suggests that after reduction, the toxin undergoes some structural change in order for the substrate to come closer to the active site which is in a deep cavity. It is also believed that the light chain will separate from the heavy chain to enter the cytosol to attack the targets. However, in a recent structure determination in our laboratory in which the protein was reduced with 10 mM DTT and crystallized in the presence of DTT, even though the Sγ- Sγ distance is more than 3.1 Å, the two chains stay together in a compact form (unpublished results). Also, there is no significant difference in the main chain fold of the molecule. We believe that reduction of disulfide alone is not enough for the catalytic domain to separate. There could still be an unidentified process required to separate the catalytic domain.

EVIDENCE FOR GANGLIOSIDE BINDING

The first step in the intoxication process is binding of neurotoxins to the neuronal cell. This takes place via gangliosides available at the surface of the neuronal cell. However, to explain the high activity of this neurotoxin, a double-receptor model—a low-affinity ganglioside and a high-affinity protein receptor—has been proposed. The toxins first bind to the neuronal cells via low-affinity gangliosides and then move laterally to bind to the high-affinity receptor, a protein. Neurotoxins bind to di- and trisialogangliosides, especially to the 1b series. GD1b and GT1b bind effectively to the neurotoxins. The structure of BoNT-B in complex with sialyl lactose defines the binding site of sialyl lactose to the C-fragment of BoNT-B. Sialyl lactose partly mimics one branch of the sugar moiety of GT1b; thus, this structure provides a model for interaction of ganglioside to the neurotoxin. The results from our studies correlate with the mutagenic and biochemical studies.

The C-terminal half of the binding domain preserves the ganglioside binding property of the neurotoxin (41). In the case of TeNT, the C-terminal residues (1281–1314) are sufficient for ganglioside binding and photo-affinity labeling occurs predominantly at His1292 (42). Also, BoNT-A tryptophan fluorescent quenching is accompanied by ganglioside binding, suggesting that tryptophans are part of the ganglioside binding site. Sequence comparison of BoNTs and TeNT reveals that there are a number of conserved tryptophan residues at the C-terminus of all neurotoxins (43). In TeNT, residues 1235–1294, containing tryptophan at 1288, are particularly critical for binding. This tryptophan corresponds to Trp1261 in BoNT-B, which is also exposed to solvent, making it more amenable for fluorescent quenching. This tryptophan is exposed in all neurotoxins for which three-dimensional structures are known. In BoNT-B, this residue is located just before the N-terminus of α25. In view of all this, it was thought that the ganglioside-binding site may include this tryptophan and residues in this site. However, the crystal structure of the complex reveals significant differences in the interactions predicted by these methods. For example, it was suggested that the two lysines close to His1292 in TeNT might bind to the negatively-charged carboxylate groups of sialic acids of GT1b (42), which suggests that three lysine residues and one arginine close to Glu1265 of BoNT-B might bind to the negatively charged carboxylate groups of sialic acids of GT1b, by analogy. There is a cleft between Trp1261 and His1240 and the sialic acid sits between these two and the sugar moiety makes several hydrogen bonds with the protein molecule. Sialic acid and the galactose make hydrogen-bonding contacts with Glu1188, Glu1189, His1240, and Tyr1262. Sialic acid also makes hydrophobic contacts with Trp1261. However, the sialic acid does not make any contact with Lys1267, Arg1268, Lys1269, or Glu1265, as proposed for TeNT (42). These resi-

dues, though close to Trp1261 in primary sequence, are spatially far from this binding site. The closest contact the sialic acid makes with a lysine is with Lys1264 at 6.4 Å. Only the terminal sialic acid and the adjacent galactose are making contacts with the protein molecule while glucose is protruding outside of the protein. Superposition of the three C-fragment models after least squares fit brings His1252 (BoNT-A), His1240 (BoNT-B), and His1270 (TeNT) spatially in the same place. Similarly Glu1202 (BoNT-A), Glu1189 (BoNT-B), and Asp1221 (TeNT) align both in sequence and space. Tryptophan and these residues form the same kind of pocket in all three structures. Because one branch of the sugar moiety of GT1b has a terminal sialic acid with the same 2→3 link with the galactose, we propose that this will provide a model for interaction for all neurotoxins. His1292, the site of photo-affinity labeling in TeNT, lies on the other side of Trp1288 relative to His1240, creating a small pocket. However, preliminary studies with other branched sugar moieties show no density in this region in the difference density map that could accommodate the other sialic acid of GT1b. Figure 3.1 shows the site where sialyl lactose binds. Sialyl lactose and the interacting protein residues form a nice lock-and-key arrangement.

As discussed earlier, the structure of the BoNT-B:sialyl lactose complex provides a model for the interaction for the sugar moiety of ganglioside GT1b and the binding domain. The residues defining this site are common to all neurotoxins; hence, the interaction of ganglioside sugar may be the same in other complexes as well. Accordingly, this binding site offers itself a target for inactivated recombinant vaccine development. If the binding of neurotoxin to the cell could be prevented, the toxicity itself could be eliminated. Recombinant vaccine must be superior to the presently available experimental vaccine, a chemically inactivated toxin.

ACKNOWLEDGEMENTS

We thank Drs. B. R. Singh, B. R. DasGupta, and M. Adler for useful discussions. We also thank Dr. D. Kumaran for his help. Research supported by the Chemical and Biological Non-proliferation Program—NN20 of the US Department of Energy under Prime Contract No. DE-AC02–98CH10886 with Brookhaven National Laboratory.

REFERENCES

1. Sathyamurthy V, Dasgupta BR. Separation, purification, partial characterization and comparison of the heavy and light chains of botulinum neurotoxin types A, B, and E. *J Biol Chem* 1985;260:10461–10466.
2. Schiavo G, Rossetto O, Montecucco C. Clostridial neurotoxins as tools to investigate the molecular events of neurotransmitter release. *Semin Cell Biol* 1994;5: 221–229.
3. Simpson LL. Molecular pharmacology of botulinum toxin and tetanus toxin. *Annu Rev Pharmacol Toxicol* 1986;26:427–453.
4. Montecucco C, Papini E, Schiavo G. Bacterial protein toxins penetrate cells via a four-step mechanism. *FEBS Lett* 1994;346:92–98.
5. Choe S, Bennett MJ, Fujii G, et al. The crystal structure of diphtheria toxin. *Nature* 1992;357:216–222.
6. Allured VS, Collier RJ, Carroll SF, et al. Structure of exotoxin A of *Pseudomonas aeruginosa* at 3.0 Angstrom resolution. *Proc Natl Acad Sci U S A* 1986;83: 1320–1324.
7. Schantz EJ, Johnson EA. Properties and use of botulinum toxin and other microbial neurotoxins in medicine. *Microbiol Rev* 1992;56:80–99.
8. Sixma TK, Kalk KH, van Zanten BA, et al. Refined structure of *Escherichia coli* heat-labile enterotoxin, a close relative of cholera toxin. *J Mol Biol* 1993;230: 890–918.
9. Stein PE, Boodhoo A, Armstrong GD, et al. The crystal structure of pertussis toxin. *Structure* 1994;2:45–57.
10. Menestrina G, Schiavo G, Montecucco C. Molecular mechanisms of action of bacterial protein toxins. *Mol Aspects Med* 1994;15:79–193.
11. Montecucco C, Schiavo G. Mechanism of action of tetanus and botulinum neurotoxins. *Mol Microbiol* 1994; 13:1–9.
12. Oguma K, Fujinaga Y, Inoue K. Structure and function of *Clostridium botulinum* toxins. *Microbiol Immunol* 1995;39:161–168.
13. Schiavo G, Rossetto O, Santucci A, et al. Botulinum neurotoxins are zinc proteins. *J Biol Chem* 1992;267: 23479–27483.
14. Blasi J, Chapman ER, Link E, et al. Botulinum neurotoxin A selectively cleaves the synaptic protein SNAP-25. *Nature* 1992;365:160–163.
15. Schiavo G, Shone CC, Rossetto O, et al. Botulinum neurotoxin serotype F is a zinc-endopeptidase specific for VAMP/synaptobrevin. *J Biol Chem* 1993;268: 11516–11519.
16. Schiavo G, Benfenati F, Poulain B, et al. Tetanus and botulinum-B neurotoxins block neurotransmitter release by a proteolytic cleavage of synaptobrevin. *Nature* 1992;359:832–835.
17. Blasi J, Chapman ER, Yamasaki S, et al. Botulinum neurotoxin C blocks neurotransmitter release by means

of cleaving HPC-1/syntaxin. *EMBO J* 1993;12: 4821–4828.
18. Schiavo G, Santucci A, Dasgupta BR, et al. Botulinum neurotoxins serotypes A and E cleave SNAP-25 at distinct COOH-terminal peptid bonds. *FEBS Lett* 1993; 335:99–103.
19. Schiavo G, Rossetto O, Catsicas S, et al. Identification of the nerve terminal targets of botulinum neurotoxin serotypes A, D, and E. *J Biol Chem* 1993;268: 23784–23787.
20. Schiavo G, Malizio C, Trimble WS, et al. Botulinum G neurotoxin cleaves VAMP/synaptobrevin at a single Ala–Ala peptide bond. *J Biol Chem* 1994;269: 20213–20216.
21. Söllner T, Whiteheart SW, Brunner M, et al. SNAP receptors implicated in vesicle targeting and fusion. *Nature* 1993;362:318–324.
22. Johnson EA, Goodnough MC. Preparation and properties of botulinum toxin type A for medical use. In: Tsui JKC, Calne DB, eds. *Handbook of dystonia.* New York: Marcel Dekkar, 1995:347–365.
23. Lacy DB, Tepp W, Cohen AC, et al. Crystal structure of botulinum neurotoxin type A and implications for toxicity. *Nat Struct Biol* 1998;5:898–902.
24. Swaminathan S, Eswaramoorthy S. Structural analysis of the catalytic and binding sites of *Clostridium botulinum* neurotoxin B. *Nat Struct Biol* 2000;7:693–699.
25. Hanson MA, Stevens RC. Cocrystal structure of synaptobrevin-II bound to botulinum neurotoxin type B at 2.0 Å resolution. *Nat Struct Biol* 2000;7:687–692.
26. Umland TC, Wingert LM, Swaminathan S, et al. Structure of the receptor binding fragment Hc of tetanus neurotoxin. *Nat Struct Biol* 1997;4:788–792.
27. Weiner M, Freymann D, Ghosh P, et al. Crystal structure of colicin Ia. *Nature* 1997;385:461–464.
28. Persson B, Argos P. Topology prediction of membrane proteins. *Protein Sci* 1996;5:363–371.
29. Lebeda FJ, Olson MA. Structural predictions of the channel-forming region of botulinum neurotoxin heavy chain. *Toxicon* 1995;33:559–567.
30. Schiavo G, Shone CC, Bennett MK, et al. Botulinum neurotoxin type C cleaves a single Lys–Ala bond within the carboxyl-terminal region of syntaxins. *J Biol Chem* 1995;270:10566–10570.
31. Holmen MA, Matthews BW. Structure of thermolysin refined at 1.6 Å resolution. *J Mol Biol* 1982;160: 623–639.
32. Pohl E, Holmes RK, Hol WGJ. Motion of the DNA-binding domain with respect to the core of the diphtheria toxin repressor (DtxR) revealed in the crystal structures of apo- and holo-DtxR. *J Biol Chem* 1998;273: 22420–22427.
33. Stams T, Nair SK, Okuyama T, et al. Crystal structure of the secretory form of membrane-associated human carbonic anhydrase IV at 2.8-Å resolution. *Proc Natl Acad Sci U S A* 1996;93:13589–13594.
34. Greenblatt HM, Almog O, Maras B, et al. *Streptomyces griseus* aminopeptidase: x-ray crystallographic structure at 1.75-Å resolution. *J Mol Biol* 1997;265:620–636.
35. Li L, Binze T, Niemann H, et al. Probing the mechanistic role of glutamate residues in the zinc-binding motif of type A botulinum neurotoxin light chain. *Biochemistry* 2000;39:2399–2405.
36. Antharavally BS, DasGupta BR. Covalent structure of botulinum neurotoxin type B; location of sulfhydryl

groups and disulfide bridge and identification of C-termini of light and heavy chains. *J Protein Chem* 1998; 17:407–415.

37. Antharavally B, Tepp W, DasGupta BR. Status of Cys residues in the covalent structure of botulinum neurotoxin types A, B, and E. *J Protein Chem* 1998;17: 187–196.

38. Ferrer-Montiel AV, Canaves JM, DasGupta BR, et al. Tyrosine phosphorylation modulates the activity of clostridial neurotoxins. *J Biol Chem* 1996;271:18322–18325.

39. Schiavo G, Matteoli M, Montecucco C. Neurotoxins affecting neuroexocytosis. *Physiol Rev* 2000;80:717–766.

40. de Paiva A, Poulain B, Lawrence GW, et al. A role for the interchain disulfide or its participating thiols in the internalization of botulinum neurotoxin A revealed by a toxin derivative that binds to ecto-acceptors and inhibits transmitter release intracellularly. *J Biol Chem* 1993; 268:20838–20844.

41. Halpern JL, Loftus A. Characterization of the receptor-binding domain of tetanus toxin. *Nature* 1993;268: 11188–11192.

42. Shapiro RS, Specht CD, Collins BE, et al. Identification of a ganglioside recognition domain of tetanus toxin using a novel ganglioside photo-affinity ligand. *J Biol Chem* 1997;272:30380–30386.

43. Thompson JD, Higgins DG, Gibson TJ. CLUSTAL W: improving the sensitivity of progressive multiple sequence alignment through sequence weighting, position-specific gap penalties and weight matrix choice. *Nucleic Acids Res* 1994;22:4673–4680.

44. Kraulis P. MOLSCRIPT: a program to produce both detailed and schematic plots of proteins. *J Appl Crystallogr* 1991;24:946–950.

Scientific and Therapeutic Aspects of Botulinum Toxin
edited by M.F. Brin, J. Jankovic, and M. Hallett
Lippincott Williams & Wilkins, Philadelphia, © 2002.

4

The Receptor Binding Domains of Clostridial Neurotoxins

J. Mark Sutton, Lindsey Spaven, Nigel J. Silman, Bassam Hallis, Oliver Chow-Worn, and Clifford C. Shone

The different clinical symptoms of botulism and tetanus poisoning mask the underlying similarity in the modes of action of the toxins (1,2). Botulinum toxins (BoNTs) act at the neuromuscular junction where they block the release of acetylcholine preventing muscle contraction and causing widespread flaccid paralysis. Tetanus toxin initially binds to the same peripheral nerves as the BoNTs but is then transported retrogradely to the central nervous system where it blocks the release of glycine by inhibitory interneurons. This results in spastic paralysis because of failure to regulate muscle contraction, a clinical symptom that appears to be directly opposite to that observed for botulinum poisoning. Biochemically, BoNTs and tetanus neurotoxin (TeNT) exert their effects via a similar pathway of intoxication. The toxins bind to receptor molecules on the surface of peripheral nerves (3). Binding is followed by internalization of the toxin, by receptor-mediated endocytosis, and release of the toxin into the nerve ending. The neurotoxins are zinc-endopeptidases that exert their effect by the specific cleavage of proteins involved in the fusion of synaptic vesicles to the neuronal membrane, preventing the release of neurotransmitters. The target and site of substrate cleavage differs for the neurotoxins. BoNT-B and TeNT cleave the same site on vesicle-associated membrane protein (VAMP), which is also cleaved by BoNT-D, BoNT-F, and BoNT-G. Synaptosomal-associated protein of 25 kDa (SNAP-25) is cleaved by BoNT-A, BoNT-E, and BoNT-C, which also cleaves syntaxin (reviewed in 2).

The clostridial neurotoxin family are all structurally conserved, consisting of a light chain (LC) of approximately 50 kDa plus a heavy chain (HC) of approximately 100 kDa linked by a disulfide bond. Biochemical data and the recent description of the crystal structure for BoNT-A (4), BoNT-B (5), and the C-terminal of TeNT/HC (6) have allowed the allocation of function to various domains within the toxin. The LC domains are responsible and sufficient for the zinc-endopeptidase activity associated with each neurotoxin. The HC is involved in receptor binding and the translocation of the LC into the nerve ending. The N-terminal 50 kDa (H_N) consists of a series of extended α-helices and is involved in translocation of the enzymatic domain from the endosome into the cell cytosol (7), whereas the C-terminal 50 kDa (H_C) is involved in receptor binding (8,9). Overall, the structures of the toxins are remarkably similar to a wide range of other bacterial toxins including diphtheria toxin which use a similar AB (activating–binding) architecture for their enzymatic and delivery domains (10).

Clostridial neurotoxins bind specifically to neuronal cells with a subnanomolar binding affinity. The eight neurotoxins do not compete with each other for binding to cell membranes (11) suggesting that there may be several distinct receptor pools which mediate the uptake of different serotypes. The identification of the receptor molecules is also complicated by a range of studies which suggest that there is both a protein and a carbohydrate moiety involved in the binding and internalization of the toxins. Several studies show that TeNT and its H_C fragment bind to polysialogangliosides of the 1b class, notably GT1b and GD1b, but do not bind to simpler monosialic gangliosides such as GM_1 (8,12). An elegant study by Williamson et al. (13) showed that treatment of neuronal cells with an agent capable of blocking ganglioside synthesis prevents both binding and intoxication by TeNT. Thus, the ganglioside component may play a key role in determining cellular specificity. Polysialogangliosides are particularly abundant on neuronal cells where they may play a role in cell differentiation and signaling (14). The precise binding affinity for individual gangliosides differs between members of the clostridial neurotoxin family (12), although all appear to be able to bind to GT1b and GD1b. Because the different serotypes are unable to cross-compete for cell binding, it is difficult to argue convincingly that gangliosides are the sole receptor for clostridial neurotoxins. This is unlike cholera in which ganglioside GM_1 is its sole receptor (15). This conclusion is supported by other studies that show that protease treatment of neuronal cells can also block binding (16). A dual receptor model with an initial binding to gangliosides followed by lateral movement to a protein receptor has been proposed (17). Alternatively, the ganglioside may bind to the H_C domain and cause a change in conformation that will allow its binding to the protein receptor. A number of protein receptors have been proposed for clostridial neurotoxins including synaptotagmin (18), β-adducin (19), and, most recently, a 15-kDa integral membrane protein (20). The latter interacts directly with the H_C domain of TeNT in cross-linking experiments (21).

Binding data for a variety of H_C fragments have begun to define the regions involved in receptor binding. Mutations in the C-terminal domain (H_{CC}) but not in the N-terminal domain (H_{CN}) affect ganglioside binding. (8). Two regions of the molecule were identified: removal of the C-terminal ten amino acids (1305–1314) abolishes both ganglioside and cell binding, while amino acids 1235–1294 were shown to be particularly important for ganglioside binding. Results from Shapiro et al. (22) also implicate the C-terminus of TeNT/H_{CC} in ganglioside

binding with the demonstration that a 34-amino acid peptide (amino acids 1281–1314) is sufficient to bind gangliosides, albeit at a low affinity. This study also showed that photoactivatable ganglioside analog specifically labeled His1292, implicating the adjacent lysine residues in interactions with the ganglioside. This same region is also implicated in BoNT-E binding, as the equivalent peptide sequence (amino acids 1223–1229) is recognized by a monoclonal antibody that blocks intoxication (23). In BoNT-A, the removal of the C-terminal 30 amino acids by trypsin treatment prevents cell binding (9). The incubation of BoNT-A with gangliosides results in the fluorescence quenching of tryptophan suggesting that there is tryptophan residue within the binding pocket (24). As there are three conserved tryptophan residues within the final 30 amino acids of the clostridial neurotoxins, the precise identity of this tryptophan-containing pocket has waited until the recent publication of crystal structures for various neurotoxin fragments.

The crystal structures of BoNT-A (4), BoNT-B (5), and TeNT-H_C (6), together with studies in which carbohydrates have been cocrystallized with carbohydrate molecules [TeNT-H_C (25); BoNT-B (5)], have been published since 1997. To date, it has not been possible to cocrystallize a toxin fragment with a complete ganglioside. However the data do provide information concerning the likely points of interaction with the carbohydrate subunits that comprise the ganglioside side chains. The H_C consists of two distinct and separate domains. The N-terminal H_{CN} domain is similar in structure to many lectins consisting of 14-stranded β-barrel structure, often referred to as a jelly roll motif. The C-terminal H_{CC} domain forms a β-trefoil motif that is similar to that found in members of the trypsin inhibitor family (4). The study of Emsley et al. (25) shows the positions adopted by lactose, galactose, sialic acid, and N-acetylgalactosamine in soaked crystals of TeNT-H_C. The binding sites are not adjacent on the surface of the crystal as might be expected for a complex carbohydrate such as a ganglioside. The lactose binding pocket with key side chains provided by N1220, S1287, D1222, T1270, Y1290, G1300, and

W1289 appears to be most closely conserved with the BoNT-A structure, where there are equivalent amino acids for all but N1220. This pocket in BoNT-A also includes a solvent exposed tryptophan residue, equivalent to W1265 in BoNT-A, which has been identified by Stevens et al. (4) as the most likely candidate for the quenched tryptophan residue proposed by Kamata et al. (24). The other carbohydrate-binding sites appear to less conserved as evidenced by the very different residues implicated in binding to free sialic acid as compared to sialic acid within sialyl lactose (5). The significance of these binding pockets will be confirmed by cocrystallization of the toxins with gangliosides and by the mutational analysis of key residues. As yet, no function has been assigned to the H_{CN} domain, although its similarity to lectins raises the intriguing possibility that it may be involved in an as yet unidentified binding interaction possibly related to intracellular trafficking.

A comparison of the sequence similarity between the toxins shows that they are relatively divergent in the H_{CC} domain (with a maximum of 30% identity) but are more conserved in the H_{CN} domain (26). There is no obvious difference between the botulinum and tetanus that might account for their different trafficking properties. The study by Ginalski et al. (26) has used the published crystal structures to model the H_{CC} domain based on the general architecture of β-trefoil domains. The identification of key residues may prove difficult given that the sequences must provide both the core structure for the conserved ability to bind cellular receptors and the diversity observed in the respective binding partners of the neurotoxins.

The study of the receptor-binding domains of the clostridial neurotoxins has been fueled in recent years by the development of a number of applications in neuronal targeting. A number of proteins [Sutton et al. unpublished; (27–29)] have been delivered using clostridial neurotoxin fragments. Such molecules clearly have a potential application in the treatment of a range of neurologic conditions, both in the periphery (BoNT) and the central nervous system (CNS) (TeNT). The delivery of DNA packages (30) and adenoviruses (31) has also raised the possibility

that clostridial neurotoxin fragments can be used as delivery vectors for neuronal gene therapy.

Our studies attempted to build on the existing biochemical and crystallography data to define the limits of the binding domain and to identify key residues within this domain. The results identify the H_{CC} region of TeNT as being responsible for binding to gangliosides and cells. Site-directed mutagenesis has identified Y1290 as being involved in the binding interaction.

METHODS

Cloning and Expression of TeNT-H_C Mutants

The TeNT-H_C gene used in these studies was a fully synthetic gene with a codon bias optimized for expression in *Escherichia coli*. All manipulations were carried out using standard methods (32). Deletion mutants were constructed by cloning of short oligonucleotide linkers into sites engineered in the original gene. Site-directed mutants were constructed by PCR or splice overlap PCR using mutagenic primers (33) and their sequences confirmed. All fragments were expressed as MBP fusions from the vector pMAL-c2x (New England Biolabs). Expression was carried out in Terrific broth essentially as outlined in the protocol manual with cultures grown to mid logarithmic phase at 30°C (86°F) before induction. Following addition of IPTG at a final concentration of 500 μmol the temperature was reduced to 25°C (77°F) and cultures grown for a further 2 hours. Purification on an amylose column was precisely as described in the protocol manual [New England Biolabs (NEB)]. Eluted protein was dialyzed against 20 mmol HEPES pH 7.4 containing 200 mmol NaCl.

Radioiodination of TeNT

TeNT, purified by ion exchange chromatography (34), was dialyzed against 0.1 M borate buffer pH 8.5 and then 100 μL containing 300 μg TeNT was reacted with dried Bolton and Hunter reagent (37 MBq; Amersham Pharmacia Biotech) for 15 minutes on ice with gentle agitation. Unreacted reagent was separated from the

^{125}I-labeled TeNT by gel filtration on Sephadex G25 (PD10 column, Pharmacia) equilibrated in 0.05 M HEPES, 0.2 M NaCl pH 7.4.

Competition Binding Assays with Rat Brain Synaptosomes

Rat brain synaptosomes were prepared as described previously (9) and diluted in 0.05 M HEPES pH 7.4 buffer to a final concentration of 2 mg mL^{-1} synaptosomal protein. Binding assays were performed in either 0.05 M HEPES pH 7.4 buffer containing 0.6% BSA (HEPES binding buffer) or HANK's pH 7.4 buffer containing 0.6% BSA (HANK's binding buffer). Binding\assay incubations (0.2 mL) contained a final concentration of 2 nmol ^{125}I-labeled TeNT and varying concentrations of TeNT-H$_C$ fragments. Assays performed in HEPES binding buffer were initiated by the addition of synaptosomal membranes to a final concentration of 1 μg mL^{-1} synaptosomal protein and those in HANK's buffer by the addition of 100 μg mL^{-1} synaptosomal protein. Assays were incubated for 2 hours at 2°C (35.6°F) and then washed twice with 1-mL aliquots of the respective binding buffer and radioactivity in the synaptosome pellet determined (9).

Binding to Gangliosides

Gangliosides GT$_{1b}$ or GM$_1$ (Research Biochemicals International) were diluted to 20 μg mL^{-1} in methanol, added to microtiter plates (50 μL/well) and allowed to dry for 16 hours at 22° C (71.6°F). Plates were then blocked with HEPES binding buffer for 1 hour at 37°C (98.6°F) before being washed six times with phosphate-buffered saline, pH 7.4. Binding assay mixtures containing 2 nmol ^{125}I-labeled TeNT and various concentrations of unlabeled TeNT-H$_C$ fragments in HEPES binding buffer were added (50 μL/well) and incubated for 1 hour at 22°C (71.6°F). Plates were then washed with 2 × 150 μL of HEPES-binding buffer and the radioactivity bound to plate wells determined.

RESULTS

Analysis of the Functional Domains of TeNT-H$_C$ Responsible for Binding to Rat Brain Synaptosomes

Deletion mutants were constructed within the H$_C$ domain to clarify conflicting data about the limits of the binding domain (Fig. 4.1A). H$_{CN}$ and H$_{CC}$ domains were expressed in isolation (amino acids 865–1140 and 1084–1315 respectively). H$_{CN}$ was disrupted by removing amino acids 865–927. The C-terminal region of H$_C$ (amino acids 1233–1315), including the 34 amino acids identified as retaining ganglioside-binding activity, was also expressed. All proteins were tested for their ability to compete for binding with ^{125}I-labeled TeNT to rat brain synaptosomes (Fig. 4.1B) or to bind to ganglioside GT1b on solid phase (Fig. 4.1C). The H$_{CC}$-long construct showed wild-type binding activity in both assays. The isolated H$_{CC}$ domain retained binding activity, although this was significantly reduced as compared to H$_C$. This suggests that either the interface between the two domains is involved in binding or that the conformation is disturbed by the removal of the H$_{CN}$ domain. Neither the H$_{CN}$ nor the C-terminal region of H$_C$ showed any binding activity.

Identification of Key Residues Within the Binding Domain of TeNT-H$_C$

Site-directed mutants were constructed in TeNT-H$_{CC}$ to try and identify key amino acids within the binding domain (Fig. 4.2). These mutants were tested in competition experiments using two different binding conditions to try to differentiate between mutants that affected ganglioside binding and mutants that might interfere with binding to the protein component of the receptor complex (16). In low ionic strength buffers, (HEPES) TeNT binds to a neuraminidase-sensitive, ganglioside-like acceptor on synaptic membranes. In physiologic buffers (HANK's), TeNT binds to a receptor site that is additionally sensitive to proteases which might suggesting an interaction with the protein acceptor component under these conditions (16).

Mutants within the C-terminal region of the

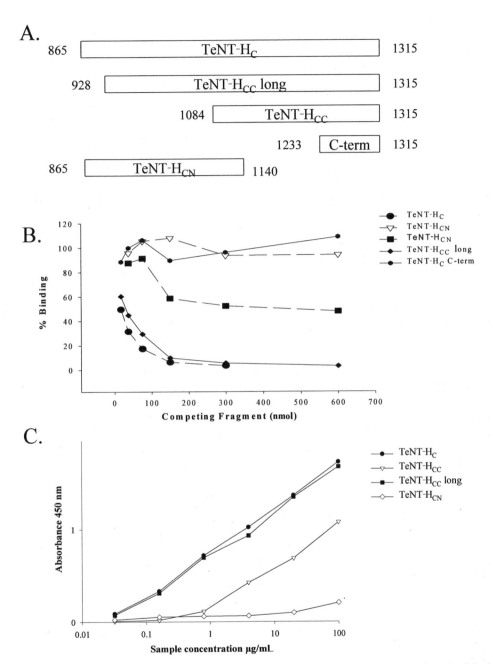

FIG. 4.1. Construction of deletion mutants of TeNT-H_C implicate the C-terminal domain (H_{CC}) in binding to gangliosides and rat brain synaptosomes. Deletions were constructed in the TeNT-H_C (*panel A*). The proteins were expressed and purified and tested for their ability to bind to gangliosides (*panel B*) and to compete with ^{125}I-labeled tetanus toxin for binding to rat brain synaptosomes (*panel C*). The disruption of the H_{CN} domain by the removal of amino acids 865–927 had no effect on either ganglioside or synaptosome binding. The isolated H_{CC} domain retained a proportion of the binding activity of the native H_C although this was reduced in both assays. Neither an isolated H_{CN} domain, nor a peptide consisting of the C-terminal amino acids 1233–1315 of H_C, showed any binding activity.

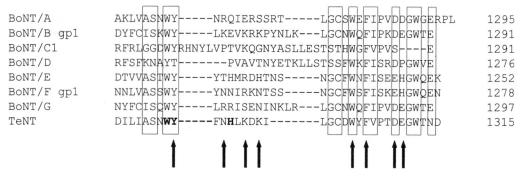

FIG. 4.2. Alignment of the C-terminal 40 amino acids of the clostridial neurotoxin family. The mutations constructed in this study are shown as arrows. Residues that are conserved in at least six of the eight serotypes are shown boxed. The amino acids H1293, Y1290, and W1289, which are implicated in ganglioside and receptor binding, are shown in bold. For the sake of clarity, only single members of each serotype are shown.

β-trefoil domain of the TeNT-H_C were tested in the binding assays. Table 4.1A shows the effects of various mutations in this region on the binding of TeNT-H_C to rat brain synaptosomes. Region 1305–1310 is apparently critical for ganglioside binding (8). Of the mutations in this region only E1310A caused a significant reduction in binding. This was more marked when binding assays were performed in HANK's buffer, which might suggest an interaction with the protein receptor component. This residue lies within

a shallow pocket on the surface of TeNT-H_C bounded by strands β17, β22, and adjacent loops on the other two sides (6). However, mutations made in these regions or conservative mutations of E1310 and the adjacent charged residue (D1309) had no effect on synaptosome binding (Table 4.1A). Together these results might indicate that mutations in this region have a conformational effect on receptor binding rather than being involved in a direct interaction.

The amino acid H1293 has been implicated

TABLE 4.1. *Binding of TeNT site-directed mutants to rat brain synaptosomes*

Hc mutant	Binding relative to native TeNT-H_C	
	HEPES buffer	HANK's buffer
A. Mutations in C-terminal Pocket		
E1310→A	34% ± 17%	9% ± 4.1%
E1310→Q	as native	as native
E1310→Q; D1309→N	as native	as native
D1309→A	as native	as native
D1309→N	as native	as native
F1305→A	as native	as native
W1303→A	as native	35% ± 8%
R1168→A	as native	32% ± 4%
R1168→K	as native	as native
Y1170→A	as native	as native
B. Mutations in Helix 5 Pocket		
Y1290→A	7.7% ± 1.5%	>1%
Y1290→F	42% ± 11%	54% ± 3.5%
Y1290→S	>3%	>1%
N1292→A	as native	as native
K1295→A	as native	as native
K1297→A	as native	as native

in ganglioside binding (22) and mutagenesis of this residue significantly reduced binding to gangliosides (35). Again this residue lies in a shallow surface pocket, on the opposite side of the β-trefoil domain to the C-terminus, adjacent to helix-5 (6). Site-directed mutants were constructed in the vicinity of H1293 (Fig. 4.2). Mutation Y1290A significantly reduced the binding to rat brain synaptosomes in low ionic strength buffer at pH 7.4 and more markedly in HANK's buffer (Table 4.1B). Additional mutants of Y1290 were constructed. Mutant Y1290F caused approximately twofold reduced binding to synaptosomes compared to wild-type TeNT-H_C, whereas Y1290S showed an even greater effect on binding than the Y1290A mutant. The possibility that these Y1290 mutations might cause gross alteration to the conformation of the H_{CC} domain was checked by measuring the CD spectra of the proteins. No significant differences in the CD spectra were observed compared to native TeNT-H_C

Ganglioside-Binding Properties of TeNT-HC Y1290 Mutants

The Y1290 mutants were analyzed in solid-phase ganglioside-binding assays to exclude any other components that might be involved in the interaction. The mutants were compared with wild-type TeNT-H_C for their ability to compete with ^{125}I-labeled TeNT for binding to GT1b (Table 4.2). The binding of Y1290 mutants to ganglioside showed a similar pattern to the results observed on rat brain synaptosomes with the binding of Y1290F>Y1290A>Y1290S. No specific binding of ^{125}I-labeled TeNT to GM_1 ganglioside was observed in similar assays.

TABLE 4.2. *Binding of Y1290 site-directed mutants to ganglioside GT1b*

H_C mutant	Binding to GT1b relative to native TeNT-H_C
Y1290→A	16.1% ± 2.9%
Y1290→F	38.0% ± 2%
Y1290→S	>1%

DISCUSSION

The results described here have begun to define the regions of the TeNT-H_C domain required for receptor binding. The C-terminal half of TeNT-H_C (H_{CC}) of TeNT toxin retains the ability to bind gangliosides and cells (21) although in our assay systems this ability is significantly reduced. We have also identified Y1290 as being essential for binding to both ganglioside and synaptosomes. This residue is conserved within the clostridial neurotoxin family (Fig. 4.2). The result is entirely consistent with the model proposed by Ginalski et al. (26) using structure-based sequence alignment. Y1290 has also been identified as one of the amino acids that interacts with the lactose in a binding pocket on the surface of TeNT-H_{CC} (25). In addition, H1293, which is also implicated in ganglioside binding (22,35), is located on the rim of this pocket. Interestingly mutations in H1293 caused significant reductions in ganglioside binding without affecting the ability of the TeNT-H_C to bind to cells (35). Our results suggest that Y1290 does affect membrane binding to rat brain synaptosomes and it will be interesting to observe the effect of this mutation on the ability of TeNT-H_C to compete with TeNT to block intoxication. Overall, the data provide direct evidence for the location of the ganglioside-binding pocket as proposed by Ginalski et al. (26) and suggest that Y1290 plays a key role in this interaction.

Clearly further analysis will be required to identify other contact points within this binding pocket and elsewhere on TeNT-H_{CC}. A comprehensive set of mutants may allow us to address the involvement of gangliosides in determining the specificity of receptor binding by clostridial neurotoxins. In turn, this will lead to a greater understanding of the mechanism of neurotoxin entry into cells and its potential applications as a delivery system for neuronal therapy.

REFERENCES

1. Niemann H. Clostridial neurotoxins. In: Alouf JE, Freer JH, eds. *Sourcebook of bacterial protein toxins.* London: Academic Press, 1991:303–348.
2. Schiavo G, Matteoli M, Montecucco C. Neurotoxins affecting neuroexocytosis. *Physiol Rev* 2000;80:717–766.

3. Dolly JO, Black J, Williams RS, et al. Acceptors for botulinum neurotoxin reside on motor nerve terminals and mediate its internalization. *Nature* 1984;307: 457–460.

4. Lacy B, Tepp W, Cohen AC, et al. Crystal structure of botulinum neurotoxin type A and implications for toxicity. *Nat Struct Biol* 1998;5:898–902.

5. Swaminathan S, Eswaramoorthy S. Structural analysis of the catalytic and binding sites of *Clostridium botulinum* neurotoxin B. *Nat Struct Biol* 2000;7:693–699.

6. Umlan TC, Wingert LM, Swaminathan S, et al. Structure of the receptor binding fragment HC of tetanus neurotoxin. *Nat Struct Biol* 1997;4:788–792.

7. Shone CC, Hambleton P, Melling J. A 50-kDa fragment from the NH$_2$-terminus of the heavy subunit of *Clostridium botulinum* type A neurotoxin forms channels in lipid vesicles. *Eur J Biochem* 1987;167:175–180.

8. Halpern JL, Loftus A. Characterization of the receptor-binding domain of tetanus toxin. *J Biol Chem* 1993;268: 11188–11192.

9. Shone CC, Hambleton P, Melling J. Inactivation of *Clostridium botulinum* type A neurotoxin by trypsin and purification of two tryptic fragments. Proteolytic action near the COOH-terminus of the heavy subunit destroys toxin-binding activity. *Eur J Biochem* 1985;151:75–82.

10. Choe S, Bennett MJ, Fujii G, et al. The crystal structure of diphtheria toxin. *Nature* 1992;357:216–222.

11. Evans DM, Williams RS, Shone CC, et al. Botulinum neurotoxin type B. Its purification, radioiodination and interaction with rat-brain synaptosomal membranes. *Eur J Biochem* 1986;154:409–416.

12. Schengrund CL, DasGupta BR, Ringler NJ. Binding of botulinum and tetanus neurotoxins to ganglioside GT1b and derivatives thereof. *J Neurochem* 1991;57: 1024–1032.

13. Williamson LC, Bateman KE, Clifford JCM, Neale EA. Neuronal sensitivity to tetanus toxin requires gangliosides. *J Biol Chem* 1999;274:25173–25180.

14. Rosner H. Significance of gangliosides in neuronal differentiation of neuroblastoma cells and neurite growth in tissue culture. *Ann N Y Acad Sci* 1998;845:200–214.

15. van Heyningen S. Binding of ganglioside by the chains of tetanus toxin. *FEBS Lett* 1976;68:5–7.

16. Pierce EJ, Davison M, Parton RG, et al. Characterization of tetanus toxin binding to rat brain membranes. Evidence for a high-affinity proteinase-sensitive receptor. *Biochem J* 1986;236:845–852.

17. Montecucco C. How do tetanus and botulinum toxins bind to neuronal membranes? *Trends Biochem Sci* 1986; 11:314–317.

18. Nishiki T, Tokuyama Y, Kamata Y, et al. The high-affinity binding of *Clostridium botulinum* type B neurotoxin to synaptotagmin II associated with gangliosides GT1b/GD1a. *FEBS Lett* 1996;378:253–257.

19. Schengrund CL, DasGupta BR, Hughes CA, et al. Ganglioside-induced adherence of botulinum and tetanus neurotoxins to adducin. *J Neurochem* 1996;66: 2556–2561.

20. Herreros J, Lalli G, Montecucco C,et al. Tetanus toxin fragment C binds to a protein present in neuronal cell lines and motoneurons. *J Neurochem* 2000;74: 1941–1950.

21. Herreros J, Lalli G, Schiavo G. C-terminal half of tetanus toxin fragment C is sufficient for neuronal binding and interaction with a putative protein receptor. *Biochem J* 2000;347:199–204.

22. Shapiro RE, Specht CD, Collins BE, et al. Identification of a ganglioside recognition domain of tetanus toxin using a novel ganglioside photo-affinity ligand. *J Biol Chem* 1997;272:30380–30386.

23. Kubota T, Watanabe T, Yokosawa N, et al. Epitope regions in the heavy chain of *Clostridium botulinum* type E neurotoxin recognized by monoclonal antibodies. *Appl Environ Microbiol* 1997;63:1214–1218.

24. Kamata Y, Yoshimoto M, Kozaki S. Interaction between botulinum neurotoxin type A and ganglioside: ganglioside inactivates the neurotoxin and quenches its tryptophan fluorescence. *Toxicon* 1997;35:1337–1340.

25. Emsley P, Fortinou C, Black I, et al. The structures of the H(C) fragment of tetanus toxin with carbohydrate subunit complexes provide insight into ganglioside binding. *J Biol Chem* 2000;275:8889–8894.

26. Ginalski K, Venclovas C, Lesyng B, et al. Structure-based sequence alignment for the beta-trefoil subdomain of the clostridial neurotoxin family provides residue level information about the putative ganglioside binding site. *FEBS Lett* 2000;482:119–124.

27. Dobrenis K, Joseph A, Rattazzi MC. Neuronal lysosomal enzyme replacement using fragment C of tetanus toxin. *Proc Natl Acad Sci U S A* 1992;89:2297–2301.

28. Francis JW, Hosler BA, Brown RH Jr, Fishman PS. CuZn superoxide dismutase (SOD-1): tetanus toxin fragment C hybrid protein for targeted delivery of SOD-1 to neuronal cells. *J Biol Chem* 1995;270: 15434–15442.

29. Francis JW, Brown RH Jr, Figueiredo D, et al. Enhancement of diphtheria toxin potency by replacement of the receptor binding domain with tetanus toxin C-fragment: a potential vector for delivering heterologous proteins to neurons. *J Neurochem* 2000;74:2528–2536.

30. Knight A, Carvajal J, Schneider H, et al. Nonviral neuronal gene delivery mediated by the HC fragment of tetanus toxin. *Eur J Biochem* 1999;259:762–769.

31. Schneider H, Groves M, Muhle C, et al. Retargeting of adenoviral vectors to neurons using the Hc fragment of tetanus toxin. *Gene Ther* 2000;7:1584–1592.

32. Sambrook J, Fritsch EF, Maniatis T, eds. *Molecular cloning, a laboratory manual, 2nd ed.* Cold Spring Harbor: Cold Spring Harbor Laboratory Press, 1989.

33. Horton RM, Hunt HD, Ho SN, et al. Engineering hybrid genes without the use of restriction enzymes: gene splicing by overlap extension. *Gene* 1989;77:61–68.

34. Shone CC, Tranter HS. Growth of clostridia and preparation of their neurotoxins. In: Montecucco C, ed. *Clostridial neurotoxins—current topics in microbiology and immunology.* Berlin: Springer-Verlag, 1995:143–160.

35. Sinha K, Box B, Lalli G, et al. Analysis of mutants of tetanus toxin Hc fragment: ganglioside binding, cell binding and retrograde axonal transport properties. *Mol Microbiol* 2000;37:1041–1051.

Scientific and Therapeutic Aspects of Botulinum Toxin
edited by M.F. Brin, J. Jankovic, and M. Hallett
Lippincott Williams & Wilkins, Philadelphia, © 2002.

5

Neurospecific Binding and Trafficking of Tetanus Toxin

Giovanna Lalli, Judit Herreros, and Giampietro Schiavo

THE PATHOPHYSIOLOGIC AND NEUROANATOMIC BASIS OF TETANUS

The dramatic effects of tetanus neurotoxin (TeNT) have been known since the beginning of medical literature, starting with Hippocrates who described a paralyzed patient with hyper-contracted skeletal muscles and first introduced the name (tetαυοσ contraction) to indicate the disease induced by this toxin. Often fatal, tetanus is caused by *Clostridium tetani,* a strictly anaerobic, sporogenic bacterium. *C. tetani* is widespread in nature in the form of spores, which can germinate under appropriate conditions of low oxygen, slight acidity and availability of nutrients (1). Such conditions are met in anaerobic wounds, where the vegetative form of the bacterium can then proliferate locally and express TeNT. Because TeNT is responsible for all clinical symptoms of tetanus, this disease can be completely prevented by antitoxin-specific antibodies (2). Toxin-neutralizing antibodies can be acquired passively by injection of purified immunoglobulins or, actively, as a result of vaccination with tetanus toxoid, which is obtained by treating TeNT with paraformaldehyde. More recently, alternative antitetanus vaccines have been developed by genetic engineering employing the binding fragment of TeNT (2).

TeNT and the closely related botulinum neurotoxins (BTX) are the most toxic substances known, with an LD_{50} in mice ranging between 0.1 and 1 ng/kg of body weight. Such high toxicity is determined both by their absolute neurospecificity and by their intracellular catalytic ac-

tivity. The time of onset of paralysis is variable depending upon species, dose, and route of entry in the body. However, a lag phase, that in the case of clinical tetanus may be longer than 1 month, is always present. The delay in appearance of the first symptoms is present also in the case of injection of purified neurotoxins and cannot be accounted for only on the basis of the time needed for spore germination and toxin expression.

After entering the general circulation, both TeNT and BTX, which together form the clostridial neurotoxin (CNT) family, bind specifically to the presynaptic membrane of neuromuscular junctions (NMJ). TeNT also binds to sensory and adrenergic neurons. The binding of both classes of CNT to NMJ is rapid, characterized by high affinity, and largely irreversible. BTX enters the cytosol and blocks the release of acetylcholine (Ach) at the NMJ, thereby causing a flaccid paralysis (3), whereas TeNT lacks any action at this level (4). By contrast, TeNT is transported retrogradely up to the spinal cord (Fig. 5.1), where it accumulates in the ventral horn of the gray matter (5). Within the spinal cord, TeNT migrates transsynaptically from the dendrites of motor neurons into coupled inhibitory interneurons and blocks the release of inhibitory neurotransmitters (4). Excitatory synapses appear not to be affected at early stages (6), but they may be inhibited at later stages (7). The specificity of TeNT for inhibitory versus excitatory synapses is maintained when TeNT is applied to organotypic preparations, but is lost in neuronal cultures (6,8), suggesting that it may be partially caused by the anatomic organization

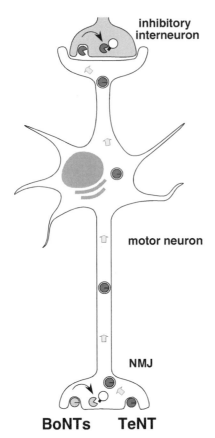

FIG. 5.1. Trafficking and differential sorting of TeNT and BoNTs. After entering the NMJ, TeNT (*right*) is retrogradely transported to the cell body of the motor neuron, where it is transsynaptically transferred and internalized by inhibitory interneurons in the spinal cord. Only at this level the L chain is translocated to the cytosol in the active state and cleaves the synaptic vesicle-associated membrane protein. In contrast, BTX (*left*) are sorted to endocytic compartments that remain at the NMJ, allowing translocation of the L chain and cleavage of their target soluble NSF (*N*-ethylmaleimide–sensitive factor) attachment receptor (SNAREs) within the NMJ.

of the tissue. This specificity for inhibitory synapses is not restricted to the spinal cord, but has been observed also for the hippocampus *in vivo* (9). This could account for the neurodegenerative and epileptogenic effects of TeNT, which mainly result from unopposed release of glutamate from excitatory synapses. During transsynaptic migration, TeNT reaches the intersynaptic

space, as demonstrated by the ability of anti-TeNT antibodies injected in the spinal fluid to neutralize its inhibitory effects (10). The blockade of spinal cord inhibitory synapses caused by TeNT impairs the neuronal circuit that ensures balanced voluntary muscle contraction, causing the spastic paralysis characteristic of tetanus (11).

The opposite clinical symptoms of tetanus and botulism result therefore from a difference in the intracellular trafficking of TeNT and BTX. The distinction between the central site of activity of TeNT and the peripheral sites of action of BTX exists, however, only at physiologic concentrations (picomolar and lower) and it is largely lost at the doses (nanomolar and higher) used in the laboratory. Under these conditions, TeNT also inhibits neurotransmitter release at peripheral synapses (12).

Morphologic examination of synapses intoxicated with TeNT reveals a consistent increase in the number of small synaptic vesicles (SSV) close to the cytosolic face of the presynaptic membrane (13). Besides this anomaly, SSV are well preserved in terms of number, size, and quantal content. At electrophysiologic level, TeNT causes a desynchronization of the quanta released after depolarization, similar to that observed upon intoxication with BTX-B, D and -F (14–17). This desynchronization and neurotransmitter release inhibition can not be relieved by treatments increasing the intrasynaptic concentrations of calcium (16). On this basis, CNTs fall into two functional groups: on one side there is TeNT together with BTX-B, -D, and -F, whereas and on the other side are BTX-A, -C, and -E, which form a second class. These findings were recently rationalized at the molecular level with the identification of the intracellular targets of CNT (see below).

STRUCTURE–FUNCTION RELATIONSHIPS

As expected from their sequence homology and similar activity at the synapse, TeNT and BTX share a closely related structural organization (18,19). TeNT is produced as an inactive polypeptide chain of 150 kDa, which is released in the culture medium only after bacterial lysis. In contrast to BTX, no accessory polypeptides are associated with TeNT. Single-chain TeNT is activated by a variety of proteases that cleave an exposed loop, generating the active di-chain form (20). This is composed by the heavy chain (H, 100 kDa) and the light chain (L, 50 kDa), which remain associated via noncovalent protein–protein interactions and a conserved interchain disulfide bond, whose integrity is essential for neurotoxicity (21). Treatment of TeNT with papain generates a C-terminal fragment, termed H_C, and a heterodimer composed of the L chain and the N-terminal portion of the H chain (22,23).

Although no crystal structure of TeNT is presently available, the analysis of the structure of the highly related BTX-A and -B confirmed the existence of three functional domains assembled together in a modular fashion (24–26). These domains are structurally distinct with the exception of a large loop in the N-terminal part of the H chain, which wraps around the perimeter of the L chain.

H_C is implicated in the neurospecific binding of CNT and in the retrograde transport of TeNT (5,22). However, its overall interaction with the neuronal membrane displays a lower affinity than the di-chain neurotoxin (20,27). The structure of the H_C of TeNT has recently been solved alone or in complex with several carbohydrate chains (28–30). H_C is composed of two distinct subdomains, rich in β-structure and of almost identical size. The N-terminal subdomain (H_{CN}) has a jelly roll fold closely similar to that present in oligosaccharide-binding proteins. The C-terminal portion (H_{CC}) of the H chain adopts a modified β-trefoil structure, which is present in several proteins involved in recognition and binding functions. The entire H_C remains completely isolated from the rest of the molecule, allowing a complete accessibility of its surfaces for binding. H_C domains from different CNTs show a similar three-dimensional structure, with the major differences being in the H_{CC} loops that are poorly conserved (18,19). The removal of the N-terminal domain from H_C does not reduce

membrane binding, whereas the deletion of only ten residues from the C-terminus abolishes neurospecific binding (31).

The N-terminal part of H chain (H_N) is implicated in the pH-dependent membrane penetration and translocation of the catalytic domain into the cytosol. It is composed of a loop interacting with the L chain and a central body whose main structural units are two amphipathic α-helices. The H_N domain exhibits a pore-forming activity *in vitro* (32,33), which is likely to involve these two α-helical structures (34).

The L chain is responsible for the intracellular activity of CNT (reviewed in 4). The catalytic site contains a zinc atom essential for the protease activity (4), which can be removed by heavy metal chelators, generating inactive apo-CNT (35–38). Insights on the common features of the L chains of CNT can be gathered from the comparison of the structures of BTX-A and BTX-B (24–26). The catalytic site is buried in the structure of the protein, being accessible from the outside only via a large channel, which accommodates the substrate. However, the precise mechanism controlling the binding of the substrate to the active site is still unclear (39,40). In BTX-A, entry to the channel is partially blocked by the large loop wrapping the L chain and by the translocation domain itself (24), whereas in BTX-B the active site is completely exposed (26). Analysis of the structure of the catalytic site shows that the zinc is held in place by two histidines located in the central and most conserved portion of CNT. These two residues reside in the sequence HExxH, which is the motif characterizing the catalytic site of metallo-endopeptidases (41,42). The glutamic acid residue present in this motif coordinates the water molecule (third ligand) necessary for the catalysis, while another glutamic acid residue more distal in the primary sequence is the fourth zinc ligand. Spectroscopic studies suggested the presence of a tyrosine residue in the vicinity of the metal atom (43), as previously observed for the members of the metzincins superfamily (44). This result was confirmed by the presence of a tyrosine residue (Y372 in BTX-B), which has an important role in the catalysis as proton donor to the cleaved peptide bond (25).

THE CELLULAR MECHANISM OF ACTION OF TENT

The mechanism adopted by TeNT and BTX to intoxicate neurons consists of four-steps:
(a) neurospecific binding;
(b) internalization;
(c) membrane translocation; and
(d) intracellular enzymatic activity.
Several reviews have recently covered the molecular basis of the intracellular activity of CNTs and of their substrates and the poorly characterized translocation step (4,16,45–47). We focus here on the interaction of TeNT with the neuronal surface and the following trafficking step.

NEUROSPECIFIC BINDING AND TARGETING

TeNT and BTX present two classes of presynaptic binding sites with subnanomolar and nanomolar affinities (5) and the available evidence suggests that the H_C domain plays a major role in the binding processes (5,22,27).

A large number of studies demonstrated the involvement of polysialogangliosides in TeNT and BTX binding (reviewed in 4,5,48). CNT show maximal binding to members of the G1b series, which are able to protect the NMJ from neurotoxin-mediated inhibition of neurotransmitter release and to partially abolish the retrograde transport of TeNT (49). Preincubation with polysialogangliosides increases the sensitivity of cultured chromaffin cells to TeNT and BTX-A (50) and inhibition of their synthesis by fumonisin B blocks the intracellular action of TeNT (51). Moreover, knockout mice for $\beta(1,4)$-N-acetylgalactosaminyl transferase and lacking complex gangliosides are less sensitive to TeNT, BTX-A and B than are wild-type animals (52).

It is unlikely, however, that the binding to polysialogangliosides totally accounts for the absolute neurospecificity of these neurotoxins (48). Experimental evidence indicates that pro-

teins may be involved in toxin binding and could be responsible for the toxicity observed in mice lacking polysialogangliosides (53–58). The presence of lectin-like and protein binding domains in the H_C fragment of TeNT and BTX (24–26,29,30) suggests that CNTs may bind to the presynaptic membrane via multiple interactions with sugar and protein-binding sites (48). Recent experiments provide strong evidence in favor of such a double receptor model by showing that TeNT interacts with an N-glycosylated glycosylphosphatidylinositol (GPI)-anchored protein in NGF-differentiated PC12 cultures, spinal cord cells, and purified motor neurons (57–59). This putative protein acceptor, which has been identified as neuronal Thy-1 in NGF-differentiated PC12 cells (58), specifically interacts with the H_C fragment of TeNT and not the analogous portions of BTX. TeNT H_C binding to the cell surface and to this protein acceptor is blocked by sialic acid-specific lectins, supporting the central role of sialic acid residues in the recognition process (57). H_{CC} is necessary and sufficient for cell binding and for the interaction with this 15-kDa protein acceptor (59). In contrast, the N-terminal half (H_{CN}) interacts very poorly with the cell surface. These results restrict the binding segment of TeNT to the β-trefoil portion of H_C, highlighting the importance of this domain for the interaction of TeNT with the neuronal surface and supporting its use as a neurospecific targeting device (see below). At the same time, these findings are pointing to a possible involvement of H_{CN} in later steps of the intoxication pathway.

Further evidence for the double-receptor model is provided by the finding that BTX-B interacts with the intravesicular domain of the SSV proteins synaptotagmin I and II in the presence of polysialogangliosides (60–62). This result was very recently extended to BTX-A and -E (63), suggesting that synaptotagmin may act as protein receptor for all BTX. However, competition experiments demonstrated that different BTX do not share the same receptor (12,64). A possible model, which recapitulates all these findings, envisages the interaction of each BTX with a different synaptotagmin isoform. The sensitivity to different BTX would then depend on the repertoire of synaptotagmins expressed on a particular cell type (65).

To reach its final site of action, TeNT has to bind and enter into two different neurons: a peripheral motor neuron and an inhibitory interneuron of the spinal cord (Fig. 5.1). The comparison of the toxicity of TeNT and its fragments at peripheral and central level indicates that TeNT binding to NMJs and to presynaptic terminals in the spinal cord is different (66,67). Niemann (68) suggested a mechanism in which polysialogangliosides act as peripheral receptors for TeNT, mediating its retrograde transport to the CNS, where the toxin would bind to a second, different acceptor. This model, however, suffers from the drawback of the low affinity and specificity of polysialogangliosides as the only TeNT receptor at peripheral level, where a high affinity interaction is necessary to account for the high toxicity of TeNT *in vivo*. Alternatively, both glycoprotein and glycolipids could be involved in the high-affinity peripheral binding of TeNT and BTX. Support for this model was recently provided by the finding that TeNT is recruited to detergent-insoluble lipid rafts on the surface of neuronal cells (58) and that the integrity of these microdomains is essential for the internalization and the intracellular activity of the toxin. BTX-B and -E bind also to lipid rafts (69), thus suggesting that, similarly to other pathogens (70), the recruitment to membrane domains enriched in cholesterol, sphingolipids, and GPI-anchored proteins could represent a general mechanism for CNT binding to neurons.

Several reports suggest that TeNT could induce protein kinase C (PKC) modulation *in vivo* and *in vitro* (71–74), arguing in favor of a possible implication of PKC pathway in TeNT neurotoxicity. Surprisingly, the activation of the signal transduction pathways involving phospholipase C1, several PKC isoforms and ERK-1/2 (75) is not dependent on the catalytic activity of TeNT and could be mimicked by the isolated HC fragment. (76). Therefore, PKC activation must be triggered by the interaction of TeNT with a surface membrane component, which may participate in TeNT binding and internalization into neuronal cells.

INTERNALIZATION

Because the catalytic activity of the L chains is directed toward intracellular targets, at least this toxin domain must reach the cytosol. *In vivo*, CNTs do not enter the cell directly via the plasma membrane, but are rather endocytosed inside acidic cellular compartments. Electron microscopic studies show that, after binding, CNTs enter the lumen of vesicular structures in a temperature- and energy-dependent process (77–85). Parton et al. (82) examined the binding and internalization of gold-labeled TeNT in dissociated spinal cord neurons. The toxin was found to accumulate in coated pits on the cell surface, followed by internalization in a variety of vesicular structures, such as endosomes, tubules, and, to a lesser extent, SSV. A recent study in hippocampal neurons (83,84) provides further insights into the internalization pathway used by TeNT. In this system, TeNT colocalizes with SSV markers following membrane depolarization, suggesting its internalization via SSV. It is well-established that nerve stimulation facilitates intoxication (reviewed in 4). A high rate of neuroexocytosis correlates with a high rate of SSV recycling, the two processes being tightly coupled (86,87). A possible explanation for the shorter onset of paralysis induced by CNT under nerve stimulation is that they enter the synaptic terminal inside the lumen of SSV, as shown for antibodies against the lumenal portion of synaptotagmin I (88,89). Despite the attractiveness of this model for the entry of CNT in CNS neurons, it is rather unlikely that this mechanism participates in the uptake of TeNT at the NMJ. In fact, three experimental findings contrast with this hypothesis. First, high-frequency stimulation increases the rate of intoxication but not the binding of TeNT to the NMJ (90). If the toxin receptor is exposed during neuroexocytosis to allow the toxin to bind and then be endocytosed, an increase of the stimulation rate should also increase the total number binding sites present at the NMJ. Second, TeNT is not active on a NMJ maintained at 18°C (64.4°F), even in the presence of high-frequency stimulation and massive neurotransmitter release, although it is fully inhibitory at 25°C (77°F) (90). Third, the uptake and retrograde transport of TeNT is perfectly functional in NMJ when neurotransmitter release is blocked by BTX-A (91). This latter fact is in agreement with the notion that retrograde transport of various ligands is not impaired in silenced NMJ (92,93). Preliminary experiments on spinal cord motor neurons show that there is indeed very limited colocalization between TeNT and SSV markers (85), indicating that the pathway of internalization and intracellular trafficking of TeNT may be different in peripheral and central neurons.

The different protein receptor complexes of TeNT and BTX might be responsible for their different targeting at the NMJ: inclusion in an endocytic carrier undergoing retrograde transport along the axon in the case of TeNT and entry inside vesicles that acidify within the NMJ for BTX (Fig. 5.1). Recent evidence indicates that the internalization of TeNT and BTX-B and -F in neurons is indeed mediated by distinct mechanisms (84). However, BTX and TeNT could share the same internalization mechanism, possibly via SSV endocytosis (83,84), in neurons in which they block neurotransmitter release (inhibitory interneurons for TeNT and NMJ for BTX).

Chimeras of TeNT H_C with superoxide dismutase (SOD) (94,95), lysosomal hydrolase (96), β-galactosidase (97), and the catalytic fragment of diphtheria toxin (98) are internalized, retrogradely transported with high efficiency, and, at least in selected cases, undergo transcytosis (97). Recombinant TeNT H_C fused with polylysine to enable binding of DNA has been recently used for nonviral gene delivery in neuroblastoma and glioma cell lines, opening the possibility for its exploitation in neuronal gene therapy (99). Hybrid proteins show long-term stability after cellular internalization, suggesting that they are probably enclosed in an endosomal compartment not targeted to lysosomes (85,100). These findings open up the possibility of using fusion proteins containing the H_C fragment or recombinant atoxic forms of TeNT (101,102), as neurospecific carriers of bioactive molecules and as tracers to study the molecular mechanism underlying retrograde transport *in vitro* (85) and to map synaptic connections *in vivo*.

TRANSLOCATION INTO THE NEURONAL CYTOSOL

After they are internalized, the L chains must cross the vesicle membrane to reach the cytosol in order to display their activity. Internalization and membrane translocation of CNT are clearly distinct steps in the process of cell intoxication, as is the case for most bacterial toxins acting in the cytoplasm (103). Compelling evidence indicates that di-chain CNT have to be exposed to a low pH step to block neurotransmitter release (reviewed in 4). However, acidic pH is not required for a direct activation of the toxin, as direct targeting of the L chain to the cytosol is sufficient to block exocytosis (4,16,45–47 and references cited therein). It is therefore likely that low pH is crucial for the process of membrane translocation of the L chain from the endocytic vesicle lumen into the cytosol, as has previously been demonstrated for several bacterial protein toxins (103). Based on this model, acidification of the endocytic carriers of BTX and TeNT should occur only in neurons in which these neurotoxins block neurotransmitter release.

The membrane interaction of CNT has been studied with model membranes, as well as with cell cultures. These studies show that low pH induces in CNT an acid conformation characterized by a higher degree of hydrophobicity. This transition enables the penetration of both the H and L chains into the hydrophobic core of the lipid bilayer (104–107). Following membrane insertion, the H_N domain of CNT is responsible for the formation of cation-selective ion channels (107–110), which are likely to allow the transit of the partially unfolded L chain across the endosomal membrane into the neuronal cytosol (103). The neutral pH of the cytosol may induce the L chain to refold, following reduction of the interchain disulfide bond. Cytosolic chaperones may be involved in facilitating the exit of the L chain from the membrane and in promoting its refolding. This process is further complicated by the essential role played by zinc in the catalytic activity of TeNT and BTX. In fact, the protonation of the histidines coordinating the zinc ion at low pH is expected to release the metal atom, which has to be acquired again in the cytosol.

INTRACELLULAR ZINC-ENDOPEPTIDASE ACTIVITY

CNTs are remarkably specific proteases. Among the many proteins and synthetic substrates assayed so far, only three targets, all members of the SNARE family, have been identified (reviewed in 4,16,45–47,111). TeNT and BTX-B, -D, -F, and -G cleave the SSV protein VAMP (vesicle-associated membrane protein). BTX-A and -E cleave the plasma membrane protein SNAP-25 (synaptosomal-associated protein of 25 kDa), whereas BTX-C targets both SNAP-25 and syntaxin, another plasma membrane SNARE (reviewed in 4,16,45–47,111).

The zinc-dependent protease activity of different CNT is directed against distinct peptide bonds in their target SNAREs, with the exception of BTX-B and TeNT that cleave VAMP at the same site. CNTs are therefore highly specific tools for the investigation of the role of SNAREs in neurotransmitter release (4), neuronal differentiation and synaptic formation (112–114), NMJ plasticity (115), and other cellular processes. Given the general role that SNAREs play in vesicular trafficking (111), the use of CNT can be extended to a variety of cell types and biochemical preparations by means of pore-forming toxins or transfection with the isolated L chains (reviewed in 116,117). In addition, targeted expression of the active domain of CNT can be used to ablate specific SNARE proteins in selected tissues, or even in entire organisms (118–120).

FUTURE PERSPECTIVES

The detailed study of TeNT and BTX has revolutionized our understanding of the process of neuroexocytosis and has promoted their use as tools in neuroscience and cell biology. The absolute neurospecificity of CNT, together with the ability of TeNT to undergo axonal retrograde transport within motor neurons, make them ideal carrier proteins for neuronal targeting. Even though the number of examples where this delivery technology has been applied is limited, their study will provide important insights on the mechanism of retrograde transport and on molecular mechanism of sorting and endocytosis at the synapse.

ACKNOWLEDGMENTS

We apologize to our colleagues whose work has been omitted because of space limitations. We thank Cesare Montecucco and members of the Molecular NeuroPathobiology Laboratory for useful discussions. Work in the laboratories of the authors is supported by the Cancer Research UK.

REFERENCES

1. Popoff MR, Marvaud J-C. Structural and genomic features of clostridial neurotoxins. In: Alouf JE, Freer JH, eds. *The comprehensive sourcebook of bacterial protein toxins, 2nd ed.* London: Academic Press, 1999: 174–201.
2. Middlebrook JL, Brown JE. Immunodiagnosis and immunotherapy of tetanus and botulinum neurotoxins. *Curr Top Microbiol Immunol* 1995;195:89–122.
3. Herreros J, Lalli G, Montecucco C, et al. Pathophysiological properties of clostridial neurotoxins. In: Freer JH, Alouf JE, eds. *The comprehensive sourcebook of bacterial protein toxins.* London: Academic Press, 1999:202–228.
4. Schiavo G, Matteoli M, Montecucco C. Neurotoxins affecting neuroexocytosis. *Physiol Rev* 2000;80: 717–766.
5. Halpern JL, Neale EA. Neurospecific binding, internalization, and retrograde axonal transport. *Curr Top Microbiol Immunol* 1995;195:221–241.
6. Bergey GK, MacDonald RL, Habig WH, et al. Tetanus toxin: convulsant action on mouse spinal cord neurons in culture. *J Neurosci* 1983;4:2310–2323.
7. Takano K, Kirchner F, Terhaar P, et al. Effect of tetanus toxin on the monosynaptic reflex. *Naunyn Schmiedebergs Arch Pharmacol* 1983;323:217–220.
8. Williamson LC, Fitzgerald SC, Neale EA. Differential effects of tetanus toxin on inhibitory and excitatory neurotransmitter release from mammalian spinal cord cells in culture. *J Neurochem* 1992;59:2148–2157.
9. Calabresi P, Benedetti M, Mercuri NB, et al. Selective depression of synaptic transmission by tetanus toxin: a comparative study on hippocampal and neostriatal slices. *Neuroscience* 1989;30:663–670.
10. Erdmann G, Hanauske A, Wellhöner HH. Intraspinal distribution and reaction in the grey matter with tetanus toxin of intracisternally injected anti-tetanus toxoid F(ab')2 fragments. *Brain Res* 1981;211:367–377.
11. Simpson LL. *Botulinum neurotoxin and tetanus toxin.* San Diego: Academic Press, 1989.
12. Habermann E, Dreyer F. Clostridial neurotoxins: han-

dling and action at the cellular and molecular level. *Curr Top Microbiol Immunol* 1986;129:93–179.

13. Hunt JM, Bommert K, Charlton MP, et al. A postdocking role for synaptobrevin in synaptic vesicle fusion. *Neuron* 1994;12:1269–1279.

14. Van der Kloot W, Molgo J. Quantal acetylcholine release at the vertebrate neuromuscular junction. *Physiol Rev* 1994;74:899–991.

15. Capogna M, McKinney RA, O'Connor V, et al. Ca^{2+} or Sr^{2+} partially rescues synaptic transmission in hippocampal cultures treated with botulinum toxin A and C, but not tetanus toxin. *J Neurosci* 1997;17:7190–7202.

16. Humeau Y, Doussau F, Grant NJ, et al. How botulinum and tetanus neurotoxins block neurotransmitter release. *Biochimie* 2000;82:427–446.

17. Jensen K, Lambert JDC, Jensen MS. Tetanus-induced asynchronous GABA release in cultured hippocampal neurons. *Brain Res* 2000;880:198–201.

18. Lacy DB, Stevens RC. Sequence homology and structural analysis of the clostridial neurotoxins. *J Mol Biol* 1999;291:1091–1104.

19. Ginalski K, Venclovas C, Lesyng B, et al. Structure-based sequence alignment for the beta-trefoil subdomain of the clostridial neurotoxin family provides residue level information about the putative ganglioside binding site. *FEBS Lett* 2000;482:119–124.

20. Weller U, Dauzenroth ME, Meyer zu Heringdorf D, et al. Chains and fragments of tetanus toxin. Separation, reassociation and pharmacological properties. *Eur J Biochem* 1989;182:649–656.

21. Schiavo G, Papini E, Genna G, et al. An intact interchain disulfide bond is required for the neurotoxicity of tetanus toxin. *Infect Immun* 1990;58:4136–4141.

22. Bizzini B, Stoeckel K, Schwab M. An antigenic polypeptide fragment isolated from tetanus toxin: chemical characterization, binding to gangliosides and retrograde axonal transport in various neuron systems. *J Neurochem* 1977;28:529–542.

23. Helting TB, Zwisler O. Structure of tetanus toxin. I. Breakdown of the toxin molecule and discrimination between polypeptide fragments. *J Biol Chem* 1977;252:187–193.

24. Lacy DB, Tepp W, Cohen AC, et al. Crystal structure of botulinum neurotoxin type A and implications for toxicity. *Nat Struct Biol* 1998;5:898–902.

25. Hanson MA, Stevens RC. Cocrystal structure of synaptobrevin-II bound to botulinum neurotoxin type B at 2.0 Angstrom resolution. *Nat Struct Biol* 2000;7:687–692.

26. Swaminathan S, Eswaramoorthy S. Structural analysis of the catalytic and binding sites of *Clostridium botulinum* neurotoxin B. *Nat Struct Biol* 2000;7:693–699.

27. Fishman PS, Parks DA, Patwardhan AJ, et al. Neuronal binding of tetanus toxin compared to its ganglioside binding fragment (Hc). *Nat Toxins* 1999;7:151–156.

28. Umland TC, Wingert LM, Swaminathan S, et al. Structure of the receptor binding fragment Hc of tetanus toxin. *Nat Struct Biol* 1997;4:788–792.

29. Emsley P, Fotinou C, Black I, et al. The structures of the HC fragment of tetanus toxin with carbohydrate subunit complexes provide insight into ganglioside binding. *J Biol Chem* 2000;275:8889–8894.

30. Fotinou C, Emsley P, Black I, et al. The crystal structure of tetanus toxin Hc fragment complexed with a

synthetic GT1b analogue suggests cross-linking between ganglioside receptors and the toxin. *J Biol Chem* 2001;276:32274–32281.

31. Halpern JL, Loftus A. Characterization of the receptor-binding domain of tetanus toxin. *J Biol Chem* 1993;268:11188–11192.

32. Hoch DH, Romero-Mira M, Ehrlich BE, et al. Channels formed by botulinum, tetanus, and diphtheria toxins in planar lipid bilayers: relevance to translocation of proteins across membranes. *Proc Natl Acad Sci U S A* 1985;82:1692–1696.

33. Gambale F, Montal M. Characterization of the channel properties of tetanus toxin in planar lipid bilayers. *Biophys J* 1988;53:771–783.

34. Oblatt-Montal M, Yamazaki M, Nelson R, et al. Formation of ion channels in lipid bilayers by a peptide with the predicted transmembrane sequence of botulinum neurotoxin A. *Protein Sci* 1995;4:1490–1497.

35. Bhattacharyya SD, Sugiyama H. Inactivation of botulinum and tetanus toxins by chelators. *Infect Immun* 1989;57:3053–3057.

36. Schiavo G, Poulain B, Rossetto O, et al. Tetanus toxin is a zinc protein and its inhibition of neurotransmitter release and protease activity depends on zinc. *EMBO J* 1992;11:3577–3583.

37. Simpson LL, Coffield JA, Bakry N. Chelation of zinc antagonizes the neuromuscular blocking properties of the seven serotypes of botulinum neurotoxin as well as tetanus toxin. *J Pharmacol Exp Ther* 1993;267:720–727.

38. Höhne-Zell B, Ecker A, Weller U, Gratzl M. Synaptobrevin cleavage by the tetanus toxin light chain is linked to the inhibition of exocytosis in chromaffin cells. *FEBS Lett* 1994;355:131–134.

39. Rupp B, Segelke B. Questions about the structure of the botulinum neurotoxin B light chain in complex with a target peptide. *Nat Struct Biol* 2001;8:663–664.

40. Stevens R, Hanson M. Questions about the structure of the botulinum neurotoxin B light chain in complex with a target peptide. *Nat Struct Biol* 2001;8:664–664.

41. Jongeneel CV, Bouvier J, Bairoch A. A unique signature identifies a family of zinc-dependent metallopeptidases. *FEBS Lett* 1989;242:211–214.

42. Vallee BL, Auld DS. Zinc coordination, function, and structure of zinc enzymes and other proteins. *Biochemistry* 1990;29:5647–5659.

43. Morante S, Furenlid L, Schiavo G, et al. X-ray absorption spectroscopy study of zinc coordination in tetanus neurotoxin, astacin, alkaline protease and thermolysin. *Eur J Biochem* 1996;235:606–612.

44. Stocker W, Bode W. Structural features of a superfamily of zinc-endopeptidases: the metzincins. *Curr Opin Struct Biol* 1995;5:383–390.

45. Roques BP, Anne C, Turcaud S, et al. Mechanism of action of clostridial neurotoxins and rational inhibitor design. *Biol Cell* 2000;92:445–447.

46. Rossetto O, Seveso M, Caccin P, et al. Tetanus and botulinum neurotoxins: turning bad guys into good by research. *Toxicon* 2001;39:27–41.

47. Linial M. Neurotoxins as tools in dissecting the exocytic machinery. In: Fuller H, ed. *Fusion of biological membrane and related problems.* New York: Kluwer Academic Press, 2000:39–72.

48. Montecucco C. How do tetanus and botulinum toxins

bind to neuronal membranes? *Trends Biochem Sci* 1986;11:315–317.

49. Stöckel K, Schwab M, Thoenen H. Role of gangliosides in the uptake and retrograde axonal transport of cholera and tetanus toxin as compared to nerve growth factor and wheat germ agglutinin. *Brain Res* 1977;132: 273–285.

50. Marxen P, Fuhrmann U, Bigalke H. Gangliosides mediate inhibitory effects of tetanus and botulinum A neurotoxins on exocytosis in chromaffin cells. *Toxicon* 1989;27:849–859.

51. Williamson LC, Bateman KE, Clifford JCM, et al. Neuronal sensitivity to tetanus toxin requires gangliosides. *J Biol Chem* 1999;274:25173–25180.

52. Kitamura M, Takamiya K, Aizawa S, et al. Gangliosides are the receptor for *C. botulinum* neurotoxin in mice. *J Neurochem* 1999;73:S64–S64.

53. Pierce EJ, Davison MD, Parton RG, et al. Characterization of tetanus toxin binding to rat brain membranes. Evidence for a high-affinity proteinase-sensitive receptor. *Biochem J* 1986;236:845–852.

54. Yavin E, Nathan A. Tetanus toxin receptors on nerve cells contain a trypsin-sensitive component. *Eur J Biochem* 1986;154:403–407.

55. Parton RG, Ockleford CD, Critchley DR. Tetanus toxin binding to mouse spinal cord cells: an evaluation of the role of gangliosides in toxin internalization. *Brain Res* 1988;475:118–127.

56. Schiavo G, Ferrari G, Rossetto O, et al. Specific cross-linking of tetanus toxin to a protein of NGF-differentiated PC12 cells. *FEBS Lett* 1991;290:227–230.

57. Herreros J, Lalli G, Montecucco C, et al. Tetanus toxin fragment C binds to a protein present in neuronal cell lines and motoneurons. *J Neurochem* 2000;74: 1941–1950.

58. Herreros J, Ng T, Schiavo G. Lipid rafts act as specialised domains for tetanus toxin binding and internalisation into neurons. *Mol Biol Cell* 2001(*in press*).

59. Herreros J, Lalli G, Schiavo G. C-terminal half of tetanus toxin fragment C is sufficient for neuronal binding and interaction with a putative protein receptor. *Biochem J* 2000; 347:199–204.

60. Nishiki T, Kamata Y, Nemoto Y, et al. Identification of protein receptor for *Clostridium botulinum* type B neurotoxin in rat brain synaptosomes. *J Biol Chem* 1994;269:10498–10503.

61. Nishiki T, Tokuyama Y, Kamata Y, et al. The high-affinity binding of *Clostridium botulinum* type B neurotoxin to synaptotagmin-II associated with gangliosides GT1b/GD1a. *FEBS Lett* 1996;378:253–257.

62. Kozaki S, Kamata Y, Watarai S, Nishiki T, Mochida S. Ganglioside GT1b as a complementary receptor component for Clostridium botulinum neurotoxins. Microb Pathog 1998;25:91–99.

63. Bal LL, Singh R. Isolation of synaptotagmin as a receptor for type A and type E botulinum neurotoxin and analysis of their comparative binding using a new microtiter plate assay. *J Nat Toxins* 1998;7:215–226.

64. Evans DM, Williams RS, Shone CC, et al. Botulinum neurotoxin type B. Its purification, radioiodination and interaction with rat-brain synaptosomal membranes. *Eur J Biochem* 1986;154:409–416.

65. Schiavo G, Osborne SL, Sgouros JG. Synaptotagmins-more isoforms than functions. *Biochem Biophys Res Commun* 1998;248:1–8.

66. Shumaker HB, Lamont A, Firor WM. The reaction of "tetanus sensitive" and "tetanus resistant" animals to the injection of tetanal toxin into the spinal cord. *J Immunol* 1939; 37:425–433.

67. Takano K, Kirchner F, Gremmelt A, et al. Blocking effects of tetanus toxin and its fragment [A-B] on the excitatory and inhibitory synapses of the spinal motoneurone of the cat. *Toxicon* 1989;27:385–392.

68. Niemann H. Molecular biology of clostridial neurotoxins. In: Alouf JE, Freer JH, eds. *A sourcebook of bacterial protein toxins.* London: Academic Press, 1991: 303–348.

69. Herreros J, Schiavo G. Lipid microdomains are involved in neurospecific binding and internalisation of clostridial neurotoxins. *Int J Med Microbiol* 2001 (*in press*).

70. Fivaz M, Abrami L, vanderGoot FG. Pathogens, toxins, and lipid rafts. *Protoplasma* 2000;212:8–14.

71. Aguilera J, Lopez LA, Yavin E. Tetanus toxin-induced protein kinase C activation and elevated serotonin levels in the perinatal rat brain. *FEBS Lett* 1990;263: 61–65.

72. Aguilera J, Yavin E. In vivo translocation and down-regulation of protein kinase C following intraventricular administration of tetanus toxin. *J Neurochem* 1990;54:339–342.

73. Aguilera J, Padros-Giralt C, Habig WH, et al. GT1b ganglioside prevents tetanus toxin-induced protein kinase C activation and down-regulation in the neonatal brain in vivo. *J Neurochem* 1993;60:709–713.

74. Gil C, Ruizmeana M, Alava M, et al. Tetanus toxin enhances protein kinase C activity translocation and increases polyphosphoinositide hydrolysis in rat cerebral cortex preparations. *J Neurochem* 1998;70: 1636–1643.

75. Gil C, Chaib-Oukadour I, Pelliccioni P, et al. Activation of signal transduction pathways involving trkA, PLCg-1, PKC isoforms and ERK-1/2 by tetanus toxin. *FEBS Lett* 2000;481:177–182.

76. Gil C, Chaib-Oukadour I, Blasi J, et al. HC fragment (C-terminal portion of the heavy chain) of tetanus toxin activates protein kinase C isoforms and phosphoproteins involved in signal transduction. *Biochem J* 2001; 356:97–103.

77. Dolly JO, Black J, Williams RS, et al. Acceptors for botulinum neurotoxin reside on motor nerve terminals and mediate its internalization. *Nature* 1984;307: 457–460.

78. Critchley DR, Nelson PG, Habig WH, Fishman PH. Fate of tetanus toxin bound to the surface of primary neurons in culture: evidence for rapid internalization. *J Cell Biol* 1985;100:1499–1507.

79. Black JD, Dolly JO. Interaction of ^{125}I-labeled botulinum neurotoxins with nerve terminals. I. Ultrastructural autoradiographic localization and quantitation of distinct membrane acceptors for types A and B on motor nerves. *J Cell Biol* 1986;103:521–534.

80. Black JD, Dolly JO. Interaction of ^{125}I-labeled botulinum neurotoxins with nerve terminals. II. Autoradiographic evidence for its uptake into motor nerves by acceptor-mediated endocytosis. *J Cell Biol* 1986;103: 535–544.

81. Staub GC, Walton KM, Schnaar RL, et al. Characterization of the binding and internalization of tetanus

toxin in a neuroblastoma hybrid cell line. *J Neurosci* 1986;6:1443–1451.

82. Parton RG, Ockleford CD, Critchley DR. A study of the mechanism of internalisation of tetanus toxin by primary mouse spinal cord cultures. *J Neurochem* 1987;49:1057–1068.

83. Matteoli M, Verderio C, Rossetto O, et al. Synaptic vesicle endocytosis mediates the entry of tetanus neurotoxin into hippocampal neurons. *Proc Natl Acad Sci U S A* 1996;93:13310–13315.

84. Verderio C, Coco S, Rossetto O, et al. Internalization and proteolytic action of botulinum toxins in CNS neurons and astrocytes. *J Neurochem* 1999;73:372–379.

85. Lalli G, Gschmeissner S, Schiavo G. Analysis of axonal retrograde transport in living motor neurons using a fluorescent fragment of tetanus neurotoxin. 2001 *(submitted)*.

86. Schweizer FE, Betz H, Augustine GJ. From vesicle docking to endocytosis: Intermediate reactions of exocytosis. *Neuron* 1995;14:689–696.

87. DeCamilli P. Molecular mechanisms in synaptic vesicle endocytosis. *J Neurochem* 1999;73:S4-S4.

88. Matteoli M, Takei K, Perin MS, et al. Exo-endocytotic recycling of synaptic vesicles in developing processes of cultured hippocampal neurons. *J Cell Biol* 1992; 117:849–861.

89. Kraszewski K, Mundigl O, Daniell L, et al. Synaptic vesicle dynamics in living cultured hippocampal neurons visualized with CY3-conjugated antibodies directed against the lumenal domain of synaptotagmin. *J Neurosci* 1995;15:4328–4342.

90. Schmitt A, Dreyer F, John C. At least three sequential steps are involved in the tetanus toxin-induced block of neuromuscular transmission. *Naunyn Schmiedebergs Arch Pharmacol* 1981;317:326–330.

91. Habermann E, Erdmann G. Pharmacokinetic and histoautoradiographic evidence for the intraaxonal movement of toxin in the pathogenesis of tetanus. *Toxicon* 1978;16:611–623.

92. Kemplay S, Cavanagh JB. Effects of acrylamide and botulinum toxin on horseradish peroxidase labelling of trigeminal motor neurons in the rat. *J Anat* 1983;137: 477–482.

93. Kristensson K, Olsson T. Uptake and retrograde axonal transport of horseradish peroxidase in botulinum-intoxicated mice. *Brain Res* 1978;155:118–123.

94. Francis JW, Hosler BA, Brown RH Jr, et al. CuZn superoxide dismutase (SOD-1):tetanus toxin fragment C hybrid protein for targeted delivery of SOD-1 to neuronal cells. *J Biol Chem* 1995;270:15434–15442.

95. Figueiredo DM, Hallewell RA, Chen LL, et al. Delivery of recombinant tetanus-superoxide dismutase proteins to central-nervous-system neurons by retrograde axonal-transport. *Exp Neurol* 1997;145:546–554.

96. Dobrenis K, Joseph A, Rattazzi MC. Neuronal lysosomal enzyme replacement using fragment C of tetanus toxin. *Proc Natl Acad Sci U S A* 1992;89:2297–2301.

97. Coen L, Osta R, Maury M, et al. Construction of hybrid proteins that migrate retrogradely and transsynaptically into the central nervous system. *Proc Natl Acad Sci U S A* 1997;94:9400–9405.

98. Francis JW, Brown RH, Figueiredo D, et al. Enhancement of diphtheria toxin potency by replacement of the receptor binding domain with tetanus toxin C-fragment: a potential vector for delivering heterologous proteins to neurons. *J Neurochem* 2000;74: 2528–2536.

99. Knight A, Carvajal J, Schneider H, et al. Non-viral neuronal gene delivery mediated by the H-C fragment of tetanus toxin. *Eur J Biochem* 1999;259:762–769.

100. Figueiredo DM, Matthews CC, Parks DA, et al. Interaction of tetanus toxin derived hybrid proteins with neuronal cells. *J Nat Toxins* 2000;9:363–379.

101. Li Y, Aoki R, Dolly JO. Expression and characterisation of the heavy chain of tetanus toxin: reconstitution of the fully-recombinant di-chain protein in active form. *J Biochem* 1999;125:1200–1208.

102. Li Y, Foran P, Lawrence G, et al. Recombinant forms of tetanus toxin engineered for examining and exploiting neuronal trafficking pathways. *J Biol Chem* 2001; 276:31394–31401.

103. Montecucco C, Papini E, Schiavo G. Bacterial protein toxins penetrate cells via a four-step mechanism. *FEBS Lett* 1994;346:92–98.

104. Boquet P, Duflot E. Tetanus toxin fragment forms channels in lipid vesicles at low pH. *Proc Natl Acad Sci U S A* 1982;79:7614–7618.

105. Montecucco C, Schiavo G, Brunner J, et al. Tetanus toxin is labeled with photoactivatable phospholipids at low pH. *Biochemistry* 1986;25:919–924.

106. Montecucco C, Schiavo G, Dasgupta BR. Effect of pH on the interaction of botulinum neurotoxins A, B, and E with liposomes. *Biochem J* 1989;259:47–53.

107. Menestrina G, Forti S, Gambale F. Interaction of tetanus toxin with lipid vesicles. Effects of pH, surface charge, and transmembrane potential on the kinetics of channel formation. *Biophys J* 1989;55:393–405.

108. Donovan JJ, Middlebrook JL. Ion-conducting channels produced by botulinum toxin in planar lipid membranes. *Biochemistry* 1986;25:2872–2876.

109. Shone CC, Hambleton P, Melling J. A 50-kDa fragment from the NH$_2$-terminus of the heavy subunit of *Clostridium botulinum* type A neurotoxin forms channels in lipid vesicles. *Eur J Biochem* 1987;167: 175–180.

110. Schmid MF, Robinson JP, DasGupta BR. Direct visualization of botulinum neurotoxin-induced channels in phospholipid vesicles. *Nature* 1993;364:827–830.

111. Jahn R, Sudhof TC. Membrane fusion and exocytosis. *Annu Rev Biochem* 1999; 68:863–911.

112. Osen Sand A, Staple JK, Naldi E, et al. Common and distinct fusion proteins in axonal growth and transmitter release. *J Comp Neurol* 1996;367:222–234.

113. Verderio C, Coco S, Bacci A, et al. Synaptic vesicle recycling is not inhibited by tetanus neurotoxin in hippocampal-neurons before synaptogenesis. *Eur J Neurosci* 1998;10:8704–8704.

114. Verderio C, Coco S, Bacci A, et al. Tetanus toxin blocks the exocytosis of synaptic vesicles clustered at synapses but not of synaptic vesicles in isolated axons. *J Neurosci* 1999;19:6723–6732.

115. Meunier FA, Herreros J, Schiavo G, et al. Molecular mechanism of action of botulinal neurotoxins and the synaptic remodeling they induce *in vivo* at the skeletal neuromuscular junction. In: Massaro EJ, ed. *Neurotoxicology handbook.* Totowa, NJ: Humana Press, 2002 *(in press)*.

116. Ahnert-Hilger G, Weller U. Application of alpha-toxin and streptolysin O in cell biology. In: Aktories K, ed.

Bacterial toxins. Tools in cell biology and pharmacology. Weinheim: Chapman and Hall, 1997:259–272.

117. Lang J, Regazzi R, Wollheim CB. Clostridial toxins and endocrine secretion: their use in insuline secreting cells. In: Aktories K, ed. *Bacterial toxins. Tools in cell biology and pharmacology.* London: Chapman & Hall, 1997:217–227.

118. Eisel U, Reynolds K, Riddick M, et al. Tetanus toxin light chain expression in Sertoli cells of transgenic mice causes alterations of the actin cytoskeleton and disrupts spermatogenesis. *EMBO J* 1993;12: 3365–3372.

119. Sweeney ST, Broadie K, Keane J, et al. Targeted expression of tetanus toxin light chain in Drosophila specifically eliminates synaptic transmission and causes behavioral defects. *Neuron* 1995;14:341–351.

120. Baines RA, Robinson SG, Fujioka M, et al. Postsynaptic expression of tetanus toxin light chain blocks synaptogenesis in Drosophila. *Curr Biol* 1999;9:1267–1270.

Scientific and Therapeutic Aspects of Botulinum Toxin
edited by M.F. Brin, J. Jankovic, and M. Hallett
Lippincott Williams & Wilkins, Philadelphia, © 2002.

6

Botulinum Neurotoxin A and Synaptic Vesicle Trafficking

Elaine A. Neale

The continuing function of the synaptic terminal depends on a constant supply of neurotransmitter-containing synaptic vesicles. With each action potential that invades a synaptic terminal, it is thought that perhaps one vesicle fuses with the presynaptic membrane of the active zone (1–5) to release its content of transmitter into the synaptic cleft where the transmitter interacts with its specific receptor on the postsynaptic membrane (Fig. 6.1A). Motor neuron terminals treated with black widow spider venom in the absence of calcium undergo a massive burst of acetylcholine release; the terminals are depleted of synaptic vesicles and the surface area of terminal membrane increases (6). Integral membrane proteins of the synaptic vesicle, not normally detectable on the terminal membrane, can be seen under these conditions by immunohistochemistry (7,8). When calcium is added back to the bathing medium, the terminal returns to normal size, regains its normal complement of synaptic vesicles, and loses evidence of vesicle proteins on its surface. Heuser and Reese (9) electrically stimulated motor nerve terminals for a brief period and then fixed terminals for electron microscopy at various times during and after the stimulation interval. With stimulation, total vesicle membrane decreased and terminal surface membrane increased. As the terminal recovered, clathrin-coated pits and coated vesicles became more numerous, membrane "cisternae" appeared in the terminal, surface membrane area returned to normal, and vesicle membrane approached normal. Throughout the course of recovery, the total amount of membrane remained constant but redistributed among the synaptic

vesicle, surface, and cisternal compartments. In a second set of experiments, the terminals were stimulated in the presence of horseradish peroxidase (HRP); washed to remove the HRP, and fixed at various times. With appropriate histochemistry, the HRP becomes electron dense. Horseradish peroxidase reaction product then marks all of the intraterminal membrane structures that were derived from the surface membrane of the terminal; i.e., were in contact with the bathing solution which contained HRP. This procedure allowed the investigators to monitor the sequence of recovery of synaptic vesicles. Indeed, in recovered terminals, a proportion of synaptic vesicles contained HRP, evidence that they were formed from the surface membrane rather than from another intraneuronal membrane source. HRP-labeled membrane cisternae formed in response to stimulation and disappeared with prolonged recovery time, suggesting their involvement in the recycling process. By examining the sequentially fixed samples, it was possible to define the progression of recovery (Fig. 6.1B). Heuser and Reese hypothesized that after fusion of the synaptic vesicle with the presynaptic membrane, the vesicle membrane collapses into the surface membrane, diffuses to a site away from the active zone, and is retrieved in the form of clathrin-coated pits and vesicles (see also Fig. 6.1C). The clathrin coat is lost and the newly endocytosed vesicles fuse to form the cisternae from which bud new synaptic vesicles. After they are refilled with transmitter, the recycled vesicles are ready to participate again in the process of transmitter release.

Although the Heuser–Reese progression re-

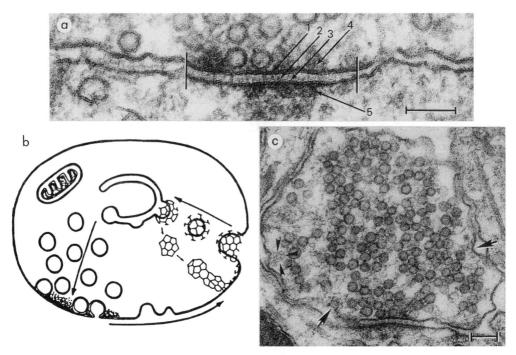

FIG. 6.1. Synaptic vesicle recycling. **A:** With each action potential that invades a synaptic terminal, it is felt that no more than one synaptic vesicle fuses with the presynaptic membrane at the active zone to release its content of neurotransmitter into the synaptic cleft. Vertical bars mark the active zone or release site. *1,* presynaptic membrane; *2,* synaptic cleft; *3,* postsynaptic membrane; *4,* presynaptic dense projection; *5,* postsynaptic density. **B:** Heuser and Reese (9) hypothesized that synaptic vesicle membrane was conserved in the motor nerve terminal by the process of recycling shown here. Upon stimulation, a synaptic vesicle fuses with and collapses into the presynaptic membrane. Vesicle membrane is retrieved, at a site distant from the active zone; vesicle membrane reuptake is mediated by clathrin-coated pits and vesicles. **C:** Synaptic terminals in spinal cord cell cultures, depolarized with potassium, also contain clathrin-coated pits (*arrows*) and empty clathrin baskets (*arrowheads*). Bars, 0.1 μm. (Figure B was modified and reproduced from Heuser JE, Reese TS. Evidence for recycling of synaptic vesicle membrane during transmitter release at the frog neuromuscular junction. *J Cell Biol* 1973;57:315–344 by permission.)

mains generally accepted, specific challenges have been mounted: that transmitter release and vesicle reformation occurs by "kiss and run" (10–14, and 15), and see (15), rather than by vesicle collapse and clathrin-mediated retrieval; that cisternae are not autonomous structures but remain connected to the surface membrane (16); and that single vesicles retain their identity and don't fuse with (i.e., become diluted into) another membrane compartment (17). What remains constant is the belief that fusion sites are specifically defined, that membrane is conserved, and that vesicle membrane is recycled. The demonstration of a strong temporal link be-

tween single action potentials and single quantum FM dye (see below) uptake suggested that unitary vesicle fusion and vesicle retrieval events were coupled closely in some way (4).

Synaptic transmission has been studied in cultures of primary dissociated spinal cord neurons (Fig. 6.2) for many years (3,18–24). Spinal cords are removed from fetal mice at 13.5 days in gestation, dissociated with trypsin and trituration, and plated as a single-cell suspension into collagen (Vitrogen-100)-coated 35-mm plastic culture dishes (18,25). The glial cells in the suspension settle onto the dish surface, divide and spread, and the neurons settle on top of this glial

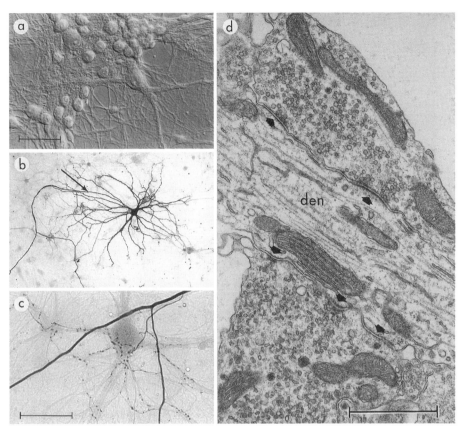

FIG. 6.2. Spinal cord neurons in cell culture for three weeks. The neurons settle on top of flattened glial cells, extend axonal and dendritic processes, and establish functional synaptic connections. **A:** Soma and dendrites of a large spinal cord neuron, several smaller neurons, and a meshwork of axonal and dendritic processes are seen in this field. Hoffman modulation contrast optics. **B:** A spinal cord neuron that, after electrophysiologic analysis, was injected with horseradish peroxidase and processed immunohistochemically 8 hours later. A number of tapering, branching dendrites emerge from the soma; only one axon (*arrow*) is extended; axonal diameter is consistent between branch points. **C:** The axon gives off a number of small branches that terminate as swellings on the surface of the soma and dendrites of another neuron. That these swellings constitute synaptic boutons has been confirmed by electron microscopy. **D:** As seen with the electron microscope, somatic and dendritic (*den*) surfaces are virtually covered with synaptic terminals. The terminal at the top contains predominantly round, clear synaptic vesicles and two synaptic active zones (*arrows*), whereas the terminal on the bottom contains flattened clear vesicles and three active zones. Bars: (**A**) and (**C**), 25 μm; (**D**), 1 μm.

layer. Considerable increases in morphologic complexity occur with time in culture (26 and Fig. 6.3). Within a few hours of plating, neurons send out processes and by 24 hours there is considerable neurite development (Fig. 6.3A). Within only a few days, synaptic interactions can be recorded (27,28). Specific labeling of neurons for developmental studies is accomplished by intracellular injection of fluorescent or opaque markers (21 and Fig. 6.3B), or by indirect immunohistochemistry using antibodies against neuron-specific enolase (29), or by the binding fragment of tetanus toxin (TeNT) and a specific anti-TeNT Fragment C antibody (30 and Fig. 6.3A). Development of identified living neurons can be followed in cultures prepared from mice that express green fluorescent protein (GFP; work in collaboration with Andres Buo-

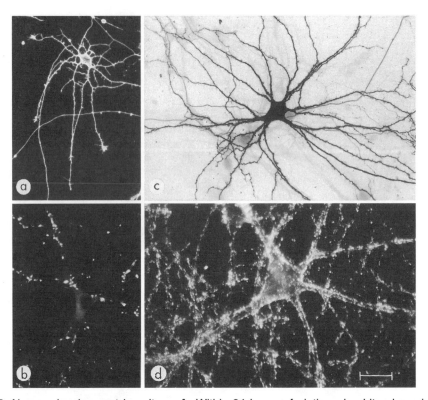

FIG. 6.3. Neuron development in culture. **A:** Within 24 hours of plating, dendrites have branched and extended for several cell diameters; the axon has grown considerably further. Process tips are marked by growth cones. This neuron was stained by indirect immunofluorescence using Fragment C of tetanus toxin and the monoclonal antibody 18.2.12.6. **B:** After 1 week in culture, immunohistochemistry for synapsin, an integral membrane protein of synaptic vesicles, shows focal fluorescence indicating aggregations of synaptic vesicles in synaptic terminals. After several weeks in culture, the complexity of the dendrite arbor (**C**) and the number of synaptic terminals (**D**) increase. Bar in (**D**), 25 μm, applies to (**B**) and (**D**).

nanno, NICHD, NIH, unpublished) or other spectral variants of GFP (31). Neurons can be stained immunohistochemically with antibodies that specifically label dendrites, axons, or synaptic terminals (32 and Fig. 6.3B and D). Several studies had described the electrophysiologic response of these spinal cord neurons to TeNT and botulinum neurotoxin (BoNT), lending validity to their use as a model system (33–35). These toxins block the occurrence of both spontaneous and evoked postsynaptic potentials, and of spontaneous action potentials. Although action potentials can be evoked in toxin-blocked neurons, the evoked potentials are not able to drive presynaptic events leading to synaptic transmission. We examined, by electron microscopy, cultures

that were electrically quiescent as a result of intoxication with TeNT and found that synaptic vesicles had accumulated in larger than usual numbers at the presynaptic active zone (30). Our interpretation was that toxin does not interfere with the movement of vesicles to the presynaptic release site, but seems to prevent vesicle fusion. This image is consistent with the now-known mechanism of toxin action. Specific brain homologs of proteins shown to be critical for vesicle docking and fusion at the yeast and mammalian Golgi apparatus are localized to either the synaptic vesicle or the axonal membrane. The catalytic domain of each of the clostridial neurotoxins is a zinc endopeptidase which acts to proteolyze one or another of these proteins (36). Toxin action is thus thought to compromise the function of these proteins, preventing fusion of synaptic vesicles with the presynaptic membrane and, consequently, preventing the release of transmitter into the synaptic cleft.

We extended our initial observation, monitoring synaptic vesicle traffic after neuron exposure to either TeNT or BoNT (37). We assayed the level of intoxication by measuring potassium-evoked neurotransmitter release (38). The assay is depicted in Fig. 6.4. Cultures are loaded with [^{3}H]glycine, exposed to potassium in the absence of calcium to establish "baseline" loss of radioactivity, and then depolarized with potassium in the presence of calcium to determine calcium-dependent release. In response to depolarization, control cultures release about 20% of the total [^{3}H]glycine present in the cells at the beginning of the assay. Toxin-treated cultures release decreasing amounts of transmitter depending on toxin concentration (38,39) and time

of exposure (38). Tetanus toxin and most of the BoNT serotypes at a concentration of 64 pM for 24 hours block potassium-evoked calcium-dependent glycine release completely (40). When transmitter release is totally blocked, the appropriate toxin substrate is proteolyzed as demonstrated by immunohistochemistry and Western blot analysis (39,40). Examination of TeNT– or BoNT-A–blocked cultures with the electron microscope confirms that toxin-induced synaptic blockade correlates with a significant increase in the number of synaptic vesicles at the presynaptic membrane (Fig. 6.5, *left*). Furthermore, in untreated cultures, the number of vesicles at the active zone can be reduced by potassium stimulation. However, under conditions of toxin-induced blockade, potassium stimulation does not alter the number of vesicles at the active zone (Fig. 6.5, *right*). It seems, then, that toxin-cleaved proteins allow synaptic vesicles to dock at the release site but do not support

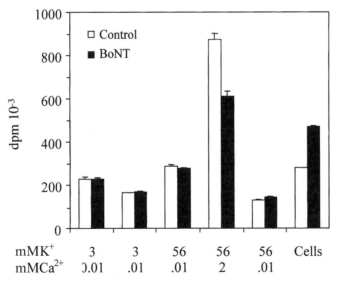

FIG. 6.4. Neurotransmitter release assay. Control and BoNT-A–treated cultures are rinsed, incubated in [^{3}H]glycine for 30 minutes at 35°C (95°F), rinsed quickly twice in HEPES-buffered salts solution containing 3 mM K$^+$/0.01 mM Ca^{2+}, and then incubated for 5-minute intervals in each of the solutions shown. Cells are dissolved in 0.2 M NaOH. Each incubation medium is collected and counted by scintillation spectrometry. Counts in the two 56/0.01 samples are averaged and taken as baseline loss of radioactivity. This value is subtracted from the counts released in 56/2 to yield K$^+$-stimulated Ca^{2+}-dependent transmitter release, which normally constitutes about 20% of total counts (the sum of all collected samples). Cultures are assayed 3 to 4 weeks after neurons are plated. In this experiment, the BoNT-A concentration and time of exposure resulted in a 40% block in glycine release.

RESTING CULTURES

DEPOLARIZED CULTURES
(5 min in 56 mM KCl / 2 mM CaCl₂)

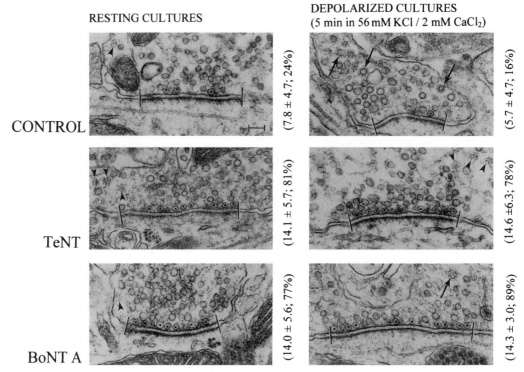

FIG. 6.5. Fine structure of the active zone. Active zones are marked by vertical bars, and "docked" synaptic vesicles (within 10 nm of the presynaptic membrane), with black squares. Resting cultures were fixed and processed for electron microscopy after toxin exposure for 16 hours (TeNT at 100 ng/mL or BoNT-A at 200 ng/mL). Sister cultures were fixed after 5 minutes of depolarization in 56 mM KCl and 2 mM CaCl₂. Ultrathin sections were tilted to observe the presynaptic membrane in cross-section, and docked synaptic were counted. The numbers beside each panel represent the mean number of docked vesicles per μm of active zone ± SD, and the percent of active zones showing more than 10 docked vesicles per μm. The number of synaptic vesicles docked at the active zone is increased in toxin-treated terminals. Fewer synaptic vesicles appear docked in stimulated control cultures than in nonstimulated but spontaneously active cultures. In contrast, when TeNT- or BoNT-A–blocked cultures are stimulated with K$^+$, the number of docked vesicles remains high. Differences between control and toxin-blocked cultures are significant; $p < .001$ (Student's t-test). *Arrows* mark clathrin-coated vesicles; *arrowheads,* empty clathrin baskets. n = 30 to 50 terminals/sample. Bar, 0.2 nm and applies to all panels. (Reproduced from Neale EA, Bowers LM, Jia M, Bateman KE, Williamson LC. Botulinum neurotoxin A blocks synaptic vesicle exocytosis but not endocytosis at the nerve terminal. *J Cell Biol* 1999;147:1249–1260 by permission.)

vesicle fusion, consistent with *in vitro* biochemical experiments (41).

An optical method for demonstrating synaptic activity (42,43) involves the use of a styryl dye, which essentially becomes fluorescent when inserted into a membrane, washes out of membrane easily, but will not cross the membrane. When synaptically inactive neuronal preparations are bathed in this dye, all surface membranes become fluorescent; fluorescence is lost when the dye is washed out. However, if the preparations are stimulated, either chemically or electrically, for several minutes in the presence of dye, fluorescently labeled surface membrane is retrieved into the interior of the synaptic terminal by the process of synaptic vesicle recycling. Subsequent washing removes surface membrane fluorescence. Synaptic terminals that respond to stimulation by synaptic vesicle fusion (exocytosis) and vesicle membrane retrieval (endocytosis) remain fluorescent because vesicles that were recycled from fluorescent surface membrane are now themselves fluorescent. FM-labeling is dependent on calcium because vesicle exocytosis requires calcium and precedes dye uptake. That the fluorescent label is on synaptic vesicles is demonstrated by loss of fluorescence with subsequent depolarization in the absence of dye. In this case, labeled vesicles fuse with the presynaptic membrane, dye diffuses into that membrane and is washed away. Figure 6.6A shows spinal cord neurons in a culture labeled with the styryl dye FM1–43. The surface of neuron somata and dendrites is encrusted with spots of fluorescence, corresponding to synaptic terminals containing some number of fluorescent synaptic vesicles. Whereas FM-staining is achieved in living cells, cultures can be fixed, permeabilized with detergent, and stained by indirect immunohistochemistry using antibodies against synaptic vesicle proteins. The pattern of FM-fluorescence is essentially identical to that in cultures stained by using an antibody against the synaptic vesicle protein synapsin (as shown in Fig. 6.3D), synaptophysin, or vesicle-associated membrane protein (VAMP, also known as synaptobrevin) (not shown).

We anticipated that toxin-quieted cultures would not recycle synaptic vesicle membrane, and therefore would not be stained with FM dyes. Figures 6.6A and B show FM staining and destaining of a control culture; both dye loading and unloading are dependent on calcium (not shown). A TeNT-blocked culture does not take up FM1–43, as expected (Fig. 6.6C). However, cultures treated with BoNT-A, at concentrations as high as 2.0 nM, continue to take up dye (Fig. 6.6D), although subsequent depolarization fails to cause dye loss (Fig. 6.6E). Thus, in BoNT-A–blocked cultures, it appears that vesicle membrane is retrieved by endocytosis in response to stimulation, but that dye loss by exocytosis does not occur.

We looked to electron microscopy for evidence of vesicle recycling in BoNT-A–blocked cultures. Nonstimulated but spontaneously active control synaptic terminals show occasional clathrin-coated membrane invaginations suggestive of membrane retrieval, whereas empty clathrin baskets are fairly common. However, potassium depolarization is associated with an increased incidence of clathrin-coated pits and coated vesicles, and an absence of empty clathrin baskets (Fig. 6.7A). Tetanus toxin-blocked terminals appear identical before and after potassium depolarization; i.e., they show a large number of vesicles apposed to the active zone and numerous empty clathrin baskets (Fig. 6.7B). BoNT-A–blocked terminals before depolarization appear identical to TeNT-treated terminals. However, after depolarization, the BoNT-A–blocked terminals have the exocytosis-related morphology of TeNT-blocked and the endocytosis-related features of control cultures; i.e., vesicles are jammed up at the active zone, but clathrin-coated pits can be found and empty clathrin baskets have disappeared (Fig. 6.7C).

The FM-dye experiments showed endocytosis of surface membrane in BoNT-A–blocked cultures, but because we could not force dye unloading by vesicle exocytosis, this technique could not provide evidence that the surface membrane was recycled ultimately to synaptic vesicles. To learn which terminal structures contained the endocytosed membrane, we stimulated cultures in the presence of HRP as done by Heuser and Reese (9). Both control and toxin-blocked cultures were depolarized with potassium in the presence of HRP for 5 minutes, washed for 30 minutes, and fixed for electron microscopy. A large proportion of synaptic vesicles in control terminals contain HRP reaction product (Fig. 6.8, *upper*). In contrast, very few vesicles are labeled in TeNT-blocked cultures (Fig. 6.8, *middle*). However, BoNT-A–blocked terminals contain a substantial number of HRP-labeled vesicles (Fig. 6.8, *lower*), suggesting that this vesicle membrane was derived from surface membrane that had been exposed to the HRP-containing medium. Botulinum neurotoxin A terminals fixed immediately after depolarization contain HRP in clathrin-coated vesicles (Fig. 6.8, *inset*), marking these as intermediates in synaptic vesicle production. The percentage of vesicles containing HRP reaction product under

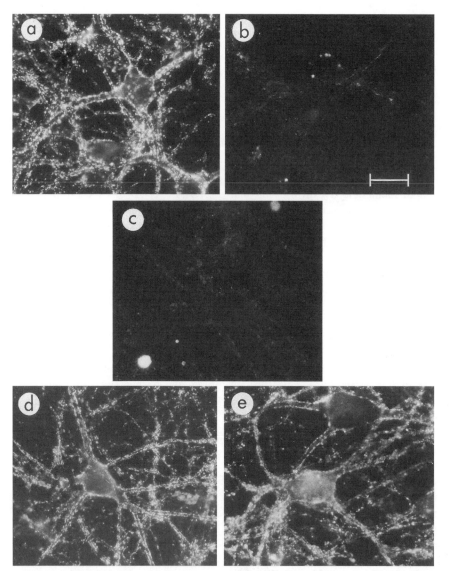

FIG. 6.6. FM1−43 staining (**A, C, D**) and destaining (**B, E**) with K$^+$ depolarization. **A, B:** Control cultures. **A:** 2 μM FM1−43 in 56 mmol KCl; 2 mM CaCl$_2$ for 5 minutes. The fluorescent image is similar to Fig. 6.3D. The labeled structures are individual active synaptic terminals containing a number of synaptic vesicles whose membranes are labeled with the fluorescent dye as a result of vesicle membrane recycling during the stimulation interval. **B:** Control culture loaded with FM1−43 as in (**A**) and subsequently depolarized with 56 mM KCl and 2 mM CaCl$_2$ in the absence of dye. There is substantial loss of FM1−43 from synaptic terminals as a result of exocytosis of labeled vesicles. **C:** FM1−43 labeling after TeNT (10 ng/mL) for 22 hours. When synaptic vesicle exocytosis is blocked by TeNT, uptake of FM1−43 is decreased substantially. **D, E:** BoNT-A (200 ng/mL; i.e., more than 20 times that required to block neurotransmitter release). **D:** FM1−43 uptake. Although fluorescence intensity is reduced from controls, FM1−43 labeling is unequivocal in cultures blocked by BoNT-A. **E:** BoNT-A−blocked culture loaded with FM1−43 as in (**D**) and subsequently incubated with 56 mM KCl and 2 mM CaCl$_2$ in an attempt to destain. In contrast to control cultures, it is not possible to destain BoNT-A−blocked cultures, providing further evidence that vesicle exocytosis cannot be stimulated. Bar, 25 μm, applies to all panels. (Reproduced in part from Neale EA, Bowers LM, Jia M, Bateman KE, Williamson LC. Botulinum neurotoxin A blocks synaptic vesicle exocytosis but not endocytosis at the nerve terminal. *J Cell Biol* 1999;147:1249−1260 by permission.)

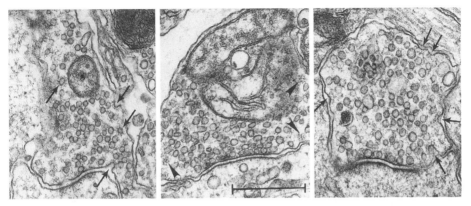

FIG. 6.7. Clathrin and synaptic vesicle recycling. **A:** K$^+$-depolarized control culture. Clathrin-coated pits and vesicles (*arrows*) are seen commonly. Empty clathrin baskets, seen frequently in resting cultures, are rare after stimulation. **B:** K$^+$-depolarized TeNT-blocked culture. K$^+$ stimulation does not cause the decrease in frequency of clathrin baskets (*arrowheads*) or increase in clathrin-coated membranes that is observed in stimulated control cultures. **C:** K$^+$-depolarized BoNT-A–blocked culture. This culture appears more similar to the stimulated control than to the stimulated TeNT-blocked culture. Empty clathrin baskets have all but disappeared and clathrin-coated membranes can be found. Toxin concentrations as in Fig. 6.5. Bar, 0.5 µm. (Reproduced in part from Neale EA, Bowers LM, Jia M, Bateman KE, Williamson LC. Botulinum neurotoxin A blocks synaptic vesicle exocytosis but not endocytosis at the nerve terminal. *J Cell Biol* 1999;147:1249–1260 by permission.)

several incubation conditions is presented in Table 6.1. As we saw with FM1–43, loading (endocytosis) and unloading (exocytosis) of HRP requires calcium. Botulinum neurotoxin A terminals contain about half the percentage of labeled vesicles after endocytosis as do controls. The HRP can be unloaded from control terminals, but not from BoNT-A–blocked terminals, again suggesting the ability of these blocked neurons to endocytose but not to exocytose.

To rule out the possibility that the 5-minute collection interval for the transmitter release assay might have caused us to miss an early transient exocytic event, patch clamp recordings were obtained from neurons during depolarization (37). Although control cells exhibited spontaneous network activity and potassium-evoked synaptic potentials, neither spontaneous nor evoked postsynaptic potentials could be detected in cultures exposed to either TeNT or BoNT-A. In addition, we modified the transmitter release assay, collecting aliquots of medium at 20-second intervals in an attempt to discriminate an early small bolus of released transmitter (37). No such bolus could be seen; loss of radioactivity from BoNT-A–blocked cultures was identi-

cal to that from TeNT-blocked cultures, and neither exceeded baseline loss. Thus, both the biochemical and electrophysiologic analyses confirmed an absence of synaptic activity (i.e., vesicle exocytosis) in BoNT-A–blocked cultures.

As a whole, the data imply that endocytosis and exocytosis are not necessarily temporally linked; that synaptic vesicles can be retrieved in the absence of immediately preceding exocytosis, that membrane endocytosis requires calcium, but perhaps a lower concentration than that required for exocytosis, and that TeNT, but not BoNT-A, interferes with membrane retrieval.

The uncoupling of exo- from endocytosis raises a number of questions, not the least of which is the source of the retrieved membrane. Is it possible that the surface of "resting" terminals contains synaptic vesicle membrane, even though immunohistochemistry fails to detect synaptic vesicle proteins (7,8,44,45)? Might such membrane be deposited as renewed supply from the soma (46–48)? Might vesicle proteins be more prominent on the surface of toxin-treated terminals because of a lower level of

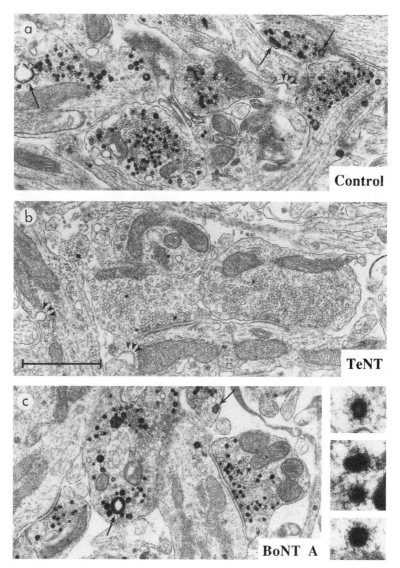

FIG. 6.8. HRP uptake stimulated by K$^+$ depolarization. **A:** Control. Recycled synaptic vesicles contain peroxidase reaction product. **B:** TeNT (10 ng/mL for 18 hours). Only occasional synaptic vesicles contain reaction product, indicating the failure of synaptic vesicles to undergo exo-/endocytosis. **C:** BoNT-A (200 ng/mL for 18 hours). A large number of synaptic vesicles contain reaction product, evidence that these vesicles have been formed by endocytosis from surface membrane. *Insets*: Reaction product labeling of clathrin-coated vesicles implicates these structures in the process of vesicle recycling. Note the larger labeled structures (*arrows*) in (**A**) and (**C**). That these structures are not seen in TeNT-exposed cultures suggests that they are an intermediate in the vesicle recycling pathway. *Arrowheads* mark coated pits associated with conventional endocytosis, which is unaffected by TeNT. These micrographs are the high-resolution equivalents of Fig. 6.6A, C, and D. Bar = 1 μm and applies to A–C. (Reproduced from Neale EA, Bowers LM, Jia M, Bateman KE, Williamson LC. Botulinum neurotoxin A blocks synaptic vesicle exocytosis but not endocytosis at the nerve terminal [In Process Citation]. *J Cell Biol* 1999;147:1249–1260 by permission.)

TABLE 6.1. *Calcium dependence of synaptic vesicle exo- and endocytosis*

		$+Ca^{2+}$*	$-Ca^{2+}$‡			$+Ca^{2+}$	$-Ca^{2+}$
	Load	10.5§	0		Load	4.8	0
Control	Unload	2.5‖	10.6	BoNT-A	Unload	5.2¶	ND

* 2 mM $CaCl_2$
‡ 0 mM $CaCl_2$ and 0.5 mM EGTA
§ Percent HRP-labeled vesicles after KCl-induced loading or unloading
‖ Significantly lower than Control, Load, plus Ca^{2+} ($p < 0.05$)
¶ Not significantly different from BoNT-A, Load, plus Ca^{2+}
Control and BoNT-A- (200 ng/mL for 18 hours) exposed cultures were rinsed in normal or Ca^{2+}-free‡; medium and incubated with HRP (8 mg/mL) for 2 minutes in medium containing 56 mM KCl with or without Ca^{2+}. Cultures were rinsed for 20 minutes in a Ca^{2+}-free buffered salts solution. Cultures loaded with HRP in the presence of Ca^{2+} were then rinsed in normal or Ca^{2+}-free salts solution and incubated for 5 minutes in 56 mM KCl with or without Ca^{2+} followed by a 10-minute wash in Ca^{2+}-free salts solution. Cultures were fixed for electron microscopy both after loading and after unloading. Vesicles were counted in micrographs at 100,000X; at least 2,000 vesicles were counted for each control sample and 5,500 for each BoNT-A sample. (Reproduced from Neale EA, Bowers LM, Jia M, Bateman KE, Williamson LC. Botulinum neurotoxin A blocks synaptic vesicle exocytosis but not endocytosis at the nerve terminal. *J Cell Biol* 1999;147:1249-1260 by permission.)

spontaneous activity and a generally lower rate of vesicle turnover? Does BoNT-A interfere with the refilling of vesicles with transmitter?

We have no evidence in spinal cord cultures to substantiate or eliminate any of the above possibilities. Early studies (49,50) indicated that neither TeNT nor BoNT-A interfered with the synthesis or storage of transmitter. A more recent study showed that TeNT inhibits the formation of synaptic vesicles from endosomal membranes in PC12 cells (51) by preventing an interaction between its protein substrate VAMP, and AP-2, an accessory protein required for recruiting clathrin to membrane prior to pit and vesicle formation. The participation of VAMP in membrane retrieval as well as vesicle fusion might help explain the finding of endocytosis in the face of a BoNT-A−, but not TeNT-, induced block in exocytosis. Two additional studies have provided evidence for a significant pool of synaptic vesicle proteins on the surface membrane of the synaptic terminal (45,52). Importantly, one of these studies demonstrates substantial vesicle endocytosis after only minimal exocytosis (52). Other experimental conditions may be used; e.g., exposure to latrotoxin (7) (the toxic component of black widow spider venom) or the manipulation of stimulation and calcium (53), to bring about a temporal separation of exo- and endocytosis. Under the latter conditions, it is clear that calcium is required for endocytosis (as with BoNT-A), and at a very low concentration

(53). Thus, it is possible to stimulate endocytosis in the absence of temporally linked exocytosis, that a pool of synaptic vesicle proteins (membrane) may persist on the terminal surface, and that VAMP but not synaptosomal-associated protein of 25 kDa (SNAP-25) may be required for synaptic vesicle retrieval.

Technical advances have allowed a more precise definition of the requirements for synaptic vesicle exocytosis and improved temporal resolution of synaptic vesicle membrane retrieval. "Kiss and run," originally envisioned by Ceccarelli (6) as the coalescence of vesicle and presynaptic membrane to form a transient fusion pore, has been redefined as a fusion event that allows transmitter release but not release of FM1–43, and is postulated to constitute ~20% of all fusion events (13,14). The more generally accepted view of transmitter release involves the collapse of vesicle membrane into the presynaptic membrane (4,9,54), recently visualized in real time with evanescent field microscopy of synaptic vesicles labeled with FM1–43 (55). Vesicle recovery after "kiss and run" is thought to comprise a simple closure of the fusion pore. Experiments using two FM dyes with different rates of dissociation from the membrane, have demonstrated two populations of synaptic vesicles characterized by recycling with half-times of 1 second versus 30 seconds (14). The rapidly recycling vesicles are felt to be "reused" rather than "reformed." The bulk of evidence to date, however, supports synaptic vesicle recycling by the clathrin-mediated endocytic process hypothesized by Heuser and Reese (9), although a rapid recycling process for collapsed vesicle membrane that does not require clathrin (56) remains a possibility. It has been proposed that the proportion of exocytic events that proceed by ''kiss and run'' versus vesicle collapse might be determined by intracellular calcium concentration (12), type of stimulus (13), or stimulus intensity (8,57). However, evidence exists that vesicle retrieval occurs by the same mechanism, most likely clathrin-mediated, after either low or high frequency stimulation (4,58). The concentration of calcium at the release site required for vesicle exocytosis may be as low as 10 μM or less (59,60). It is thought that lower concentrations of calcium are required for vesicle endocytosis than for exocytosis (52,53). Intracellular calcium levels were shown to regulate the speed of endocytosis to a maximum rate of one vesicle per second in cultures of hippocampus; no faster endocytic process was detected by an extremely sensitive assay (61,62). It was not possible in those experiments to predict the affinity of the calcium sensor critical for endocytosis. However, it was clear that endocytosis proceeded at a constant rate, regardless of stimulus size, and that vesicle retrieval is maintained for tens of seconds after the cessation of exocytosis. Thus, endocytosis may not necessarily be tightly coupled to exocytosis (61).

The clostridial neurotoxins have been accepted as tools to probe the cell biology of neurosecretion and a variety of other membrane fusion events. We have confirmed a significant botulinum neurotoxin type C1-induced neurotoxicity, evident initially at the nerve ending (32). BoNT-C1 cleaves both syntaxin and SNAP-25, although both BoNT types A and E cleave SNAP-25, these latter two toxins don't produce the same neural degeneration. Electron microscopy after BoNT-C1 exposure reveals a swelling of synaptic terminals and the accumulation of large membranous sacs within the terminals, suggestive of a membrane trafficking abnormality. Additionally, BoNT-C1 exposure was associated with increased calcium influx (32), possibly a result of toxin interference with

the association of syntaxin and calcium channels (63–66). Recent studies indicate that modulation of calcium currents is blocked by BoNT-C1 (67–69), providing improved understanding of the role of syntaxin in neural function. Studies on differences between the potency and duration of action of BoNT-A and E, despite their action on the same protein substrate, promise to add to our knowledge of the cell biology of SNAP-25 (39,70).

Obviously, the process of synaptic vesicle recycling is complicated and tightly regulated. Membrane retrieval appears to be driven by something other than membrane incorporation. What additional role BoNT-A may play in dissecting synaptic vesicle recycling remains to be seen. Further studies aimed at understanding how synaptic vesicle endocytosis occurs during BoNT-A and not during TeNT blockade will undoubtedly provide insight into this basic mechanism and may lead to the identity of the trigger and the cascade of events it initiates.

SUGGESTED READING

Bauerfeind R, David C, Grabs D, et al. Recycling of synaptic vesicles. *Adv Pharmacol* 1998;42:253–257.

Chen YA, Scheller R. Snare-mediated membrane fusion. *Nat Rev Mol Cell Biol* 2001;2:98–106.

Cremona O, De Camilli P. Synaptic vesicle endocytosis. *Curr Opin Neurobiol* 1997;7:323–330.

Jahn R, Südhof TC. Membrane fusion and exocytosis. *Annu Rev Biochem* 1999;68:863–911.

Lin RC, Scheller RH. Mechanisms of synaptic vesicle exocytosis. *Annu Rev Cell Dev Biol* 2000;16:19–49.

Mundigl O, De Camilli P. Formation of synaptic vesicles. *Curr Opin Cell Biol* 1994;6:561–567.

Slepnev VI, De Camilli P. Accessory factors in clathrin-dependent synaptic vesicle endocytosis. *Nat Rev Neurosci* 2000;1:161–172.

ACKNOWLEDGMENTS

Contributors to this work include Dr. Lura C. Williamson, Linda M. Bowers, and Karen E. Bateman. Their efforts are greatly appreciated, as are our collaborations with Drs. William H. Habig (FDA), J. Edward Brown (USAMRIID), and Cesare Montecucco (University of Padova).

REFERENCES

1. Triller A, Korn H. Transmission at a central inhibitory synapse. III. Ultrastructure of physiologically identified

and stained terminals. *J Neurophysiol* 1982;48: 708–736.

2. Neale EA, Nelson PG, Macdonald RL, et al. Synaptic interactions between mammalian central neurons in cell culture. III. Morphophysiological correlates of quantal synaptic transmission. *J Neurophysiol* 1983;49: 1459–1468.

3. Pun RY, Neale EA, Guthrie PB, et al. Active and inactive central synapses in cell culture. *J Neurophysiol* 1986;56:1242–1256.

4. Ryan TA, Reuter H, Smith SJ. Optical detection of a quantal presynaptic membrane turnover. *Nature* 1997; 388:478–482.

5. Schikorski T, Stevens CF. Quantitative ultrastructural analysis of hippocampal excitatory synapses. *J Neurosci* 1997;17:5858–5867.

6. Ceccarelli B, Hurlbut WP, Mauro A. Turnover of transmitter and synaptic vesicles at the frog neuromuscular junction. *J Cell Biol* 1973;57:499–524.

7. Valtorta F, Jahn R, Fesce R, et al. Synaptophysin (p38) at the frog neuromuscular junction: its incorporation into the axolemma and recycling after intense quantal secretion. *J Cell Biol* 1988;10:2717–2727.

8. Torri-Tarelli F, Villa A, Valtorta F, et al. Redistribution of synaptophysin and synapsin I during alpha-latrotoxin–induced release of neurotransmitter at the neuromuscular junction. *J Cell Biol* 1990;110:449–459.

9. Heuser JE, Reese TS. Evidence for recycling of synaptic vesicle membrane during transmitter release at the frog neuromuscular junction. *J Cell Biol* 1973;57:315–344.

10. Fesce R, Grohovaz F, Valtorta F, et al. Neurotransmitter release: fusion or "kiss-and-run"? *Trends Cell Biol* 1994;4:1–4.

11. Klingauf J, Kavalali ET, Tsien RW. Kinetics and regulation of fast endocytosis at hippocampal synapses. *Nature* 1998;394:581–585.

12. Fesce R, Meldolesi J. Peeping at the vesicle kiss. *Nat Cell Biol* 1999;1:E3–E4.

13. Stevens CF, Williams JH. "Kiss and run": exocytosis at hippocampal synapses. *Proc Natl Acad Sci U S A* 2000; 97:12828–12833.

14. Pyle JL, Kavalali ET, Piedras-Renteria ES, et al. Rapid reuse of readily releasable pool vesicles at hippocampal synapses. *Neuron* 2000;28:221–231.

15. Abenavoli A, Montagna M, Malgaroli A. Calcium: the common theme in vesicular recycling. *Nat Neurosci* 2001;2:117–118.

16. Takei K, Mundigl O, Daniell L, et al. The synaptic vesicle cycle: a single-vesicle budding step involving clathrin and dynamin. *J Cell Biol* 1996;133:1237–1250.

17. Murthy VN, Stevens CF. Synaptic vesicles retain their identity through the endocytic cycle. *Nature* 1998;392: 497–501.

18. Ransom BR, Neale EA, Henkart M, et al. Mouse spinal cord in cell culture. I. Morphology and intrinsic neuronal electrophysiologic properties. *J Neurophysiol* 1977;40: 1132–1150.

19. Ransom BR, Christian CN, Bullock PN, et al. Mouse spinal cord in cell culture. II. Synaptic activity and circuit behavior. *J Neurophysiol* 1977;40:1151–1162.

20. Ransom BR, Bullock PN, Nelson PG. Mouse spinal cord in cell culture. III. Neuronal chemosensitivity and its relationship to synaptic activity. *J Neurophysiol* 1977; 40:1163–1177.

21. Neale EA, Macdonald RL, Nelson PG. Intracellular

horseradish peroxidase injection for correlation of light and electron microscopic anatomy with synaptic physiology of cultured mouse spinal cord neurons. *Brain Res* 1978;152:265–282.

22. Macdonald RL, Pun RY, Neale EA, Nelson PG. Synaptic interactions between mammalian central neurons in cell culture. I. Reversal potential for excitatory postsynaptic potentials. *J Neurophysiol* 1983;49:1428–1441.

23. Nelson PG, Marshall KC, Pun RY, et al. Synaptic interactions between mammalian central neurons in cell culture. II. Quantal Analysis of EPSPs. *J Neurophysiol* 1983;49:1442–1458.

24. Wang FZ, Nelson PG, Fitzgerald SC, et al. Cholinergic function in cultures of mouse spinal cord neurons. *J Neurosci Res* 1990;25:312–323.

25. Fitzgerald SC. Dissociated spinal cord-dorsal root ganglion cultures on plastic tissue culture dishes and glass coverslips and wells. In: Shahar A, deVellis J, Vernadakis A, et al., eds. *A dissection and tissue culture manual of the nervous system.* New York: Alan R. Liss, 1989:219–222.

26. Neale EA, Bowers LM, Smith TG Jr. Early dendrite development in spinal cord cell cultures: a quantitative study. *J Neurosci Res* 1993;34:54–66.

27. Westbrook GL, Brenneman DE. The development of spontaneous electrical activity in spinal cord cultures. In: Caciagli F, Giacobini E, Paoletti R, eds. *Developmental neuroscience: physiological, pharmacological and clinical aspects.* New York: Elsevier Science, 1984: 11–17.

28. Jackson MB, Lecar H, Brenneman DE, et al. Electrical development in spinal cord cell culture. *J Neurosci* 1982;2:1052–1061.

29. Brenneman DE, Neale EA, Foster GA, et al. Nonneuronal cells mediate neurotrophic action of vasoactive intestinal peptide. *J Cell Biol* 1987;104:1603–1610.

30. Neale EA, Habig WH, Schrier BK, et al. Applications of tetanus toxin for structure-function studies in neuronal cell cultures. In: Nisticò G, Bizzini B, Bytchenko B, et al., eds. *Eighth international conference on tetanus (Leningrad).* Rome: Pythagora Press, 1989:58–65.

31. Feng G, Mellor RH, Bernstein M, et al. Imaging neuronal subsets in transgenic mice expressing multiple spectral variants of GFP. *Neuron* 2000;28:41–51.

32. Williamson LC, Neale EA. Syntaxin and 25-kDa synaptosomal-associated protein: differential effects of botulinum neurotoxins C1 and A on neuronal survival. *J Neurosci Res* 1998;52:569–583.

33. Bergey GK, Macdonald RL, Habig WH, et al. Tetanus toxin: convulsant action on mouse spinal cord neurons in culture. *J Neurosci* 1983;3:2310–2323.

34. Bergey GK, Bigalke H, Nelson PG. Differential effects of tetanus toxin on inhibitory and excitatory synaptic transmission in mammalian spinal cord neurons in culture: a presynaptic locus of action for tetanus toxin. *J Neurophysiol* 1987;57:121–131.

35. Bigalke H, Dreyer F, Bergey G. Botulinum A neurotoxin inhibits noncholinergic synaptic transmission in mouse spinal cord neurons in culture. *Brain Res* 1985; 360:318–324.

36. Montecucco C, Schiavo G. Structure and function of tetanus and botulinum neurotoxins. *Q Rev Biophys* 1995;28:423–472.

37. Neale EA, Bowers LM, Jia M, et al. Botulinum neurotoxin A blocks synaptic vesicle exocytosis but not endo-

cytosis at the nerve terminal. *J Cell Biol* 1999;147: 1249–1260.

38. Williamson LC, Fitzgerald SC, Neale EA. Differential effects of tetanus toxin on inhibitory and excitatory neurotransmitter release from mammalian spinal cord cells in culture. *J Neurochem* 1992;59:2148–2157.

39. Keller JE, Neale EA. The role of the synaptic protein SNAP-25 in the potency of botulinum neurotoxin type A. *J Biol Chem* 2001;276:13476–13482.

40. Williamson LC, Halpern JL, Montecucco C, et al. Clostridial neurotoxins and substrate proteolysis in intact neurons. Botulinum neurotoxin C acts on synaptosomal-associated protein of 25 kDa. *J Biol Chem* 1996;271: 7694–7699.

41. Schiavo G, Stenbeck G, Rothman JE, et al. Binding of the synaptic vesicle v-SNARE, synaptotagmin, to the plasma membrane t-SNARE, SNAP-25, can explain docked vesicles at neurotoxin-treated synapses. *Proc Natl Acad Sci U S A* 1997;94:997–1001.

42. Betz WJ, Bewick GS. Optical analysis of synaptic vesicle recycling at the frog neuromuscular junction. *Science* 1992;255:200–203.

43. Cochilla AJ, Angleson JK, Betz WJ. Monitoring secretory membrane with FM1–43 fluorescence. *Annu Rev Neurosci* 1999;22:1–10.

44. von Wedel RJ, Carlson SS, Kelly RB. Transfer of synaptic vesicle antigens to the presynaptic plasma membrane during exocytosis. *Proc Natl Acad Sci U S A* 1981;78: 1014–1018.

45. Mundigl O, Verderio C, Krazewski K, et al. A radioimmunoassay to monitor synaptic activity in hippocampal neurons in vitro. *Eur J Cell Biol* 1995;66:246–256.

46. Li JY, Jahn R, Dahlström A. Axonal transport and targeting of the t-SNAREs SNAP-25 and syntaxin 1 in the peripheral nervous system. *Eur J Cell Biol* 1996;70: 12–22.

47. Nakata T, Terada S, Hirokawa N. Visualization of the dynamics of synaptic vesicle and plasma membrane proteins in living axons. *J Cell Biol* 1998;140:659–674.

48. Ahmari SE, Buchanan J, Smith SJ. Assembly of presynaptic active zones from cytoplasmic transport packets. *Nat Neurosci* 2000;3:445–451.

49. Collingridge GL, Davies J. Reversible effects of low doses of tetanus toxin on synaptic inhibition in the substantia nigra and turning behaviour in the rat. *Brain Res* 1980;185:455–459.

50. Gundersen CB. The effects of botulinum toxin on the synthesis, storage and release of acetylcholine. *Prog Neurobiol* 1980;14:99–119.

51. Salem N, Faundez V, Horng JT, et al. A v-SNARE participates in synaptic vesicle formation mediated by the AP3 adaptor complex. *Nat Neurosci* 1998;1:551–556.

52. Marks B, McMahon HT. Calcium triggers calcineurin-dependent synaptic vesicle recycling in mammalian nerve terminals. *Curr Biol* 1998;8:740–749.

53. Gad H, Low P, Zotova E, et al. Dissociation between Ca^{2+}-triggered synaptic vesicle exocytosis and clathrin-mediated endocytosis at a central synapse. *Neuron* 1998; 21:607–616.

54. Kraszewski K, Mundigl O, Daniell L, et al. Synaptic vesicle dynamics in living cultured hippocampal neurons visualized with CY3-conjugated antibodies directed against the lumenal domain of synaptotagmin. *J Neurosci* 1995;15:4328–4342.

55. Zenisek D, Steyer JA, Almers W. Transport, capture and exocytosis of single synaptic vesicles at active zones. *Nature* 2000;406:849–854.

56. Artalejo CR, Henley JR, McNiven MA, et al. Rapid endocytosis coupled to exocytosis in adrenal chromaffin cells involves Ca^{2+}, GTP, and dynamin but not clathrin. *Proc Natl Acad Sci U S A* 1995;92:8328–8332.

57. Torri-Tarelli F, Bossi M, Fesce R, et al. Synapsin I partially dissociates from synaptic vesicles during exocytosis induced by electrical stimulation. *Neuron* 1992; 9:1143–1153.

58. Shupliakov O, Gad H, Löw P, et al. Calcium requirement in early stages of clathrin-mediated synaptic vesicle endocytosis. *Soc Neurosci* 1997;23:2274 (abstr #887.16).

59. Schneggenburger R, Neher E. Intracellular calcium dependence of transmitter release rates at a fast central synapse. *Nature* 2000;406:889–893.

60. Bollmann JH, Sakmann B, Borst JG. Calcium sensitivity of glutamate release in a calyx-type terminal. *Science* 2000;289:953–957.

61. Sankaranarayanan S, Ryan TA. Calcium accelerates endocytosis of vSNAREs at hippocampal synapses. *Nat Neurosci* 2001;2:129–136.

62. Sankaranarayanan S, Ryan TA. Real-time measurements of vesicle-SNARE recycling in synapses of the central nervous system. *Nat Cell Biol* 2000;2:197–204.

63. O'Connor VM, Shamotienko O, Grishin E, et al. On the structure of the "synaptosecretosome." Evidence for a neurexin/synaptotagmin/syntaxin/Ca^{2+} channel complex. *FEBS Lett* 1993;326:255–260.

64. Bezprozvanny I, Scheller RH, Tsien RW. Functional impact of syntaxin on gating of N-type and Q-type calcium channels. *Nature* 1995;378:623–626.

65. Sheng ZH, Rettig J, Takahashi M, et al. Identification of a syntaxin-binding site on N-type calcium channels. *Neuron* 1994;13:1303–1313.

66. Sheng ZH, Rettig J, Cook T, et al. Calcium-dependent interaction of N-type calcium channels with the synaptic core complex. *Nature* 1996;379:451–454.

67. Stanley EF, Mirotznik RR. Cleavage of syntaxin prevents G-protein regulation of presynaptic calcium channels. *Nature* 1997;385:340–343.

68. Bergsman JB, Tsien RW. Syntaxin modulation of calcium channels in cortical synaptosomes as revealed by botulinum toxin C1. *J Neurosci* 2000;20:4368–4378.

69. Degtiar VE, Scheller RH, Tsien RW. Syntaxin modulation of slow inactivation of N-type calcium channels. *J Neurosci* 2000;20:4355–4367.

70. Keller JE, Neale EA, Oyler G, et al. Persistence of botulinum neurotoxin action in cultured spinal cord cells. *FEBS Lett* 1999;456:137–142.

Scientific and Therapeutic Aspects of Botulinum Toxin
edited by M.F. Brin, J. Jankovic, and M. Hallett
Lippincott Williams & Wilkins, Philadelphia, © 2002.

7

Molecular Basis of the Unique Endopeptidase Activity of Botulinum Neurotoxin

Bal Ram Singh

Seven different serotypes (A–G) of botulinum neurotoxin (BoNT) are produced by various strains of *Clostridium botulinum.* Each BoNT consists of a 50-kDa light (L) chain and a 100-kDa heavy (H) chain linked through a disulfide bond. Each serotype of BoNT is synthesized as a single polypeptide chain of about 150 kDa, which is nicked into an L and an H chain either by endogenous or exogenous protease. Crystallographic structures for BoNT-A and BoNT-B were recently published (1,2), and show three distinct domains corresponding to the L chain and the two halves (H_N and H_C) of the H chain (Fig. 7.1) (3).

BoNT is secreted from the bacterium along with one or more proteins, which are referred to as neurotoxin-associated proteins (NAPs). The actual role of NAPs in botulism is not clearly understood, although the idea of a BoNT-protective role has been advanced for these proteins.

The mode of action of BoNT can be divided into four steps: ingestion and intestinal absorption; binding to neuronal membranes; internalization; and blockade of neurotransmitter release. Because it is the preformed BoNT, rather than the organism, that is the pathogenic agent, the first step in the toxico-infection process is the ingestion and absorption of the BoNT at the intestinal wall. NAPs play a critical role in protecting the BoNT from the acidity and proteases of the gastrointestinal tract. NAPs have also been proposed to help BoNT anchor to the intestinal wall and to translocate it across the mucosal layer (4,5), although there are reports that contradict this assertion (6). In any case, a clear understanding of the mechanism involved in this step is lacking.

The C-terminus of the H chain (H_C) of BoNT binds to trisialoganglioside (presumably through its H_C2 domain (see Fig. 7.1), and protein receptors on the presynaptic membranes (Fig. 7.2) of neuromuscular junctions (7–9). After internalization through endocytosis, the H chain is believed to form a channel in the endosomal membrane and enables the translocation of the L chain through the endosomal membrane into the cell cytoplasm (Fig. 7.2). The L chain then acts at nerve endings by catalyzing the proteolysis of its substrate resulting into the blockade of acetylcholine release (8).

The intracellular substrates of L chains of different types of BoNT vary. These substrates are components of the synaptic vesicle docking and fusion complex: vesicle-associated membrane protein (VAMP, also called synaptobrevin) is the substrate for BoNT-B, BoNT-D, BoNT-F, and tetanus neurotoxin (TeNT); synaptosomal-associated protein of 25 kDa (SNAP-25) is the substrate for BoNT-A and BoNT-E; and Hpc-1/syntaxin is the substrate for BoNT-C1 (10–14).

Although BoNTs possess a Zn^{2+}-endopeptidase activity against a select group of neuronal proteins involved in the exocytosis process, which causes the blockage of acetylcholine release resulting in a flaccid muscle paralysis (for reviews, see references 15,16), the endopeptidase activity of the purified BoNT under *in vitro* conditions is observed only when the disulfide bond between the two subunits of BoNT is reduced (8,17–19). Another unique feature of the BoNT endopeptidase activity is that while each

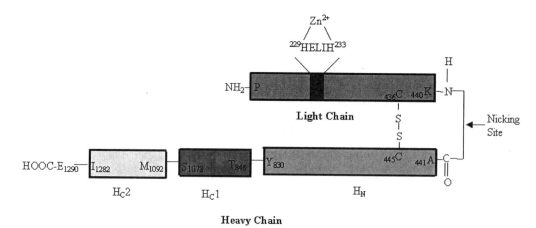

FIG. 7.1. Drawing of BoNT-B showing different structural domains.

of the seven BoNT serotypes contain an identical Zn^{2+}-binding motif in their active sites, their substrates are either entirely different proteins, or the cleavage site on the substrate is different for each serotype. Each of the BoNT endopeptidases is extremely selective for substrate (except for BoNT-C1), and has an exclusive cleavage site. Furthermore, only entire substrate proteins or their large polypeptide segments are recognized for cleavage by BoNT endopeptidases. All the BoNT endopeptidases recognize one or more (in the case of BoNT-C1) of the three SNARE [soluble NSF (*N*-ethylmaleimide–sensitive factor) attachment receptor] proteins involved in exocytosis. Other unique features of BoNT endopeptidase include a dual (structural and catalytic) role of the bound Zn^{2+}, strict topographic requirement of active-site amino acid residues, and activation of the endopeptidase activity by a group of proteins (NAPs) (19–21). BoNTs are being regarded as a new class of metalloproteases (22).

An understanding of the molecular mechanism of the unique endopeptidase activity of BoNT is an important step in discerning the comprehensive mechanism of BoNT action, which is essential to design preventive measures against occurrence of botulism.

STRUCTURAL BASIS OF UNIQUE BOTULINUM NEUROTOXIN ENDOPEPTIDASE ACTIVITY

The unique features of BoNT endopeptidase activity must originate at the structural level. A unique structural feature noted in the crystallographic structure of BoNT-A is that the catalytic domain (zinc-binding motif) is buried 20- to 24-Å deep into the protein matrix, and the N-terminal H chain peptide wraps around the L chain (1). However, this feature can perhaps explain only one of the unique features of the BoNT-A endopeptidase activity; namely, the disulfide bond reduction-mediated enhancement of the

FIG. 7.2. A: Synaptic vesicles containing neurotransmitters dock with plasma membrane through SNARE [soluble NSF (*N*-ethylmaleimide–sensitive factor) attachment receptor] proteins [synaptobrevin, syntaxin, and synaptosomal-associated protein of 25 kDa (SNAP-25)] ready to release the neurotransmitter through a Ca^{2+}-triggered fusion process. SNARE proteins remain in random coil structures until associated in the SNARE complex at docking, where they form a helical bundle. **B:** Botulinum or tetanus toxin binds to the presynaptic membrane through gangliosides and a protein receptor *(step 1)*, is internalized through endocytosis *(step 2a)*, and its L chain is translocated across the membrane *(step 2b)*. The L chain acts as a specific endopeptidase against synaptobrevin (on synaptic vesicle), syntaxin (plasma membrane), or SNAP-25 (plasma membrane). BoNTs (or tetanus neurotoxin) cleave their substrates before the SNARE complex is formed.

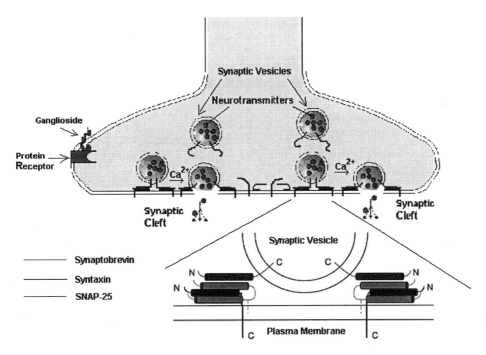

(a)

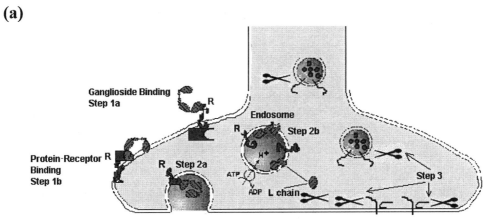

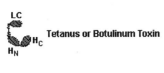

(b)

endopeptidase activity. This is explained by suggesting that disulfide bond reduction will allow release of the L chain by the H chain, thus making the 20- to 24-Å–deep active site accessible to the substrate. This idea is partially supported by a change in the tryptophan topography of BoNT-A upon the reduction of its disulfide bond (19). Specifically, the peptide segments containing tryptophan residues become more flexible upon reduction of the disulfide bond. However, this feature alone is inadequate to explain other unique characteristics of BoNT endopeptidase or toxic activity. First of all, the N-terminal wraparound peptide (N-WRAP) of H chain does not universally (for example, in BoNT-B) block the active-site crevice (2). Second, reduction of the disulfide bond does not seem to change much of the active-site structure, at least in BoNT-B (S. Swaminathan, personal communication). Third, there are other conditions, irrespective of the disulfide bond reduction, under which the toxicity/endopeptidase activity of BoNT is expressed or enhanced. Examination of structural features under these conditions holds the key to the understanding of the molecular basis of the BoNT activity.

An interesting feature of the BoNT activity is its activation under several conditions: (a) Upon nicking of the single polypeptide chain into dichain, mouse toxicity of BoNT-E increases by about 100-fold (4); (b) Disulfide bond reduction increases BoNT activity in the blockade of neurotransmitter release in cell cultures (23,24), and enhances its endopeptidase activity (17–19); (c) Endopeptidase activity of BoNT-A associated with NAPs even under nonreducing conditions is as high as that of pure BoNT-A under reducing conditions (19); (d) A 33-kDa hemagglutinin component of NAPs (Hn-33) enhances the activity of BoNT-A by about fivefold (25); (e) The endopeptidase activity of single chain BoNT-E is dramatically increased upon its nicking, even under nonreducing conditions (26); (f) At a concentration of 0.1 μM or more, BoNT-A exists as a dimer, and its monomerization enhances the endopeptidase activity by about fivefold (27). Activation of BoNT under the above conditions (generally relevant to natural physiologic conditions) provides a serendipitous opportunity to understand the difference between the unactivated and activated forms of the toxin to elucidate molecular features that could play critical roles in its biologic activity. Current knowledge about the above aspects is examined in this chapter.

UNIQUE STRUCTURAL FEATURES OF BOTULINUM NEUROTOXINS

Structural features presented by the groups of Stevens and Swaminathan support a common structural construction in at least two members (BoNT-A and BoNT-B) of this class in terms of three distinct domains and general structural features. Within 8 Å of the zinc-binding motif, BoNT-A and BoNT-B have virtually identically structural features (2). However, differences set in at a 15-Å radius point, which could lead to differences in substrate specificity.

As a unique feature noted in the structures of both BoNT-B and BoNT-A, the catalytic domain (zinc-binding motif) is buried 15 (BoNT-B) and 20 to 24 (BoNT-A) Å deep into the protein matrix, and an N-terminal H chain peptide belt wraps around the L chain (1,2). While in BoNT-A, the belt occludes the active site, it leaves the active site clearly accessible in BoNT-B. The belt, at least in BoNT-A, can perhaps explain one of the unique features of the BoNT-A endopeptidase activity; namely, the disulfide bond reduction-mediated expression of the endopeptidase activity. The disulfide bond reduction can release the L chain by the H chain belt, making the active site accessible to the substrate. However, it may not be a universal molecular feature of all BoNTs, as BoNT-B belt does not occlude its active site. In this regard, Hanson and Stevens (28) have discovered additional features by identifying three sets of loops in BoNT-B L chain, which seem to change upon separation of L and H chains and/or upon binding with synaptobrevin II. The displacement of loops 50 and 200 in BoNT-B is quite dramatic, especially in view of the difference in the topography of loop 200 between BoNT-B and BoNT-A (Fig. 7.3). When BoNT-B holotoxin, rather than BoNT-A, is used as a reference point, the displacement of loop 200 is even larger than the 13

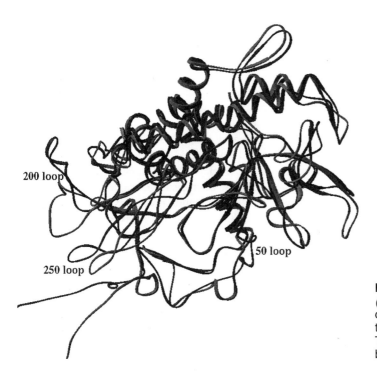

200 loop

250 loop

50 loop

FIG. 7.3. Overlay of BoNT-A *(red)* and BoNT-B *(green)* L chains using coordinates of their respective holotoxins. The figure was kindly provided by S. Swaminathan.

Å predicted by Hanson and Stevens (28). Chain separation is known to introduce changes in polypeptide folding of even BoNT-A (29). Quite significantly, it seems loops 200 and 250 in BoNT-B L chain are displaced owing to the loss of their interaction with the H_N. It is argued that movements of these loops are critical to the catalytic activity. Does that mean that the chain separation is required for the endopeptidase activity? The requirement of disulfide bond reduction points in that direction. However, it is well known that the disulfide bond reduction alone does not result in the chain separation, and BoNTs are enzymatically active without separation of their chains. It is possible that the presence of the substrate displaces the H_N interaction at least under *in vitro* conditions. Under physiologic conditions, the L chain is believed to separate from the H chain at the endosomal membrane (Fig. 7.2).

ROLES OF CYS AND DISULFIDE BOND IN BOTULINUM NEUROTOXIN ACTION

BoNT-A contains three cysteines in LC and seven in HC, while BoNT-E contains three cys-

teines in LC and five in HC. Cys residues are not always conserved, except for those at the C-terminus of the LC and N-terminus of HC participating in the disulfide bridge. Proteolysis studies of BoNT-A and BoNT-E by trypsin and pepsin revealed only one interchain disulfide bond between LC and HC (30,31). Cys1234 and Cys1279 within BoNT-A HC domain form an intrachain disulfide bond (32–34), while the intrachain disulfide in BoNT-E links Cys1196 and Cys1237 (31). The remaining cysteines in BoNT-A and BoNT-E do not participate in any disulfide bridge. Alkylation of free cysteine residues in BoNT-A did not influence the toxification either by bath application or by injection (36). It is, therefore, believed that SH-groups play no role in binding, translocation or intracellular toxicity of clostridial neurotoxins.

The expression of toxicity in the whole animal requires the HC and LC to be disulfide-linked (37), while full potency is achieved by reduction of the disulfide bond in BoNT when permeabilized cell preparation is employed to allow a free access of toxins into the interior of the cell (23,38). A simplistic explanation of the requirement of interchain disulfide-intact BoNT for mouse lethality would be the need for the two chains to be together for binding and translocation into neuronal cells. However, it has been observed that the *in vitro* endopeptidase activity of purified BoNTs is expressed only after their interchain disulfide bonds are reduced (16–18), which could explain the need for disulfide reduction in permeabilized cells. The molecular basis of the disulfide reduction-mediated enhancement of endopeptidase activity, or the mechanism by which it occurs in physiologic conditions in animal nerve cells, is not understood as yet. A recent study (39) concerning the role of disulfide bond cleavage on the enhanced endopeptidase activity reveals that nonreduced BoNT-A is more resistant to cleavage by endoproteinase Glu-C than its reduced form. Spectroscopic measurements of reduced and nonreduced BoNT-A reveal dramatic difference in the topography of aromatic amino acid residues (19). These results reinforce the notion that disulfide cleavage of BoNT-A leads to an altered structure, but the exact nature of structural change is not understood.

ROLES OF DIFFERENT DOMAINS OF THE NEUROTOXIN

Although reduction is required for maximum endopeptidase activity of the neurotoxin, no information exists about the cellular processing of toxin and no direct evidence indicates that the two chains are separated inside the cell. It remains a puzzling question as to whether the HC transverses the membrane along with the LC, or it is left behind when the disulfide bond is cleaved. Based on the requirement of HC for expression of toxicity of LC in *Aplysia* neurons (40), it can be speculated that translocation of HC domain along with the LC may also occur in vertebrate neurons. However, the LCs of TeNT and BoNT-A inhibit exocytosis on their own when applied to cytolysin-permeabilized chromaffin cells or mechanically ''cracked'' PC12 cells (23,41,42). These results strongly suggest that the isolated L chain of clostridial neurotoxins is not structurally different from the form of the L chain when it is connected to the H chain in native BoNT or TeNT. On the other

hand, spectroscopic analyses of BoNT-A reveal significant alterations in the LC and HC structure at the secondary and tertiary level upon their separation (29,43). Indirect evidence of conformational changes induced by chain separation has also come from differential proteolytic fragmentation patterns of LC and HC in intact and separated forms (39). Separated LC has activated endopeptidase activity, which is at the same level as the LC associated with HC in BoNT-A after disulfide reduction (18). Therefore, the activation process is not a result of the separation, but is, instead, a consequence of the disulfide bond reduction-induced structural alteration. Structural change in the LC without its separation from the HC has not been examined.

NAPS: THE PROTEINS AND THEIR RELATIONSHIP TO BOTULINUM NEUROTOXIN AND ITS TOXICITY

Types and Biologic Activity

Historically, the crystalline form of the type A neurotoxin was first prepared by Lamanna et al. (44). The crystalline toxin was estimated to have a molecular weight of 900,000, with no clue, at that time, that it was a complex of the neurotoxin and hemagglutinin (45). The complex nature of BoNT-A was first discovered in 1966 (46), which has been proven since then to be the nature of all the serotypes (A to G) of BoNT (4,47–49). In the complex, the 150-kDa neurotoxin part combines with one or more proteins resulting in a complex.

BoNTs produced in fluid culture or in food are complexes of BoNT (7S) and one or more NAPs, resulting in molecular sizes of 12S or larger, 16S, and 19S (50–52). The 16S complex is referred to as ''large'' or L toxin, and 19S is referred as ''extra large'' or LL toxin. BoNT-A complex can exist in three forms: M, L, or LL. BoNT-B, -C, -D, and -E complexes exist in two forms: L and M (4,53,54). So far, BoNT-F complex is known to exist only in M form, and BoNT-G complex exists only in L form (55). Some of BoNT-A and BoNT-B types, which cause infant botulism, also exist in M form only (56). The size of BoNT-A and BoNT-B complexes apparently depends on the medium for bacterial growth (57). NAPs, other than the 120-kDa neurotoxin-binding protein (NBP); (58) which has no known biologic activity, may (types A, B, C, and D) or may not (types E, F, and G) possess hemagglutinating activity (HA). NAPs with HA have not been individually purified, except in the case of type A *C. botulinum,* and are referred to as HAx, where x refers to their molecular mass in kDa. Recently, individual components of type C BoNT complex have been chromatographically separated (59). However, HA of the individual components has not been demonstrated. In case of type A *C. botulinum,* a 33-kDa protein was recently purified, which is referred to as Hn-33 (60). It has been clearly demonstrated that the toxic component responsible for botulism is the 7S toxin of 150-kDa protein (4,61,62). The question is then raised as to what is the role of the NAPs?

It seems that for the bacteria to produce the NAPs simultaneously with the BoNT, NAPs must have important role(s) to play in the intoxication process. Although roles such as their assistance in the translocation of the BoNT across the intestinal mucosal layer have been speculated, solid experimental evidence only suggests that the NAPs protect the BoNT against acidity and proteolytic attack of the enzymes of gastric juice. Such a conclusion has been drawn based on data that suggest drastically enhanced oral toxicity of the BoNT complex as compared to the purified BoNT (63–65). In addition, it has been observed that BoNT, found in the rat lymph after being administered in its complex form into the duodenum, is more toxic relative to the one administered in the purified form (66). There is also evidence that the BoNT does not dissociate in the digestive tract even at pH 7.0 (4). However, molecular dissociation occurs in the lymphatics (67). It may be noted that TeNT, which has greater than 35% sequence homology with BoNTs, is not a food poison. Incidentally, it also lacks NAPs, which further suggests a crucial role of NAPs in protecting the BoNT against digestive system (68).

So far, there is no direct evidence that NAPs play any significant role beyond the intestinal absorption of the BoNT. However, these proteins play a substantial role in protecting the BoNT against the digestive system (4,5). To the best of our knowledge, this is the only known natural system where a protein is protected by another protein from digestive proteases and acidity. An understanding of such a process at the molecular level could provide crucial insight into the development of methods for oral administration of vaccines including those against botulism and tetanus.

Genomic Organization

The genomic organizations of BoNTs and their associated proteins have been suggested by researchers (55,69–71), and are summarized in Fig. 7.4. No characteristic signal peptide sequences are observed in any of the BoNT or NAP genes. The genes of BoNTs and NAPs are closely grouped as operons on the chromosome, phage, or plasmid. The NBP gene is located only 17 base pairs (bp) (type C) or 26 bp (type A) upstream of the BoNT gene. There are two promoter regions for these genes. One overlaps the C-terminal end of NBP genes and the other is shared with the NBP genes, controlling cotranscription of the two genes. The neurotoxin genes are either transcribed alone or along with NBP genes via a polycistronic mRNA, and thus these two genes form an operon. HA gene clusters form another operon transcribed in the opposite directions from the BoNT and NBP genes. HA gene clusters are located 262 bp (in type C) or 930 bp (in type A) upstream of the NBP gene, respectively. Each HA gene contains its own transcription terminator which is predicted to form a stem-and loop structure in the mRNA.

The hemagglutinin genes HA33, HA17, and HA70 from type C *C. botulinum* were first sequenced by Hauser et al. (70). The three genes, which are closely linked and form an operon, are transcribed alone or together in the opposite direction to that of NBP and BoNT genes. The HA17 gene encoding 146 amino acids is located between the HA33 and HA70 genes. The HA70 is cleaved to a predicted 22-kDa protein and to a 48-kDa protein after translation, which correspond to the HA20–23 and HA53–57 bands from type A and C on sodium dodecyl sulfate-

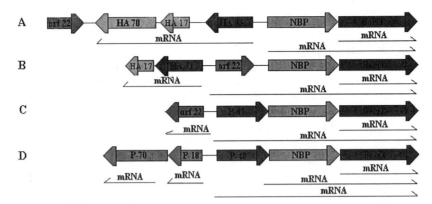

FIG. 7.4. Genomic organizations of *C. botulinum* (**A**) type C, (**B**) types A and B, (**C**) type F, and (**D**) type E. (From Li B, Qian X, Sarkar HK, Singh BR. Molecular characterization of type E *C. botulinum* and comparison with other types of *Clostridium botulinum. Biochim Biophys Acta* 1998;1395:21–27, with permission.)

polyacrylamide gel electrophoresis (SDS-PAGE) (55,72). Homology among the HA33 genes ranges between 36% and 92%.

NAP-Enhancement of BoNT Endopeptidase Activity

We recently reported that NAPs also potentiate the Zn^{2+}-endopeptidase activity of BoNT-A in an *in vitro* assay by using its known intracellular target protein, SNAP-25, as a substrate (19). While isolated BoNT-A exhibited no protease activity prior to reduction with dithiothreitol (DTT), BoNT-A complex exhibited a high endopeptidase activity even in its nonreduced form (Table 7.1). Our results suggest that the bacterial production of NAPs along with BoNT is designed for the NAPs to play an accessory role

TABLE 7.1. *Endopeptidase activity (cleavage of SNAP-25) of BoNT-A and BoNT-A complex with NAPs before and after reduction (+DTT, dithiothreitol) of its disulfide bond*

Condition	BoNT-A	BoNT-A complex
No DTT	4%	66%
+DTT	69%	80%

Data taken from Cai S, Singh BR. A correlation between differential structural features and the degree of endopeptidase activity of type A botulinum neurotoxin in aqueous solution. *Biochemistry* 2001;40:4693–4702.

in the BoNT function, in contrast to their previously known limited role in protecting the neurotoxin in the gastrointestinal tract and in the external environment.

NICKING-MEDIATED ACTIVATION OF BOTULINUM NEUROTOXIN

A major feature of BoNT is its activation by endogenous or exogenous proteolytic nicking (4,73), or by reduction of the disulfide bond between its L and H chains (15–19). BoNT is produced as a single polypeptide chain in bacterial cultures, and is nicked endogenously [e.g., BoNT-A (73)], or it can be nicked by exogenous protease such as trypsin [e.g., BoNT-E (74)]. The nicked form of the toxin is up to 100-fold more toxic than the unnicked form in mouse lethality tests (4,75). The nicked (di-chain) form of BoNT is still linked through a disulfide bond, which is needed to be maintained for its mouse lethality, as in this form, the nerve membrane binding domain (H chain) can carry the toxic domain (L chain) to its site of action. A simplistic explanation for nicking-mediated increase in the toxic activity of BoNT is argued to stem from the facilitation of the L chain translocation across the endosomal membrane after nicking, as the nicking allows the L chain to separate from the membrane-integrated H chain. In cellular assay systems in which di-chain BoNT is directly introduced into cells by permeabilizing the cell membranes either mechanically (PC12 cells) or by digitonin (chromaffin cells), it has been observed that reduction of the disulfide bond is required for the biologic activity (blockade of neurotransmitter release) of BoNT (23,24). These observations provided the first indication that the nicking- and disulfide reduction-mediated increase in toxicity might be dependent on more than just a facilitated translocation of the L chain.

CORRELATION BETWEEN THE QUATERNARY STRUCTURE AND BOTULINUM NEUROTOXIN ENDOPEPTIDASE ACTIVITY

The quaternary structures of proteins play important roles in the stabilization of native proteins (76,77), and are closely related to their biologic functions (78). The recently released crystallographic structure of BoNT-A obtained under conditions in which its interchain disulfide bond remains intact has revealed that BoNT-A exists as a monomer in the crystalline state (1). There is about 23% α-helical structure and 17% β-sheet structure in the toxin. The crystallographically derived β-sheet structure is dramatically different from estimates of 36% based on prediction from primary structure (79), or 44% based on far-UV circular dichroism (CD) analysis of BoNT-A in solution (43). Therefore, it is possible that there is a major difference between crystal and solution structures. The structure of BoNTs in solution has not been examined in any systematic detail, especially at the quaternary level. In fact, limited studies carried out so far have revealed conflicting observations (80). For BoNT-A, an aggregated species corresponding to trimer/tetramer was observed on native gel electrophoresis (34,81). The crystalline structure of BoNT-A had initially indicated a dimeric species (82), but is now believed to be a monomeric species (1). BoNT-A in aqueous solution was found to be a dimer as revealed by dynamic light scattering (83).

The quaternary structure derived from x-ray crystallography, however, is not reliable, because under crystallization conditions the quaternary structure may change (84,85). The secondary structure resolved from x-ray crystallography is different from the solution structure in certain other proteins also (85). A clear understanding of the structure of BoNTs in solution is essential, not only because of conflicting reports, but also because it could hold the key to the understanding of the molecular basis of unique Zn^{2+}-endopeptidase activity, as well as translocation of the neurotoxin across the neuronal membrane.

The low LD_{50} of BoNTs indicates that an extremely low concentration of BoNT is active under physiologic conditions (10^{-15} to 10^{-16} M range in the animal body fluids) (8). It is estimated that after the toxin gets into the neuronal cytosol, a single molecule of enzymatically active toxin is sufficient to intoxicate a synapse (86). The effective concentration for BoNT-A to block neurotransmitter release on a neuromuscular junction has been determined as 10^{-8} to 10^{-9} M (87). Thus, an understanding of BoNT's structure in solution at physiologic concentration is essential to provide detailed mechanism involved in its action. However, all structural information about BoNTs so far is based on relatively high protein concentration.

In a recent study, we, for the first time, systematically investigated the structure of BoNT-A in solution state using different biophysical techniques. We also investigated the quaternary structure of BoNT-A at a concentration lower than 5 nM, using fluorescence anisotropy. BoNT-A exists as a dimer in solution. The dimeric form of BoNT-A self-dissociates into monomeric form at concentrations below 50 nM. The conclusion of a transition from dimeric to monomeric form of BoNT-A at a concentration of 50 to 75 nM suggests that BoNT-A exists in a monomeric form under physiologic conditions. Examination of the endopeptidase activity of dimeric and monomeric forms of BoNT-A under reducing conditions, by measuring the cleavage of its intracellular target protein, SNAP-25, revealed that the enzymatic activity (catalytic efficiency) of the monomeric form is about fourfold higher than that of its dimeric form (27).

ENZYMATIC ACTIVITY DIFFERENCE BETWEEN THE TWO STRUCTURAL FORMS OF BOTULINUM NEUROTOXIN-A

Differences in the biologic activity of BoNT-A in its different structural states can help resolve its molecular mechanism of action, which is important to BoNT's clinical application, and for developing antidotes against botulinum. Because the existence of monomeric and dimeric forms of BoNT-A in aqueous solution depends on its concentration, it became readily possible to test any differences in the biologic activity of the two types of BoNT-A structure.

The endopeptidase activity difference between dimeric and monomeric forms of BoNT-A (Table 7.2) indicates that dimeric form of BoNT-A even under reducing conditions only partially opens its active site, whereas the active site is fully accessible in the monomeric form of BoNT-A under reducing conditions (Fig. 7.5). This reveals a novel mechanism of activation of an endopeptidase. Inhibition of endopeptidase activity by disulfide-linked multimerization has been shown in the rat testicular endopeptidase EC 3.4.24.15 (88). Our observation with BoNT presents the first example in which enzymatic activity of an endopeptidase can be enhanced by self-dissociation of its oligomeric form into monomeric form.

The physiologic role of the quaternary structure of BoNT-A could be also related to its translocation into the nerve cell. As part of its mode of action, BoNT-A is known to form a membrane pore in endosomes at low pH. It has been proposed that the oligomeric species of BoNT-A is involved in the pore formation (80,89). The observation of dimeric and monomeric species of BoNT-A in solution suggests a possible equilibrium between them, which could change under different pH conditions. It is possible that the oligomeric species of BoNTs are formed in the membrane to form the pore (90), while the pore is only large enough to translocate the monomeric form of BoNTs (or their L chains) into the neuronal cytosol (91). A physiologic observation relevant to this suggestion is BoNT-A's differential effect on mouse phrenic diaphragm at different concentrations (92,93).

SUMMARY AND HYPOTHESIS FOR FUTURE RESEARCH

We suggest a hypothesis (Fig. 7.5) encompassing all of the above observations. Our hypothesis is that the NAPs play an accessory role directly in the BoNT's biologic (endopeptidase) activity, in addition to their role in protecting the BoNT in the gastrointestinal tract and in the external environment. Protein–protein interaction in the native BoNT complex may change the BoNT structure making its active site more accessible to its substrates. We believe that purified BoNT exists as a dimer in solution at normal concentrations used in biochemical and biophysical measurements. As a dimer the disulfide-linked di-chain, BoNT has its active site occluded. Interaction with NAPs or reduction of the disulfide bond alters the tertiary structure of BoNT L chain to expose the active-site motif for interaction with SNAP-25. Nicking of the single-chain BoNT in the presence of NAPs (e.g., endogenous nicking of BoNT-A) introduces a different type of structural change in its folding compared to the nicking of purified BoNT (e.g., BoNT-E), as a result of the constraints imposed by bound NAPs. Purification of endogenously nicked BoNT (e.g., BoNT-A) results in tertiary and qua-

TABLE 7.2. *Enzyme kinetic parameters of dimeric and monomeric forms of BoNT-A under reducing conditions*

Enzyme	K_m (μmol)	k_{cat} (min^{-1})	k_{cat}/K_m (μmol^{-1} min^{-1})
Dimeric form	106$\pm$12	251$\pm$32	2.3
Monomeric form	51$\pm$15	603$\pm$68	12

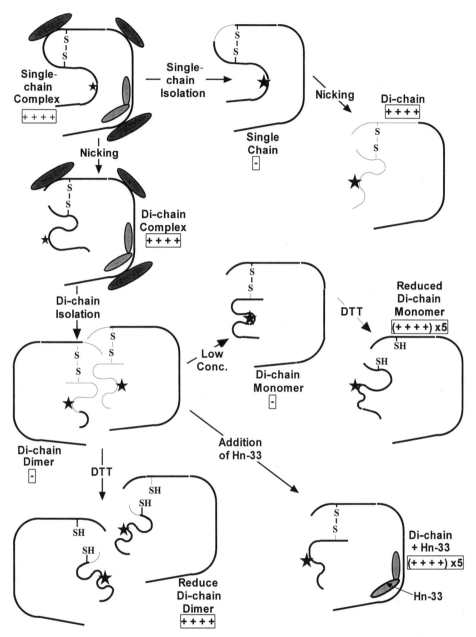

FIG. 7.5. Representation of the activation pathways of BoNT-A and possibly BoNT-E. *Left side:* BoNT-A is synthesized as a single polypeptide, and is associated with NAPs. A similar complex is envisaged for BoNT-E (53,54). The active site denoted by * is exposed and the BoNT is in monomeric form. Its endopeptidase activity is high *(+ + + +)* even without disulfide reduction. Nicking of the single-chain BoNT-A into di-chain endogenously retains its activity level. Separation of the di-chain BoNT-A from its NAPs yields a dimeric form of the toxin with little endopeptidase activity *(-)*. This dimeric BoNT-A can be activated *(+ + + +)* by disulfide reduction, by Hn-33 (a component of NAPs) binding, or by monomerization (at low concentration). *Right side:* when the single-chain BoNT-E is separated from its NAPs, it remains monomeric (could also be dimeric) with no endopeptidase activity *(-)*. The single chain BoNT-E can be activated *(+ + + +)* by nicking even when its disulfide bond is intact. Note: This schematic is just a representation of possible structures. Other possibilities also exist.

ternary structural changes, which suppress the endopeptidase activity needing activation through disulfide bond reduction. The tertiary structural changes introduced by these factors (nicking, disulfide reduction, NAPs) are partially additive, and perhaps affect the equilibrium between the dimeric and monomeric forms. In the dimeric form, the polypeptide segment covering the active site motif is at the interface of the two molecules, and therefore constrains the exposure of the active site. Transformation of the dimeric form to monomer (e.g., by lowering the concentration) allows exposure of the active site readily, thus enhancing its activity.

ACKNOWLEDGMENTS

The work was supported, in part, by grants from NIH (NS33740) and from the Camille and Henry Dreyfus Foundation. The author is thankful to Dr. S. Swaminathan for providing Fig. 7.3 and other unpublished information.

REFERENCES

1. Lacy DB, Tepp W, Cohen AC, DasGupta BR, Stevens RC. Crystal structure of botulinum neurotoxin type A and implications for toxicity. *Nat Struct Biol* 1998;5: 898–902.
2. Swaminathan S, Easwaramoorthy S. Structural analysis of the catalytic and binding sites of *Clostridium botulinum* neurotoxin B. *Nat Struct Biol* 2000;7:693–699.
3. Singh BR. Intimate details of the most poisonous poison. *Nat Struct Biol* 2000;7:617–619.
4. Sakaguchi G. *Clostridium botulinum* toxins. *Pharmacol Ther* 1983;19:165–194.
5. Fujinaga Y, Inoue K, Watanabe S, et al. The haemagglutinin of *Clostridium botulinum* type C progenitor toxin plays an essential role in binding of toxin to the epithelial cells of guinea pig small intestine, leading to the efficient absorption of the toxin. *Microbiology* 1997; 143:3841–3847.
6. Maksymowych AB, Reinhard M, Malizio CJ, et al. Pure botulinum neurotoxin is absorbed from the stomach and small intestine and produces peripheral neuromuscular blockade. *Infect Immun* 1999;67:4708–4712.
7. Nishiki T, Kamata Y, Nemoto Y, et al. Identification of protein receptor for *Clostridium botulinum* type B neurotoxin in rat brain synaptosomes. *J Biol Chem* 1994; 269:10498–10503.
8. Ahnert-Hilger G, Bigalke H. Molecular aspects of tetanus and botulinum neurotoxin poisoning. *Prog Neurobiol* 1995;46:83–96.
9. Canal JM, Arribas M, Ruiz-Avila L, et al. Characterization of a rabbit serum raised against a botulinum toxin type A binding protein from presynaptic plasma membranes from Torpedo electric organ. *Toxicon* 1995;33: 507–514.
10. Ferro-Novick S, Jahn R. Vesicle fusion from yeast to man. *Nature* 1994;370:191.
11. Shone CC, Roberts AK. Peptide substrate specificity and properties of the zinc-endopeptidase activity of botulinum type B neurotoxin. *Eur J Biochem* 1994;225: 263–270.
12. Bark IC, Hahn KM, Ryabinin AE, et al. Differential expression of SNAP-25 protein isoforms during divergent vesicle fusion events of neural development. *Proc Natl Acad Sci U S A* 1995;92:1510–1514.
13. McMahon HT, Sudhof TC. Synaptic core complex of synaptobrevin, syntaxin and SNAP25 forms high affinity α-SNAP binding site. *J Biol Chem* 1995;270: 2213–2217.
14. van Weert A, Dunn KW, Geuze HJ, et al. Transport from late endosomes to lysosomes, but not sorting of integral membrane proteins in endosomes, depends on the vacular proton pump. *J Cell Biol* 1995;130:821–834.
15. Montecucco C, Schiavo G. Tetanus and botulism neurotoxins: A new group of zinc proteases. *Trends Biochem Sci* 1993;18:324–327.
16. Li L, Singh BR. Structure-function relationship of clostridial neurotoxins. *Toxin Rev* 1999;18:95–112.
17. Schiavo G, Benfenati F, Poulain B, et al. Tetanus and botulinum B neurotoxins block neurotransmitter release by a proteolytic cleavage of synaptobrevin. *Nature* 1992;359:832–835.
18. Blasi J, Chapman ER, Link E, et al. Botulinum neurotoxin A selectively cleaves the synaptic protein SNAP-25. *Nature* 1993;365:160–163.
19. Cai S, Sarkar HK, Singh BR. Enhancement of the endopeptidase activity of botulinum neurotoxin by its associated proteins and dithiothreitol. *Biochemistry* 1999;38: 6903–6910.
20. Fu FN, Lomneth RB, Cai S, et al. Role of zinc in the toxic structure and activity of botulinum neurotoxin. *Biochemistry* 1998;37:5267–5278.
21. Li L, Binz T, Niemann H, et al. Probing the mechanistic role of glutamate residue in the HExxH zinc-binding motif of type A botulinum neurotoxin light chain. *Biochemistry* 2000;39:2399–2405.
22. Tonello F, Morante S, Rosetto O, et al. Tetanus and botulism neurotoxins: a novel group of zinc-endopeptidases. *Adv Exp Med Biol* 1996;389:251–260.
23. Lomneth R, Martin TFJ, DasGupta BR. Botulinum neurotoxin light chain inhibits norepinephrine secretion in PC12 cells at an intracellular membranous or cytoskeletal site. *J Neurochem* 1991;57:1413–1421.
24. Erdal E, Bartels F, Binschek T, et al. Processing of tetanus and botulinum A neurotoxins in isolated chromaffin cells. *Naunyn Schmiedebergs Arch Pharmacol* 1995; 351:67–78.
25. Sharma SK, Singh BR. Functional role of Hn-33: enhanced cleavage of synaptic protein SNAP-25 by *C. botulinum* neurotoxin type A. Presented at the 216th National Meeting of the American Chemical Society, Boston, August 23–27, 1998.
26. Sharma SK, Singh BR. Nicking-mediated enhancement in the endopeptidase activity of type E botulinum neurotoxin. *Protein Sci* 1999;8 (Suppl 1):383M(abstr).
27. Cai S, Singh BR. A correlation between differential structural features and the degree of endopeptidase ac-

tivity of type A botulinum neurotoxin in aqueous solution. *Biochemistry* 2001;40:4693–4702.

28. Hanson MA, Stevens RC. Cocrystal structure of synaptobrevin-II bound to botulinum neurotoxin type B at 2.0 Å resolution. *Nat Struct Biol* 2000;7:687–692.

29. Singh BR, DasGupta BR. Changes in the molecular topography of the light and heavy chains of type A botulinum neurotoxin following their separation. *Biophys Chem* 1989;34:259–267.

30. Krieglstein KG, DasGupta BR, Henschen AH. Covalent structure of botulinum neurotoxin type A: location of sulfhydryl groups, and disulfide bridges and identification of C-termini of light and heavy chains. *J Protein Chem* 1994;13:49–57.

31. Antharavally BS, DasGupta BR. Covalent structure of botulinum neurotoxin type E: location of sulfhydryl groups, and disulfide bridges and identification of C-termini of light and heavy chain. *J Protein Chem* 1997; 16:787–799.

32. DasGupta BR, Rasmussen S. Role of amino groups in the structure and biological activity of botulinum neurotoxin types A and E. *Biochem Biophys Res Commun* 1981;101:1209–1215.

33. Shone CC, Hambleton P, Melling J. Inactivation of *Clostridium botulinum* type A neurotoxin by trypsin and purification of two tryptic fragments. Proteolytic action near the COOH-terminus of the heavy subunit destroys toxin-binding activity. *Eur J Biochem* 1985;151:75–82.

34. Gimenez JA, DasGupta BR. Botulinum type A neurotoxin digested with pepsin yields 132, 97, 72, 45, 42, and 18 kD fragments. *J Protein Chem* 1993;12:351–363.

35. de Paiva A, Poulain B, Lawrence GW, et al. A role for the interchain disulfide or its participating thiols in the internalization of botulinum neurotoxin A revealed by a toxin derivative that binds to ecto-acceptors and inhibits transmitter release intracellularly. *J Biol Chem* 1993; 268:20838–20844.

36. DasGupta BR. Structure and biological activity of botulinum neurotoxin. *J Physiol Paris* 1990;84:220–228.

37. Singh BR. Structure-function relationship of botulinum and tetanus neurotoxins. In: DasGupta BR, ed. *Botulinum and tetanus neurotoxins: neurotransmission and biomedical aspects.* Orlando, FL: Plenum Press, 1993: 377–392.

38. Stecher B, Gratzl M, Ahnert-Hilger G. Reductive chain separation of botulinum A toxin—a prerequisite to its inhibitory action on exocytosis in chromaffin cells. *FEBS Lett* 1989;248:23–27.

39. Beecher D J, DasGupta BR. Botulinum neurotoxin type A: limited proteolysis by endoproteinase Glu-C and alpha-chymotrypsin enhanced following reduction; identification of the cleaved sites and fragments. *J Protein Chem* 1997;16:701–712.

40. Poulain B, Wadsworth JD, Maisey EA, et al. Inhibition of transmitter release by botulinum neurotoxin A. Contribution of various fragments to the intoxication process. *Eur J Biochem* 1989;185:197–203.

41. Ahnert-Hilger G, Weller U, Dauzenroth ME, et al. The tetanus toxin light chain inhibits exocytosis. *FEBS Lett* 1989;242:245–248.

42. Sanders D, Habermann E. Evidence for a link between specific proteolysis and inhibition of [³H]-noradrenaline release by the light chain of tetanus toxin. *Naunyn Schmiedebergs Arch Pharmacol* 1992;355:409–415.

43. Singh BR, DasGupta BR. Structure of heavy and light chain subunits of type A botulinum toxin analyzed by circular dichroism and fluorescence measurements. *Mol Cell Biochem* 1989;85:67–73.

44. Lamanna C, MacElroy OE, Eklund HW. The purification and crystallization of *Clostridium botulinum* type A toxin. *Science* 1946;103:613–614.

45. Lamanna C. Haemagglutination by botulinal toxin. *Proc Soc Exp Biol Med* 1948;69:332–336.

46. Boroff DA, Townend R, Fleck U, et al. Ultracentrifugation analysis of the crystalline toxin and isolated fractions of Clostridium toxin type A. *J Biol Chem* 1966; 241:5165–5167.

47. Kitamura M, Sakaguchi S, Sakaguchi G. Dissociation of *Clostridium botulinum* type E toxin. *Biochem Biophys Res Commun* 1967;29:892–897.

48. Fujii N, Kimura K, Tsuzuki N, et al. Construction and expression of genes for neurotoxin and non-toxic components of *C. botulinum* types C and E. In: DasGupta BR, ed. *Botulinum and tetanus neurotoxins.* New York: Plenum Press, 1993:405–420.

49. Nukina M, Mochida Y, Miyata T, et al. Purification, characterization and oral toxicity of botulinum type G progenitor toxin. In: DasGupta BR, ed. *Botulinum and tetanus neurotoxins.* Orlando, FL: Plenum Press, 1993: 401–404.

50. Schantz EJ, Spero L. Molecular size of *C. botulinum* toxins. In: Ingram M, Roberts TA, eds. *Botulism 1966.* London: Chapman and Hall, 1967:296–301.

51. Sakaguchi G, Sakaguchi S, Kozaki S, et al. Cross-reaction in reversed passive hemagglutination between *Clostridium botulinum* type A and B toxins and its avoidance by the use of anti-toxic component isolated by affinity chromatography. *Jpn J Med Sci Biol* 1974;27:161–172.

52. Sugii S, Sakaguchi G. Molecular construction of *Clostridium botulinum* type A toxins. *Infect Immun* 1975; 12:1262–1270.

53. Zhang Z, Singh, BR. A novel complex of type E *Clostridium botulinum. Protein Sci* 1995;4(Suppl 2): 110(abstr).

54. Li L, Li B, Parikh SN, et al. A novel type E *Clostridium botulinum* neurotoxin progenitor complex. *Protein Sci* 1997;6(Suppl 2):139T(abstr).

55. Fujita R, Fujinaga Y, Inoue K, et al. Molecular characterization of two forms of nontoxic-nonhemagglutinin components of *Clostridium botulinum* type A progenitor toxins. *FEBS Lett* 1995;376:41–44.

56. Cordoba JJ, Collins MD, East AK. Studies on the genes encoding botulinum neurotoxin type A of *Clostridium botulinum* from a variety of sources. *Syst Appl Microbiol* 1994;18:13–22.

57. Schantz EJ, Johnson EA. Properties and use of botulinum toxin and other microbial neurotoxins in medicine. *Microbiol Rev* 1992;56:80–89.

59. Kouguchi H, Sagane Y, Watanabe T, et al. Isolation of the components of progenitor toxin produced by *Clostridium botulinum* type C strain Stockholm. *Jpn J Electroph* 2000;44:27–34.

60. Fu FN, Sharma SK, Singh BR. A protease-resistant novel hemagglutinin purified from type A *Clostridium botulinum. J Protein Chem* 1998;17:53–60.

61. Simpson LL, ed. *Botulinum neurotoxin and tetanus toxin.* San Diego: Academic Press, 1989.

62. DasGupta BR, ed. *Botulinum and tetanus neurotoxins: neurotransmission and biomedical aspects.* Orlando, FL: Plenum Press, 1993.

63. Sakaguchi G, Sakaguchi S. Oral toxicities of *Clostridium botulinum* type E toxins of different forms. *Jpn J Med Sci Biol* 1974;27:241–244.

64. Ohishi I, Sugii S, Sakaguchi G. Oral toxicities of *Clostridium botulinum* toxins in response to molecular size. *Infect Immun* 1977;16:107–109.

65. Ohishi I, Sakaguchi G. Oral toxicities *of Clostridium botulinum* type C and D toxins of different molecular sizes. *Infect Immun* 1980;28:303–309.

66. Sugii S, Ohishi I, Sakaguchi G. Correlation between oral toxicity and *in vitro* stability of *Clostridium botulinum* type A and B toxins of different molecular sizes. *Infect Immun* 1977;16:910–914.

67. Kitamura M, Sakaguchi S, Sakaguchi G. Significance of 12S toxin of *Clostridium botulinum* type E. *J Bacteriol* 1969;98:1173–1178.

68. Singh BR, Li B, Read D. Botulinum versus tetanus neurotoxins: why is botulinum neurotoxin a food poison but not tetanus? *Toxicon* 1995;33:1541–1547.

69. East AK, Stacey JM, Collins MD. Cloning and sequencing of a hemagglutinin component of the botulinum neurotoxin complex encoded by *Clostridium botulinum* types A and B. *Syst Appl Microbiol* 1994;17:306–312.

70. Hauser D, Eklund MW, Boquet P, et al. Organization of the botulinum neurotoxin C1 gene and its associated non-toxic protein genes in *Clostridium botulinum* C 468. *Mol Gen Genet* 1994;243:631–640.

71. Li B, Qian X, Sarkar HK, Singh BR. Molecular characterization of type E *C. botulinum* and comparison with other types of *Clostridium botulinum*. *Biochim Biophys Acta* 1998;1395:21–27.

72. Tsuzuki K, Kimura K, Fujii N, et al. The complete nucleotide sequence of the gene coding for the non-toxic nonhemagglutinin component of *Clostridium botulinum* type C progenitor toxin. *Biochem Biophys Res Commun* 1992;183:1273–1279.

73. Dekleva ML, DasGupta BR. Nicking of single-chain *Clostridium botulinum* type A by an endogenous protease. *Biochem Biophys Res Commun* 1989;162: 767–772.

74. Singh BR, DasGupta BR. Conformational changes associated with the nicking and activation of botulinum neurotoxin type E. *Biophys Chem* 1990;38:123–130.

75. DasGupta BR. The structure of botulinum neurotoxin. In: Simpson LL, ed. *Botulinum neurotoxin and tetanus toxin.* San Diego: Academic Press, 1989:53–67.

76. Cashikar AG, Rao NM. Unfolding pathway in red kidney bean acid phosphatase is dependent on ligand binding. *J Biol Chem* 1996;271:4747–4746.

77. Philo JS, Rosenfeld R, Arakawa T, et al. Refolding of brain-derived neurotrophic factor from guanidine hydrochloride: kinetic trapping in a collapsed form which is incompetent for dimerization. *Biochemistry* 1993;32: 10812–10818.

78. Mei G, Di Venere A, Buganza M, et al. Role of quaternary structure in the stability of dimeric proteins: the case of ascorbate oxidase. *Biochemistry* 1997;36: 10917–10922.

79. Lebeda, FJ, Olson, MA. Secondary structural predictions for the clostridial neurotoxins. *Proteins* 1994;20: 293–300.

80. Singh BR. Critical aspects of bacterial protein toxins. In: Singh BR, Tu AT, eds. *Natural toxins 2: structure, mechanism of action, and detection.* New York: Plenum Press, 1996:63–84.

81. Ledoux DN, Be XH, Singh BR. Quaternary structure of botulinum and tetanus neurotoxins as probed by chemical cross-linking and native gel electrophoresis. *Toxicon* 1994;32:1095–1104.

82. Stevens RC, Evenson ML, Tepp W, et al. Crystallization and preliminary x-ray analysis of botulinum neurotoxin type A. *J Mol Biol* 1991;222:877–880.

83. Stevens RC. Low-resolution model of botulinum neurotoxin type A. In: DasGupta BR, ed. *Botulinum and tetanus neurotoxins.* New York: Plenum Press, 1993: 393–395.

84. Lubkowski J, Bujacz G, Boque L, et al. The structure of MCP-1 in two crystal forms provides a rare example of variable quaternary interactions. *Nat Struct Biol* 1997; 4:64–69.

85. Singh BR, Fu FN, Ledoux DN. Crystal and solution structures of superantigenic staphylococcal enterotoxins compared. *Nat Struct Biol* 1994;1:358–360.

86. Schiavo G, Rossetto O, Tonello F, et al. Intracellular targets and metalloprotease activity of tetanus and botulism neurotoxins. *Curr Top Microbiol Immunol* 1995; 195:257–274.

87. Coffield JA, Bakry N, Zhang RD, et al. Characterization of a vertebrate neuromuscular junction that demonstrates selective resistance to botulinum toxin. *J Pharmacol Exp Ther* 1997;280:1489–1498.

88. Shrimpton CN, Glucksman MJ, Lew RA, et al. Thiol activation of endopeptidase EC 3.4.24.15. A novel mechanism for the regulation of catalytic activity. *J Biol Chem* 1997;272:17395–17399.

89. Singh BR, Lebeda F. Membrane channel activity and translocation of tetanus and botulinum neurotoxins. *J Toxicol Toxin Rev* 1999;18:45–76.

90. Schmid MF, Robinson JP, DasGupta BR. Direct visualization of botulinum neurotoxin-induced channels in phospholipid vesicles. *Nature* 1993;364,827–830.

91. Donovan JJ, Middlebrook JL. Ion-conducting channels produced by botulinum toxin in planar lipid membranes. *Biochemistry* 1986;25:2872–2876.

92. Bandyopadhyay S, Clark AW, DasGupta BR, et al. Role of heavy and light chains of botulinum neurotoxin in neuromuscular paralysis. *J Biol Chem* 1987;262: 2660–2663.

93. Maisey EA, Wadsworth JDF, Poulain B, et al. Involvement of the constituent chains of botulinum neurotoxins A and B in the blockage of neurotransmitter release. *Eur J Biochem* 1988;177:683–691.

PHARMACOLOGY OF
BOTULINUM NEUROTOXINS

Scientific and Therapeutic Aspects of Botulinum Toxin
edited by M.F. Brin, J. Jankovic, and M. Hallett
Lippincott Williams & Wilkins, Philadelphia, © 2002.

8

Insights into the Extended Duration of Neuroparalysis by Botulinum Neurotoxin A Relative to the Other Shorter-Acting Serotypes: Differences Between Motor Nerve Terminals and Cultured Neurons

J. Oliver Dolly, Godfrey Lisk, Patrick G. Foran, Frederic Meunier,
Nadiem Mohammed, G. O'Sullivan, and Anton de Paiva

A multiphasic mechanism for the neuromuscular paralytic action (1) of the seven serotypes (A to G) of botulinum neurotoxin (BoNT) has been documented by (a) their saturable, high-affinity binding to ecto-acceptors distinct for each toxin (2,3), which are located exclusively on peripheral cholinergic nerve endings (4,5); (b) acceptor-mediated, temperature-sensitive, and energy-dependent endocytotic uptake; (c) translocation from acidic endosomal compartments into the cytosol (6,7); and (d) inhibition of acetylcholine release as a result of cleavage (reviewed in 8) of SNAREs [soluble NSF (*N*-ethylmaleimide–sensitive factor) attachment receptors, proteins essential for regulated exocytosis], by the metalloendoprotease activities of light chain of BoNTs (9–12). It is reassuring that the recently resolved three-dimensional structures of BoNT-A and -B pinpointed distinct domains responsible for these sequential steps (13,14). The preferential susceptibility to BoNTs of cholinergic synapses in the peripheral nervous system is attributed to their possession of the productive ecto-acceptors, because intracellular administration of the toxins leads to inhibition of the release of all neurotransmitters tested (15,16), including peptides (17). Another notable feature of these toxins' actions is their amazing specificity—no presynaptic compo-

nents or mechanisms are affected other than regulated exocytosis. At least in the case of BoNT-A, the constitutive process remains unaltered, a feature that helps avoid atrophy of the motor nerve, even months after chemodenervating with toxin (18).

Although all the toxin serotypes have similar multistep modes of intoxication, it is not surprising that they cause distinct patterns of neuromuscular paralysis because each cleaves a different SNARE or different peptide bond within a given SNARE (reviewed in 8): synaptosomal-associated protein of 25 kDa (SNAP-25) (cleaved by BoNT-A, -E and -C1), syntaxin1 (-C1) and synaptobrevin (-B, -D, -F, and -G).

This study examines how the various toxin-truncated targets, as well as the nature of the different BoNT serotypes, can influence the duration of reduced neuronal activity. In particular, the turnover of their products and life-times of the various BoNT proteases were measured, with the aim of deciphering a basis for an amazingly long duration of paralysis caused by BoNT-A in human (19) and rodent muscles (18,20) in relation to that of other serotypes. It emerges that the relative contributions of different factors (i.e., longevity of BoNT-A and life-time of the truncated SNAP-25) to its duration of action are dictated by specialized features of highly differentiated motor nerve endings and, thus, deviate from the situation in cultured neurons or neuroendocrine cells. Such novel findings are highly pertinent to the successful and widespread clinical use of type A toxin for the treatment of numerous disorders resulting from hyperactivity of cholinergically innervated muscles (21).

RESULTS

The Duration of BoNT-A–Induced Neuromuscular Paralysis Far Exceeds that Caused by -B, -F, or -E: Nerve Sprouting Is Related Reciprocally to the Time Courses of Exocytosis Blockade

Intramuscular injection of a therapeutic dose of BoNT-A into the hind leg of mice resulted in a paralysis, as measured by the loss of toe-spread reflex (TSR, score of 5 = maximal block) that lasted for ~30 days (Fig. 8.1A). In contrast BoNT-E, which cleaves off 26 residues (rather than the 9 by BoNT-A) from the C-terminal of SNAP-25, gave a transient inhibition with return of the normal TSR (score = 0) within 4 to 5 days (Fig. 8.1A). BoNT-F and -B (not shown) which proteolyze the vesicular SNARE, synaptobrevin, at different bonds abolished neuromuscular transmission for 7.5 (Fig. 8.1A) and ~18 days, respectively. This rank order of durations (A>>B>F>E) accords with those found for human muscles (19,22,23) except for the absolute times being shorter in mice; such a discrepancy is partly the result of the TSR score which reflects the initial phase of partial resumption of function rather than the complete recovery seen after ~3 months (18).

To gain further insights into the basis of these distinct time courses for each toxin, we undertook repeated *in vivo* imaging of the same individual nerve endings in the sternomastoid muscle of living mice (18) to monitor functional and morphologic changes throughout the course of botulinization. Presynaptic uptake of a green dye, 4di-2ASP, visualized the terminals, while depolarization-dependent labeling of synaptic vesicles with the red fluorescent dye FM1–43 gave a measure of endocytosis (and exocytosis when prelabeling was carried out). Dual labeling

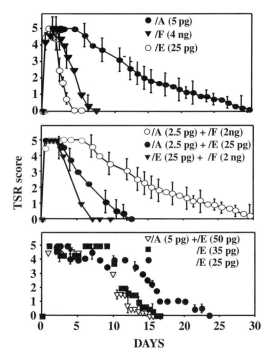

FIG. 8.1. Time courses for recovery from neuromuscular paralysis induced by BoNT-A, -E, or -F following injection into mouse leg muscles. **A:** BoNT-A, -E, or -F at the stated doses was injected into the right hind leg of mice and the loss of toe-spread reflex (TSR) in the affected limb was monitored until a complete restoration of TSR had ensued. The level of paralysis was scored on a scale of 0 to 5, 0 representing a complete absence of paralysis and 5 representing a total loss of TSR. Recovery in type E and F botulinized mice is faster than that seen with type A. **B:** Coapplication of BoNT-E, but not -F, with type A toxin shortened the duration of neuromuscular paralysis caused by the latter. **C:** Sequential administration of increasing amounts of BoNT-E following a 3-day prior injection of -A hastened recovery in a dose-dependent manner.

of control nerve endings at day 0 showed colocalization of the green and red vital dyes, resulting in a yellow fluorescence (Fig. 8.2A–C). Within 2 days of administering BoNT-A, the latter staining diminished (18) and a network of sprouts (→) appeared by days 3 to 5, continuing to grow at days 14 and 28 (Fig. 8.2A) and reaching a maximum length of ~150 μm at day 42. These nerve outgrowths quickly acquired endo- and exocytotic activity as revealed by the yellow

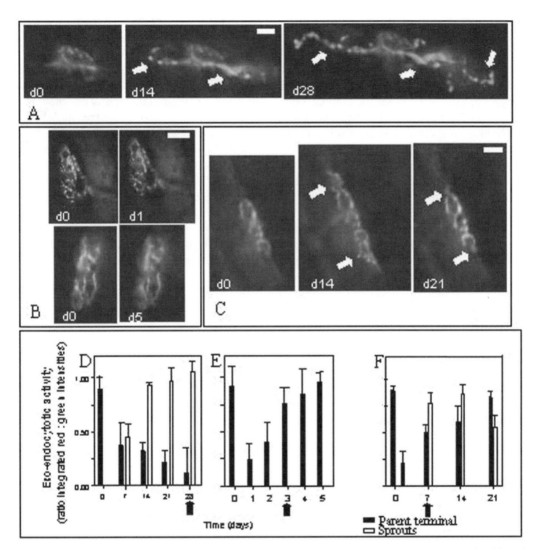

FIG. 8.2. *In vivo* imaging of mouse sternomastoid endplates after localized injections of sublethal amounts of BoNT-A and -F, but not -E, reveals extensive nerve terminal remodeling and switching in synaptic activity between the original nerve endings and their sprouts. Synaptic plasticity induced by BoNT-A was less pronounced with BoNT-F poisoning and not detectable after type E. Injection of 0.5 pg of BoNT-A into mouse sternomastoid muscle resulted in a loss of the ability of the original endplates, stained with 4-di-2-ASP (green) to exo-endocytose FM1–43 (red) on stimulation with 60 mM K^+ (**A** and filled bars in **D**) and elicited sprouts (*arrows*) capable of stimulated uptake of this dye (**A** and empty bars in **D**). Although a depletion of FM1–43 uptake in BoNT-E (5 pg) poisoned terminals was evident after 1 day (**B** and **E**), recovery of endo-/exocytosis occurred by day 3 (**E**) and no sprouts were elicited. Within 1 day of injecting 0.4 ng of BoNT-F, FM1–43 uptake was dramatically reduced at the terminals (**C** and **F**); from day 7, short sprouts capable of stimulated FM1–43 endocytosis were seen and uptake into the original endings started to resume, which was complete at d21. ⬆ indicate the time of initial onset of nerve-induced muscle tension; scale bars represent 20 μm. Color images available at www.wemove.org/toxins book/

fluorescence therein and by the presence of the SNAREs, synaptotagmin, and voltage-activated Ca^{2+} channels (18,24,25). Quantitation of the integrated luminance values for several endplates demonstrated that vesicle recycling had dropped to a minimal level at the original terminal by day 28, the earliest time when the initial return of nerve-evoked muscle twitch could be detected (Fig. 8.2D). As the intensity of FM1–43 labeling had peaked in the sprouts at this time point (Fig. 8.2D), this sole source of synaptic activity must underlie the first phase of recovery; accordingly, acetylcholine receptors were found to be clustered then on the muscle membrane adjacent to the sprout contacts (18). Full resumption of the normal level of synaptic function only occurs after ~90 days when the parent nerve endings have recovered completely and the then-redundant sprouts retracted (18).

Injection of an equivalent effective dose of BoNT-E also diminished FM1–43 uptake within 24 hours but by day 3, near-complete recovery had occurred in the original terminal and nerve-induced muscle twitch became detectable (Fig. 8.2B, E); resumption of vesicle recycling was complete by day 5. Most importantly, no sprouts were detectable after exposure to BoNT-E, a result very different to that seen for type A. Finally, BoNT-F produced an intermediate pattern, with the inhibition of FM1–43 uptake at the parent terminals (Fig. 8.2C) recovering more slowly and sprouts were present at day 7; these started to retract by 21 days (Fig. 8.2F) and had vanished by 4 weeks. These novel findings collectively demonstrate an inverse relationship between the duration of inhibition of neurotransmitter release and the degree of synapse remodeling. They also reveal the remarkable plasticity of motor nerve endings and a requirement of 72-hour paralysis to trigger the remodeling process.

The Extended Blockade of Neuromuscular Transmission by BoNT-A is Shortened Upon Co- or Sequential Administration of BoNT-E

To establish whether a persistence of BoNT-A protease is important for its long-lasting effect at the neuromuscular junction, type E toxin was coinjected with BoNT-A into mouse leg muscles, followed by measurement of TSR. Strikingly, the recovery time was reduced to 12.5 days (Fig. 8.1B), from the 30 days seen with BoNT-A alone (Fig. 8.1A), and the nerve sprouting normally induced by type A was prevented by type E (not shown). Similarly, applications of various doses of BoNT-E 3 days following type A, to allow the latter to induce paralysis, yielded recovery at approximately the same number of days (after the second injection) as with type E on its own (Fig. 8.2A, C). Thus, the acceleration of recovery by BoNT-E cannot be a result of its prevention of type A internalization; accordingly, BoNT-F proved unable to hasten appreciably the resumption of neurotransmission in BoNT-A-chemodenervated muscle (Fig. 8.2A, B). The results of this series of experiments concur with ability of type E to speed up the reappearance of function in type A-treated human muscle (22), again using therapeutic doses (discussed later). On the other hand, when BoNT-F and -E were coapplied, the recovery was dictated by the time course of the longer-acting F toxin (Fig. 8.2B). Hence, it can be deduced that an adequate fraction of the minimal effective dose of BoNT-A used was not retained within the terminals to sustain paralysis under experimental conditions resembling its clinical usage.

BoNT-A–Truncated SNAP-25 (SNAP-25$_A$) Persists in Motor Nerve Terminals Whereas the Cleavage Product of Type E is Short-lived: BoNT-E Accelerates the Disappearance of SNAP-25$_A$

To assess the contributions of the lifetimes of the toxins' products to the disparate durations of action, these were monitored using affinity-purified IgGs shown to be specific for SNAP-25$_A$ (26) or SNAP-25$_E$ in conjunction with confocal microscopy. Initially, murine nerve endings, from control muscle samples and BoNT-A–treated sternomastoid at various times after exposure, were labeled with IgG reactive exclusively with SNAP-25$_A$ and counterstained with rhodamine-conjugated α-bungarotoxins to pinpoint the nicotinic receptors and endplate regions. SNAP-25$_A$ was not detectable in the control, as expected, but it appeared within 6 days of treatment with BoNT-A and, remarkably, persisted to day 40 before disappearing (Fig. 8.3A). Notably, the A-truncated SNARE could only be visualized within the endplate area demarcated by the receptor staining (Fig. 8.3A), with its apparent absence in the functionally active sprouts. In stark contrast, SNAP-25$_E$ was seen at nerve terminals within 2 days of exposure to BoNT-E but had vanished by day 7 (Fig. 8.3B), consistent with its transient action noted earlier.

Considering these very different lifetimes of SNAP-25$_A$ and SNAP-25$_E$, together with the demonstrated cleavage by BoNT-E of an additional 17 residues from SNAP-25$_A$ (27), BoNT-E was applied 3 days later to BoNT-A–treated nerve muscle preparations. Confocal microscopy revealed that SNAP-25$_A$ could be detected at day 11 but had diminished 4 days later (Fig. 8.4A) rather than at 50 days observed for A alone (Fig. 8.3A). Clearly, treatment with BoNT-E greatly accelerated the disappearance of SNAP-25$_A$, although not at the same rate as SNAP-25$_E$ which was seen at day 5 but not at day 11 (Fig. 8.4B). Furthermore, more detailed analysis of the micrographs suggested that BoNT-E

treatment induces a translocation of SNAP-25$_A$ from the presynaptic membrane to a more "cytosolic-like" location, consistent with triggering of its trafficking and eventual disposal. In conclusion, it seems that deleting residues 181–197 from SNAP-25$_A$ with BoNT-E increases its turnover, thereby, promoting removal of SNAP-25$_A$ from the terminal and affording resumption of transmitter release there. Although SNAP-25$_A$ appears to be a major hindrance to the recovery of exocytosis at the original nerve endings, more in-depth information was sought by determining the half-lives of both BoNT-A and its truncated target in cultured cells, that allow such biochemical measurements.

Distinct Durations of Inhibition of Exocytosis by BoNT Serotypes from Cerebellar Granule Neurons Correspond to Their Protease Lifetimes

Our earlier experiments on cultured chromaffin cells showed a very slow recovery of evoked catecholamine secretion after treating with BoNT-A (26). This was found to be largely caused by a persistence of its protease activity because expression of the transfected gene for wild-type SNAP-25 failed to rescue exocytosis

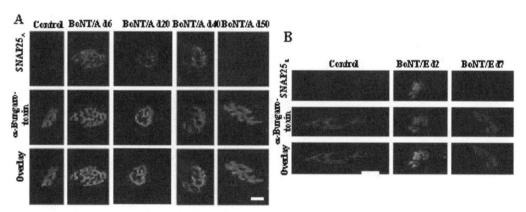

FIG. 8.3. Persistence of SNAP-25$_A$ and rapid clearance of SNAP-25$_E$ in murine motor nerve terminals treated with BoNT-A or -E. Control and toxin-treated endplates were dual-labeled with rhodamine-conjugated α-bungarotoxin and anti-SNAP-25$_A$ or SNAP-25$_E$ antibodies, followed by FITC-conjugated secondary IgGs; fluorescent images were recorded by confocal microscopy. **A:** In control sternomastoid muscle, SNAP-25$_A$ could not be detected, whereas immunostaining was found after BoNT-A-treatment and it resided within areas occupied by the nAChR (days 16 to 40), as revealed by the overlaid images. **B:** Staining of SNAP-25$_E$ was apparent in nerve terminals and in preterminal axons 2 days after BoNT-E injection, but became undetectable by day 7 postinjection. Bars = 10 μm. Color images available at www.wemove.org/toxins book/

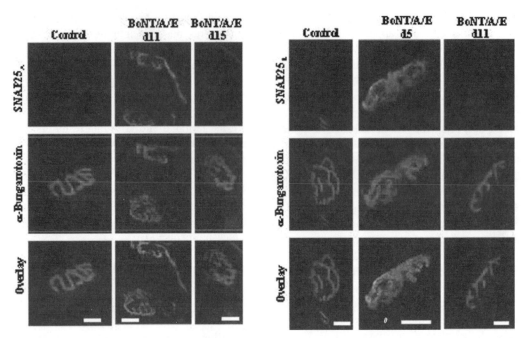

FIG. 8.4. Fate of SNAP-25$_A$ and SNAP-25$_E$ at motor nerve endings upon sequential injection of BoNT-E 3 days after injection of type A. Muscle fibers from the control and BoNT-A-treated mouse sternomastoid followed (after 3 days) in the latter case by injection of BoNT-E were dual-labeled by rhodamine-conjugated α-bungarotoxin and either anti-SNAP-25$_A$ or -SNAP-25$_E$ IgGs with subsequent visualization using FITC-conjugated secondary antibodies. Confocal microscopy revealed that SNAP-25$_A$ was detectable up to 11 days after BoNT-E injection in a few branches of the motor nerve terminals and preterminal axons; this staining was no longer seen 4 days later (day 15). SNAP-25$_E$ was present at day 5 but invisible 11 days after BoNT-E injection. Scale bars represent 10 μm. Color images available at www.wemove.org/toxins book/

even 3 weeks after intoxication of the cells, but BoNT-A–resistant mutants recovered secretion. As these endocrine cells give slower exocytosis of large dense-core granules than the fast release of neurotransmitters from small synaptic vesicles, rat cerebellar neurons were employed. These proved a convenient *in vitro* cell model (28) because of affording quantitation of transmitter release and monitoring of the SNAREs by Western blotting, throughout the course of intoxication. Concentrations of each toxin serotype were chosen to inhibit ~ 90% of K$^+$-elicited Ca^{2+}-dependent glutamate release from the cultured neurons under the conditions used (Fig. 8.5). BoNT-A gave the most prolonged blockade, with no resumption of neuroexocytosis apparent 35 days after the initial exposure to toxin (the maximum length of the experiment); recovery from type B was appreciably faster but slower than that for types F or E (Fig. 8.5). Ali-

quots of the same cells were subjected to sodium dodecyl sulfate-polyacrylamide gel electrophoresis (SDS-PAGE), followed by Western blotting with antibodies specific for the intact [SNAP-25 or synaptobrevin (Sbr)] or cleaved (SNAP-25$_A$ or -25$_E$) SNAREs. In each case (Fig. 8.5), near-complete cleavage by the toxins of the requisite target occurred (day 0) and, notably, the times taken for reappearance of the intact substrates correspond to the rank order of duration of inhibition of transmitter release (BoNT-A>>B>F>E). Measurements were made of the extents of inhibition of exocytosis caused by various toxin concentrations at different times after exposure of the cells (Fig. 8.6). Rightward shifts were observed in the concentration of each toxin required to give 50% inhibition of transmitter release with increasing time after treatment. From this extensive data, the half-lives of the toxins' inhibitory activities were calculated

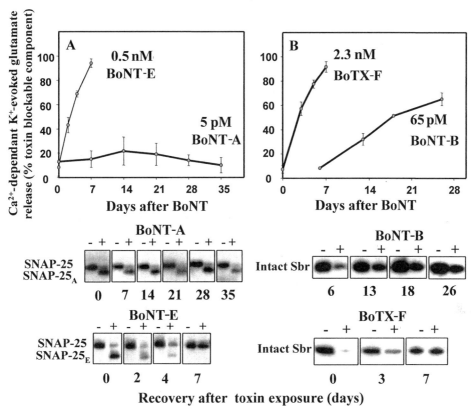

FIG. 8.5. Distinct durations of blockade of neuroexocytosis in cultured neurons by BoNT-A, -B, -E, and -F; correspondence with proteolysis of SNAP-25 or synaptobrevin 2. Rat cerebellar granule cells were exposed for 24 hours in the absence or presence of the specified toxin concentrations and maintained in culture by regular changes of medium. At the postintoxication periods indicated, the abilities of control and toxin-treated neurons to undergo evoked exocytosis were determined. Protein samples from all experiments were immunoblotted with appropriate IgGs to determine the amounts of intact and toxin-cleaved SNAREs.

(Fig. 8.6). These ranged from less than 24 hours for BoNT-E to 2 and 10 days for BoNT-F and -B; values for BoNT-A and -C1 exceeded the lengths of these experiments. It must be emphasized that such times are composite values and do not reveal the relative contribution from persistence of the toxins' protease and/or their products. Therefore, to distinguish these parameters, the longevity of BoNT-A and -B proteases were determined directly by [^{35}S]-methionine pulse-chase labeling of the cells at various times after intoxication, followed by immunoisolation of SNAP-25 and Sbr2 (Fig. 8.7). Western blotting established that the majority of the latter targets had been cleaved by BoNT-A and -B; virtually

no full-length SNAP-25 was observed up to 20 days, but partial replenishment of Sbr had occurred after 18 days, consistent with the time course of recovery of function shown earlier (Fig. 8.6). In the case of Fig. 8.7A, decrease in intact SNAP-25 and the appearance of SNAP-25$_A$ were measured, whereas for BoNT-B (Fig. 8.7B) diminished immunoreactivity of Sbr reflected its cleavage. Importantly, the newly synthesized ^{35}S-labeled SNAP-25 continued to be efficiently cleaved at up to 20 days after exposure to BoNT-A, especially after the additional 14-hour chase period (Fig. 8.7A). As both intact and A-truncated SNAP-25 have t$_{1/2}$ ~1 to 2 days in the cultured neurons (data not shown), the

BoNT serotype	Days
E	~0.8
F	~2
B	~10
C1	>>18*
A	>>31*

* No detectable recovery

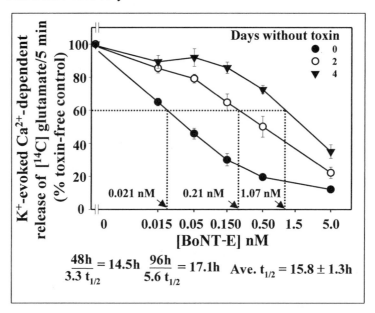

$$\frac{48h}{3.3\ t_{1/2}} = 14.5h \quad \frac{96h}{5.6\ t_{1/2}} = 17.1h \quad \text{Ave. } t_{1/2} = 15.8 \pm 1.3h$$

FIG. 8.6. Determination of the half-lives of inhibition of neuroexocytosis from cerebellar granule neurons by BoNTs after 1 day of exposure. The $t_{1/2}$ of inhibition by the different BoNTs were assessed by monitoring the reductions in the extent of exocytosis inhibition caused by an initial toxin concentration after various times of recovery. Toxin concentrations yielding equivalent blockades of exocytosis at different postintoxication periods were extrapolated from dose-dependency curves (example shown) and subjected to first-order decay analysis.

pulse-chase data established that prolonged inhibition of neuroexocytosis by BoNT-A results from persistence of its protease. In the case of cerebellar granule neurons exposed 18 days earlier to BoNT-B, cleavage of radiolabeled, newly synthesized Sbr could only be detected after a 16-hour pulse (Fig. 8.7B). Considering that the toxin cleaved products of Sbr are rapidly degraded in these cells, and the full-length protein has $t_{1/2}$ ~5 days (data not shown), the demonstrated persistence of BoNT-B protease for at least 2 weeks indicates that this is the major factor underlying its duration of inhibition of neuroexocytosis (Fig. 8.6).

Features of BoNT-A Chemodenervation at Motor Nerve Terminals not Shared with Cultured Neurons: A Unified Hypothesis

To examine the differences observed in the apparent lifetime of BoNT-A protease in peripheral cholinergic nerve endings and cultured neu-

A

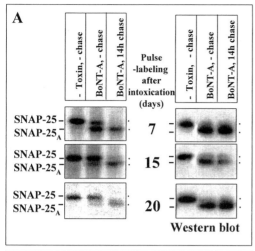

B Pulse-labeling after intoxication (days)

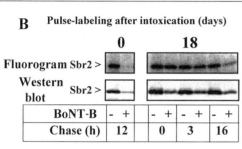

FIG. 8.7. BoNT-A and -B proteases persist for weeks in cerebellar granule cells as revealed by [^{35}S]-methionine pulse-labeling and immunopre-cipitation of SNAP-25 and synaptobrevin 2. The rat neurons were exposed for 24 hours in the absence or presence of either 10 pM BoNT-A or 100 pM BoNT-B and then maintained in culture without toxin for the periods indicated, prior to a 4 hour [^{35}S]-methionine pulse-labeling (with or without the specified chases) and immunoprecip-itation of SNAP-25 or synaptobrevin 2, using suitable IgGs. Immunoadsorbed SNAREs were frac-tionated by SDS-PAGE, Western blotted, and the newly synthesized radiolabeled proteins ana-lyzed by fluorography.

rons or neuroendocrine cells, we monitored cleavage of SNAP-25 in mouse phrenic nerve diaphragms by BoNT-A, -E, or both using con-centrations that abolished neuromuscular trans-mission. Selective immunoprecipitation was employed to enrich the sparse amounts of this SNARE in the endplate regions of diaphragm and in the phrenic nerve. By using this method, it proved possible to quantify reliably full-length as well as SNAP-25$_A$ or SNAP-25$_E$ in the dia-phragm (Fig. 8.8). A notable absence of trun-cated SNAP-25 in the nerve trunk is indicative of the lack of diffusion of active toxin. Impor-tantly, minimal cleavage occurred, relative to the content of SNAP-25 in each sample, when either toxin was used alone or the two together to in-duce paralysis. Achieving blockade of synaptic transmission when such a small fraction of the total SNAP-25 pool had been proteolyzed strongly suggests preferential cleavage of a sub-population of this protein that is primarily re-sponsible for transmitter release and, thus, prob-ably positioned at the active zones (Fig. 8.9). Subsequent dilution of the toxin by diffusion seems likely to occur, so the level of active pro-tease could drop below the minimal effective dose; at least exposure of nerve-stimulated dia-phragm to a higher BoNT-A and/or -E concen-tration produced cleaved SNAP-25 in the phre-nic nerve.

In summary, therefore, based on these collec-tive findings from the multiple experimental strategies employed, it is reasonable to postulate a model (Fig. 8.9) that reconciles the data on BoNT-A and -E for the major target tissue (i.e., neuromuscular junctions *in vivo* and *ex vivo*) and *in vitro* cultured cells. Intramuscular injection of low quantities of BoNT-A causes limited and localized production of SNAP-25$_A$, thereby blocking transmitter release before being dimin-ished by dilution/diffusion, albeit still active. The resultant truncated protein could form exo-cytotic-incompetent, relatively stable complexes with the partnering SNAREs (Sbr, syntaxin1), as demonstrated by *in vitro* studies (29). Such interactions of a relatively high local concentra-tion of SNAP-25$_A$ would reduce participation of any intact SNAP-25 in the vicinity that had escaped cleavage by toxin. Also, these might en-able SNAP-25$_A$ to squat near the release sites; furthermore, with endocytosis coupled to exo-cytosis having been inhibited, its removal would be retarded. Similar entry of BoNT-E could cleave any remaining intact SNAP-25 and SNAP-25$_A$ when transiently dissociated from SNARE complexes, as shown in Fig. 8.8. Our experimental results indicate that cleavage of an additional 17 residues from SNAP-25$_A$ pre-cludes such complex formation (29) and, hence,

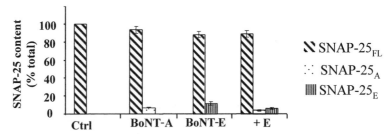

FIG. 8.8. Limited proteolysis of SNAP-25 by BoNT-A or -E accompanies complete neuromuscular paralysis. Mouse phrenic nerve-hemidiaphragms were incubated at 37°C (98.6°F) in aerated Krebs ringer containing either 2 nM BoNT-A, 0.5 nM type E, or both. Nerves were stimulated (0.2 Hz, 1.5–2.5v) and the extent of evoked muscle twitch recorded. Following 110 minutes of nerve stimulation, the tissues were washed, the phrenic nerve carefully dissected from the diaphragm and all samples immunoprecipitated. SNAP-25 precipitates from control and paralyzed diaphragms, or the nerves, were immunoblotted using an anti guinea pig antibody raised against recombinant GST-linked SNAP-25 that reacts equally well with intact and toxin-truncated SNAP-25s. Blots of diaphragm were densitometrically scanned to determine the extents of intact A-truncated or E-cleaved protein (means ± SD; n = 2/3 experiments).

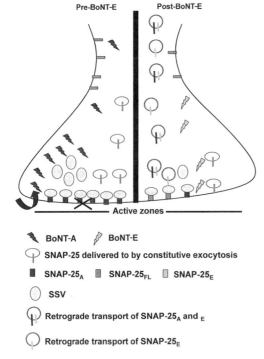

FIG. 8.9. A model to explain how BoNT/E could shorten the duration of BoNT/A-induced paralysis of the motor nerve terminals. BoNT/A causes a localised production of exocytosis-incompetent SNAP-25$_A$ before being rapidly diminished by dilution or degradation. The inhibitory SNAP-25$_A$ 'squats' at release sites, presumably due to binding partnering SNAREs which could retard its removal, thus, interfering with exocytosis. Removal of 17 additional C-terminal residues from SNAP-25$_A$ by BoNT/E creates a product, SNAP-25$_E$, that is readily removed from the nerve endings. Thus, BoNT/E treatment can accelerate recovery of neuromuscular transmission after blockade by BoNT/A of acetylcholine release. Color images available at www.wemove.org/toxins book/

hastens the removal of the nonfunctional truncated SNAP-25, allowing incorporation of the intact protein (Fig. 8.9) and culminating in a resumption of regulated exocytosis. Clearly, highly specialized features of differentiated motor terminals, whose synapses lie long distances from the cell body in the spinal cord, contribute to the extraordinary persistent action of BoNT-A, which is highly desirable for clinical/therapeutic purposes. In contrast, the maintenance of higher intracellular toxin concentrations in cultured cerebellar granule neurons (this study), spinal cord neurons (30), neuroendocrine cells (26), or, indeed, sciatic nerve (31) over prolonged periods would sustain an adequate quantity of protease to cause prolonged cleavage of SNAP-25 and the observed inability of BoNT-E to overcome this activity.

ACKNOWLEDGMENTS

This work is supported by Allergan Inc., BBSRC, and University of London studentships (to G.L. and G. O'S) and an EEC fellowship (to F.M.).

REFERENCES

1. Simpson LL. Molecular pharmacology of botulinum toxin and tetanus toxin. *Ann Rev Pharmacol Toxicol* 1986;26:427–453.
2. Dolly JO, de Paiva A, Foran P, et al. Probing the process of transmitter release with botulinum and tetanus neurotoxins. *Semin Neurosci* 1994;6:149–158.
3. Ashton AC, de Paiva AM, Poulain B, et al. Factors underlying the characteristic inhibition of the neuronal release of transmitters by tetanus and various botulinum toxins. In: Das Gupta, B.R., ed. *Botulinum and tetanus neurotoxins: neurotransmission and biomedical aspects.* New York: Plenum Publishing, 1993:191–213.
4. Dolly JO, Black J, Williams RS, et al. Acceptors for botulinum neurotoxin reside on motor nerve terminals and mediate its internalization. *Nature* 1984;307:457–460.
5. Black JD, Dolly JO. Interaction of ^{125}I-labelled botulinum neurotoxins with nerve terminals. I. Ultrastructural autoradiographic localization and quantitation of distinct membrane acceptors for types A and B on motor nerves. *J Cell Biol* 1986a;103:521–534.
6. Simpson LL, DasGupta BR. Botulinum neurotoxin type E: studies on mechanism of action and on structure-activity relationships. *J Pharmacol Exp Ther* 1983;224:135–140.
7. Black JD, Dolly JO. Interaction of ^{125}I-labelled botulinum neurotoxin with nerve terminals. II. Autoradio-

graphic evidence for its uptake into motor nerves by acceptor-mediated endocytosis. *J Cell Biol* 1986;103:535–544.
8. Schiavo G, Matteoli M, Montecucco C. Neurotoxins affecting neuroexocytosis. *Physiol Rev* 2000;80:717–766.
9. de Paiva A, Dolly JO. Light chain of botulinum neurotoxin is active in mammalian motor nerve terminals when delivered via liposomes. *FEBS Lett* 1990;277:171–174.
10. de Paiva A, Ashton AC, Foran P, et al. Botulinum A like type B and tetanus toxins fulfills criteria for being a zinc-dependent protease. *J Neurochem* 1993;61:2338–2341.
11. Raciborska DA, Trimble WS, Charlton MP. Presynaptic protein interactions *in vivo*: evidence from botulinum A, C, D, and E action at frog neuromuscular junction. *Eur J Neurosci* 1998;10:2617–2628.
12. Kalandakanond S, Coffield JA. Cleavage of intracellular substrates of botulinum toxins A, C, and D in a mammalian target tissue. *J Pharmacol Exp Ther* 2001;296:749–755.
13. Lacy DB, Stevens RC. Unraveling the structures and modes of action of bacterial toxins. *Curr Opin Struct Biol* 1998;8:778–784.
14. Swaminathan S, Eswaramoorthy S. Structural analysis of the catalytic and binding sites of *Clostridium botulinum* neurotoxin B. *Nat Struct Biol* 2000;7:693–699.
15. Ashton AC, Dolly JO. Characterization of the inhibitory action of botulinum neurotoxin type A on the release of several transmitters from rat cerebrocortical synaptosomes. *J Neurochem* 1988;50:1808–1816.
16. Bigalke H, Heller L, Bizzini B, et al. Tetanus toxin and botulinum A toxin inhibit release and uptake of various transmitters, as studied with particulate preparations from rat brain and spinal cord. *Naunyn Schmiedebergs Arch Pharmacol* 1981;316:244–251.
17. McMahon HT, Foran P, Dolly JO, et al. Tetanus toxin and botulinum toxins type A and type B inhibit glutamate, γ-aminobutyric acid, aspartate, and met-enkephalin release from synaptosomes—clues to the locus of action. *J Biol Chem* 1992;267:21338–21343.
18. de Paiva A, Meunier FA, Molgó J, et al. Functional repair of motor endplates after botulinum neurotoxin A poisoning: bi-phasic switch of synaptic activity between nerve sprouts and their parent terminals. *Proc Natl Acad Sci U S A* 1999;96:3200–3205.
19. Sloop RR, Cole BA, Escutin RO. Human response to botulinum toxin injection: type B compared with type A. *Neurology* 1997;49:189–194.
20. Adler M, Macdonald DA, Sellin LC, et al. Effect of 3,4-diaminopyridine on rat extensor digitorum longus muscle paralyzed by local injection of botulinum neurotoxin. *Toxicon* 1996;34:237–249.
21. Brin MF. Botulinum toxin: chemistry, pharmacology, toxicity, and immunology. *Muscle Nerve* 1997:S146–S168.
22. Eleopra R, Tugnoli V, Rossetto O, et al. Different time courses of recovery after poisoning with botulinum neurotoxin serotypes A and E in humans. *Neurosci Lett* 1998;256:135–138.
23. Mezaki T, Kaji R, Kohara N, et al. Comparison of therapeutic efficacies of type A and F botulinum toxins for blepharospasm: a double-blind, controlled study. *Neurology* 1995;45:506–508.

24. Angaut-Petit D, Molgo J, Comella JX, et al. Terminal sprouting in mouse neuromuscular junctions poisoned with botulinum type A toxin: morphological and electrophysiological features. *Neuroscience* 1990;37:799–808.

25. Angaut-Petit D, Juzans P, Molgó J, et al. Mouse motor-nerve terminal immunoreactivity to synaptotagmin II during sustained quantal transmitter release. *Brain Res* 1995;681:213–217.

26. O'Sullivan GA, Mohammed N, Foran PG, et al. Rescue of exocytosis in botulinum toxin A-poisoned chromaffin cells by expression of cleavage-resistant SNAP-25: identification of the minimal essential C-terminal residues. *J Biol Chem* 1999;274:36897–36904.

27. Lawrence GW, Foran P, Mohammed N, et al. Importance of two adjacent C-terminal sequences of SNAP-25 in exocytosis from intact and permeabilized chromaffin cells revealed by inhibition with botulinum neurotoxins A and E. *Biochemistry* 1997;36:3061–3067.

28. Foran PGP, Mohammed N, Lisk GO, et al. Evaluation of the therapeutic usefulness of botulinum neurotoxin/ B,C1,/E and /F compared to the long-lasting type A: Basis for distinct durations of inhibition of exocytosis in central neurons. 2002 (submitted).

29. Hayashi T, McMahon H, Yamasaki S, et al. Synaptic vesicle membrane fusion complex: action of clostridial neurotoxins on assembly. *EMBO J* 1994;13:5051–5061.

30. Keller JE, Neale EA, Oyler G, et al. Persistence of botulinum neurotoxin action in cultured spinal cord cells. *FEBS Lett* 1999;456:137–142.

31. Adler M, Keller JE, Sheridan RE, et al. Persistence of botulinum neurotoxin A demonstrated by sequential administration of serotypes A and E in rat EDL muscle. *Toxicon* 2001;39:233–243.

Scientific and Therapeutic Aspects of Botulinum Toxin
edited by M.F. Brin, J. Jankovic, and M. Hallett
Lippincott Williams & Wilkins, Philadelphia, © 2002.

9

Immunologic and Other Properties of Therapeutic Botulinum Toxin Serotypes

K. Roger Aoki

Botulinum neurotoxin (BTX) type A (BTX-A) is used worldwide for the treatment of focal dystonias, cerebral palsy, adult spasticity, and many other conditions (1). Type A is one of seven different BTX serotypes, which are referred to alphabetically as types A, B, C1, D, E, F, and G. Until recently, the only commercially available BTX products were based on the A serotype (BOTOX from Allergan and DYSPORT from Ipsen). However, a product containing botulinum neurotoxin type B (BTX-B) was recently approved for the treatment of cervical dystonia (MYOBLOC from Elan), and a preparation containing type F has been examined in several patient populations (2,3).

The development of new BTX therapies is valuable because each product is unique and is likely to be useful in a particular subset of patients. For instance, a BTX preparation with a short duration may allow physicians to preview the effects of surgical interventions for the treatment of cerebral palsy. Additionally, patients who develop neutralizing antibodies to one BTX serotype may benefit from other serotypes for a period of time.

This chapter considers some of the differences among BTX preparations that are likely to affect their clinical profiles. Particular attention is given to immunologic properties because patients who develop neutralizing antibodies to the toxin may no longer obtain clinical benefit from their injections. Clearly, if patients can no longer respond to a particular product, all the other properties of that product are moot. The ability

of patients to respond over the long-term is especially critical in BTX therapy because many of the conditions for which it is used are chronic and require repeated treatment over the course of many years.

IMMUNOLOGIC CONSIDERATIONS

Neutralizing Versus Nonneutralizing Antibodies

All BTX serotypes are produced as protein complexes that contain a 150-kDa neurotoxin protein and one or more nontoxin proteins, hemagglutinin (HA) and nontoxin nonhemagglutinin (NTNH). The 150-kDa protein is the active portion of the complex. The nontoxin proteins help to maintain the neurotoxin's structure and to protect it from degradation (4,5).

Although the structure of the 150-kDa neurotoxin is similar for all serotypes, the overall protein complex size differs as a result of the particular nontoxin proteins present (Table 9.1). Type A is the only serotype that forms the 900-kDa complex, originally called the LL form (6). Type A, together with types B, C1, and hemagglutinin-positive D, also forms the 500-kDa complex (originally called the L form) and 300-kDa complex (originally called the M form), but types E, F, and hemagglutinin-negative D only form the 300-kDa complex (7,8).

Under certain conditions, humans may form antibodies to either the 150-kDa neurotoxin, the nontoxin proteins, or both. Antibodies formed against the nontoxin proteins do not affect the activity of the neurotoxin and are called nonneutralizing antibodies (9). Antibodies formed

K. Roger Aoki is an employee of Allergan, Inc.

TABLE 9.1. *Neurotoxin complex sizes formed by the various botulinum toxin serotypes*

Serotype	≈300 kDa	≈500 kDa	≈900 kDa
A	√	√	√
B	√	√	
C_1	√	√	
D (HA+)	√	√	
D (HA−)	√		
E	√		
F	√		

HA, hemagglutinin

against the 150-kDa neurotoxin are the most clinically important; these blocking antibodies can interfere with, or neutralize, the toxin's biologic activity, and are therefore called neutralizing antibodies (9). Currently, the only methods that can definitively test for the presence of neutralizing antibodies are biologic assays such as the mouse protection assay (MPA) and the mouse hemidiaphragm assay (10,11).

Relationship Between Protein Load and Antigenicity

Animal studies show that, in general, the more antigen to which an organism is exposed, the greater the antibody response (12). For BTXs, this means that increasing the amount of neurotoxin complex protein is likely to increase the risk of antibody formation (13). This is precisely what we found in a preclinical study that compared the antigenicity of two BTX-A preparations with different protein loads (14).

In this experiment, rabbits received monthly intramuscular injections (3.0 U/kg) with one of two BTX-A (BOTOX) preparations that contained different amounts of neurotoxin complex protein per unit dose. Serum samples taken 1 week after the eighth monthly injection were tested for neutralizing antibodies in the MPA. The two BTX-A preparations had equal muscle-weakening potency in mice, as determined by the digit abduction scoring assay (14). However, one preparation contained approximately 25 ng of neurotoxin complex protein per 100 U (original BOTOX from Allergan), whereas the other contained approximately 5 ng of neurotoxin complex protein per 100 units (current BOTOX from Allergan).

Following eight monthly intramuscular injections, eight of nine rabbits that received the higher protein formulation had neutralizing antibodies. In contrast, only one of nine rabbits that received the lower protein formulation had neutralizing antibodies at this time point (Fig. 9.1) (14). From these results, we concluded that the lower protein formulation was less antigenic than the higher protein formulation in rabbits.

Preliminary data suggest that this difference in antigenic potential may also be seen in humans. Historically, approximately 5% to 10% of

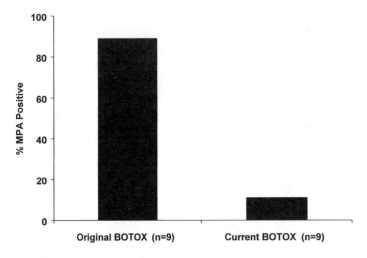

FIG. 9.1. Comparison of the antigenic potential of original and current BOTOX in rabbits after 8 monthly injections. Data represent percent of rabbits that had neutralizing antibodies as detected by the MPA.

cervical dystonia patients treated with the original formulation of BTX-A developed neutralizing antibodies (13,15,16). In contrast, a preliminary analysis of 83 cervical dystonia patients who have been treated exclusively with the current low-protein formulation for up to 19 months (average of 9 months) found that all patients who were available for follow-up were continuing to respond (17). This preliminary analysis suggests that few patients have developed neutralizing antibodies, although serum antibody testing and objective documentation of response will be required before this conclusion can be drawn. However, thus far, these data are consistent with the results of our preclinical research.

COMPARISON OF THE ANTIGENIC POTENTIAL OF BOTULINUM NEUROTOXIN SEROTYPES

BoNT serotypes differ in activation level, potency, and duration of action. Some of these properties may differ even between different preparations that contain the same serotype. Therapeutic preparations in which these properties are not optimal will expose patients to more neurotoxin complex protein, which might increase the risk of antibody formation.

Activation

For BTXs to exert their muscle relaxing activity, they must be nicked or activated to form the di-chain moiety (light chain linked to a heavy chain by a disulfide bond). Some of the serotypes are inherently activated, meaning that they are nicked by proteases endogenous to the bacterial strain. For example, BTX-A is recovered from cultures more than 95% nicked (18). In contrast, type E is completely unnicked and must be exposed to exogenous proteases such as trypsin in order to be activated. For other serotypes, such as type B, only a portion of the neurotoxin molecules are nicked (19). Therapeutic BTX preparations containing unnicked or partially nicked serotypes are often subjected to a step designed to increase the percentage of nicked toxin during the production process. Even with this step,

however, there is a limit to the amount of neurotoxin that can be nicked because the process will eventually affect the structure of the neurotoxin protein itself.

Unnicked toxin will not contribute to muscle-weakening activity but will increase the protein load of the neurotoxin complex preparation. In this way, the unnicked neurotoxin may act as a toxoid, increasing the patient's overall neurotoxin protein exposure and potentially increasing antigenicity potential of the preparation. Presumably, the antibodies would be directed against the unnicked and nicked forms of the toxin. Because the vast majority of the toxin epitopes will remain (between nicked and unnicked), the probability of creating neutralizing antibodies against the toxin might be increased. Antibodies against the other protein components (NTNH and HA) are not neutralizing (9) and are therefore not clinically relevant in reducing the therapeutic effect of a botulinum toxin-based product.

Unnicked neurotoxin may also compete with nicked toxin for binding sites, reducing the muscle-weakening potency of the preparation. When the toxin is formed by the clostridia, it is in the fully folded form. When the bacteria undergoes its autolysis, the toxin is exposed to a "soup" of proteases (which vary among the serotypes) to clip the region between the light and heavy chains. This clipping is the nicking action. Therefore, it is logical to assume that the unnicked version is a good antagonist because the tertiary structure is preserved. A related piece of supporting information is the publication by Prof. Oliver Dolly's laboratory, which reported the creation of both tetanus and botulinum toxin derivatives with point mutations of the light chain that rendered the material "nontoxic." They demonstrated that the inactive derivative was a much more efficient antagonist against native toxin than just free heavy chain. They concluded that the light chain and heavy chain work together to place the toxin in a higher affinity conformation than does the free heavy chain alone (49). For all of these reasons, it is important for the percentage of nicked neurotoxin to be as high as possible in a therapeutic BTX preparation.

Potency

Unit doses. Potency usually refers to the units needed to produce muscle weakness. Even though all BTX preparations use the same definition of a unit (intraperitoneal LD50 in mice), some require much higher doses than others to produce a clinical effect. For instance, clinical doses of the two BTX-A products differ, with doses of one product (BOTOX) being three to five times lower than the other (DYSPORT) (20–22). Similarly, clinical doses of the product containing BTX-B (MYOBLOC) are several orders of magnitude higher than the type A products (23,24). It is likely that these differences are partly caused by variations in the way the LD_{50} tests are performed (25). However, it is also well accepted that species differ in their sensitivity to the various neurotoxin serotypes. For example, the rat neuromuscular junction requires 1 to 20 units of BTX-A to inhibit activity but more than 1,200 units of BTX-B to inhibit activity (25a).

Specific potency. Another important potency consideration is the specific potency of the preparation, which is sometimes referred to as specific activity. Specific potency is the number of units per weight of neurotoxin complex protein and is usually given as units per nanogram. By dividing the specific potency into the unit dose used clinically, it is possible to calculate the amount of neurotoxin complex protein that patients receive per treatment. However, specific potency alone is an inappropriate comparator for the different preparations because of differences in species sensitivity and the way the LD_{50} tests are performed.

Neurotoxin complex protein per dose. Animal experiments support the proposition that the total amount of neurotoxin complex protein per effective dose is an important factor in determining the antigenic potential of a BTX preparation. We conducted an experiment in rabbits to compare the antigenic potential of commercial BTX-A (BOTOX) and an experimental preparation of BTX-B (from WAKO Chemicals). The experi-

mental preparation of type B (WAKO) had a higher neurotoxin complex protein load and was therefore expected to show a higher antigenic potential.

Preclinical comparison of serotypes. In this experiment, rabbits were injected monthly with BTX-A (current BOTOX; 0.10 ng/kg) or an experimental preparation of type B (WAKO; 1.7 or 7.3 ng/kg). The unit doses of these two preparations that were needed to produce comparable muscle weakness in mice were not significantly different (mean ED_{50} values from six experiments with ten mice per dose: BOTOX, 6.2 U/kg; WAKO B, 11.8 U/kg) (51). Consequently, we used comparable unit doses of the two preparations in the antigenicity experiments (3.0 U/kg of BOTOX; 2.0, 8.7, or 20.0 U/kg of WAKO B). Rabbits treated with 20.0 U/kg of type B (WAKO) did not survive the first injection. For the other groups, serum samples taken 1 week after each monthly injection were tested in the MPA for neutralizing antibodies against the appropriate serotype.

After three monthly injections, all of the four rabbits treated with the high dose and two of the four rabbits treated with the low dose of BTX-B (WAKO) showed neutralizing antibodies (Fig. 9.2). All rabbits treated with the high dose continued to be antibody-positive at every subsequent month in the 8-month study. After seven monthly injections, three of four rabbits treated with the lower dose of type B (WAKO) had neutralizing antibodies. In contrast, only one of nine rabbits treated with BOTOX had neutralizing antibodies after seven monthly injections. It may be noted that adjustment of the relevant doses between serotypes and across species, as necessitated in this experiment, makes unequivocal interpretation of the results difficult. However, these results are consistent with previous clinical research showing that higher neurotoxin complex protein loads are associated with a higher incidence of neutralizing antibody formation (13,16).

Clinical comparison of serotypes. The type B product available for clinical use (MYOBLOC) has a different neurotoxin complex protein load than the one used in the previous preclinical experiments. The amount of neurotoxin complex

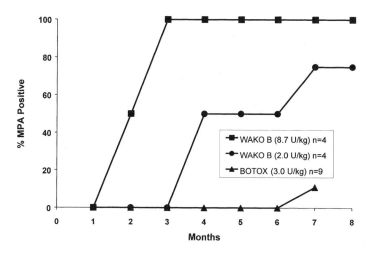

FIG. 9.2. Comparison of the antigenic potential of botulinum toxin type A (BOTOX) and an experimental preparation of botulinum toxin type B (WAKO Chemicals) in rabbits. Data represent percent of rabbits with neutralizing antibodies as determined by the MPA.

protein per dose administered to cervical dystonia patients is shown in Fig. 9.3 for all of the commercial products. If it is true that increased protein exposure directly correlates with increased antigenicity, it could be predicted that the type B preparation (MYOBLOC) would result in the highest incidence of neutralizing antibody formation, followed by the Ipsen type A preparation (DYSPORT), and, finally, by the Allergan type A preparation (BOTOX).

Information about the antigenicity of BTX-B (MYOBLOC) and the original preparation of BTX-A (original BOTOX from Allergan) has become publicly available since the Toxin '99 meeting (46,47). Both products were recently approved for the treatment of cervical dystonia

and the product inserts contain data on percentages of patients with neutralizing antibodies, as required by the United States Food and Drug Administration (FDA). A study of cervical dystonia patients with average disease duration of 11 years who had received multiple treatments with the original, higher protein, BTX-A product (original BOTOX from Allergan) found that 17% of the patients had neutralizing antibodies (46). A subsequent analysis of the BOTOX antibody-positive patients showed no significant improvement in head position, as compared to placebo, supporting that the MPA assay appropriately identified clinical nonresponding patients. The results of prospective antigenicity studies with the current preparation of BTX-A

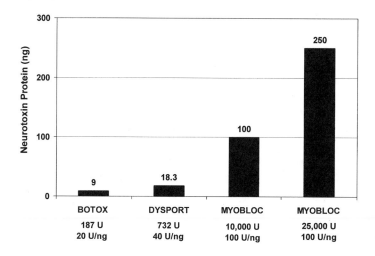

FIG. 9.3. Neurotoxin complex protein exposure with the various BTX products at doses used to treat cervical dystonia. Doses were taken from references 24, 39, and 48. Note that the specific potency varies depending on the vehicle used for reconstitution of BTX-A. For instance, the specific potency of BTX-A (BOTOX) is 34 U/ng when reconstituted with gelatin phosphate buffer, as in the initial phases of production, and 20 U/ng when reconstituted with saline, as in the final stage of production.

(current BOTOX from Allergan), which contains 80% less neurotoxin complex protein, are not yet available. However, preclinical (13,14) and retrospective clinical data (17) suggests that the antigenic potential of the current Allergan preparation is likely to be substantially lower than the original preparation. According to the product insert, the estimated incidence of neutralizing antibody formation in cervical dystonia patients treated with the commercial BTX-B preparation (MYOBLOC) is 10% for 1 year and 18% after 18 months (47). Because this was an interim analysis, the final BTX-B antigenicity rate remains to be established. Both companies are currently prospectively evaluating the neutralizing antibody formation rate in patients naïve to their serotype.

Duration

For BTX preparations that are used to treat chronic conditions, a long duration of action is important because it minimizes the number of treatments needed per year. This reduces the cumulative amount of neurotoxin protein to which patients are exposed, and consequently, may help to reduce antigenic potential. This preserves the ability of patients to respond to long-term therapy. A long duration also reduces the annual cost of physician visits and medication and is more convenient for patients.

Measuring duration. Many clinical studies have attempted to measure the duration of the therapeutic BTX products. However, the duration obtained depends critically on the end point selected for study and the measurement method used. Different methods can result in very different estimates of duration for any given BTX preparation. For example, the time it takes patients to return to baseline is longer than the duration of peak benefit. Also, patients may return for reinjection before their condition has returned to pretreatment levels. Therefore, when considering the duration of action for any given BTX preparation, it is important to consider the end point being measured and the methods used to obtain the data.

Direct comparisons of BTX serotypes. The

most accurate way to compare the durations of different BTX preparations is to study them in the same experiment. Only in this case are the experimental conditions, methods, and outcome measures the same for both preparations. Therefore, only in this case can a conclusion be made that one preparation has a longer duration than another, because extraneous variables are held constant and any difference in the results can be attributed to differences in the preparations being tested.

Comparison of serotypes A and B. Dolly and colleagues compared the *in vitro* duration of action of BTX types A and B (gift from C. Shone) in adrenal chromaffin cells (26). Cells were exposed to 6.6 nM of BTX-A or 66.0 nM of BTX-B. Fifty-six days after exposure to BTX-A, evoked norepinephrine release was still inhibited by 64%. In contrast, release was inhibited by 10% at this time point following treatment with BTX-B. The authors concluded that BTX-A had a longer duration of effect than type B in this system. There was no influence of any differential binding of BTX-A and BTX-B on the chromaffin cells because mild permeabilizing conditions were used to deliver the BTX to the cell interior.

A study by Sloop and colleagues compared the duration of BTX-A (BOTOX) and type B (MYOBLOC) in humans without neuromuscular disorders (27). Volunteers received injections of type A or B into opposite extensor digitorum brevis muscles and electromyographic (EMG) measures were used to assess muscle-weakening effects. The doses of each product that produced maximal EMG responses in a previous dose-response study were compared (10 units BOTOX vs 480 units MYOBLOC). Results showed that the duration of effect of the type B preparation (MYOBLOC) was nearly identical across all doses, with a full return to baseline by 11 weeks postinjection as measured by EMG. In contrast, the higher doses of the type A preparation (BOTOX) still showed 65% of their original EMG effect at 11 weeks postinjection. In fact, type A (BOTOX) showed 22% of its original muscle weakness at 57 weeks after injection. The authors concluded that BTX-A (BOTOX) had a longer duration of action than BTX-B (MYOBLOC) in this study.

Since the Toxins '99 meeting, the duration of action of BTX-A (BOTOX) and BTX-B (MYOBLOC) was compared in the murine digit abduction score (DAS) assay. Doses of the preparations were selected to obtain a local near maximal peak response (29 U/kg BOTOX vs 67 U/kg MYOBLOC). The duration of action of BTX-A was longer than that of BTX-B, 36 versus 14 days, respectively (50). Thus, the *in vitro,* preclinical, and normal human muscle EMG results consistently demonstrate the duration of action differences between BTX-A and BTX-B. The duration of action comparison of the two serotypes in cervical dystonia or other disease conditions remains to be established. The product inserts of each product suggest that clinical efficacy lasts 12 to 16 weeks, although the clinical trials of both products were not designed to determine their duration of action.

Comparison of types A and F. Botulinum toxin types A and F were directly compared in a double-blind trial of nine patients with blepharospasm (3). Patients received injection of type A toxin (Chiba) on one side and the same units of type F toxin (Chiba) on the other side. The two preparations showed a similar onset of effect, maximal benefit, and adverse event profile. However, the duration of clinical effect was significantly shorter with type F as determined by the time until patients returned to the clinic following recurrence of symptoms in one eye. The authors concluded that the shorter duration of type F might limit its usefulness for chronic conditions such as blepharospasm.

Summary. Percentage of nicked neurotoxin, neurotoxin complex protein per dose, and duration may all contribute to the antigenicity potential of a therapeutic BTX preparation. BTX preparations and products clearly differ in these factors. Because of the importance of BTX therapy in a wide variety of conditions, it is important to preserve the ability of patients to respond over the long-term. As a result, preparations that optimize these three important features are preferable for conditions that require repeated treatment.

Cross-Reactivity

Historically, BTXs were classified into different serotypes based on their lack of cross-neutralization in animals (28). This study and others were invaluable in forming our early understanding of BTX. However, research conducted during the past 10 years that used more modern and sensitive techniques have found that cross-reactivity among serotypes does occur. This is an important observation because it suggests that patients who develop antibodies may not simply be switched to a different serotype without consequences. Cross-reactivity is the *in vitro* binding of antibodies found in patient sera to the primary antigen, as expected, and to another unexpected antigen. Cross-neutralization is the ability of the sera to block the activity of the second antigen (toxin in this context) from having a biologic effect, even though the patient was never exposed to the second antigen. Cross-reactivity would be expected to occur before any cross-neutralization is observed because the *in vitro* methods are more sensitive than the *in vivo* measurement of toxin neutralization. However, the presence of cross-reactive antibodies would predict that the patient would be immunologically primed to exposure with a second neurotoxin and would thus develop an immune response faster than a naïve patient. To date, no clinical studies have shown that such priming has led to faster development of antibodies in patients. Additional experience with the BTX-B preparation is needed to determine if this expected priming response will be observed in patients.

In one study, mice were injected with various fragments of the BTX-A protein, using an immunization protocol (29). Serum samples were then tested to determine if they contained any cross-reacting antibodies. Results showed that certain fragments of the type A protein stimulated the production of antibodies that reacted with serotypes B, C, D, E, and F.

Atassi and colleagues have also found some evidence for cross-reactivity (30,31). These investigators immunized mice with peptides from the heavy chain of BTX-A that contained T-cell or antibody epitopes (30). Serum samples from the mice were subsequently tested for reactivity with the C-terminal portion of the type A heavy chain (HC). Results showed that some of the peptides induced the production of antibodies that reacted with HC. Many of these cross-reacting peptides had five or more continuous residues that were identical or similar to sequences in one or more of the other BTX serotypes (31). This finding suggests that the antibodies directed against specific type A protein fragments will recognize those same protein fragments in other serotypes. These results indicate that there is a sound biochemical/immunologic basis for cross-reactivity among BTX serotypes.

Research also shows that certain BTXs can cross-react with tetanus toxin. In one study, mice were injected with various tetanus toxin peptides (32). Serum samples were tested for cross-reactivity with BTX serotypes A, B, C1, and E using immunoblots. Results showed cross-reactivity between one of the tetanus toxin peptides and BTX serotypes B and C1, and to a lesser extent, type E. Type A did not cross-react with this peptide, probably because of its lower sequence similarity to tetanus toxin in this region (32).

These preclinical studies raise the possibility that cross-reactivity may occur in the clinic. To date, only a few clinical studies have addressed this issue. In two studies of patients treated with BTX-A for movement disorders, *in vitro* tests showed that approximately one-third of patients had cross-reactive antibodies against BTX-B despite never having been treated with the B serotype (33,34).

Because these studies were performed *in vitro*, the biologic significance of the data remains to be determined. However, if cross-reactivity and subsequent cross-neutralization does occur in patients, it is possible that some patients who develop antibodies type A may not respond to type B or may become nonresponsive after only a few injections. The reverse case is also a concern, and theoretically more likely to occur because of increased protein load; namely, if patients develop antibodies to BTX-B, they may not respond to type A or may become resistant more quickly than expected. Because it is so critical to preserve long-term clinical responsive-

ness, it is important to minimize the potential for antibody development. This strongly suggests that patients should always be treated initially with the BTX preparation that produces clinical efficacy with the lowest protein load.

Safety

A distinct advantage of BTX-A over oral pharmacologic treatments is its safety profile (35). Adverse events that occur with BTX-A are typically mild, transient, and localized, even in conditions such as cervical dystonia that require higher dose injections into large muscles (21,36). The safety of BTXs depends on their ability to remain relatively localized to the site of injection. Diffusion to nearby muscles is thought to underlie many of the most frequent adverse events observed with BTX-A, such as ptosis following injection into extraocular muscles and dysphagia following injection into the sternocleidomastoid. Diffusion out of the muscle into the systemic circulation could potentially lead to additional side effects not commonly seen with BTX-A.

Because of differences in BTX serotypes and formulations, the well-established safety profile of BTX-A cannot be assumed for other BTX serotypes. Differences may even be found between BTX products containing the same serotype. For example, although several studies found a similar adverse event profile of the two type A products (Allergan and Ipsen) (37,38), other studies found a higher incidence of adverse events with the Ipsen preparation (39,40).

Preclinical comparison of the type A products. We used an animal model to directly compare the tendency of the two type A products to diffuse out of the injected muscle (34). Mice were given a single intramuscular injection of either the Ipsen (DYSPORT, 0 to 200 units) or Allergan (BOTOX, 0 to 50 units) BTX-A product into the hind limb. The safety margin was calculated as the ratio of the weight-loss dose (WLD) to the ED_{50} dose in the digit abduction scoring assay (34). The WLD was defined as the first dose that caused a statistically different group mean weight from the vehicle control group ($p < 0.05$, *t*-test). The ED_{50} was the dose that produced a half-maximal muscle weakening score of 2 in the digit abduction scoring assay.

This margin describes the separation between the dose needed for muscle-weakening efficacy and the dose that diffuses out of the muscle into the systemic circulation, leading to weight loss. Thus, this experiment was meant to model clinical muscle relaxation (ED_{50}) and adverse events caused by systemic circulation of the toxin (WLD). A higher safety margin is desirable because it indicates a greater separation between these two doses.

The WLD for the Allergan preparation was 30 U/kg, whereas the WLD for the Ipsen preparation was 50 U/kg (Table 9.2). In line with the doses used clinically, the ED_{50} of the Allergan preparation was lower than the ED_{50} of the Ipsen preparation. The Allergan toxin also had a higher safety margin, suggesting that the Ipsen preparation may have a greater tendency to leave the site of injection and enter the systemic circulation, although alternative explanations cannot be ruled out. If this tendency also occurs clinically, it may explain the higher incidence of certain side effects with the Ipsen preparation found in some studies (39,40). Since the report of this WLD-based safety margin, these results were confirmed comparing the safety margin based on the murine intramuscular LD_{50}/ED_{50} (51).

Dysphagia. All of the commercial BTX products have been studied for the treatment of cervical dystonia and all are associated with dysphagia in a percentage of patients. Controlled studies of the Allergan product given at approximately 150 to 250 U have found a 7% to 19% incidence of dysphagia (41,42). Controlled studies of the Ipsen product given at 450 to 1,000 U have found a 15% to 40% incidence of dysphagia (22,43). Similarly, controlled studies of

the type B product from Elan given at 10,000 U, the most effective dose reported, have found a 22% to 28% incidence of dysphagia (23,24).

Because none of the previous studies directly compared the incidence of dysphagia associated with the different products, strong comparative conclusions cannot be made. However, these results suggest that the two type A preparations may be associated with different rates of dysphagia. This apparent difference may be related to product formulation. Type B also appears to have a somewhat higher rate of dysphagia than one of the type A products, which may be caused by product formulation or the much higher doses. With higher doses, there are more molecules of toxin, which would be expected to diffuse to a greater extent. However, the smaller size of the type B neurotoxin complex protein—500 to 700 kDa in contrast to the 900-kDa complex size of the type A preparations—may also be a factor.

Dry mouth. When used for the treatment of cervical dystonia, the type B preparation (MYOBLOC) clearly results in a higher incidence of dry mouth than is observed with the type A products. The incidence of dry mouth with the commercial type B product has ranged from 24% to 44% for the 10,000 U dose in controlled studies (20,44). In contrast, dry mouth is reported by approximately 3% to 4% of patients treated with either BTX-A (BOTOX) or placebo in general clinical use, with an even lower incidence reported in controlled studies (36,42). Several studies found that the incidence of dry mouth with the Ipsen type A product may be somewhat higher than is typically reported for the Allergan product (22,45).

The immediate cause of dry mouth following BTX injection is unclear. It may represent local diffusion to autonomic targets, but it may also be a systemic effect. It is also possible that serotype B may have a greater affinity for autonomic targets, but this hypothesis remains to be tested.

TABLE 9.2. *Safety margins (WLD/DAS ED_{50}) for the two botulinum toxin type A products*

	DAS ED_{50} (U)	WLD (U)	Safety margin
BOTOX	3.5	30	8.6
DYSPORT	15.2	50	3.3

Ten mice per dose group. The two products were compared in the same experiment.

DISCUSSION

The important clinical properties of BTXs can be viewed as a triangle of efficacy, safety, and antigenicity. When these three points are balanced, the therapeutic BTX preparation becomes extremely useful for a wide variety of disorders. It should show good clinical efficacy with a low incidence of adverse events and a low risk of antibody formation. However, if this balance is not realized, the utility of the BTX preparation is compromised. For instance, if clinical doses must be increased in an attempt to achieve efficacy, safety is likely to decrease and antigenic potential to increase.

As a result of differences in potency, duration of action, and formulation, some BTX preparations require higher doses than do other preparations. The data discussed in this chapter suggests that these preparations do have a higher incidence of adverse events. Preclinical data also suggest a higher risk of antibody formation. Alternatively, preparations with a high neurotoxin complex protein load may need to be used at extremely low doses in order to avoid antibody formation. However, efficacy may then be suboptimal. Taken together, this information provides support that BTX doses are unique and must not be converted between products.

According to the triangle model of balance among efficacy, safety, and antigenicity, certain BTX preparations should be superior to others as a first-line therapy. Other preparations, particularly those based on different BTX serotypes, may be useful in treating patients who become resistant because of neutralizing antibodies. This will allow patients to receive the maximum benefit from BTX therapy, while holding a viable treatment option in abeyance in case of future nonresponse.

REFERENCES

1. Jankovic J, Brin MF. Botulinum toxin: historical perspective and potential new indications. *Muscle Nerve Suppl* 1997;6:S129–S145.
2. Greene PE, Fahn S. Use of botulinum toxin type F injections to treat torticollis in patients with immunity to botulinum toxin type A. *Mov Disord* 1993;8:479–483.
3. Mezaki T, Kaji R, Kohara N, et al. Comparison of therapeutic efficacies of type A and F botulinum toxins for blepharospasm: a double-blind, controlled study. *Neurology* 1995;45:506–508.
4. Schantz EJ, Johnson EA. Properties and use of botulinum toxin and other microbial neurotoxins in medicine. *Microbiol Rev* 1992;56:80–99.
5. Chen F, Kuziemko GM, Stevens R. Biophysical characterization of the stability of the 150-kilodalton botulinum toxin, the nontoxic component, and the 900-kilodalton botulinum toxin complex species. *Infect Immun* 1998;66:2420–2425.
6. Sugiyama S, Sakaguchi G. Molecular construction of *Clostridium botulinum* type A toxins. *Infect Immun* 1975;12:1262–1270.
7. Sakaguchi G, Kozaki S, Ohishi I. Structure and function of botulinum toxins. In: Alouf JE, ed. *Bacterial protein toxins.* London: Academic Press, 1984:435–443.
8. Melling J, Hambleton P, Shone CC. *Clostridium botulinum* toxins: nature and preparation for clinical use. *Eye* 1998;2:16–23.
9. Goschel H, Wohlfarth K, Frevert J, et al. Botulinum A toxin therapy: neutralizing and nonneutralizing antibodies—therapeutic consequences. *Exp Neurol* 1997;147: 96–102.
10. Pearce LB, First ER, MacCallum RD, et al. Pharmacologic characterization of botulinum toxin for basic science and medicine. *Toxicon* 1997;35:1373–1412.
11. Wohlfarth K, Goschel H, Frevert J, et al. Botulinum A toxins: units versus units. *Naunyn Scmiedebergs Arch Pharmacol* 1997;355:335–340.
12. Rosenberg JS, Middlebrook JS, Atassi MZ. Localization of the regions on the C-terminal domain of the heavy chain of botulinum toxin A recognized by T lymphocytes and by antibodies after immunization of mice with pentavalent toxoid. *Immunol Invest* 1997;26:491–504.
13. Hatheway CL, Dang C. Immunogenicity of neurotoxins of *Clostridium botulinum.* In: Jankovic J, Hallett M, eds. *Therapy with botulinum toxin.* New York: Marcel Dekker, 1994:25:93–107.
14. Aoki R, Garrett M, Spanoyannis A, et al. BOTOX (botulinum toxin type A) purified neurotoxin complex prepared from the new bulk toxin retains the same preclinical efficacy as the original but with reduced immunogenicity. *Neurology* 1999;52(6 Suppl 2): A521–522(abst).
15. Greene P, Fahn S, Diamond B. Development of resistance to botulinum toxin type A in patients with torticollis. *Mov Disord* 1994;9:213–217.
16. Jankovic J, Schwartz K. Response and immunoresistance to botulinum toxin injections. *Neurology* 1995;45: 1743–1746.
17. Brin MF, Comella C, O'Brien C, et al. An interim analysis of the clinical status of patients receiving current BOTOX (lot 2024 or subsequent lots) for the treatment of cervical dystonia (CD). *Mov Disord* 2000;15(Suppl 2):28–29(abstr).
18. DasGupta BR, Sathyamoorthy V. Purification and amino acid composition of type A botulinum neurotoxin. *Toxicon* 1984;22:415–424.
19. DasGupta BR, Sugiyama H. Molecular forms of neurotoxins in proteolytic *Clostridium botulinum* type B cultures. *Infect Immun* 1976;14:680–686.
20. Brin MF, Blitzer A. Botulinum toxin: dangerous terminology errors. *J Roy Soc Med* 1993;86:493–494.
21. Brashear A, Truong D, Charles D. A randomized double-blind, placebo-controlled study of intramuscular Botox for the treatment of cervical dystonia (CD). *Mov Disord* 1998;13(Suppl 2):276(abstr).
22. Poewe W, Deuschl G, Nebe A, et al. What is the optimal dose of botulinum toxin A in the treatment of cervical

dystonia? Results of a double-blind, placebo-controlled, dose-ranging study using Dysport. *J Neurol Neurosurg Psychiatry* 1998;64;13–17.

23. Brashear A, Lew MF, Dykstra DD, et al. Safety and efficacy of NeuroBloc (botulinum toxin type B) in type A-responsive cervical dystonia. *Neurology* 1999;53: 1439–1446.

24. Brin MF, Lew MF, Adler CH, et al. Safety and efficacy of NeuroBloc (botulinum toxin type B) in type A-resistant cervical dystonia. *Neurology* 1999;53:1431–1438.

25. Zbinden G, Flury-Roversi M. Significance of the LD_{50}-test for the toxicological evaluation of clinical substances. *Arch Toxicol* 1981;47:77–99.

25a.Sellin, LC, Thesleff S, DasGupta BR. Different effects of type A and B botulinum toxin on transmitter release at the rat neuromuscular junction. *Acta Physiol Scand* 1983;119:127–133.

26. O'Sullivan GA, Mohammed N, Foran PG, et al. Rescue of exocytosis in botulinum toxin A-poisoned chromaffin cells by expression of cleavage-resistant SNAP-25. *J Biol Chem* 1999;274:36897–36904.

27. Sloop RR, Cole BA, Escutin RO. Human response to botulinum toxin injection: type B compared with type A. *Neurology* 1997;49:189–194.

28. Burke GS. Notes on *Bacillus botulinus*. *J Bacteriol* 1919;4:555–565.

29. Dertzbaugh MT, West MW. Mapping of protective and cross-reactive domains of the type A neurotoxin of *Clostridium botulinum*. *Vaccine* 1996;14:1538–1544.

30. Oshima M, Middlebrook JL, Atassi MZ. Antibodies and T cells against synthetic peptides of the C-terminal domain (Hc) of botulinum neurotoxin type A and their cross-reaction with Hc. *Immunol Sci Lett* 1998;60:7–12.

31. Atassi MZ, Oshima M. Structure, activity, and immune (T and B cell) recognition of botulinum neurotoxins. *Crit Rev Immunol* 1999;19:219–260.

32. Halpern JL, Smith LA, Seamon KB, et al. Sequence homology between tetanus and botulinum toxins detected by an antipeptide antibody. *Infect Immun* 1989; 57:13–22.

33. Doellgast GJ, Brown JE, Koufman JA, et al. Sensitive assay for measurement of antibodies to *Clostridium botulinum* neurotoxins A, B, and E: use of hapten-labeled antibody elution to isolate specific complexes. *J Clin Microbiol* 1997;35:578–583.

34. Aoki KR. Preclinical update on BOTOX (botulinum toxin type A)-purified neurotoxin complex relative to other botulinum neurotoxin preparations. *Eur J Neurol* 1999;6(Suppl 4):S3–S10.

35. Brans JW, Lindeboom R, Snoek JW, et al. Botulinum toxin versus trihexyphenidyl in cervical dystonia: a prospective, randomized, double-blind controlled trial. *Neurology* 1996;46:1066–1072.

36. Tsui JKC, Eisen A, Stoessl AJ, et al. Double-blind study of botulinum toxin in spasmodic torticollis. *Lancet* 1986;2:245–247.

37. Sampaio C, Ferreira JJ, Simoes F, et al. DYSBOT: a single-blind, randomized parallel study to determine whether any differences can be detected in the efficacy and tolerability of two formulations of botulinum toxin

type A—Dysport and Botox—assuming a ratio of 4:1. *Mov Disord* 1997;12:1013–1018.

38. Odergren T, Hjaltason H, Kaakkola S, et al. A double-blind, randomised, parallel group study to investigate the dose equivalence of Dysport and Botox in the treatment of cervical dystonia. *J Neurol Neurosurg Psychiatry* 1998;64:6–12.

39. Dodel RC, Kirchner A, Koehne-Volland R, et al. Costs of treating dystonias and hemifacial spasm with botulinum toxin A. *Pharmacoeconomics* 1997;12:695–706.

40. Nussgens Z, Roggenkamper P. Comparison of two botulinum-toxin preparations in the treatment of essential blepharospasm. *Graefes Arch Clin Exp Ophthalmol* 1997;235:197–199.

41. Greene P, Kang U, Fahn S, et al. Double-blind, placebo-controlled trial of botulinum toxin injections for the treatment of spasmodic torticollis. *Neurology* 1990;40: 1213–1218.

42. Hauser RA, Comella C, Brashear A, et al. A randomized, multicenter, double-blind, placebo-controlled study of original Botox (botulinum toxin type A) purified neurotoxin complex for the treatment of cervical dystonia. *Mov Disord* 2000;15(Suppl 2):30–31(abstr).

43. Blackie JD, Lees AJ. Botulinum toxin treatment in spasmodic torticollis. *J Neurol Neurosurg Psychiatry* 1990; 53:640–643.

44. Lew MF, Adornato BT, Duane DD, et al. Botulinum toxin type B: a double-blind, placebo-controlled, safety and efficacy study in cervical dystonia. *Neurology* 1997; 49:701–707.

45. Kessler KR, Skutta M, Benecke R, et al. Long-term treatment of cervical dystonia with botulinum toxin type A: Efficacy, safety, and antibody frequency. *J Neurol* 1999;246:265–274.

46. FDA Center for Biologics Evaluation and Research. Botulinum toxin type A (BOTOX), Allergan, Inc., product approval information—licensing action [online] 2000a. Available at: www.fda.gov/cber/products/botaller122100.htm (accessed January 11, 2001).

47. FDA Center for Biologics Evaluation and Research. Botulinum toxin type B (MYOBLOC), Elan Pharmaceuticals product approval information—licensing action [online] 2000b. Available at: www.fda.gov/cber/products/botelan120800.htm (accessed January 11, 2001).

48. Toxin '99 Presentations. The International Conference of Basic and Therapeutic Aspects of Botulinum and Tetanus Toxins. Orlando, FL: November 15–19, 1999.

49. Zhou L, de Paiva A, Liu D, et al. Expression and purification of the light chain of botulinum neurotoxin A: a single mutation abolishes its cleavage of SNAP-25 and neurotoxicity after reconstitution with heavy chain. *Biochemistry* 1995;34:15175–15181.

50. Aoki KR. Botulinum neurotoxin serotypes A and B preparations have different safety margins in preclinical models of muscle weakening efficacy and systemic safety. *Toxicon* accepted for publication January 2002.

51. Aoki KR. A comparison of the safety margins of botulinum neurotoxin serotypes A, B, and F in mice. *Toxicon* 2001;39:1815–1820.

Scientific and Therapeutic Aspects of Botulinum Toxin
edited by M.F. Brin, J. Jankovic, and M. Hallett
Lippincott Williams & Wilkins, Philadelphia, © 2002.

10

Production, Quality, and Stability of Botulinum Toxin Type B (MYOBLOC™) for Clinical Use

James E. Callaway and Andrew J. Grethlein

To date, seven immunologically distinct serotypes of botulinum toxin (designated A through G) have been isolated and characterized (1). All may act as extremely potent toxins, with lethal doses as small as 0.05 to 0.1 μg (2). The type A serotype (Oculinum, Botox) was the first to be investigated clinically, and after two decades of developmental work, gained approval in the United States in 1989 for the treatment of strabismus, blepharospasm, and hemifacial spasm. It is currently produced as a sterile, lyophilized preparation of crystalline type A protein complexes that must be reconstituted in 0.9% sodium chloride solution prior to injection.

Despite the success of botulinum toxin type A in therapy, many concerns have been raised specifically with regard to its production and the ultimate quality of the toxin (3). Current type A preparations undergo lyophilization or vacuum-drying during the manufacturing process, which has been reported to inactivate toxin and increase the amount of denatured protein in the final product (4). Inactive toxin and denatured proteins can serve as toxoids that promote the development of neutralizing antibodies in patients (5). Reports on the incidence of antibodies directed against the type A toxin in patients undergoing repeated botulinum toxin type A therapy range from 3% to 57% (6,7). This wide range is partly the result of the use of many different assays. In addition, current type A prepa-

rations are reconstituted into a neutral or a slightly alkaline saline solution prior to injection. This process has been associated with loss of potency (4).

In 2000, 11 years following FDA approval of the type A toxin, botulinum toxin type B (MYOBLOC) was approved for the treatment of cervical dystonia. Clinical efficacy in cervical dystonia has been demonstrated in both type A-responsive and type A-resistant patients (8,9). Its usefulness in other neurologic syndromes, such as spasticity and pain, is currently being investigated. In the development of this new toxin, the goal was to produce a highly purified and stable liquid formulation that would avoid the lyophilization and reconstitution processes necessary with type A preparations. In this chapter, we review the characteristics of the purified type B toxin complex and then discuss the undertakings to optimize the production process for a highly purified and stable liquid formulation of botulinum toxin type B.

CHARACTERIZATION OF DRUG SUBSTANCE

Botulinum toxin type B is isolated from bacterial fermentation culture medium as part of a large multimeric protein complex. The molecular weight of the complex is estimated by size exclusion chromatography to be 700 kDa and is composed of the 150 kDa neurotoxin moiety noncovalently bound to at least five nontoxin proteins, some of which may have hemagglutinating ac-

James Callaway and Andrew Grethlein are employees of Elan Corporation.

tivity (10,11). The nontoxin proteins do not contribute to the activity of the neurotoxin, but are believed to stabilize the three-dimensional structure of a labile neurotoxic protein (12). In clinical use, injection of purified forms of these complexes may help to reduce the potential diffusion of toxin to adjoining noninjected muscles (3,5). As with other botulinum toxin serotypes, the stability of these large protein complexes is preserved under mildly acidic conditions (pH 5 to 7) (13,14). The complexes dissociate in basic conditions (pH > 7) (15,16).

By itself, the type B neurotoxin is a single-chain polypeptide that is 1,290 amino acid residues long (17). In this form, the neurotoxin has limited potency. During fermentation of *Clostridium botulinum,* bacterially produced proteases cleave or "nick" the single chain neurotoxin into an active di-chain polypeptide (18). The nicking occurs at a distinct cleavage site approximately one-third of the way from the N-terminus, and results in two chains, a heavy chain (100 kDa) and light chain (50 kDa), held together by a single disulfide bond. The heavy chain determines cholinergic specificity and facilitates entry of the light chain into the cytosol of the neuron, whereas the light chain contains the catalytic domain effecting neurotoxicity (19). The commercial manufacturing process for botulinum toxin type B results in a majority of the toxin being cleaved during fermentation. As a result, the type B neurotoxin presents as three polypeptides of 150 kDa (intact), 100 kDa (heavy chain), and 50 kDa (light chain) when analyzed by reducing sodium dodecyl sulfate-polyacrylamide gel electrophoresis (SDS-PAGE).

The clinical preparation of botulinum toxin type B is a liquid formulation containing highly purified type B complexes. It is formulated in slightly acidic solution (pH 5.6) to ensure that the toxin complexes remain intact and stable before and during injection. The solution contains a mixture of single chain (unnicked) and enzymatically cleaved, di-chain (nicked) toxin. The nicked form constitutes approximately 75% of the total toxin. After it is injected into the muscle, the neurotoxin dissociates from the complex to inhibit acetylcholine release and to induce muscle paralysis in the target muscle.

TYPE B TOXIN PRODUCTION

Commercial-scale production of purified botulinum toxin type B complexes consists of three stages: fermentation, recovery, and purification. Importantly, the production process for botulinum toxin type B does not include lyophilization or vacuum-drying. Lyophilization of type A toxin preparations has been associated with inactivation of toxin (3,4,20). It is not known, however, what impact this inactivation has on the overall clinical experience.

Fermentation

The fermentation process is initiated using a frozen culture of the type B strain of *C. botulinum,* and under anaerobic conditions, proceeds through two successive seed cultures (S1 and S2). The S2 seed cultures are used as inocula for the production culture (S3), which is grown in a liquid medium of casein hydrolysate, yeast extract, and glucose for more than 3 days. During S3, there is a period of rapid cell growth during which the pH decreases about one pH unit, followed by little or no stationary growth, and then cell lysis during which the pH increases slightly. The toxin complex is released from the bacterium during cell lysis, and nicking of the neurotoxin occurs throughout the lytic and postlytic phases of the fermentation cycle (21).

Recovery

Following fermentation, the S3 culture is chilled within the fermenter to below 20°C (68°F) and then harvested in an acidic environment to precipitate the crude toxin complex. The precipitated toxin is washed with water to remove trapped contaminants and then centrifuged to produce a pellet, which is weighed prior to resuspension in buffer. During recovery, the precipitated toxin is resuspended in buffer and purified by a series of ammonium salt precipitations. The final pellet is resuspended, diafiltered, and then dead-end filtered.

Purification

Purification is achieved with diethylaminoethane anion exchange (DEAE) and size-exclusion chromatography (SEC), each followed by

0.2 μm filtration. The DEAE efficiently binds nucleic acid as the toxin complex flows through, ensuring that only those fractions with significant levels of protein and low levels of nucleic acid remain for purification by SEC. SEC is performed subsequent to the DEAE step to further increase the purity and consistency of the toxin complex. The sterile product is diluted to a final concentration of 5000 U/mL (approximately 50 ng/mL) in a slightly acidic solution (pH 5.6) containing 10 nM sodium succinate, 100 nM sodium chloride, and 0.5 mg/mL human serum albumin.

ROBUSTNESS OF PRODUCTION PROCESS

The robustness of the production process for botulinum toxin type B complex was determined by subjecting each stage of the process (i.e., fermentation, recovery, purification) to prespecified "worst" and "extreme" case operating conditions (Table 10.1). Four separate production runs were carried out, and analytical tests were conducted on the in-process and final preparations to determine the effects of altering critical operating procedures on key quality attributes of the toxin complex. For fermentation,

the worst-case condition consisted of altering parameters that would minimize cell growth and toxin production. Under the extreme-case condition, the opposite end of the range for the same parameters was used to maximize cell growth and toxin production. The last two sets of fermentations were carried out under normal operating conditions, and were used to challenge the process parameters during recovery and purification that affect toxin purity.

Key quality attributes of the toxin include purity, complex integrity, specific activity, and percent nicking. These physicochemical and biologic tests used to define these attributes are described in the next section. Data from these tests show that despite broad deviations from normal operating conditions, all four production runs yielded highly purified and intact toxin complex (Table 10.2). In one lot operated under worst-case fermentation conditions, the toxin product had a percent nicking value of 59%. The lower percent nicking was attributed to experimental conditions of early harvest, high pH, and reduced concentrations of nutrients. Considering that multiple parameters were altered during fermentation of this lot, however, the worst-case condition still resulted in an acceptable toxin product. Taken together, these results demon-

TABLE 10.1. *Production conditions used to test the robustness of the commercial production process*

Production stage	Run 1	Run 2	Run 3	Run 4
Fermentation	Worst ↑ pH of fermentation early harvest ↓ incubation temperature ↓ incubation time ↓ medium concentration	Extreme ↓ pH of fermentation late harvest ↑ incubation temperature ↑ incubation time ↑ medium concentration	Normal	Normal
Recovery	Normal	Normal	Worst ↓ centrifugation speed ↓ centrifugation time	Extreme ↑ centrifugation speed ↑ centrifugation time
Purification	Normal	Normal	Worst ↑ column load ↑ column flow rate, DEAE ↑ mobile phase pH ↓ column flow rate, SEC	Extreme ↓ column load ↓ column flow rate, DEAE ↓ mobile phase pH ↑ column flow rate, SEC

TABLE 10.2. *Effects of altering critical process parameters on key toxin attributes:*
results from four production runs

Parameter	Run 1	Run 2	Run 3	Run 4
Protein purity	Conforms	Conforms	Conforms	Conforms
Percentage nicking	59%	69%	70%	73%
Specific activity	84 U/ng	121 U/ng	109 U/ng	81 U/ng
Complex integrity	Conforms	Conforms	Conforms	Conforms

strate that the production process for botulinum toxin type B complex is extremely resilient and robust.

QUALITY OF TOXIN

Three consecutive manufacturing lots were carried out under normal operating conditions to assess the quality (e.g., purity, complex integrity, specific activity, percent nicking), consistency, and stability of botulinum toxin type B preparations.

Purity

Purity of the botulinum toxin type B preparations was assessed using SDS-PAGE, a technique that reduces, denatures, and separates the toxin complex into its individual peptides. In this assay, the disassembled type B toxin complex presented as eight bands separated according to relative molecular weights (Fig. 10.1) (22). The neurotoxin itself was represented by three bands: intact toxin (150 kDa), heavy chain (100 kDa), and light chain (50 kDa). The percentage of nicked neurotoxin, or toxin in its active di-chain form, was calculated by the ratio of heavy and light chains relative to the amount of total toxin (heavy chains + light chains + intact toxin). These percentages were consistent among the three lots, ranging between 74% and 78%. Five nontoxin proteins were also resolved by SDS-PAGE, and ranged in molecular weight from 17 kDa to 116 kDa. Complex consistency was determined visually by comparing to a reference standard to assure that all of the polypeptides that comprise the complex were present and at the correct level relative to the reference stan-

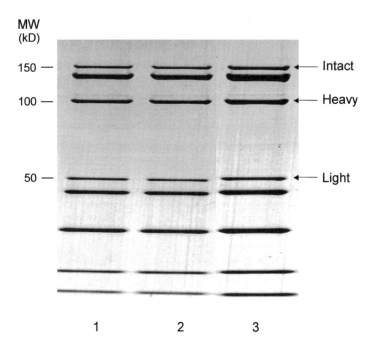

MW
(kD)

150 — ← Intact

100 — ← Heavy

50 — ← Light

1   2   3

FIG. 10.1. SDS-PAGE of the three batches (lanes 1 to 3) of botulinum toxin type B liquid formulation demonstrated the purity and consistency of the protein complex from batch to batch. (From Setler P. The biochemistry of botulinum toxin type B. *Neurology* 2000; 55(Suppl 5):S22–S28, with permission.)

dard. Electrophoretic profiles were found to be comparable for each of the three manufacturing lots.

Further confirmation of structure and purity was determined through N-terminal sequencing of the protein bands resolved by electrophoresis and eluted from the gel. Ten amino acids from the N-terminus were sequenced, and results were compared with the expected amino acid sequence from the genetic code of the type B strain of *C. botulinum* (17). Matching closely with published sequences, the data confirmed the identity of the intact, heavy, and light chain proteins of botulinum toxin type B and affirmed the high fidelity of nicking at the lysine-alanine scissile bond (residues 440–441). The eight polypeptides of the toxin complex were all present, and the contaminating proteins had been effectively and reproducibly removed.

Complex Integrity

Botulinum toxin type B is characterized structurally as the native protein complex by SEC. In a solution of pH 5.5 (similar to that used to formulate the purified toxin complex, pH 5.6), the toxin complex eluted as a single peak with a molecular weight of 700 kDa (Fig. 10.2A) (22). In this slightly acidic environment, the neurotoxin was present as a uniform, intact, and stable complex. Results were similar for each of the three manufacturing lots. As indicated previously, the pH of the solution is an important determinant of whether the toxin complex remains intact or dissociates. Botulinum toxins are most stable in slightly acidic solution and dissociate in neutral or alkaline solution (10). When an identical botulinum toxin type B sample was dialyzed overnight in a solution of pH 7.8, the toxin complex dissociated and eluted as two peaks on the SEC assay, with one eluting as free neurotoxin and the other representing the complex proteins (Fig. 10.2B).

Specific Activity

The potency of botulinum toxin type B is determined using the standard mouse intraperitoneal (IP) LD_{50} potency assay (23). Results are ex-

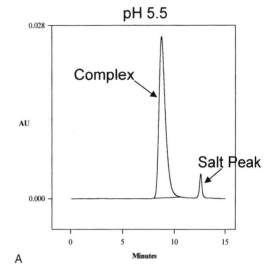

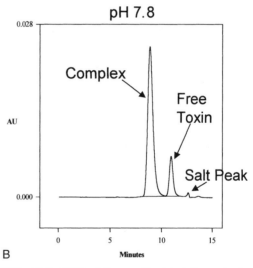

FIG. 10.2. SEC of the purified botulinum toxin type B complexes. **A:** At acidic pH 5.5, the complex eluted as a single entity, indicating that the toxin was uniform and intact. **B:** In alkaline pH 7.8, a second peak appeared, indicating that the complex had dissociated. Botulinum toxin type B is prepared as a slightly acidic (pH 5.6) liquid formulation. (From Setler P. The biochemistry of botulinum toxin type B. *Neurology* 2000;55(Suppl 5):S22–S28, with permission.)

TABLE 10.3. *Drug product specific activities from three consecutive manufacturing runs*

Batch	Protein concentration (ng/mL)*	Mouse LD_{50} potency (U/mL)	Specific activity (U/ng)**
1	5.0×10^4	4.5×10^6	90
2	1.23×10^5	12.4×10^6	101
3	1.22×10^5	13.0×10^6	107

*Determined by A_{280}.
**Calculated as the ratio of mouse LD_{50} potency units to protein concentration.

pressed as units (U), with one unit equivalent to the amount required to produce lethality in 50% of the mice injected. Specific activity represents the potency of the toxin in mouse units by weight, and is calculated as the ratio of mouse LD_{50} potency (U/mL) to concentration of toxin (ng/mL). Ultraviolet light absorbency at a wavelength of 280 nm (A_{280}) is used to determine toxin concentration using a validated extinction coefficient of 2.087 $AUmg^{-1}cm^{-2}$. A high level of specific activity is desirable to minimize the amount of toxin needed to achieve therapeutic effect and assure no generation of inactive or denatured toxin. For the three manufacturing lots, specific activities were 90, 101, and 107 U/ng, respectively (Table 10.3). These values are the highest reported in literature for botulinum toxin type B (24–26).

A distinguishing feature of this botulinum toxin is that the high specific activity is retained as it is formulated into drug product for pharmaceutical use. To prepare pharmaceutical quality botulinum toxin type B, the concentrated toxin is diluted approximately 1,000-fold with 0.5 mg/mL of human serum albumin in saline at pH 5.6 and sterile filtered before aseptic filling. Data from the formulation of three distinct drug product lots from two separate preparations of concentrated toxin are presented in Table 10.4.

TABLE 10.4. *Botulinum toxin type B specific activity comparison*

Lot ID	Drug product specific activity (U/ng)*	Final product specific activity (U/ng)**
Lot A	88	92
Lot B	88	88
Lot C	87	95

*Determined by IP potency and A_{280} methods.
**Determined by IP potency and enzyme-linked immunoassay (ELISA) methods.

Given that only nanogram amounts of toxin are present in each vial of product, an enzyme-linked immunoassay (ELISA) method that used an antibody specific for properly folded type B toxin was validated for toxin quantification and used to determine the toxin levels in drug product. These data show no drop in specific activity through the process of drug-product manufacturing and confirm that the toxin retains full activity. This is in contrast to the type A toxin (Botox), which is reported to drop 40% (from 34 U/ng for the purified toxin to 20 U/ng for the reconstituted product) following freezing and vacuum-drying (28,29).

STABILITY

Stability tests under varying pH and temperature conditions have been conducted on the liquid formulation of botulinum toxin type B. Stability was confirmed using the ELISA method previously described. At the elevated temperature of 40°C (104°F), the toxin was extremely stable for 4 weeks when incubated in slightly acidic solution of pH 5.0 or pH 5.5 (Fig. 10.3A) (22). As expected, however, some loss of toxin was observed over time as the pH of the storage solution was increased to pH 6.0 or pH 6.5. When stored at room temperature (25°C/77°F) for prolonged periods in slightly acidic solution of pH 5.6, the potency of the purified botulinum toxin type B (as measured by the mouse LD_{50} assay) was stable for 9 months (Fig. 10.3B), and at refrigerated temperature (2° to 8°C/35.6° to 46.4°F), potency was retained for more than 36 months (Fig. 10.3C). The recommended storage condition for botulinum toxin type B solution is currently 2° to 8°C (35.6° to 46.4°F).

Production of botulinum toxin type B as a slightly acidic liquid formulation (pH 5.6) there-

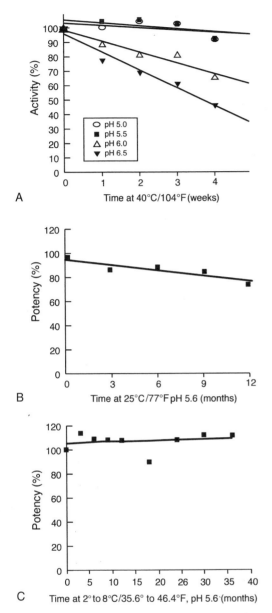

FIG. 10.3. Stability of botulinum toxin type B drug product. **A:** At elevated temperature (40°C/104°F), botulinum toxin type B was stable for at least 4 weeks in acidic solution. **B:** At room temperature (25°C/77°F) in pH 5.6, it was stable for 9 months. **C:** At refrigerated temperature (2° to 8°C/35.6° to 46.4°F) in pH 5.6, it was stable for at least 36 months. (Figure A is from Setler P. The biochemistry of botulinum toxin type B. *Neurology* 2000;55(Suppl 5):S22–S28, with permission.)

fore ensures that the stability, integrity, and activity of the toxin complex are preserved before and during injection. Vacuum-dried preparations of the type A toxin require the use of 0.9 mg sodium chloride and 0.5 mg human serum albumin per vial. The commercially available type A toxin reconstitutes to a pH of 7.3 and rapidly loses potency, such that within 12 hours a statistically significant loss of potency has occurred, even when stored at refrigerated temperatures (27). The cause of this highly perishable potency for the type A toxin has been attributed to the instability of the toxin complex at neutral pH and the damage done to the toxin as the result of vacuum-drying, as reflected in a loss in specific activity from 34 to 20 U/ng (28,29). Injection of the toxin as the intact complex form instead of the dissociated subunits may potentially reduce the diffusion rate of toxin into adjoining, non-injected muscles (3,4).

CONCLUSIONS

Botulinum toxin type B (MYOBLOC) is a new botulinum toxin formulated as a sterile solution and recently approved for use in patients with cervical dystonia. The type B toxin is a complex of several proteins including the neurotoxin moiety. Purified forms of these complexes help to stabilize the neurotoxin during its production and upon injection into the patient. In the development of a new toxin, the objective was to produce a liquid formulation containing highly purified type B toxin complexes with high specific activity and adequate long-term stability. These factors are concerns with current commercial type A preparations that are vacuum-dried during the purification process and must be reconstituted prior to injection.

The production process for botulinum toxin type B has been determined to be extremely robust. This was determined in a series of production runs that were subjected to variations in operating conditions in the different stages of production (i.e., fermentation, recovery, purification). Final toxin product in all cases was highly purified with high specific activities. Biochemical analyses on the type B toxin from three separate manufacturing runs have shown that the process consistently delivers highly purified, intact, and stable type B complexes. The uniformity and potency of the product were consistent from batch to batch. Developed as a liquid formulation in a solution of pH 5.6, the type B preparation avoids the lyophilization and reconstitution processes associated with inactivation and perishable potency of type A preparations. In addition, the new liquid formulation of botulinum toxin type B exhibits long-term stability and can be kept in refrigerated temperatures (2° to 8°C/35.6° to 46.4°F) for at least 3 years or at room temperature (25°C/77°F) for 9 months.

REFERENCES

1. Sugiyama H. *Clostridium botulinum* neurotoxin. *Microbiol Rev* 1980;44:419–448.
2. Cherington M. Clinical spectrum of botulism. *Muscle Nerve* 1998;21:701–710.
3. Johnson EA, Goodnough MC. Preparation and properties of botulinum toxin for medical use. In: Tsui JKC, Calne DB, eds. *Handbook of dystonia.* New York: Marcel Dekker, 1995:346–365.
4. Schantz EJ, Johnson EA. Quality of botulinum toxin for human treatment. In: DasGupta BR, ed. *Botulinum and tetanus neurotoxins.* New York: Plenum Press, 1993: 657–659.
5. Baffi RA, Garnick RL. Quality control issues in the analysis of lyophilized proteins. *Develop Biol Standard* 1991;74:181–184.
6. Siatkowski RM, Tyunikov ABAW. Serum antibody production to botulinum A toxin. *Ophthalmology* 1993; 100:1861–1866.
7. Zuber M, Sebald M, Bathien N, et al. Botulinum antibodies in dystonic patients treated with type A botulinum toxin: frequency and significance. *Neurology* 1993; 43:1715–1718.
8. Brashear A, Lew MF, Dykstra DD, et al. Safety and efficacy of NeuroBloc (botulinum toxin type B) in type A-responsive cervical dystonia. *Neurology* 1999;53: 1439–1446.
9. Brin MF, Lew MF, Adler CH, et al. Safety and efficacy of NeuroBloc (botulinum toxin type B) in type A-resistant cervical dystonia. *Neurology* 1999;53:1431–1438.
10. Sakaguchi G. *Clostridium botulinum* toxins. *Pharmacol Ther* 1983;19:165–194.
11. Somers E, DasGupta BR. *Clostridium botulinum* type A, B, C1 and E produce proteins with or without hemagglutinating activity: do they share common amino acid sequences and genes? *J Protein Chem* 1991;10: 415–425.
12. DasGupta BR, Sugiyama H. Molecular forms of neurotoxins in proteolytic *Clostridium botulinum* type B cultures. *Infect Immun* 1976;14:680–686.
13. Bonventre PF, Kempe LL. Physiology of toxin production by *Clostridium botulinum* types A and B. III: Effect of pH and temperature during incubation on growth, autolysis, and toxin production. *Appl Microbiol* 1959; 7:374–377.
14. Ohye DF, Christian JHB. Combined effects of temperature, pH and water activity on growth and toxin production by *C. botulinum* types A, B and E. In: Ingram M, Roberts TA, eds. *Botulism 1966.* London: Chapman & Hall, 1967:217–223.
15. Townsend CT, Yee L, Mercer WA. Inhibition of the growth of *Clostridium botulinum* by acidification. *Food Res* 1954;19:1–7.
16. Wagman J. Isolation and sedimentation study of low molecular weight forms of type A botulinum toxin. *Arch Biochem Biophys* 1954;50:104–112.
17. Whelan SM, Elmore MJ, Bodsworth NJ, et al. Molecular cloning of the *Clostridium botulinum* structural gene encoding the type B neurotoxin and determination of its entire nucleotide sequence. *Appl Environ Microbiol* 1992;58:2345–2354.
18. Kozaki S, Oga Y, Kamada Y, Sakaguchi G. Activation of *Clostridium botulinum* type B and E derivative toxins with lysine specific proteases. *FEMS Microbiol Lett* 1985;27:149–154.
19. Montecucco C, Schiavo G. Structure and function of tetanus and botulinum neurotoxins. *Q Rev Biophys* 1995;28:423–472.
20. DasGupta BR, Boroff DA. Separation of toxin and hemagglutinin from crystalline toxin of *Clostridium botulinum* type A by anion exchange chromatography and determination of their dimensions by gel filtration. *J Biol Chem* 1968;5:1065–1072.
21. Siegel LS, Metzger JF. Effect of fermentation conditions on toxin production by *Clostridium botulinum* type B. *Appl Environ Microbiol* 1980;40:1023–1026.
22. Setler P. The biochemistry of botulinum toxin type B. *Neurology* 2000;55(Suppl 5):S22–S28.
23. Hatheway CH, Dang C. Immunogenicity of the neurotoxins of *Clostridium botulinum*. In: Jankovic J, Hallett M, eds. *Therapy with botulinum toxin.* New York: Marcel Dekker, 1994:93–107.
24. Beers WH, Reich E. Isolation and characterization of *Clostridium botulinum* type B toxin. *J Biol Chem* 1969; 244:4473–4479.
25. Kozaki S, Miyazaki S, Sakaguchi G. Development of antitoxin with each of two complementary fragments of *Clostridium botulinum* type B derivative toxin. *Infect Immun* 1977;18:761–766.
26. Ohishi I, Sakaguchi G. Activation of botulinum toxins in the absence of nicking. *Infect Immun* 1977;17:402–407.
27. Gartlan MG, Hoffman, HT. Crystalline preparation of botulinum toxin type A (Botox): Degradation in potency with storage. *Otolaryngol Head Neck Surg* 1993;108: 135–140.
28. BOTOX Product Monograph. *BOTOX botulinum toxin type A purified neurotoxin complex.* Irvine, CA: Allergan, Inc., 1998.
29. BOTOX Package Insert. *BOTOX (botulinum toxin type A) purified neurotoxin complex.* Irvine, CA: Allergan, Inc., 2000.

Scientific and Therapeutic Aspects of Botulinum Toxin
edited by M.F. Brin, J. Jankovic, and M. Hallett
Lippincott Williams & Wilkins, Philadelphia, © 2002.

11

Spread of Paralysis to Nearby and Distant Noninjected Muscles in a Monkey Hand Model: Comparison of BoNT-B and BoNT-A

Joseph C. Arezzo, Mona S. Litwak, Florence A. Caputo, Kathleen E. Meyer, and George M. Shopp

Botulinum neurotoxins (BoNTs) are produced by bacteria of the genus *Clostridium,* and exist as at least seven antigenically distinct serotypes, designated A, B, C1, D, E, F, and G. These neurotoxins are closely related in macromolecular structure, and cause paralysis by inhibiting the release of acetylcholine from cholinergic nerve terminals at the neuromuscular junction (1). The mechanism of action of botulinum toxins is believed to be a three-step process (2,3). The first step involves the extracellular binding of the toxin to serotype-specific acceptors on cholinergic motor nerve terminals. The toxin is then internalized via endocytosis and released into the cytosol of the nerve terminal. It then binds to its specific intracellular protein target, leading to disruption of the exocytotic process and inhibition of acetylcholine release from the nerve terminal.

The initial clinical use of BoNT was limited to the treatment of strabismus and blepharospasm (e.g., reference 4); however, the therapeutic use of this toxin has grown exponentially in the past decade (references 5 to 9 are recent reviews). This remarkable expansion has been driven by four principal factors: (a) the clear empirical demonstration that BoNT is effective in treating multiple disorders characterized by excessive contraction of skeletal and smooth muscle (e.g., cervical dystonia, achalasia); (b) the continued

exploration of the effects of BoNT in novel conditions linked to cholinergic activity (e.g., headache, focal hyperhidrosis); (c) the growing demand for the use of BoNT in dermatology (e.g., hyperfunctional facial lines); and (d) the dramatic increase in the use of BoNT for the treatment of movement disorders in children (e.g., spasticity).

The expanded therapeutic use of BoNT is also predicated on the fact that treatment has proven ''relatively safe'' and is well tolerated. In spite of the fact that BoNT is one of the most deadly substances known to man (10), and that there is unquestionable evidence that, at therapeutic doses, the toxin is not confined to the injection site (11), there are few reports of serious or sustained adverse reactions. Safety issues may, however, become increasingly important as higher doses are used to treat conditions such as cerebral palsy, and as the effects of exposure are determined in a more heterogeneous group of patients.

In BoNT therapy, safety is a function of the degree to which the compound ''spreads'' from the site(s) of injection to nearby and remote cholinergic neurons. Nearby spread of the direct effects of BoNT is most likely caused by the diffusion of unbound toxin through extracellular space, driven by the concentration gradient and the dynamics of the injection. Shaari and colleagues (12) used a glycogen-depletion model to demonstrate that BoNT easily spreads across fascia to affect noninjected adjacent muscles. A

Kathleen Meyer and George Shopp are employees of Elan Corporation.

dose-dependent "spread" of the effects of BoNT to nearby muscles has been reported in experimental animals using acetylcholinesterase staining (11,13) and in situ muscle twitch properties (14). These findings have been confirmed in humans by using a rating scale for weakness (15) and by electrophysiology (16–18). In one study treating writer's cramp, weakness in nearby noninjected muscles of the forearm was observed in 63% of patients (15). Many of the classic side effects of BoNT therapy, for instance, dysphagia following injections to pharyngeal muscles, are most likely related to local diffusion of BoNT (11).

In contrast, remote "spread," in which the effects of BoNT are observed at a considerable distance from the injection site (e.g., contralateral muscle or intrinsic muscle of the foot following injection in the neck), cannot be fully explained by diffusion. If these effects are a result of altered release of acetylcholine at the distant muscle, they most likely involve vascular or lymphatic transport of the toxin. In spite of earlier reports regarding the use of ^{125}I-labeled BoNT (19), there is little, or no, current evidence for the retrograde transport of BoNT in neurons as a mechanism of spread. Increased temporal jitter in single-fiber electromyography (EMG) and alteration in the turns pattern in the quantitative EMG signal are the most common evidence of remote spread (20–27), but the loss of muscle fibers at sites distant from the BoNT injection have also been reported (28). The remote effects are generally subclinical; however, symptoms of generalized weakness have been described in a few BoNT-treated patients (29,30).

Recently, the B serotype of botulinum toxin (BoNT-B) was proven safe and effective in the treatment of cervical dystonia (31,32) and has become a commercially available product (MY-OBLOC). This compound differs from the commercial forms of serotype A (BoNT-A) by virtue of distinct acceptor sites (therefore a unique mechanism of entry into the neuron) and its ability to cleave different target proteins in the vesicle docking and fusion complex. Synaptobrevin (also known as vesicle-associated membrane protein or VAMP) is the target protein cleaved by BoNT-B, while synaptosomal-associated protein of 25 kDa (SNAP-25) is the target protein cleaved by BoNT-A. The commercial forms of botulinum toxin also differ in formulation and stability, the pH of the solution to be injected, and potentially in the percentage of free toxin per unit volume of injected product (references 33 and 34 are recent reviews). The addition of a new BoNT treatment option mandates comparison of the effectiveness of the products in inducing the desired paresis of the injected muscle and comparison of the relative safety of each treatment option as judged by "spread" of the direct effect to nearby and remote muscles.

The present study had two specific goals: (a) to develop an objective, reliable, and sensitive primate model to quantify the degree of muscle paralysis induced by botulinum toxins, and (b) to compare the "spread" of paralysis induced by BoNT-B and BoNT-A in nontreated muscles (i.e., both nearby and remote) at doses resulting in equivalent effects in the injected muscle.

MATERIALS AND METHODS

Study Subjects

Sixty-two adult female cynomolgus monkeys (*Macaca fascicularis*) weighing between 1.7 kg and 4.5 kg were evaluated. Housing, dosing, and electrophysiologic testing were conducted at the Sierra Biomedical, Inc. facility (Sparks, Nevada); all procedures were reviewed by the Animal Care and Use Committee at this facility. Cynomolgus monkeys represent the closest feasible model of the human neuromuscular system (35) and, more specifically, the intrinsic muscles of their hand are similar in relative size and functioning to human hands. In addition, cynomolgus monkeys exhibit similar mechanistic and pharmacologic responses to botulinum toxin (36,37). Female monkeys were evaluated to minimize size differences across comparison groups. Animals were housed individually in stainless steel cages in accordance with USDA regulations, and were under veterinary supervision for the duration of the study. At all doses tested, both BoNT-B and BoNT-A were well tolerated. No treatment-related clinical adverse effects were observed, and all animals survived the study.

Test Articles

BoNT-A was obtained from commercially available stocks (BOTOX) supplied as lyophilized powder. To achieve desired doses, BoNT-A was reconstituted in 0.9% sodium chloride (NaCl) and diluted to a final concentration with 0.5 mg/mL human serum albumin in 0.9% NaCl. As per labeling instructions, BoNT-A was stored in a freezer at or below $-7°C$. BoNT-B was supplied as a clear liquid formulation, and was diluted with a solution consisting of 100 mM NaCl, 10 mM succinate, and 0.5 mg/mL human serum albumin. BoNT-B was stored refrigerated between $2°C$ ($35.6°F$) and $8°C$ ($46.4°F$). Freshly prepared diluted toxin solutions were used for each dosing day.

Monkey Hand Model

The direct effects of BoNT-B and BoNT-A were compared by injecting the toxin into the abductor pollicis brevis (APB) muscle of the hand and then measuring the degree of induced change in the compound muscle action potential (CMAP) of this muscle. The peak amplitude of the CMAP response (i.e., M wave) is a well-established experimental and clinical electrophysiologic measure; its reduction has been reported as the "most consistent electrophysiologic effect" in botulism (38). Although the relationship between the force of contraction and intramuscular electrical activity is often complex (e.g., reference 39), the surface-recorded CMAP is generally sensitive to the number of activated motor units, the synchrony of their activation, and the strength of contraction (Fig. 11.1). This measure has been validated as an index of BoNT-induced paralysis in both rats and monkeys (40,41).

In a separate series of studies (see below), the "spread" effects of the two toxins were determined by also examining the change in CMAP amplitudes in the noninjected nearby first dorsal interosseous (FDI) muscle and in the relatively remote abductor digiti minimi (ADM) muscle. The FDI is adjacent to the APB, but located on the back of the hand; the ADM is located on the opposite side of the hand (Fig. 11.2). Neither of these muscles is innervated by the median nerve that innervates the APB, eliminating retrograde transport of the toxin as a possible source of spread.

In all studies, the volume of injection was held constant at 100 μL and a single injection was made in each APB muscle. The induced change in the CMAP was determined by comparing values at baseline (immediately preceding the injec-

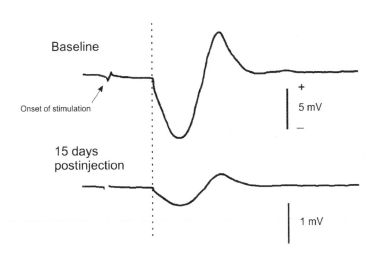

BoNT-B induced reduction of the CMAP

Baseline

Onset of stimulation

15 days
postinjection

+

5 mV

−

1 mV

FIG. 11.1. Compound muscle action potential (CMAP or M wave). Recorded from the surface of the muscle, this response represents the summed depolarization of distributed motor units driven by supramaximal stimulation of the associated nerve. Its onset is a measure of maximal motor nerve conduction and the delay in neuromuscular transmission; its peak reflects the number and synchrony of activated extrafusal motor fibers. BoNT injection results in a reduction in the peak amplitude of the CMAP, with no change in onset latency. Note the change in calibration between baseline and postinjection recordings (positive is up).

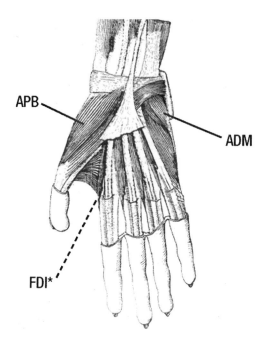

FIG. 11.2. Diagram of the monkey hand. The APB muscle is the direct site of botulinum toxin injection. The FDI muscle is adjacent to the APB, but is innervated by a different nerve (i.e., deep branch of the ulnar nerve for FDI; median for APB). The ADM muscle is relatively distant, sharing neither a nerve nor fascial boundary with the injected APB. ADM, abductor digiti minimi; APB, abductor pollicis brevis; FDI, first dorsal interosseous.

tion) and 14 days postinjection. Throughout injection and recording, the investigators always remained "blinded" as to the dose and nature of the compound injected into each APB.

Measurement Procedures

Electrophysiologic testing was conducted using a portable EMG/EP instrument (Teca TD-10), in compliance with the US FDA Good Laboratory Practice regulations. Animals were fasted and anesthetized with 10 mg/kg Ketaset (IM), followed by 12 to 15 mg/kg sodium pentobarbital (IV). Stimulation was achieved using a constant voltage square pulse (0.05- to 0.2-msec duration) isolated from ground. The stimulating cathode was positioned overlying the appropriate nerve (i.e., median for APB; ulnar for FDI and

ADM), approximately 1.0 cm from the distal wrist crease, with the anode 1.5 cm further proximal. The CMAP was monitored as the stimulation intensity (both voltage and duration) was systematically increased to ensure production of the maximal CMAP amplitude; onset latency was continuously monitored to avoid overstimulation of the nerve and consequent shifting of the effective site of activation. Recording and stimulation sites were marked to facilitate consistent electrode placement. Throughout testing, animals were positioned on a heating pad connected to a circulating water bath and rectal and skin temperatures were maintained above 34°C (93.2°F) and 32°C (89.6°F), respectively.

For the APB muscle, the CMAP was recorded using a 5-mm diameter surface electrode positioned overlying the "belly of the muscle" with reference to a ring electrode placed on the second digit. At each time point, three separate records of the CMAP were obtained, with the active lead repositioned approximately 2 mm off the center point between measurements (i.e., spatial sampling). The mean of the three responses determined the peak amplitude used in calculating BoNT effects. For smaller signals (e.g., after BoNT injection), the CMAP was averaged three to five times at each placement prior to scoring peak amplitude. Because of their size, orientation, and the presence of surrounding muscles, the CMAP in the FDI and ADM muscles were recorded using a low-impedance subcutaneous electrode positioned on the surface of the target muscle. For each muscle, the CMAP was again measured at three closely placed sites and averaged for small signals. The electrodes and spatial sampling procedures were extensively piloted prior to the onset of these experiments to optimize the repeat measure reliability of the recording and to minimize the influence of activity in surrounding muscles.

RESULTS

Determination of Minimum Effective Dose

The minimum effective dose (MED) is defined as the dose of BoNT that produces a reduction in the CMAP of 70% to 75% (e.g., 8.0 mV signal at baseline reduced to approximately 2.2 mV signal 14 days after BoNT injection). The MED was selected as a key study end point for three reasons: (a) it represents a level of BoNT-induced change in muscle function that clearly corresponds to a "clinically evident" deficit; (b) it avoids the asymptotes of the dose-response curve; (c) targeting a 70% change allows exploration of experimental circumstances that might increase or decrease the effectiveness of the BoNT treatment selected.

An initial series of studies was designed to determine the MED for both BoNT-B and BoNT-A following a single 100-μL injection into the APB. Dose-response curves were determined in separate studies for each compound using four doses and four monkeys per group (total $n = 16$ per compound). Each subject was treated with either BoNT-B or BoNT-A in the APB muscle bilaterally (total of eight muscles per dose). The doses selected for examination were based on previous pilot studies and included 0.05, 0.16, 0.50, and 1 U for BoNT-B and 0.005, 0.023, 0.108, and 0.500 U for BoNT-A. Analysis of the dose-response curves (Fig. 11.3) determined that the MED for BoNT-B was 0.44 U and the equivalent MED for BoNT-A was 0.09 U. The range of doses examined for each compound differed (i.e., 20-fold range for BoNT-B vs a 100-fold range for BoNT-A), as did the apparent slope in the dose regions evalu-

ated. Following standard practice, the MED is expressed in "mouse units" (i.e., one unit equals amount of toxin that will kill half of the IP injected mice); the substantial difference in the absolute value of MEDs reflects the relative potency of each compound in mice versus monkey.

Comparison of "Spread" Effects for BoNT-A and BoNT-B

Both the direct effects (change in injected muscle) and spread effects (change in nearby and relatively remote muscles) were examined in a series of monkeys treated with BoNT-B in one APB muscle and BoNT-A in the contralateral APB muscle. A total of 30 adult female monkeys were examined, divided into three doses per compound and ten monkeys per dose group. The side injected with each compound was randomized to avoid possible laterality effects. The doses selected were multiples of the MED for each compound, established in the earlier study. Because "spread" was a target, relatively large doses were administered, including: MED (BoNT-B, 0.44 U; BoNT-A, 0.09 U), 5xMED (BoNT-B, 2.11 U; BoNT-A, 0.43 U), and 25xMED (BoNT-B, 10.1 U; BoNT-A, 2.06 U) for each compound. The volume was maintained at 100 μL and a single injection was used in each treated muscle. Comparing the effects of

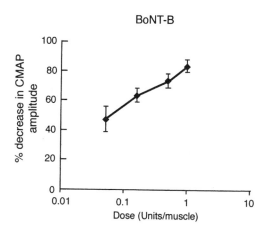

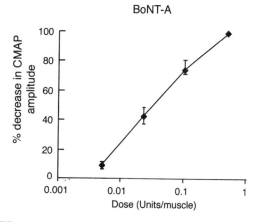

FIG. 11.3. Dose-response curves for the injected APB muscle. These response curves were determined separately for BoNT-B and BoNT-A. The estimated MED (dose at which the CMAP is reduced by 70% to 75%) is 0.44 U for BoNT-B and 0.09 U for BoNT-A.

multiples of the MED is potentially problematic if the slope of the dose-response curves differs for the two compounds. Therefore, the direct effect in the injected muscle was determined for each dose used in the evaluation of spread and shown to be equivalent for BoNT-B and BoNT-A (Table 11.1).

APB: Administration of the calculated MED for BoNT-B produced a 77.4% decrement in the injected APB muscle, whereas the MED for BoNT-A produced a 77.8% in this response. At 5x and 25x the MED, both compounds caused nearly complete paralysis of the APB muscle, characterized by a reduction of the CMAP of greater than 95% compared to baseline values. In spite of these profound changes in postsynaptic activity, the onset latency of the residual CMAP (when detectable) and the direct distal measurement of median nerve conduction velocity were unaffected by either BoNT-B or BoNT-A.

Nearby Muscle (FDI): Following an injection confined to the APB muscle, the CMAP in the nearby FDI muscle demonstrated a dose-dependent reduction in peak amplitude for each compound evaluated (Fig. 11.4). At the MED, both compounds induced minimal paralysis (less than 25% reduction in CMAP amplitude). However, at 5xMED, the percent reduction in CMAP after 2 weeks was significantly greater with BoNT-A than BoNT-B (72.0% vs 52.7%, respectively; $p = 0.033$) and even more so at 25xMED (92.8% vs 56.1%, respectively; $p = 0.002$).

Distant Muscle (ADM): The spread of para-

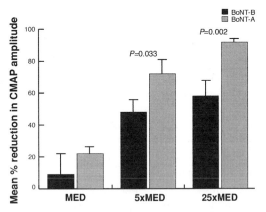

FIG. 11.4. Mean percent reduction in CMAP induced by BoNT-B and BoNT-A in the nearby FDI muscle from baseline to 14 days postinjection. A dose-dependent response is observed for both agents; however, BoNT-B exhibits less spread to a nearby, noninjected muscle.

lytic effects of BoNT-B and BoNT-A were profoundly different in the relatively remote ADM muscle (Fig. 11.5). This muscle is located across the hand from the injection site and does not share a fascial boundary or nerve with the treated muscle. No decrease in the CMAP from baseline to day 14 was observed with BoNT-B at the MED or at 5 times the MED; at 25xMED, BoNT-B produced only a 5.5% reduction in CMAP amplitude. In contrast, a dose-response effect was observed with BoNT-A; percent reductions in CMAP at the MED, 5xMED, and 25xMED, were 9.8%, 27.5%, and 54.8%, respectively. Differences between BoNT-A and

TABLE 11.1. *Direct effect of BoNT-B and BoNT-A at the injected APB muscle*

Dose group	Mean CMAP (mV)		% Reduction in CMAP amplitude
	Baseline	14 Days postinjection	
MED			
0.44 U BoNT-B	7.0	1.6	77.4
0.09 U BoNT-A	6.9	1.5	77.8
5xMED			
2.11 U BoNT-B	8.0	0.3	95.7
0.43 U BoNT-A	6.8	0.0	99.3
25xMED			
10.1 BoNT-B	8.2	0.1	98.9
2.06 BoNT-A	7.5	0.0	99.8

BoNT-A, botulinum toxin type A; BoNT-B, botulinum toxin type B; CMAP, compound muscle action potential; MED, minimum effective dose.

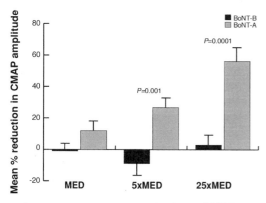

FIG. 11.5. Mean percent reduction in CMAP amplitude of BoNT-B and BoNT-A in the relatively distant ADM muscle from baseline to 14 days postinjection. A dose-dependent response is observed at this distant site for BoNT-A. BoNT-B exhibited minimal spread, even at 25 times the MED.

BoNT-B were significant at both 5x and 25x the MED ($p < 0.001$ and 0.0001, respectively). An analysis of the pattern of induced change in individual muscles is instructive (Fig. 11.6). The highest degree of change in the ADM induced by BoNT-B was one muscle with an approximate 40% loss in muscle strength. In contrast,

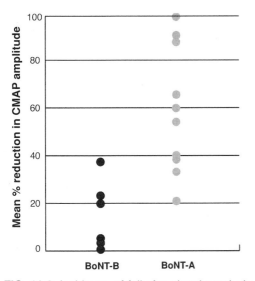

FIG. 11.6. Incidence of fully functional paralysis in the relatively distant ADM muscle at 25xMED for both BoNT-B and BoNT-A.

seven of the ten muscles injected with BoNT-A had a reduction of amplitude exceeding 40%, with three of ten muscles demonstrating functional paralysis (greater than 80% loss of amplitude). Injections of each compound into opposing APB muscles in the same animals minimized the impact of subjective variables (e.g., animal-to-animal differences in sensitivity to BoNT) and anthropometric variables (e.g., weight, activity level).

DISCUSSION

The key finding of the present study is that there is less ''spread'' of the paralytic effects for BoNT-B than is observed for BoNT-A. There are three requirements for the above statement to be clinically meaningful: (a) The cross-compound comparison of spread must have been determined at doses of each compound producing equivalent direct effects in the injected muscle. For a small muscle of the hand (i.e., APB) in the monkey, the equivalent MED doses of BoNT-A (specifically BOTOX) and BoNT-B (specifically MYOBLOC) have a ratio of approximately 1:5. This ratio should not be directly generalized to human studies or to larger muscles. In the present study, spread was always examined using equal multiples of the MED for each compound. (b) Spread effects must have been determined using a dose range similar to that used in therapy. The mid-dose of BoNT-A used in the present study corresponds to a dose of approximately 10 U of BOTOX in humans after correcting for differences in cross-species muscle mass. This dose overlaps the clinical usage of BOTOX for the injected APB muscle. (c) The assessment of induced change in noninjected muscles must have been measured by using a technique that is both sensitive to relatively subtle deficits and specific to alterations in neuromuscular transmission. A parametric reduction in the amplitude of the CMAP, coupled with normal conduction parameters in distal motor axons, meets each of these criteria and is a well-accepted clinical measure.

Spread as a Safety Concern

The greater spread associated with BoNT-A is evident in both nearby and relatively remote muscles, but the differences across compounds are especially clear for the more distant sites. Both BoNT-B and BoNT-A exhibited a dose-dependent spread of partial paralytic effects to a nearby, noninjected muscle. This type of spread may be desirable in some clinical circumstances; for instance, in treatment of spasticity. However, in most therapeutic uses, spread can have substantial negative consequences. For instance, in the treatment of blepharospasm, the toxin can spread to the levator muscle to cause ptosis or to the extraocular muscles to induce a vertical strabismus (42,43). In a similar manner, injections targeting various muscles in the neck can cause unwanted "side effects" reflecting changes in pharyngeal and laryngeal muscles (e.g., reference 44). The reduced spread associated with BoNT-B may be especially appreciated in the cosmetic use of BoNT, where fine control and the ability to accurately predict the spatial limits of the induced effect are of paramount value.

Spread of BoNT effects to relatively distant sites is never desirable in clinical practice. Generalized weakness is a rare occurrence in BoNT therapy; however, a recent report highlighted case histories of three patients that developed generalized muscle weakness consistent with mild botulism following treatment with BoNT-A (30). Denervation in distant muscles was confirmed on biopsy in one of these patients. In a large survey of patients treated for idiopathic cervical dystonia (45), generalized weakness was reported as an adverse event in 2.3% of patients (16 of 685) following treatment with BoNT-A (DYSPORT); "neck muscle weakness" was reported in 17.2% of these subjects. In contrast, neither generalized weakness nor focal neck weakness was reported as an adverse event in the two recent clinical trials examining BoNT-B (MYOBLOC) for the treatment of cervical dystonia (31,32).

Evidence of subclinical changes in distant muscles following BoNT therapy is cause for concern when considering the treatment of patients with possible disease-related preexisting loss of neurotransmission. The safety margin in these patients may be reduced and they may be at increased risk for the remote spread of botuli-

num toxin. Consistent with these concerns, Erbguth et al. (46) discussed a patient with Lambert-Eaton myasthenic syndrome that developed pelvic and shoulder muscle weakness after being treated with BoNT-A for blepharospasm, while Mezaki et al. (47) reported the development of generalized weakness in a patient with amyotrophic lateral sclerosis treated with BoNT-A for spasticity in the lower limbs. The marked reduction in remote spread observed in the present study strongly suggests that BoNT-B may be advantageous in the treatment of "at risk" subjects.

Factors that Influence Spread of BoNT

Injection characteristics: Early studies in the primate established that at a fixed dose, smaller injection volumes resulted in less spread of the toxin to surrounding tissues (48). This has been confirmed in clinical practice, but the optimal volume/dose relationship is often complex, reflecting the need for effective diffusion within a muscle and the desire to minimize the number of injection sites. The bore of the needle, the speed of injection, and the degree of local tissue damage determine the immediate distribution of toxin surrounding the needle tip. The closer the needle is to dense arrays of local cholinergic motor neurons at the motor endplate region, the more effective the paralysis (49) and, presumably, the less unbound toxin is available to spread to noninjected sites. These considerations suggest that the use of EMG-guided injections may impact "spread" as well as accuracy.

Subject characteristics: There are relatively few studies, but as in the adult, BoNT therapy appears to be well tolerated in children (50). However, children may be especially vulnerable to the effects of systemic BoNT spread. Notably, the treatment of multimuscular diseases such as spasticity requires relatively large total doses of BoNT when considered on a unit per kilogram basis. Furthermore, patients with existing conditions, such as pseudobulbar palsy, are especially at risk. Preliminary studies suggest that even when the injection volume is reduced by 50%, the effects of both BoNT-B and BoNT-A exhibit greater spread from a single intramuscular injection in juvenile monkeys compared to adult monkeys (51). On the other end of the spectrum, minimizing "spread" may be an important consideration in BoNT therapy of older subjects. Neuromuscular transmission, as measured by EMG characteristics, is affected by age (e.g., references 52 and 53), and the "safety margin" of transmission may also be influenced by normal aging and by an age-related increase in prevalence of subclinical neuromuscular disorders. Activity level within the injected muscle has also been shown to interact with the degree of paralysis in BoNT therapy (54,55), presumably by increasing local binding of the toxin molecules. Thus, greater activity may minimize the quantity of BoNT compound available for "spread." Finally, a history of previous injections may also influence the degree of BoNT spread. Erdal and colleagues (27) report that activity in the noninjected sternocleidomastoid muscle showed EMG changes after multiple treatments that were not evident during the initial injection cycle. These "long-term" changes in noninjected muscles could reflect an alteration in a central motor program, as suggested by the authors, or, alternatively, they could represent an increase in "spread" secondary to muscle atrophy and a reduction in binding sites in the repetitively injected contralateral muscle.

Toxin characteristics: As evident from the data presented in this study, the specific compound used may significantly alter the nearby and distant spread effects of BoNT therapy. There is no definitive study of the properties of BoNT-B and BoNT-A following intramuscular injection, but there are important biochemical differences in these compounds (reviewed in references 33 and 34). In their natural state, both BoNT-B and BoNT-A exist as a complex, formed by the active neurotoxin and one or more nontoxic proteins. The nontoxic proteins normally serve to protect the toxin when it is ingested orally. For each serotype, the BoNT complex is only stable at slightly acidic pH. The lyophilized preparation of BOTOX (BoNT-A) is usually reconstituted at a pH of 7.3, at which level the botulinum toxin complex may begin to dissociate into subunits of differing molecular weight (i.e., some isolated neurotoxin, some

neurotoxin still in complex). In contrast, MYOBLOC (BoNT-B) is maintained at a pH of 5.6 to ensure the complex remains stable and intact (i.e., uniform molecular weight) during injection. The relatively wide range of molecular weights of the subunits of BOTOX, as compared to the consistent molecular weight of the intact complex for MYOBLOC, may account for the observed differences in their spread patterns (56).

CONCLUSIONS

BoNT therapy is an important option in the treatment of a wide variety of motor and pain disorders. Safety in this form of therapy is related to the degree to which the unbound toxin molecules spread from the injection to surrounding sites and possibly systemically to distant regions. Whereas spread to nearby noninjected muscles may be beneficial in certain clinical circumstances, spread to relatively distant muscles is clearly an adverse effect that impacts the safety of BoNT therapy. In a primate hand model, BoNT-B exhibits less spread of paralytic activity to both nearby and relatively remote muscles than does BoNT-A when the compounds are evaluated at doses producing the same direct effect in the injected muscle. Reduction in spread may be especially important in clinical circumstances requiring substantial control, as well as when treating children and patients with compromised neuromuscular function.

ACKNOWLEDGMENTS

I would like to thank Tina Lin, Shirley Seto, and Linda O'Donnell for their efforts and contributions to this paper.

REFERENCES

1. Burgen ASV, Dickens F, Zatman LJ. The action of botulinum toxin on the neuro-muscular junction. *J Physiol* 1949;109:10–24.
2. Simpson LL. Kinetic studies on the interaction between botulinum toxin type A and the cholinergic neuromuscular junction. *J Pharmacol Exp Ther* 1980;212:16–21.
3. Habermann E, Dreyer F. Clostridial neurotoxins: handling and action at the cellular and molecular level. *Curr Top Microbiol Immunol* 1986;129:93–179.

4. Scott AB, Kennedy KG, Stubbs HA. Botulinum toxin injection as a treatment for blepharospasm. *Arch Ophthalmol* 1985;103:347–350.

5. Jankovic J. Botulinum toxin in movement disorders. *Curr Opin Neurol* 1994;7:358–366.

6. O'Brien CF. Clinical applications of botulinum toxin: implications for pain management. *Pain Dig* 1998;8: 342–345.

7. Mahant N, Clouston PD, Lorentz IT. The current use of botulinum toxin. *J Clin Neurosci* 2001;7:389–394.

8. Simpson DM. Treatment of spasticity with botulinum toxin. *Muscle Nerve* 2000;23:447–449.

9. Grahram HK, Aoki KR, Autti-Rämö I, et al. Recommendations for the use of botulinum toxin type A in the management of cerebral palsy. *Gait Posture* 2000;11: 67–79.

10. Lamanns C. The most poisonous poison. *Science* 1969; 130:763–772.

11. Borodic GE, Joseph M, Fay L, Cozzolino D, et al. Botulinum A toxin for the treatment of spasmodic torticollis: dysphagia and regional toxin spread. *Head Neck* 1990; 12:392–398.

12. Shaari CM, George E, Wu BL, et al. Quantifying the spread of botulinum toxin through muscle fascia. *Laryngoscope* 1991;101:960–964.

13. Borodic GE, Ferrants R, Pearce LB, et al. Histologic assessment of dose-related diffusion and muscle fiber response after therapeutic botulinum A toxin injections. *Mov Disord* 1994;9:31–39.

14. Dodd SL, Rowell BA, Vrabas IS, et al. A comparison of the spread of three formulations of botulinum neurotoxin A as determined by effects on muscle function. *Eur J Neurol* 1998;5:181–186.

15. Ross MH, Charness ME, Sudarsky L, et al. Treatment of occupational cramp with botulinum toxin: diffusion of toxin to adjacent noninjected muscles. *Muscle Nerve* 1997;20:593–598.

16. Buchman AS, Comella CL, Stebbins GT, et al. Quantitative electromyographic analysis of changes in muscle activity following botulinum toxin therapy for cervical dystonia. *Clin Neuropharmacol* 1993;16:205–210.

17. Eleopra R, Tugnoli V, Caniatti L, et al. Botulinum toxin treatment in the facial muscles of humans: evidence of an action in untreated near muscles by peripheral local diffusion. *Neurology* 1996;46:1158–1160.

18. Girlanda P, Quartone A, Sinicropi S, et al. Unilateral injection of botulinum toxin in blepharospasm: single-fiber electromyography and blink reflex study. *Mov Disord* 1996;11:27–33.

19. Weigand H, Erdmann G, Welhöner HH. ^{125}I-labelled botulinum A neurotoxin: Pharmacokinetics in cats after intramuscular injection. *Naunyn Schmiedebergs Arch Pharmacol* 1976;292:161–165.

20. Sanders DB, Massey EW, Buckley EC. Botulinum toxin for blepharospasm: single-fiber EMG studies. *Neurology* 1986;36:545–547.

21. Lange DJ, Brin MF, Warner CL, et al. Distant effects of locally injected botulinum toxin. *Muscle Nerve* 1987; 10:552–555.

22. Lange DJ, Rubin M, Greene PE, et al. Distant effects of locally injected botulinum toxin: double-blind study of single-fiber EMG changes. *Muscle Nerve* 1991;14: 672–675.

23. Olney RK, Aminoff M, Gell DJ, et al. Neuromuscular effects distant from site of botulinum neurotoxin injection. *Neurology* 1988;38:1780–1783.

24. Lange DJ, Brin MF, Fahn S, et al. Distant effects of locally injected botulinum toxin: incidence and course. *Adv Neurol* 1988;50:609–613.

25. Girlanda P, Guiseppe V, Niclosi C, et al. Botulinum toxin therapy: distant effect on neuromuscular transmission and autonomic nervous system. *J Neurol Neurosurg Psychiatry* 1992;55:844–845.

26. Garner CG, Straube A, Witt JN, et al. Time course of distant effects of local injections of botulinum toxin. *Mov Disord* 1993;8:33–37.

27. Erdal J, Østergaard L, Fuglsang-Frederiksen A, et al. Long-term botulinum toxin treatment of cervical dystonia—EMG changes in injected and noninjected muscles. *Clin Neurophysiol* 1999;110:1650–1654.

28. Ansved T, Odergren T, Borg K. Muscle fiber atrophy in leg muscles after botulinum toxin type A treatment of cervical dystonia. *Neurology* 1997;48:1440–1442.

29. Bakheit AMO, Ward CD, McLellian DL. Generalised botulism-like syndrome after intramuscular injections of botulinum toxin type A: a report of two cases. *J Neurol Neurosurg Psychiatry* 1997;62:198.

30. Bhatia KP, Münchau A, Thompson PD, et al. Generalised muscular weakness after botulinum toxin injections for dystonia: a report of three cases. *J Neurol Neurosurg Psychiatry* 1999;67:90–93.

31. Brashear A, Lew MF, Dykstra DD, et al. Safety and efficacy of NeuroBloc (botulinum toxin type B) in type A-responsive cervical dystonia. *Neurology* 1999;53: 1439–1446.

32. Brin MF, Lew MF, Adler CH, et al. Safety and efficacy of NeuroBloc (botulinum toxin type B) in type A-resistant cervical dystonia. *Neurology* 1999;53:1431–1438.

33. Setler P. The biochemistry and preclinical pharmacology of botulinum toxin B. *Neurology* 2000;55(Suppl): S22–S28.

34. Callaway JE, Arezzo JC, Grethlein AJ. Botulinum toxin type B: an overview of its biochemistry and preclinical pharmacology. *Semin Cutan Med Surg* 2001;2: 127–136.

35. Lui J, Lau HK, Pereira BP, et al. Terminal nerve branch entries (motor points) of forearm muscles: a comparative study between monkey and human. *Acta Anat* 1996; 155:41–49.

36. Herrero BA, Ecklund AE, Street CS, et al. Experimental botulism in monkeys: a clinical pathological study. *Exp Mol Pathol* 1967;6:84–95.

37. Scott AB, Suzuki D. Systemic toxicity of botulinum toxin by intramuscular injection in the monkey. *Mov Disord* 1988;3:333–335.

38. Cherington M. Clinical spectrum of botulism. *Muscle Nerve* 1998;21:701–710.

39. Christensen H, LoMonaco M, Dahl K, et al. Processing of electrical activity in human muscle during a gradual increase in force. *Electroencephal Clin Neurophysiol* 1984;58:230–239.

40. Cichon JV Jr, McCaffrey TV, Litchy WJ, et al. The effects of botulinum toxin type A injection on compound muscle action potential in an in vivo rat model. *Laryngoscope* 1995;2:144–148.

41. Moyer ED, Stephens EA, Esch F, et al. Effects of intramuscular injection of botulinum toxin type B in nonhuman primates. In: DasGupta BR ed. *Botulinum and teta-*

nus neurotoxins. New York: Plenum Press, 1993: 655–656.

42. Scott AB, Kennedy RA, Stubbs HA. Botulinum A toxin as a treatment for blepharospasm. *Arch Ophthamol* 1985;103:347–350.

43. Jankovic J. Botulinum A toxin in the treatment of blepharospasm. *Adv Neurol* 1988;49:467–472.

44. Jankovic J, Schwartz K. Botulinum toxin injections for cervical dystonia. *Neurology* 1990;40:277–280.

45. Kessler KR, Skutta M, Benecke R, for the German Dystonia Study Group. Long-term treatment of cervical dystonia with botulinum toxin A: efficacy, safety, and antibody frequency. *J Neurol* 1999;246:265–274.

46. Erbguth F, Claus D, Engelhart A, et al. Systemic effect of local botulinum toxin injections unmasks subclinical Lambert-Eaton myasthenic syndrome. *J Neurol Neurosurg Psychiatry* 1993;56:1235–1236.

47. Mezaki T, Kaji R, Kohara N, et al. Development of general weakness in a patient with amyotrophic lateral sclerosis after focal botulinum toxin injection. *J Am Acad Neurol* 1996;46:845–846.

48. Scott A. Botulinum toxin injection of eye muscles to correct strabismus. *Trans Am Ophthalmol Soc* 1981;79: 734–770.

49. Shaari CM, Sanders I. Quantifying how location and dose of botulinum toxin injections affect muscle paralysis. *Muscle Nerve* 1993;9:964–969.

50. Boyd RN, Graham JEA, Nattras GR, et al. Medium term outcome-response characterization and risk factors analysis of botulinum toxin type A in the management of spasticity in children with cerebral palsy. *Eur J Neurol* 1999;6(Suppl 4):S37–S45.

51. Arezzo JC, Litwak MS, Caputo FA, et al. Spread of paralytic activity of NeuroBloc (botulinum toxin type B) and BOTOX (botulinum toxin type A) in juvenile monkeys: an electrophysiology model. *Eur J Neurol* 2000;7(Suppl):18.

52. Bischoff C, Machetanz J, Conrad B. Is there an age-dependent continuous increase in the duration of the motor unit action potential? *Electroencephal Clin Neurophysiol* 1991;81:304–311.

53. Davidson B, Ludlow CL. Long-term effects of botulinum toxin injections in spasmodic dysphonia. *Ann Otol Rhinol Laryngol* 1996;105:33–42.

54. Eleopra R, Tugnoli V, De Grandis D. The variability in the clinical effect induced by botulinum toxin type A: the role of muscle activity in humans. *Mov Disord* 1997; 12:89–94.

55. Chen R, Karp BI, Goldstein SR, et al. Effects of muscle activity immediately after botulinum toxin injection for writer's cramp. *Mov Disord* 1999;14:307–312.

56. Schantz EJ, Johnson EA. Quality of botulinum toxin for human treatment. In: DasGupta BR, ed. *Botulinum and tetanus neurotoxins.* New York: Plenum Press, 1993; 657–659.

Scientific and Therapeutic Aspects of Botulinum Toxin
edited by M.F. Brin, J. Jankovic, and M. Hallett
Lippincott Williams & Wilkins, Philadelphia, © 2002.

12

The Glycogen Depletion Assay and the Measurement of Botulinum Toxin Injections

Asif Amirali and Ira Sanders

The systemic effects of botulinum toxin A (BTX-A) were first recognized more than 100 years ago (18). However, it was not until 1981 that BTX-A was used as a therapeutic modality by Scott (15). Since then the number of applications of BTX-A has grown significantly. The current range of conditions being treated with intramuscular injection of BTX-A include focal dystonias (blepharospasm; oromandibular-facial-lingual dystonia; cervical dystonia; laryngeal dystonia; task-specific dystonia), various forms of involuntary movement disorders (hemifacial spasm; palatal myoclonus; tics), certain forms of inappropriate contractions (strabismus; nystagmus; myokymia; bruxism; stuttering; achalasia; pelvirectal spasms; spasticity) and some other applications (protective ptosis, cosmetic) (7).

Currently, two major brands of BTX-A are available for clinical purposes. One is marketed under the name BOTOX (botulinum toxin type A purified neurotoxin complex), is manufactured by Allergan Inc. (Irvine, CA) and is licensed worldwide. The other is manufactured by Ipsen (France) and marketed under the name DYSPORT (*Clostridium botulinum* type A toxin-hemagglutinin complex), and is licensed in Europe and Asia. The original and older batch of BOTOX (batch #79–11–83) has been replaced completely by the new batch (batch #CGB-023) during the past 2 to 3 years.

The measure of BTX-A dosage is the "unit," the amount that is lethal to 50% of female Swiss-Webster mice (18 to 20 g) when injected intraperitoneally (LD_{50}) (6). In theory, both BOTOX and DYSPORT should have the same clinical effects when injected at equal doses (LD_{50} units). In practice, however, this is not the case. For example, DYSPORT requires three to four times the dose needed for BOTOX to have a similar therapeutic benefit for torticollis (3,11). In blepharospasm, the standard recommended dose per site for DYSPORT is 20 to 40 LD_{50} units whereas for BOTOX it is 2.5 to 5.0 LD_{50} units (3). Brin and Blitzer (4) had previously suggested a DYSPORT/BOTOX equivalency ratio of approximately 4–5:1. Based on these findings, it can be concluded that the mouse LD_{50} assay fails to accurately predict the relative biologic strength of the toxin after intramuscular injection.

ALTERNATIVES TO THE MOUSE LD_{50} ASSAY

In addition to the mouse LD_{50} assay, there are few techniques available to quantify the distribution of the paralytic effect of BTX-A in an animal model. Scott (15) had used the injection of saline and vital blue mixed with BTX-A into the extraocular muscles of cats and primates to study the diffusion characteristics of BTX-A. Quantification of paralytic effect involved observation of the animal's ocular motion for evidence of paralysis. Pearce et al. (10) have used the technique of hind limb paralysis in mice. In their experiments, the gastrocnemius muscle of mice were injected with different dilutions of BTX-A. Quantification of paralysis was based on visual observation of "complete paralysis," defined as inability of the hind limb to support the weight of mice or use it to escape. Each dilution tested was injected into groups of ten mice. The percentage of mice paralyzed by each dilution was plotted against the log dose and probit analysis was used to define the "median paralysis unit" (MPU). Although useful, this technique still relies on visual observation of "complete paralysis." Wohlfarth et al. (19) used a phrenic nerve-hemidiaphragm preparation in an *in vitro* model. Their method relied on diffusion of the BTX-A in an organ bath containing the phrenic nerve-hemidiaphragm preparation as opposed to being injected as is done under clinical circumstances. Even though this technique has been used reliably in assessing clostridial toxicity, the technique could not be used to quantify the *in vivo* clinical activity of BTX-A.

THE GLYCOGEN-DEPLETION TECHNIQUE

The glycogen-depletion technique quantitates BTX-A activity *in vivo* by histologic methods. The technique of glycogen depletion was first applied by Shaari and Sanders (16) to study diffusion parameters of BTX-A in an animal model. It was subsequently used to study the effects of location, dose and two-dimensional area of BTX-A injection on the paralysis of the guinea pig tibialis anterior (TA) muscle (17), and to compare the biologic effect of various preparations of BOTOX and DYSPORT (Amirali et al. submitted for review).

The basic rationale for the technique is that prolonged electrical stimulation of the nerve to a muscle causes depletion of glycogen within muscle fibers (5). Neuromuscular blockade by BTX-A at the motor endplate blocks neuromuscular transmission to those muscle fibers, hence preserving their glycogen. By measuring the area of preserved glycogen, the site of effective BTX-A action can be inferred.

The technique involves injection of the toxin into the middle of the TA motor endplate band of a rat. A 24-hour delay allows the toxin injection to diffuse within the muscle, bind to motor endplates, and produce neuromuscular blockade. Then the nerve to the TA (common peroneal nerve) is dissected and electrically stimulated until all the glycogen within stimulated muscle

fibers is exhausted. The muscle is then rapidly excised and frozen by immersion in liquid nitrogen, cryosectioned and stained for glycogen with the periodic acid–Schiff reagent (PAS). The fibers that retain their glycogen are assumed to have been paralyzed by the toxin and appear dark in stained sections. The area of dark-stained muscle fibers can be measured using computer analysis software.

The rat TA muscle was chosen because of its large size, surgical accessibility, simple longitudinal arrangement of muscle fibers in its midsection, and homogenous content of type II (fast twitch) muscle fibers, and because glycogen-depletion experiments have been successful using this muscle (5). In addition, the muscle has a simple motor endplate (MEP) band that lies approximately at the level of the midsection of the muscle (17,18) and its location in relation to external landmarks has been clearly defined by staining whole mounts of the muscle for acetylcholinesterase (16,17).

THREE COMMERCIALLY AVAILABLE PREPARATIONS OF BTX-A COMPARED BY USING THE GLYCOGEN-DEPLETION TECHNIQUE

The glycogen-depletion technique was used to compare the currently marketed form of BOTOX (CGB-023), the originally marketed form of BOTOX (79–11–23), and DYSPORT. The experimental procedure is similar to the one employed by Shaari et al. (16,17) and is described in detail below.

The procedure involved injecting a known volume of toxin at a predefined unit concentration into the TA muscle of the rat. Both BOTOX and DYSPORT were received in the marketed form and were reconstituted with normal saline prior to injection to achieve a unit concentration of 0.01 U/μL. The animal was anesthetized using a combination of ketamine (85 mg/kg) and xylazine (15 mg/kg) injected intraperitoneally. The leg to be injected was shaved and immobilized using stereotaxic apparatus. The skin was dissected to expose the midbelly of the muscle. Based on the acetylcholine (ACh) E experiments, the MEP band was located 2 cm below the inferior border of the patella. This landmark was chosen for injection of the BTX-A in all the experiments conducted by Shaari and Sanders (16,17), and Amirali et al. (submitted for review). A small slit was opened in the perimysium at the site of the MEP to facilitate the entrance of the needle for injection. A 10 μL Hamilton syringe (Hamilton Company, Reno, Nevada) was used to inject 5 μL (0.05 U) of each preparation. The value of 0.05 U was chosen after a dose-response study using BOTOX (batch #79–11–83) was conducted to find an amount that caused approximately 50% paralysis. The injection site was 2 cm below the inferior border of the patella, halfway between the medial and lateral borders of the muscle and at a depth of 3 mm from the surface of the muscle. The toxin was injected over a period of 1 minute and the needle left in place for another 10 minutes to allow the toxin to diffuse away from its tip.

After injection the leg was sutured and the toxin allowed to spread in the muscle for a period of 24 hours. After this waiting period, the animal was reanesthetized and the TA was exposed. Using microsurgical equipment the common peroneal nerve to the TA was dissected. A section of the nerve was dissected free from surrounding tissue and placed on bipolar electrodes. The nerve was then stimulated using a Grass S88 stimulator at 3 mA and 20 Hz using biphasic pulses for a total of 20 minutes. Following stimulation, the muscle was immediately excised and fast frozen by using isopentane and dry ice. The animal was sacrificed with a 1 mL dose of phenobarbital. The muscle was then sectioned at 20 μm through the region of the MEP and stained for glycogen using PAS (Sigma Chemical Co., St. Louis, MO). The stained sections were digitally photographed using a Spot-100 digital camera coupled to a Zeiss Axiophot photomicroscope. The muscle fibers where the BTX-A had diffused in sufficient quantities to cause neuromuscular blockade were paralyzed and appeared dark upon staining. Photographs of sections taken through the MEP area were used to measure the area of paralysis.

Nine BOTOX #79–11–83, ten BOTOX #CGB-023, and six DYSPORT injected TA were available for analysis. One rat was used as a control. The right TA of the control rat was injected with normal saline and stimulated as above. Because none of the muscle fibers were paralyzed, all were stimulated and appeared white upon staining. The left TA of the control rat was dissected and stained without any injection or stimulation. All of these fibers retained their glycogen and appeared dark upon staining. The digital images for each BTX-A injected TA as well as the control rat were imported into Sigma Scan PRO, an image analysis software program for area measurement of each photographed section. The average stained area for each TA was then calculated as area of action of BTX-A in the plane of section.

RESULTS

Of the two control TA muscles, the left TA, which was neither injected nor stimulated, appeared completely dark upon staining showing all its muscle fibers contained glycogen (Fig. 12.1A). The right TA, which was injected with normal saline and then stimulated after 24 hours appeared pale after staining, showing that all its muscle fibers had depleted their glycogen (Fig. 12.1B). The staining of BTX-A injected TA appeared somewhere between these two extremes, depending on the BTX-A used.

The mean areas of BTX-A action on the TA and their standard deviations are shown in Table 12.1. Figure 12.2 shows the PAS-stained cross-sections taken from the three BTX-A injected rat TA muscles.

BOTOX VERSUS DYSPORT

The current batch of BOTOX (Fig. 12.2A), batch #CGB-023, appeared to have diffused the most and had the largest area of paralysis, 32.30 mm^2 (SD ± 6.03, $n = 10$). By contrast, DYSPORT (Fig. 12.2C) paralyzed the smallest cross-sectional area of the three tested preparations, equal to 14.60 mm^2 (SD ± 1.44, $n = 6$). The area paralyzed by the original batch of BOTOX (79–11–83) (Fig. 12.2B) lay roughly between these values (23.52, SD ± 4.80, $n = 9$).

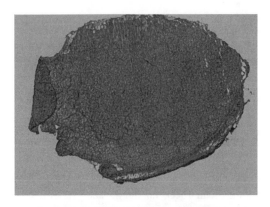

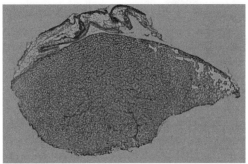

FIG. 12.1. Control rat. (Top) Figure shows a section taken through the left tibialis anterior (TA) muscle in a control rat. The left TA was neither injected not stimulated. (Bottom) Section taken through the right TA muscle in the same rat. This side was injected with saline and the nerve to TA was stimulated as in experimental rats.

CURRENT BOTOX VERSUS ORIGINAL BOTOX

Based upon these experimental conditions, the current batch of BOTOX (CGB-023) has 37% greater diffusion (area of 32.3 mm²) as compared to the original batch (79–11–23) (area of 23.52 mm²). The difference in diffusion activity between the two batches of BOTOX, manufactured by the same company, presumably follow-

ing similar protocols, may be a significant finding.

DISCUSSION

The new batch of BOTOX (batch #CGB-023) appears to have a relatively greater diffusion of the biologic effect at the same unit concentration when compared with DYSPORT, with a BOTOX/DYSPORT equivalency area ratio of 2.2. This does not necessarily translate into greater clinical potency, although a larger dose of DYSPORT is required to achieve similar ther-

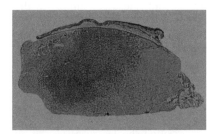

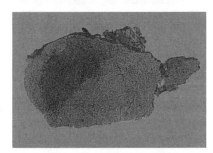

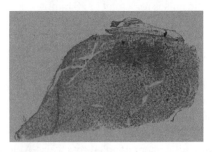

FIG. 12.2. Representative sections taken from the three groups of rats that were injected with either BOTOX batch # CGB 023 (top), BOTOX batch # 79–11–83 (center) or DYSPORT (bottom). Fibers that were paralyzed by the botulinum toxin did not twitch upon stimulation of the nerve to the TA and hence retained their glycogen. These appeared dark upon staining. The average areas of toxin effected paralysis are shown in Table 12.1.

TABLE 12.1. *Area of BTX-A action (mm²)*

	BOTOX# 79–11–83	BOTOX# CGB 023	DYSPORT
Mean	23.52	32.30	14.60
Standard Deviation	4.80	6.03	1.44

apeutic benefits in various clinical conditions. A closer look at the pharmacokinetics of the two preparations may help explain the observed differences.

The pharmacokinetics of the toxin depends to a large extent on the method of producing and refining the toxin. BTX-A is obtained from cultures of *Clostridium botulinum* grown in a fermenter and then harvested by centrifugation after acidification (13,14). The toxin is then solubilized and purified and the solution is checked for contamination, protein content, and potency. The desired amount of toxin is diluted in a medium containing human serum albumin, and then vacuum-dried (BOTOX) or freeze-dried (DYSPORT) and sealed in vials. The toxin is supplied in this lyophilized dry form and has to be reconstituted with saline prior to injection (12–14). Differences in relative biologic activity between the two different batches of BOTOX and DYSPORT may be attributable to variations in the production and purification of the toxin, or the variability within the experimental procedure.

The clinical relevance of these studies is questioned. This is particularly the case because the dose of DYSPORT used in these experiments represents a fraction of the comparable clinically effective dose as compared to BOTOX. In other words, while the dose of BOTOX and DYSPORT used in these experiments is the same, the dose of DYSPORT used in clinical practice is about four to five times the dose of BOTOX (4).

One factor that may account for the difference between BOTOX and DYSPORT is the technique that is used to dilute the toxins during potency testing. During the potency testing stage, DYSPORT is solubilized using gelatin phosphate buffer that is known to increase the potency of BTX-A compared to saline (8). BOTOX on the other hand is tested with saline. Both are reconstituted with saline under clinical settings prior to injection.

Another factor that may explain the apparent difference in the biologic strengths of the two preparations is the amount of albumin present in the lyophilisate. DYSPORT is supplied in vials that contain 500 units of BTX-A, 125 μg

of albumin, and 2.5 mg of lactose (1). On the other hand BOTOX vials supplied for clinical use contain 100 units of BTX-A, 500 μg of albumin, and 0.9 mg NaCl (1). According to Bigalke et al. (1), packaging the finished products with a larger amount of albumin can increase the bioavailability of DYSPORT. The rationale for this is that more protein in the vial prevents the BTX-A (itself a protein) from sticking to the glassware or plastic during the dilution stage, thus making more of the toxin available for injection. In fact, Wohlfarth et al. (19) compared BOTOX and DYSPORT using same dose (units) of toxin, containing the same amount of albumin, at equal concentration and volume, and found no difference in the potencies of the two preparations. That study was performed using the phrenic nerve-hemidiaphragm preparation noted above and tested BOTOX (batch #CGB 001/10/97) and DYSPORT (batch #114/05/97). Our results, however, show a distinct difference between the two preparations, although we used a different batch of BOTOX and DYSPORT. However, Wohlfarth also found a difference in compound muscle action potential (CMAP) of the extensor digitorum brevis muscle in healthy human volunteers after injecting BOTOX (CGB 001/10/97) and DYSPORT (114/05/97) using similar experimental protocols. BOTOX produced a higher amplitude of the CMAP at a lower dose (5 units) of the toxin. The dose of the toxin used in our experiments was 0.05 units, 100 times less than the dose used by Wohlfarth et al. Thus, albumin alone may not fully explain the difference in potencies of the two preparations, especially at lower doses. However, no other study groups, including ours, have addressed this issue.

It is important to evaluate the efficacy of the glycogen-depletion technique because technical aspects of the method could have played a role in the observed differences. The technique used to quantify paralysis in this experiment physiologically traces BTX-A activity. A simple comparison of the BTX-A injected TA muscles with their noninjected counterparts (Fig. 12.1) shows that the technique appears to accurately reflect the activity of the muscle fibers at the extremes of the assay conditions; i.e., when there is no toxin injected and when a maximal dose of toxin is administered. A muscle that has not been injected or actively stimulated would be expected to retain most of its glycogen. This appears to be the case with one TA muscle that was sectioned and stained specifically for this purpose (Fig. 12.1A). On the other hand, the TA muscle without any neuromuscular blockade would recruit all activated muscle fibers upon stimulation, thus losing all of its glycogen (Fig. 12.1B). Shaari et al. used the technique to extensively study the effect of varying the dose and volume of BTX-A on muscle paralysis (17) and found the technique to be very reliable.

One limitation of the technique is that it probably underestimates the actual spread of toxin within the muscle. In any given experiment the toxin undoubtedly would have spread beyond the dark margins seen on the sections. But the quantity of the toxin may not have been sufficient to completely block neural transmission of these muscle fibers. Therefore the stained regions represent the minimum extent of BTX-A induced paralysis and a clinically relevant paralysis may involve more of the muscle (16,17). In our experiment, this factor probably affected all three BTX-A preparations and is the only effect of the toxin that could not be accounted for with this technique. In addition, the area of effect will vary depending on the location of the tissue cross-section studied, and should be normalized to the total cross-section of the muscle section. Furthermore, a full dose-response curve has not been performed. For these reasons, the results should be considered preliminary.

Pearce et al. (8,9) have suggested what they have called the "median paralysis unit" as a more accurate measure of biologic activity of the toxin than the mouse LD_{50} unit. Their method involves quantifying paralysis by using a regional chemodenervation assay, but, as noted earlier, relies on visual observation for complete paralysis. The phrenic nerve-hemidiaphragm technique used by Wohlfarth et al. (19) measures the activity of the toxin in vitro. Besides, as they themselves pointed out, the technique cannot be used to define or quantify the unit; it can only serve as a tool for comparing different preparations. The glycogen-depletion assay used in our study also relies on regional chemodenervation and was also effective in reflecting biologic activity of the different preparations of the BTX-A, but could not indicate the efficacy in other more complex muscle types.

Although our study did not try to define a "unit" for BTX-A activity, an arbitrary cross-sectional area of the TA may be chosen to represent the unit. For example, the rat TA "glycogen-depletion assay unit" (GDU) may equal the amount of toxin which, when injected into the TA of an adult male Sprague-Dawley rat weighing 250 to 300 g, causes chemodenervation of an area equal to 25 mm^2 after a 24-hour period. The 25 mm^2 was arbitrarily chosen because it lies roughly between the average values obtained with DYSPORT (14.6 mm^2) and the new batch of BOTOX (32.3 mm^2). All new preparations of BTX-A could be measured using this assay to define the unit, which would more closely reflect their biologic activity diffusion after the production stage. Further work is needed to establish a dose-response study to determine the dose of each product to achieve a target area of effect for a more accurate comparison.

REFERENCES

1. Bigalke H, Wohlfarth K, Irmer A, et al. Botulinum A toxin: DYSPORT improvement of biological availability. *Exp Neurol* 2001;168:162–170.
2. Deleted in proof.
3. Brin MF. Botulinum toxin: chemistry, pharmacology, toxicity, and immunology. *Muscle Nerve* 1997;Suppl 6: 129–145.
4. Brin MF, Blitzer A. Botulinum toxin: dangerous terminology errors. *J R Soc Med* 1993;86:493–494.
5. Edstrom L, Kugelberg E. Histochemical composition, distribution of fibres and fatiguability of single motor units: Anterior tibial muscle of the rat. *J Neurol Neurosurg Psychiatry* 1968;31:424–433.
6. Hatheway CG, Dang C. Immunogenicity of the neurotoxins of *Clostridium botulinum*. In: Jankovic J, Hallett M, eds. *Therapy with botulinum toxin*. New York: Marcel Dekker, 1994:93–108.
7. Jankovic J, Brin MF. Botulinum toxin. Historical perspective and potential new indications. *Muscle Nerve* 1997;Suppl 6:129–145.
8. Mclellan K, Das RE, Ekong TA, et al. Therapeutic botulinum type A toxin: factors affecting potency. *Toxicon* 1996;34:975–985.
9. Pearce LB, Borodic GE, First ER, et al. Measurement of botulinum toxin activity: evaluation of the lethality assay. *Toxicol Appl Pharmacol* 1994;128:69–77.

10. Pearce LB, Borodic GE, Johnson EA, et al. The median paralysis unit: a more pharmacologically relevant unit of biologic activity for botulinum toxin. *Toxicon* 1995; 33:217–227.

11. Poewe W, Schelosky L, Kleedorfer B, et al. Treatment of spasmodic torticollis with local injections of botulinum toxin. One-year follow-up in 37 patients. *J Neurol* 1992;239:21–25.

12. Schantz EJ, Johnson EA. Dose standardisation of botulinum toxin. *Lancet* 1990;335:421.

13. Schantz EJ, Johnson EA. Properties and use of botulinum toxin and other microbial neurotoxins in medicine. *Microbiol Rev* 1992;56:80–99.

14. Schantz EJ, Johnson EA. Preparation and characterization of botulinum toxin type A for human treatment. In: Jankovic K, Hallet M, eds. *Therapy with botulinum toxin.* New York: Marcel Dekker, 1994:41–49.

15. Scott AB. Botulinum toxin injection of eye muscles to correct strabismus. *Trans Am Ophthalmol Soc* 1981;79: 734–770.

16. Shaari CM, George E, Wu BL, et al. Quantifying the spread of botulinum toxin through muscle fascia. *Laryngoscope* 1991;101:960–964.

17. Shaari CM, Sanders I. Quantifying how location and dose of botulinum toxin injections affect muscle paralysis. *Muscle Nerve* 1993;6:964–969.

18. van Ermengem E. Classics in infectious diseases. A new anaerobic bacillus and its relation to botulism. (Originally published as "Ueber einen neuen anaeroben Bacillus und seine Beziehungen zum Botulismus" in *Zeitschrift fur Hygiene und Infektionskrankheiten* 1897;26: 1–56.) *Rev Infect Dis* 1979;1:701–719.

19. Wohlfarth K, Goschel H, Frevert J, et al. Botulinum A toxins: units versus units. *Naunyn Schmiedebergs Arch Pharmacol* 1997;355:335–340.

CLINICAL DISEASES

Scientific and Therapeutic Aspects of Botulinum Toxin
edited by M.F. Brin, J. Jankovic, and M. Hallett
Lippincott Williams & Wilkins, Philadelphia, © 2002.

13

Clinical Botulism

Stephen S. Arnon

Clinical botulism is the acute, flaccid paralysis caused by the neurotoxins of *Clostridium botulinum,* or, rarely, by an equivalent neurotoxin produced by unique strains of *C. butyricum* or *C. baratii.* Five forms of human botulism are known: infant (intestinal) botulism, foodborne (classical) botulism, wound botulism, inhalational botulism, and iatrogenic botulism. Each form of human botulism has a different pathogenesis and epidemiology.

C. botulinum is a gram-positive, spore-forming obligate anaerobe whose natural habitat worldwide is soil, dust, and marine sediments. Hence, it is frequently found in a wide variety of fresh, as well as cooked, agricultural products. Spores of some *C. botulinum* strains can endure boiling for several hours, which enables the organism on occasion to survive heat-based food preservation techniques. In contrast, botulinum toxin is heat-labile and is easily destroyed by heating at 80°C (176°F) or above for 10 minutes. Little is known about the ecology of neurotoxigenic strains of *C. butyricum* and *C. baratii.*

Botulinum toxin exists in seven antigenic toxin types, arbitrarily assigned the letters A to G. These seven toxin types can be distinguished by the inability of protective (neutralizing) antibody raised against one toxin type to protect against poisoning by a different toxin type (e.g., anti-A antitoxin does not protect against toxins B to G). The seven toxin types are often used as convenient clinical and epidemiologic markers. Neurotoxigenic *C. butyricum* strains produce a type E-like toxin, whereas neurotoxigenic *C. baratii* strains produce a type F-like toxin. Toxin types A, B, E, and F are well-established causes of human botulism, whereas types C and D cause

illness in other animals. Type G was discovered in an Argentinian cornfield in 1970, and has not been established as a cause of either human or animal disease.

Botulinum toxin is the most poisonous substance known (1). Its potency derives from its ability to block neuromuscular transmission and cause death through paralysis of airway and respiratory musculature. As described elsewhere in this volume, the phenomenal, and for two centuries mysterious, potency of botulinum toxin was finally explained by discovery of its enzymatic basis: the seven "light" chains are Zn^{2+}-endopeptidases whose substrates are one or more of three protein components of the "docking complex" by which synaptic vesicles fuse with the terminal cell membrane and release acetylcholine into the synaptic cleft. Of these three substrates, synaptobrevin is cleaved by toxin types B, D, F, and G; SNAP-25 (synaptosomal-associated protein of 25 kDa) is cleaved by toxin types A, C, and E, and syntaxin is cleaved only by toxin type C (2).

PATHOGENESIS

All five forms of human botulism result from a final common disease pathway: botulinum toxin is carried by the bloodstream to peripheral cholinergic synapses, where it binds irreversibly, blocking acetylcholine release and causing impaired autonomic and neuromuscular transmission. Infant (intestinal) botulism is an infectious disease that results from ingesting the spores of any of the three botulinum-toxin–producing clostridial strains, with subsequent spore germination, multiplication, and production of botulinum toxin in the large intestine (3). Although rare, older children and adults also are susceptible to intestinal botulism, which has occurred in the context of either a Meckel's diverticulum or a surgically altered intestinal anatomy, sometimes accompanied by treatment with broad-spectrum antibiotics (4). Foodborne botulism is an intoxication that results from swallowing botulinum toxin already contained in an improperly preserved food (5). Wound botulism results from spore germination and colonization of traumatized tissue by *C. botulinum*; it is the analog of tetanus, but much rarer (6). Inhalational botulism results from accidental or intentional aerosolization of botulinum toxin while attempting to weaponize it or defend against its weaponization; three human cases have been reported (7). Iatrogenic botulism occurs rarely, after therapeutically injected botulinum toxin causes a sustained localized or generalized weakness. Two patients who had preexisting, underlying neurologic diseases (i.e., multiple sclerosis, amyotrophic lateral sclerosis) have been reported in the literature (8,9). One report suggested the possibility that the toxin might have been inadvertently injected into the venous circulation (9). There is also clinical experience with toxin diffusion causing dysphagia severe enough to require intubation and hospital admission in some toxin-treated cervical dystonia patients.

CLINICAL MANIFESTATIONS

All forms of botulism manifest clinically as a symmetric flaccid paralysis that affects and descends from the muscles of the head, face, mouth, and throat. It is not possible to have botulism without having bulbar palsies. This evolution of clinical signs is thought to result from the bloodborne distribution of botulinum toxin and the large relative blood flow and high density of innervation in the cranial nerve musculature. However, in infants, such symptoms as poor feeding, weak suck, feeble cry, drooling, and even obstructive apnea are often not recognized as being bulbar in origin. Patients with evolving illness may already have generalized weakness and loss of muscle tone in addition to cranial nerve palsies when first seen.

In older children with foodborne or wound botulism, the onset of neurologic symptoms follows a characteristic pattern of diplopia, blurred vision, ptosis, dry mouth, dysphagia, dysphonia, and dysarthria, with decreased gag and corneal reflexes. Paresthesias are not seen in botulism except when a patient hyperventilates from anxiety. The sensorium remains clear, but this may be difficult to ascertain because of slurred speech.

Foodborne botulism often begins with gastrointestinal symptoms of nausea, vomiting, and diarrhea. These symptoms are thought to result from metabolic byproducts of growth of *C. botulinum* or from the presence of other toxic contaminants in the food (10), as gastrointestinal distress is not seen in wound botulism. However, constipation is common in foodborne botulism once flaccid paralysis becomes evident. Illness usually begins 12 to 36 hours after ingestion of the contaminated food, but can range from as little as 2 hours to as long as 8 days. The incubation period in wound botulism is 4 to 14 days. Fever may be present in wound botulism but is absent in foodborne botulism unless a secondary infection (e.g., pneumonia) is present. The three natural forms of botulism display a wide spectrum in their clinical severity, ranging from the very mild with minimal ptosis, flattened facial expression, and minor dysphagia and dysphonia, to the fulminant, with rapid onset of extensive paralysis, respiratory distress, and sudden apnea. Fatigability with repetitive muscle activity is the clinical hallmark of botulism.

Infant botulism differs in apparent initial symptoms of illness only because the infant cannot articulate them. Usually, the first indication of illness is constipation (defined as 3 or more days without defecation), although this sign is often overlooked by both parents and physicians. Parents typically notice lethargy, listlessness, poor appetite, weak cry, and diminished activity. Dysphagia may show itself as secretions drooling from the mouth. Gag, suck, and corneal reflexes diminish as the paralysis advances. Oculomotor palsies may be evident only with sustained observation. Paradoxically, the pupillary light reflex may be unaffected until the child is severely paralyzed, or it may be initially sluggish. Loss of head control is typically a prominent sign as the weakness becomes generalized. Respiratory arrest may occur suddenly from airway obstruction by unswallowed secretions or by obstructive flaccid pharyngeal musculature. Occasionally, the diagnosis of infant botulism is suggested by a respiratory arrest that occurs after the infant is positioned for lumbar puncture.

In mild cases, or in the early stages of illness, the physical signs of infant botulism may be subtle and easily missed. Eliciting cranial nerve palsies and fatigability of muscular function requires careful examination. It is common for patients to be seen by several physicians over successive days until the paralysis has become sufficiently evident to suggest the diagnosis. Ptosis may not be seen unless the head of the child is kept erect. The presence of decreased anal sphincter tone may suggest a generalized neuromuscular disease.

The classical picture of botulism is the acute onset of (a) a flaccid descending paralysis with (b) a clear sensorium, and (c) no fever. The rarity of foodborne and wound botulism makes them easily confused with other diseases. Routine laboratory studies, including the cerebrospinal fluid, are normal in botulism unless dehydration or starvation ketosis is present. Electromyography (EMG) may demonstrate a defect in neuromuscular transmission, and the typical EMG finding in foodborne and wound botulism is facilitation (potentiation) of the evoked muscle action potential at high frequency (50 Hz) stimulation. In infant botulism a characteristic pattern, known by the acronym BSAP (brief, small, abundant motor-unit action potentials), is present in clinically weak muscles (11).

The diagnosis of botulism is established by demonstrating the presence of botulinum toxin in serum, or of *C. botulinum* toxin or organisms in wound material or feces. *C. botulinum* is not part of the normal resident intestinal flora of humans, and its presence in the setting of acute flaccid paralysis is diagnostic. Suspected botulism represents a medical and public health emergency that is required to be reported immediately in virtually all United States health jurisdictions. An epidemiologic diagnosis of foodborne botulism can be made when *C. botulinum* organisms and toxin are found in a food item incriminated by ingestion history.

Management of botulism rests on four principles: (a) fatigability with repetitive muscle activity is the clinical hallmark of the disease; (b) complications are best avoided by anticipating them; (c) meticulous supportive care is necessary; and (d) botulinum antitoxin should be given as quickly as possible. Correct positioning (as illustrated in reference 1) is especially important in nonintubated patients in order to protect the airway and improve respiratory mechanics.

A rising PCO_2 signals alveolar hypoventilation and irreversible muscle fatigue. Endotracheal intubation should be done prophylactically to maintain airway patency and to avoid aspiration. About one-half of hospitalized patients will need intubation. Tracheostomy is seldom required because with proper positioning, patients with flaccid paralysis of their pharyngeal musculature (and its reflexes) can tolerate intubation for weeks or months without permanent sequelae.

Feeding should be done by nasogastric or nasojejunal tube until sufficient oropharyngeal strength and coordination has returned to enable oral feedings. Tube feeding also assists in the restoration of peristalsis, a nonspecific but probably essential part of eliminating *C. botulinum* from the intestinal flora. Intravenous feeding (hyperalimentation) is discouraged because of the potential for infection and the advantages of tube feeding.

Antibiotic therapy is not part of the treatment of uncomplicated intestinal or foodborne botulism because the toxin is primarily an intracellular molecule that is released into the intestinal lumen with vegetative bacterial cell death and lysis. Antibiotics should be reserved for the treatment of secondary infections, and in this setting, a nonclostridiocidal antibiotic such as trimethoprim/sulfamethoxazole or nalidixic acid is preferred. Aminoglycoside antibiotics should be avoided because they may potentiate the blocking action of botulinum toxin at the neuromuscular junction.

Equine botulinum antitoxin is indicated for the treatment of foodborne and wound botulism. Wound botulism also requires aggressive treatment with antibiotics and surgical débridement in a manner analogous to tetanus. The current commercially available botulinum antitoxin is a horse serum-derived product that has side effects of serum sickness, anaphylaxis, and potential life-long sensitization to equine proteins. A human-derived botulinum antitoxin specifically for the treatment of infant botulism, formally known as Botulism Immune Globulin Intravenous (Human) (BIG-IV), demonstrated encouraging results in its pivotal clinical trial in California (mean hospital stay was shortened by more than 3 weeks) (3). BIG is now available in the United States for the treatment of infant botulism under a US Food and Drug Administration-approved Treatment Investigational New Drug protocol. BIG-IV may be obtained by telephoning the California Department of Health Services (510-540-2646 day or night) (12). A licensure application for BIG-IV was submitted to the Food and Drug Administration in mid-2001.

Prevention of the complications of botulism is best accomplished by anticipatory avoidance. The best such efforts notwithstanding, some critically ill paralyzed patients who spend weeks or months on ventilators in intensive care units inevitably develop complications. Patients with botulism display little daily variation while their nerve endings regenerate, and medical staff need to guard against complacency. Infant botulism does not have a relapsing course, and suspected "relapses" usually reflect premature hospital discharge or an undiscovered underlying complication, such as pneumonia.

The healing process in botulism occurs through sprouting of temporary new terminal unmyelinated motoneurons that substitute for the paralyzed nerve terminal. Movement then resumes. Clinically and in experimental animals, this process averages about 4 weeks. A longer-term reinnervation by the parent nerve terminal eventually occurs, with dying back of the temporary sprouts (13).

In the United States, the case:fatality ratio for hospitalized infant botulism is less than 1%, a tribute to the availability and high quality of intensive care. In other countries, the experience has not been as fortunate. The case:fatality ratio in foodborne and wound botulism varies by age, with younger patients having the best prognosis. Some adults with botulism have reported chronic weakness and fatigue as sequelae.

Without BIG-IV treatment, hospital stay in infant botulism averages approximately 1 month. However, length of hospital stay differs significantly by toxin type, with type B cases hospitalized a mean of 3.7 weeks and type A cases a mean of 5.6 weeks. Infant botulism is also a costly illness. For all California patients in the years 1984–1994, hospital costs averaged $2,700 per day in constant 1995 dollars (physician fees not included). Twenty-five percent of patients had hospital stays costing $100,000 or more; the most expensive case was hospitalized for 10 months at a cost in excess of $890,000.

PREVENTION OF CLINICAL BOTULISM

Foodborne botulism is best prevented by adhering to safe methods of home canning (pressure cooker and acidification), by avoiding suspicious foods, and by heating all home-canned foods to 80°C (176°F) for at least 10 minutes. Wound botulism is best prevented by thorough cleansing and surgical débridement of contaminated traumatic injuries with provision of appropriate antibiotics and by avoiding illicit drugs.

Circumstantial evidence suggests that most infant botulism patients first inhaled and then swallowed airborne clostridial spores; such cases are presently unpreventable. The one identified, avoidable source of C. botulinum spores for infants is honey, and all major pediatric and public health agencies in the United States have recommended that honey not be fed to an infant younger than 1 year old. Corn syrups were once thought to be a possible source of botulinum spores, but recent evidence indicates otherwise (3). Breast-feeding appears to slow the onset of infant botulism and to diminish the risk of respiratory arrest in infants in whom the disease develops (3), most probably through its influence on the composition of the intestinal flora and through the immune factors that it contains.

Immunization to prevent botulism can be accomplished through use of botulinum toxoid, an Investigational New Drug that is used mainly to protect laboratory personnel against accidental exposure to botulinum toxin. Botulinum toxoid was also used to immunize Allied troops during the 1991 Gulf War because intelligence reports had identified the production capability for botulinum toxin in Iraq (1,14,15). After the war this capacity was confirmed by the United Nations inspection teams, to whom Iraq admitted to having produced at least 19,000 L of concentrated botulinum toxin, of which approximately 10,000 L had been placed in missiles and artillery shells (14,15). Iraq is just one of several nations believed to be weaponizing botulinum toxin (1). The emergence of botulinum toxin as a therapeutic agent (see elsewhere in this volume) provides a compelling reason to immunize only those persons who need botulinum toxoid for their occupational safety, in that immunity to a particular toxin type deprives a person of ever receiving the therapeutic benefit of that toxin type.

THERAPEUTIC USES OF BOTULINUM TOXIN

However paradoxical it may have once seemed, botulinum toxin over the past decade has risen to the status of "wonder drug" (16,17). As this volume describes, it is used to treat a variety of diseases characterized by spasm or overactivity, or a particular muscle or group of muscles. In many of these illnesses, the muscular hyperactivity is the primary disorder (e.g., cervical dystonia), while in other illnesses it is secondary to another disease (e.g., multiple sclerosis). In most of these conditions, intramuscular injection of botulinum toxin is the treatment of choice and has replaced previous and much-less–satisfactory surgical or pharmacologic alternatives. Clinically effective paralysis with botulinum toxin typically lasts from several weeks to several months (16,17).

The widespread applicability of botulinum toxin's ability to relax tense muscles originates in the work of two investigators. Alan Scott was the ophthalmologist who pioneered preclinical evaluation of botulinum toxin in monkeys and its subsequent clinical use in patients with strabismus (wandering eye) and blepharospasm. Edward Schantz was the protein chemist who had crystallized botulinum toxin type A and provided it on request to Scott (16). Botulinum toxin type A was licensed by the US Food and Drug Administration (FDA) in December 1989 for the treatment of blepharospasm and strabismus, thus culminating more than a decade of collaborative effort by Scott and Schantz. In December 2000, FDA licensed both types A and B botulinum toxins for the treatment of cervical dystonia.

Once the effectiveness of botulinum toxin had become evident to clinicians, its application to other disorders of muscle contraction and movement quickly followed (16,17). The list of disorders for which botulinum toxin is being evaluated continues to lengthen and now includes smooth-muscle (gastrointestinal, genitourinary) disorders as well as a variety of skeletal muscle conditions that are the subject of other chapters in this book. Botulinum toxin has even found extensive cosmetic use in the removing of frown lines and "crow's feet" wrinkles on the face and in blocking excessive axillary sweating.

The clinical use of botulinum toxin is not without its problems. There are several side-effects. Unwanted paralysis of adjacent muscles (e.g., ptosis obscuring vision, dysphagia resulting in aspiration) results from the diffusion of toxin away from the injection site. This complication limits the amount of toxin that can be injected at a given treatment session. Other side effects include a transient "influenza-like" syndrome suggestive of an allergic reaction and the development of neutralizing antibodies that render the patient resistant to further treatment.

Clinical experience with botulinum toxin continues to accumulate rapidly, and international conferences on its use now occur with regularity. Even so, further refinement and improvement in its usefulness can be expected in the years ahead. It is likely that additional botulinum toxin serotypes will come into widespread use, including type C toxin, which uniquely of the eight clostridial neurotoxins has syntaxin as its substrate. Also, various combinations of toxins will likely be tried in order to prolong the duration of desired weakening or of frank paralysis (e.g., a mixture of toxins A, B, and C would sever the three different substrates), and the problem of neutralizing antibody formation will probably be solved (12). Finally, molecular engineering of the toxins may improve their duration of action or permit delivery of the light chain to other cell types, where it could block unwanted secretory activity.

The paradoxical emergence of the world's most poisonous substance as a therapeutic marvel during the very years that at least one nation was preparing to use it as a weapon of mass destruction illustrates again the constant potential for the perversion of scientific knowledge. This paradox reemphasizes the need for humanitarian principles always to prevail in the use of such knowledge, as well as the need for leadership in ensuring that such weapons will never be used.

REFERENCES

1. Arnon SS, Schechter R, Inglesby TV, et al. Botulinum toxin as a biological weapon: medical and public health management. Consensus Statement of the Working Group on Civilian Biodefense. *JAMA* 2001;285; 1059–1070.
2. Schiavo G, Rossetto O, Tonello F, et al. Intracellular targets and metalloprotease activity of tetanus and botulism neurotoxins. *Curr Top Microbiol Immunol* 1995; 195:257–274.
3. Arnon SS. Infant botulism. In: Feigin RD, Cherry JD, eds. *Textbook of pediatric infectious diseases, 4th ed.* Philadelphia: WB Saunders, 1998:1570–1577.
4. Fenicia L, Franciosa G, Pourshaban M, et al. Intestinal toxemia botulism in two young people, caused by *Clos-tridium butyricum* type E. *Clin Infect Dis* 1999;29: 1381–1387.
5. Shapiro RL, Hatheway C, Swerdlow DL. Botulism in the United States: a clinical and epidemiologic review. *Ann Intern Med* 1998;129:221–228.
6. Werner SB, Passaro D, McGee J, et al. Wound botulism in California, 1951–1998: recent epidemic in heroin injectors. *Clin Infect Dis* 2000;31:1018–1024.
7. Holzer VE. Botulism from inhalation [in German]. *Med Klin* 1962:57:1735–1738.
8. Mezaki T, Kaji R, Kohara N, et al. Development of general weakness in a patient with amyotrophic lateral sclerosis after focal botulinum toxin injection. *Neurology* 1996;46:845–846.
9. Bakheit AMO, Ward CD, Mclellan CL. Generalised botulism-like syndrome after intramuscular injections of botulinum toxin type A: a report of two cases. *J Neurol Neurosurg Psychiatry* 1997;62:198.
10. Smith LDS. *Botulism: the organism, its toxins, the disease.* Springfield, IL: Charles C Thomas Publisher, 1977.
11. Johnson RO, Clay SA, Arnon SS. Diagnosis and management of infant botulism. *Am J Dis Child* 1979;133: 586–593.
12. Arnon SS. Clinical trial of human botulism immune globulin. In: DasGupta BR, ed. *Botulinum and tetanus neurotoxins: neurotransmission and biomedical aspects.* New York: Plenum Press, 1993:477–482.
13. de Paiva A, Meunier FA, Molgo J, et al. Functional repair of motor endplates after botulinum neurotoxin type A poisoning: biphasic switch of synaptic activity between nerve sprouts and their parent terminals. *Proc Natl Acad Sci U S A* 1999;16;96:3200–3205.
14. Zilinskas RA. Iraq's biological weapons: the past as future? *JAMA* 1997;278:418–424.
15. Shoham D. Iraq's biological warfare agents: a comprehensive analysis. *Curr Rev Microbiol* 2000;263: 179–204.
16. Jankovic J, Hallet M, eds. *Therapy with botulinum toxin.* New York: Marcel Dekker, 1994.
17. Moore P, ed. *Handbook of botulinum toxin treatment.* Oxford: Blackwell Science, 1995.

Scientific and Therapeutic Aspects of Botulinum Toxin
edited by M.F. Brin, J. Jankovic, and M. Hallett
Lippincott Williams & Wilkins, Philadelphia, © 2002.

14

Clinical Aspects of Tetanus

John C. Morgan and Thomas P. Bleck

The first recorded description of tetanus involved an ancient Egyptian patient who developed nuchal rigidity and trismus (lockjaw) following a penetrating skull wound (1,2). Hippocrates and his Greek contemporaries were also keenly aware of the clinical manifestations of tetanus and the mortality associated with the disease (3). In 1888, approximately two millennia later, Sir William Gowers (4) provided an eloquent description of tetanus:

Tetanus is a disease of the nervous system characterized by persistent tonic spasm, with violent brief exacerbations. The spasm almost always commences in muscles of the neck and jaw, causing closure of the jaws (trismus, lockjaw), and involves muscles of the trunk more than those of the limbs. It is always acute in onset, and a very large proportion of those who are attacked die.

Four years prior to Gower's description, Nicolaier (5) identified a strychnine-like toxin produced by anaerobic soil bacteria. Work published in 1890 by Behring and Kitasato (6) demonstrated that immunization with an inactivated extract of this bacteria (*Clostridium tetani*) prevented tetanus. This led to passive tetanus immunization of United States military personnel in World War I and active tetanus immunization during World War II, which resulted in a substantial decrease in tetanus in this population (7,8). Widespread immunization has reduced reported tetanus cases to approximately 40 to 60 per year in the United States and 12 to 15 cases per year in Great Britain over the last decade (9). Despite marked reduction of tetanus cases in developed countries with national immunization programs, tetanus continues to afflict approxi-

mately one million people annually worldwide (8).

While the morbidity and mortality for treatment of tetanus has declined over the past 50 years, the costs of treating patients with this disease has increased as a consequence of the expensive and intensive care they require. The proper use of worldwide immunization strategies could help to eliminate the needless loss of lives and massive expenditure of resources to treat these patients.

EPIDEMIOLOGY

Today there are between 800,000 and 1 million deaths caused by tetanus annually throughout the world (8,10), suggesting a mortality rate of approximately 16 per 100,000 population per year. This number, however, has a high degree of uncertainty because reported cases of tetanus are significantly lower than this estimate. In 1981, the mortality rate for Africa was estimated at 28 per 100,000 population; in Asia 15 per 100,000 population; in Europe, 0.5 per 100,000 population; and in North America less than 0.1 per 100,000 population (11). While the number of reported cases in the United States has dropped from approximately 500 per year in the late 1940s to around 30 to 40 per year currently (Fig. 14.1), there are 120,000 deaths annually in Africa from neonatal tetanus alone, and it can account for 10% to 30% of infant mortality in many countries (12). Neonatal tetanus accounts for about half of the total number of cases worldwide and has a mortality rate between 80% and 90% (13,14). Approximately 80% of the worldwide neonatal tetanus cases occur in Africa and southeast Asia (15). There were an estimated

Tetanus Cases in the United States
1947–2000

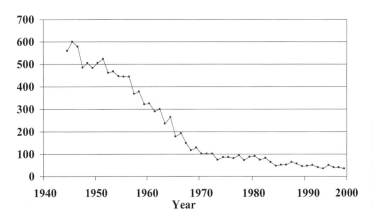

FIG. 14.1. Reported cases of tetanus in the United States from 1947 to 2000. (Data from the annual Summaries of Notifiable Diseases, published by the US Centers for Disease Control and Prevention.)

500,000 worldwide deaths from neonatal tetanus in 1994; however, since the 1980s it is estimated that the number of deaths from neonatal tetanus has been reduced by half through vaccination, before or during pregnancy, and with clean delivery and cord care (16).

TABLE 14.1. *Etiology of US tetanus cases, 1972–1989 excluding neonates*[a]

Etiologic factor	Number of patients	Percentage
Acute injuries	996	78
Type of injury		
Punctures	349	35
Lacerations	329	33
Other or unknown	318	32
Cause of wound		
Outdoor injury	268	21
Indoor injury	370	29
Animal-related	38	3
Surgical wound	38	3
Major trauma	51	4
Unknown circumstances	230	18
Not acute injury-related	268	22
Chronic wound	179	15
Parenteral drug abuse	26	2
No apparent source	65	5

[a] Data from the US Centers for Disease Control and Prevention. Table 14.1 was adapted from Bleck TP, Brauner JS. Tetanus. In: Scheld WM, Whitley RJ, Durack DT, eds. *Infections of the Central Nervous System, 2nd ed.* Philadelphia: Lippincott-Raven, 1997:629–653.

Adults who contract tetanus are predominantly male; presumably because of greater exposure of men to injuries that can lead to tetanus (17–19). The populations at risk today in the United States are the young (persons younger than 20 years of age), the elderly (persons older than 60 years of age), immigrants, and intravenous drug abusers (20–22). The etiologies of reported tetanus cases in the United States are categorized in Table 14.1. In underdeveloped countries, those at highest risk are newborns and agricultural workers (11).

PATHOGENESIS

Clostridium tetani is an obligately anaerobic gram-positive bacillus that produces spores found throughout indoor and outdoor environments. When the redox potential of inoculated tissue is low, these spores germinate into bacteria and proliferate. *C. tetani* produces two exotoxins: tetanospasmin (''tetanus toxin'') and tetanolysin. Tetanolysin has unclear clinical significance; however, it may aid in the damage of viable tissue near the wound site, lowering the redox potential, and allowing for continued growth of anaerobes, perhaps by disrupting membrane channels (23,24).

Tetanospasmin causes all the typical clinical manifestations of tetanus. It is synthesized as a single 151 kDa polypeptide (25,26) that is cleaved by a bacterial protease into a heavy chain (100 kDa) and a light chain (50 kDa) (27), connected by a disulfide bridge (28). These chains are thought to be involved in different phases of toxin binding, cell entry and toxicity. The main action of tetanospasmin is inhibition of neurotransmitter release at the presynaptic nerve terminal (29), which accounts for the clinical presentation of tetanus. The toxin first binds to the presynaptic membrane (30) and then passes through the cell membrane by an unknown mechanism; perhaps through uncoated vesicles or by making pores in cell membranes (31). The toxin then appears to enter the cytoplasm via an acidic vacuole (similar to diphtheria toxin) (32). Once in the cytoplasm of the presynaptic nerve terminal, tetanospasmin cleaves synaptobrevin (33), an essential protein for docking neurotransmitter-filled vesicles to the membrane. Cleavage of synaptobrevin prevents vesicular fusion with the synaptic membrane and subsequent neurotransmitter release.

Retrograde and transsynaptic transport of tetanospasmin from the neuromuscular junction (NMJ) near the site of inoculation, to the spinal cord, and ultimately to the brain, explains its widespread effects on the nervous system (34). The heavy chain of the toxin is necessary for the retrograde transport of the toxin to the soma. Given these unique properties, portions of tetanus toxin have been used extensively in neuroanatomical studies and as a vehicle for delivery of neurotrophic factors (35) or lysosomal enzymes (36) to neurons. Tetanospasmin also is hematogenously spread, but must enter the nervous system via retrograde transport in neurons (37). Extraneuronal tetanus toxin is potentially accessible to circulating antibodies, however, toxin which is intraneuronal or intraaxonal is not, and this helps explain the delay in improvement for several days after initiation of treatment.

Once transported to the spinal cord or brainstem, tetanospasmin prevents glycine or gamma-aminobutyric acid (GABA) release from presynaptic inhibitory neurons (38). Without this inhibitory input, alpha motor neurons increase their resting firing rate, leading to muscle rigidity. Normal relaxation of antagonist muscles is subsequently impaired, and the motor system responds to an afferent stimulus with an intense, sustained contraction of a wide range of muscles characteristic of a tetanic spasm.

Autonomic dysfunction caused by tetanus presents with tachycardia; labile hypertension; cardiac arrhythmias; peripheral vasoconstriction; pyrexia; profuse perspiration; increased carbon dioxide output; and increased urinary catecholamine excretion (39). Tetanospasmin disinhibits sympathetic reflexes at the spinal cord level (40); however, possible hypothalamic involvement is supported by the development of the syndrome of inappropriate antidiuretic hormone secretion (SIADH) (41). There are usually signs of a hypersympathetic state in patients with tetanus near the end of the first week or developing in the second week (42). Patients with tetanus occasionally develop bradycardia and hypotension (43), as well as disruptions in gastric motility (44), raising the likelihood that parasympathetic function is also disrupted.

Blockade of the NMJ in tetanus was demonstrated more than 60 years ago (45). More recent single-fiber electromyography studies demonstrate a presynaptic defect in the release of acetylcholine similar in quality to botulism (46). The NMJ may be permanently disabled by tetanospasmin and the return of muscle fiber function appears dependent on axonal sprouting and formation of new synapses (47). Occasionally, significant weakness and decreased muscle tone in tetanus is present and tetanospasmin's effect on the NMJ is a possible cause.

CLINICAL MANIFESTATIONS OF TETANUS

Tetanus infection often follows a local inoculation through a puncture wound, burn, postpartum infection of the uterus, umbilical stump of newborns, compound fracture, or nonsterile intramuscular injection (48). In up to 30% of patients, however, there are no identifiable routes of infection (49). The time it takes for patients to develop their first symptom after inoculation with *C. tetani* spores is termed the *incubation period*. The length of the incubation period appears to be directly related to the distance of the inoculation site from the central nervous system (CNS); i.e., wounds inoculated in the foot usually have a longer incubation period than do wounds of a more proximal site. This period can range from 24 hours to months and an incubation period of less than 1 week is associated with a poor prognosis (44). The time it requires for patients to progress from their first symptom to their first reflex spasm is the *period of onset.* A period of onset that is less than 48 hours also implies a poor prognosis (44).

The clinical description of tetanus syndromes preceded the determination of tetanus' pathophysiology and so distinctions between clinical entities do not reflect differences in mechanisms. They do reflect variations in the site of tetanus toxin action, however, as the toxin acts at the neuromuscular junction predominantly in some forms and predominantly in central inhibitory systems in others. The terminology defined below has remained in use because these clinical classifications are prognostically useful.

Generalized tetanus is the most commonly recognized form of the disease. Patients with this form of the disease demonstrate trismus (lockjaw), diffuse muscular rigidity, and generalized muscle spasms. They may also complain of pain and headache in addition to these symptoms. Trismus—the inability to fully open the mouth because of rigidity of the masseter muscles—is the most common presenting sign. Trismus often results in the classic finding of *risus sardonicus* (Fig. 14.2), a facial expression that consists of lateral extension of the corners of the mouth, raised eyelids, and wrinkling of the forehead. This may be a subtle finding requiring comparison to old photographs of the patient to be distinguishable. Involvement of other muscle groups can follow the onset of trismus; first the neck, then the thorax and abdomen, and finally the extremities. Generalized spasms resemble opisthotonus (Fig. 14.3), decerebrate posturing or even seizures and are elicited by both external (noises, drafts of air, touching the patient) and internal (full bladder, coughing) stimuli. The spasms are extremely painful, last for a few seconds to minutes and occur at irregular intervals. Full consciousness is retained during the spasms, which helps to differentiate them from

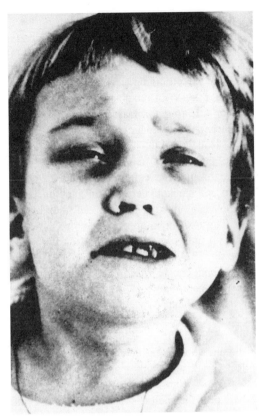

FIG. 14.2. Risus sardonicus in a child. (From Veronesi R, Focaccia R. The clinical picture. In: Veronesi R, ed. *Tetanus: Important New Concepts.* Amsterdam: Excerpta Medica, 1981;183–206, with permission.)

seizures or decerebrate posturing. It is interesting to note that tetanospasmin is epileptogenic in experimental models, (50) however, true epileptic seizures in tetanus are rare except in the setting of hypoxia.

Early in the course of generalized tetanus respiratory compromise is the most serious problem. Spasms can lead to laryngeal obstruction and death by asphyxiation. Abdominal rigidity can result in apnea and this is a distinguishing feature in differentiating tetanus from strychnine poisoning. Deep-tendon reflexes are usually hyperactive. Autonomic dysfunction, usually occurring within a week of the first generalized spasm, is the leading cause of death in tetanus patients (51) since the advent of mechanical ventilation and modern respiratory care. The disease

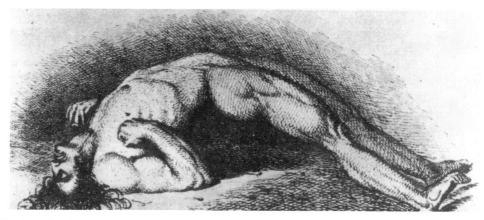

FIG. 14.3. Sir Charles Bell's sketch of a soldier with typical opisthotonic posturing associated with tetanus. (From Bell C. *Essays on the Anatomy and Physiology of Expression, 2nd ed.* London: J Murray, 1824.)

may continue to progress over 10 to 14 days, reflecting the time required for the toxin to be transported into the central nervous system. Recovery usually begins by the second or third week, and often requires up to 4 weeks to become complete. Without antitoxin, tetanus can persist for as long as the toxin is produced. Patients who survive tetanus have little in the way of natural immunity and recurrent tetanus is well documented, because the quantity of tetanospasmin produced in tetanus is usually insufficient to stimulate an immune response (52,53).

There are multiple acute complications of tetanus, including rhabdomyolysis, hyperthermia, autonomic dysfunction usually manifested by a hypersympathetic response, and vertebral fractures (especially in older patients) (54). Barring the psychiatric effects of an episode of tetanus, long-term complications are uncommon. Rarely calcifications and contracture may occur in damaged muscles (55), and compressive neuropathies and compartment syndromes have also been described.

With the advent of modern mechanical ventilation and respiratory care, the mortality of tetanus has decreased from greater than 90% over a century ago to approximately 26% in the United States today (56,57). Although autonomic complications are the most common cause of death today, infections and pulmonary thromboembolism also remain important.

Localized tetanus is characterized by painful fixed rigidity of the muscles at or near the site of *C. tetani* inoculation. This may be mild and remain localized for weeks or months, and usually resolves spontaneously. Deep-tendon reflexes are often brisk and tetanospasmin may affect the NMJ, causing weakness, as well as rigidity. Partial immunity may prevent hematogenous spread and generalized tetanus; however, unless treated, localized tetanus frequently evolves into the generalized form.

Cephalic tetanus occurs with injuries to the head or neck and it is frequently associated with concomitant *C. tetani* and aerobic bacterial infection in otitis media (58,59). Patients on presentation usually have facial paresis and occasionally dysphagia (60) or ophthalmoparesis (61) can occur. The incubation period is usually brief (1 to 2 days) and this unusual form of tetanus can evolve into the generalized form if left untreated.

Neonatal tetanus is a generalized form of the disease and is far more common in Third World countries than in the developed world. In the eighteenth century, neonatal tetanus was termed the "7-day disease" in the Americas (62) and was known as the "9-day fits" in Dublin, Ireland (63). By 1887, it was known that the umbilical stump was the major portal of entry for *C. tetani* in this form of the disease (64). A variety of childbirth practices can result in contamination of the umbilical stump with *C. tetani* spores, including application of manure, soil, banana extracts, coffee or tobacco (65,66). Of diseases that are preventable by vaccination, tetanus is only second to measles as a cause of childhood mortality (67). Lack of maternal immunity to tetanus is necessary for the development of this form of the disease as mothers who are immune or immunized during pregnancy confer immunity to the infant for several weeks by transfer of maternal antibody. Four factors play a role in developing neonatal tetanus: (a) the cleanliness of the environment; (b) the cleanliness of the instruments and dressings; (c) the length of the stump (a shorter stump appears to increase risk); and (d) the care with which the cord is ligated (68). The incubation period averages approximately 1 week; however it can range from 1 day to as long as 4 weeks. The mortality rate is between 80% and 90% with the largest numbers of deaths in the first week of the disease. The infants usually present during the second week of life with irritability, weakness, and a poor suck. Typical opisthotonic posturing associated with tetanic spasms occurs later, and it is important to differentiate tetanus from neonatal seizures or other metabolic abnormalities which cause posturing in this age group. A hypersympathetic state (as described above) is frequently the cause of death. Unlike the usual full neurologic recovery in adults or children who survive a bout of tetanus, neonates may have permanent motor neuron loss (69) and developmental delay (70).

DIAGNOSIS

Tetanus remains a clinical diagnosis, and a clinical picture of trismus, muscle rigidity, stimulus-induced tetany, and a history of a wound or injury within the last 3 weeks are highly suggestive of the disease. Neonatal tetanus should be suspected in a newborn with poor feeding and increased muscle rigidity and spasms, especially in the setting of poor umbilical hygiene or in an unimmunized mother. In countries where tetanus is common, the diagnosis is usually made in a timely fashion; however, diagnosis in the developed world is often delayed, presumably

because of the infrequent presentation of the disease (71). In the United States today, it is important to suspect tetanus in the elderly population because of waning immunity and lack of reimmunization (21,72). Electromyography may demonstrate denervation, reinnervation and increased alpha motor neuron excitability (73). *C. tetani* is rarely cultured from wounds, blood/serum studies are usually normal or nonspecific, and cerebrospinal fluid studies are also usually normal. Laboratory studies in the diagnosis of tetanus primarily exclude other conditions and help to determine the patient's immune status.

Table 14.2 illustrates considerations in the differential diagnosis of tetanus. Strychnine is a direct antagonist at the glycine receptor and most closely mimics tetanus (74). A differentiating factor between strychnine intoxication and tetanus is a usual lack of abdominal muscle rigidity between spasms in strychnine poisoning and trismus frequently occurs later with strychnine. A history of strychnine ingestion may aid in the diagnosis, and biochemical analysis may reveal the toxin in body fluids. Dystonic reactions induced by antipsychotics or other dopamine antagonists can be confused with tetanus. Torticollis and oculogyrate crisis are dystonic reactions seen with these drugs; however, they do not occur in tetanus. Treatment of the dystonic reaction with an anticholinergic agent, such as benztropine or diphenhydramine, can further differentiate dystonia from tetanus. Meningismus and nuchal rigidity associated with meningitis can also be rarely confused with tetanus, but the history and cerebrospinal fluid analysis should help clinicians differentiate between the two conditions. Hypocalcemic tetany is often accompanied by Chvostek's sign (spasm in the facial muscles elicited by tapping the facial nerve in the region of the parotid gland) and Trousseau's phenomenon (tapping the palm and eliciting a muscle spasm). Tetany caused by hypocalcemia is exacerbated by hyperventilation and is easily confirmed by routine serum chemistries. Hypocalcemic tetany is further distinguished from tetanus in that it usually involves the extremities rather than the axial musculature and trismus is less common. Generalized tonic-clonic seizures can be confused with tetanus; however, patients

TABLE 14.2. *Differential diagnosis of tetanus*[a]

Possible diagnosis	Distinctions from tetanus
GABA antagonist intoxication (e.g., strychnine)	Lack of rigidity between spasms; biochemical analysis
Dystonic reaction to dopamine blockade (e.g., haloperidol)	Oculogyric crisis; lateral head turning; biochemical analysis; rapid response to anticholinergic treatment
Meningitis (producing nuchal rigidity)	Severe headache; rigidity confined to the neck; Kernig's and Brudzinski's signs; cerebrospinal fluid analysis
Alveolar abscess (mimicking trismus)	Local pain and tenderness; dental radiographs
Generalized convulsive status epilepticus	Loss of consciousness; clonic movements; electroencephalogram
Acute abdominal pathology (producing abdominal rigidity)	Nausea and vomiting; rebound tenderness; abdominal distention or ileus
Hypocalcemic tetany	Chvostek's and Trousseau's signs; exacerbation by hyperventilation; predominance of extremity rather than axial symptoms; biochemical analysis
Stiff-person syndrome	Insidious course; late (or no) lower cranial involvement; absence of trismus; relaxation during sleep
Psychogenic ("pseudotetanus")	Complex or inconsistent posturing; lack of rigidity; distractability; secondary gain may be evident

[a] Adapted from Bleck TP. Clincal aspects of tetanus. In: Simpson LL, ed. *Botulinum Neurotoxin and Tetanus Toxin*. San Diego: Academic Press, 1989:379–398.

with tetanus have preservation of consciousness unlike the former. Both of these conditions do respond to benzodiazepines. Rarely, acute abdominal pathology can cause abdominal rigidity and orofacial infections can mimic trismus. "Stiff-person syndrome" (75) is distinguished from tetanus by an insidious onset, lack of lower cranial nerve involvement usually, absence of trismus and relaxation during sleep. "Pseudotetanus" is a conversion disorder in which the patients movements resemble tetanus. These patients are often easily distracted, they have inconsistent complex movements or postures, and there may be an element of secondary gain.

Determination of immunity to tetanus by obtaining an adequate immunization history is usually sufficient as the failure rate of immunization when properly administered is approximately 4 per 100 million immunocompetent persons (76). Serum concentrations of antitetanus antibodies should be determined in all patients with suspected tetanus, not as an initial diagnostic or management tool, as these assays may take days, but to help retrospectively exclude the diagnosis. An antitoxin level of 10 mIU/mL is usually considered protective, however there are reports of cases of tetanus with higher serum concentrations of antibody, even up to 160 mIU/mL (77). A recent population-based study demonstrated

that antibody levels wane with aging (20), however, it is extremely rare for a person to contract tetanus after completion of a primary tetanus series (78).

TREATMENT

Patients with generalized or neonatal tetanus often require mechanical ventilation and intensive care to survive. A review of 335 consecutive tetanus patients prior to the establishment of an intensive care unit (ICU) revealed a mortality rate of 44% (79). After organization of an ICU, the subsequent mortality rate was reduced to 15% in 306 consecutive tetanus patients (79). Prevention of deaths as a result of acute respiratory failure was the major improvement in this study. The mainstays of therapy include: (a) neutralizing existing toxin before it enters the nervous system; (b) inhibiting further production of tetanus toxin; (c) muscle relaxation and sedation; (d) controlling autonomic instability; and (e) ventilatory, nutritional, and general ICU support. Table 14.3 illustrates a protocol for treatment of generalized tetanus. Neonatal tetanus should also be managed using this protocol, recognizing that the autonomic therapies have not been extensively studied in infants and active

TABLE 14.3. *Management protocol for generalized tetanus*[a]

Diagnosis and stabilization: first hour after presentation

A. Assess airway and ventilation. If necessary, prepare for endotracheal intubation and NMJ blockade (e.g., ve-curonium, 0.1 mg/kg).
B. Obtain samples for antitoxin level; strychnine and dopamine antagonist assays; electrolytes; blood urea nitrogen; creatinine; creatine kinase; and urinary myoglobin determination. If meningitis is part of the patient's differential diagnosis, perform a lumbar puncture.
C. Determine the portal of entry, incubation period, period of onset, and immunization history.
D. Administer 1 to 2 mg of intravenous (IV) benztropine or 50 mg of IV diphenhydramine to aid in excluding a dystonic reaction (see text).
E. Administer an IV benzodiazepine (diazepam in 5-mg increments or lorazepam in 2-mg increments) to control spasms and to decrease rigidity. Initially employ a dose adequate to produce sedation and minimize reflex spasms. If this dose compromises the airway or ventilation, intubate using a short-acting neuromuscular blocking agent before transferring the patient to a quiet, darkened area of the ICU.

Early management phase: first 24 hours
A. Administer human tetanus immunoglobulin (HTIG) 500 units intramuscularly (IM).
B. At a different site, administer IM an adsorbed tetanus toxoid such as tetanus-diphtheria vaccine (0.5 mL) or diphtheria-tetanus-pertussis vaccine (0.5 mL) as appropriate for age. Adsorbed tetanus toxoid without diphtheria toxoid is available for patients with a history of reaction to diphtheria toxoid; otherwise, the correct combination for the patient's age should be employed.
C. If intrathecal administration of antitoxin is being considered, it should be administered at this point (not the standard of care in the United States).
D. Begin IV metronidazole 500 mg given every 6 hours for 7 to 10 days.
E. Perform a tracheostomy after placement of an endotracheal tube and under NMJ blockade if spasms produce any degree of airway compromise, or if dysphagia or difficulty managing secretions occurs.
F. Débride the wound if this is indicated for its own management (this has no apparent effect on the course of tetanus).
G. Place a soft, small-bore orogastric feeding tube or a central venous hyperalimentation catheter.
H. Administer benzodiazepines as needed to control spasms and produce sedation. If adequate control is not achieved, institute long-term NMJ blockade (e.g., with a vecuronium infusion or intermittent pancuronium injections). Continue benzodiazepines for sedation with electroencephalographic monitoring to ensure somnolence.
I. Initiate physical therapy for pulmonary toilet and passive range or motion as soon as the patient has been stabilized pharmacologically. Additional sedation should be given before each treatment, and again during the treatment if the therapy provokes spasms.

Intermediate management phase: next 2 to 3 weeks
A. Treat sympathetic hyperactivity with IV labetalol (0.25 to 1.0 mg/min) or morphine (0.5 to 1.0 mg/kg/h). Consider epidural blockade with local anesthetics. Avoid diuretics for blood pressure control, because volume depletion will worsen autonomic instability.
B. If hypotension is present, place a pulmonary artery catheter and an arterial line, and administer fluid boluses, dopamine, or norepinephrine.
C. Sustained bradycardia usually requires a pacemaker. Atropine or isoproterenol may be useful during pacemaker placement. External pacing should be avoided unless the patient is under NMJ blockade.
D. Begin prophylactic subcutaneous heparin and/or sequential compression devices to help prevent pulmonary embolism.
E. Use a flotation bed, if possible, to prevent skin breakdown and peroneal nerve palsies. Otherwise, ensure frequent turning and employ antirotation boots.
F. Maintain benzodiazepines until NMJ blockade, if employed, is no longer necessary, and the severity of spasms has diminished substantially. Taper the dose over 14 to 21 days.
G. Begin rehabilitation planning.

Convalescent stage: 2 to 6 weeks
A. When spasms are no longer present, begin physical therapy. Many patients require supportive psychotherapy.
B. Before discharge, administer another dose of the appropriate tetanus toxoid combination.
C. Schedule a third dose of toxoid to be given 4 weeks after the second dose is given.

[a] Adapted from Bleck TP, Brauner JS. Tetanus. In: Scheld WM, Whitley RJ, Durack DT, eds. *Infections of the Central Nervous System, 2nd ed.* Philadelphia: Lippincott-Raven, 1997:629–653.

immunization should not be administered to infants before 6 weeks of age.

Once the clinical diagnosis of generalized tetanus is made, treatment should begin with intravenous diazepam or lorazepam to control spasms and to reduce rigidity. Endotracheal intubation should be performed if necessary to maintain airway control and early tracheostomy is advocated by some authors (80). Patients should receive a single intramuscular injection of 500 IU of human tetanus immunoglobulin (HTIG) (81) to help neutralize circulating tetanospasmin that has not entered the nervous system. While 250 units of intrathecal HTIG was superior to 1,000 IU administered intramuscularly in one study (82), other studies have failed to demonstrate benefit (83,84). Intrathecal HTIG therapy is not approved by the United States Food and Drug Administration and preparations available here often contain preservatives that may be toxic by this route (54). Equine antitetanus serum may be more readily available in underdeveloped regions, but there is a much higher incidence of hypersensitivity reactions (20%) with this preparation. It is usually dosed at 500 to 1,000 IU/kg intravenously or intramuscularly and has a half-life of only 2 days as compared to HTIG, which has a half life of 24.5 to 31.5 days (9).

Wound débridement helps to prevent secondary infection, but does not change the course of the disease. If no portal of entry is readily identified, the patient should be carefully examined for otitis media, uterine infections, needle marks, and foreign bodies. Antibiotic treatment should be initiated at presentation, and one study demonstrated that metronidazole is superior to penicillin, allowing significantly less progression of the disease, shorter hospitalization, and improved survival (7% mortality with metronidazole vs 24% with penicillin) (85). A more recent randomized trial in Viet Nam involving more than 1,000 tetanus patients treated with metronidazole or penicillin failed to demonstrate a difference in mortality (86). Patients who received metronidazole, however, appeared to require fewer muscle relaxants and sedatives (86). Five hundred mg of metronidazole should be administered intravenously for 7 to 10 days to complete treatment. If metronidazole is not available, 100,000 to 200,000 IU/kg/d of penicillin should be administered intramuscularly or intravenously for 7 to 10 days.

Muscle relaxation is best accomplished with benzodiazepines or baclofen, which act as GABA-receptor agonists. Diazepam and lorazepam are most commonly used; however, midazolam is also effective. Large doses of these agents may be required for treatment of spasms and rigidity—occasionally, greater than 500 mg/d of diazepam, 200 mg/d of lorazepam, or a continuous infusion of 0.1 to 0.3 mg/kg/h of midazolam may be required. Intrathecal administration of baclofen is also effective for spasms (87,88). If benzodiazepines or baclofen are unsuccessful in controlling muscle spasms, then neuromuscular blockade is necessary. Vecuronium (6 to 8 mg/h) is often the agent of choice because it is less likely to cause autonomic instability (89). Pancuronium bromide (bolus of 0.1 mg/kg, then infusion of 0.3 to 0.6 µg/kg/min) can also be used when vecuronium is not available; however, this drug is associated with hypertension, tachycardia, and elevated cardiac output (90), which is often confused with autonomic instability caused by tetanus. Rocuronium was ineffective in controlling tetany and spasms in a recent case report (91).

Autonomic instability is managed by a variety of agents. The treatment of choice in the hypersympathetic state of tetanus is combined alpha- and beta-adrenergic blockade with intravenous labetalol (92). Esmolol, clonidine, morphine sulfate, atropine, and magnesium sulfate may be useful alternatives; however, agents that predominantly act as beta-blockers should be avoided because of unopposed alpha-adrenergic vasoconstriction (48). Spinal or epidural bupivacaine also improves hemodynamic instability in some cases. Bradycardia may necessitate placement of a temporary pacemaker and hypotension may require fluid boluses and treatment with pressors.

The nutritional requirements of tetanus patients can be extraordinary. With adequate sedation, control of spasms, and suppression of autonomic hyperactivity, however, the nutritional requirements in these patients are similar to other critically ill patients. The protein and calories required to maintain adequate nutrition may exceed the maximal tolerable daily volume of enteral formulas (93). Gastric emptying may be impaired and central venous hyperalimentation may be necessary.

Common acute complications of tetanus infection today include respiratory and urinary tract infections related to mechanical ventilation and use of indwelling catheters, respectively (94). Other common complications include rhabdomyolysis with subsequent renal failure (95), vertebral compression fractures in older patients (96), developmental delay in neonatal cases (97), and psychological after-effects in up to 40% of patients who survive (98). As described earlier, autonomic instability is the main cause of mortality in locales where ICU care is available.

PREVENTION

Tetanus has been described as an "inexcusable disease" (99) because of our ability to effectively prevent the condition by active immunization with formaldehyde-treated tetanus toxoid. The health care costs of treating one case of generalized tetanus equals the cost of immunizing several thousand people (100). Three intramuscular injections of alum-adsorbed tetanus toxoid (ten lyophilized units, 0.5 mL) provide almost complete immunity for 5 years. Routine immunization in the infant usually begins between 6 weeks and 2 months of age followed by two subsequent immunizations at 1- to 2-month intervals. A fourth vaccination should be given 1 year after the third, and a fifth vaccination should be given between 4 and 7 years of age. Children younger than 7 years of age should receive the combined diphtheria-tetanus-acellular pertussis (DTaP) vaccine, whereas individuals

older than 7 years of age should receive tetanus-diphtheria (Td) vaccine lacking the pertussis component (Advisory Committee on Immunization Practices guidelines). Patients older than 7 years of age who have not received a primary immunization series should receive Td vaccine on three occasions, with the second dose being administered 1 to 2 months after the first, and the third dose being administered 6 months to 1 year after the second. The complete series must be given in order to ensure adequate antibody titers and routine boosters should be administered every 10 years thereafter.

Neonatal tetanus remains a significant problem in the Third World because of large numbers of nonimmune women of child-bearing age. Recently, a single dose of tetanus toxoid was administered in the third trimester to pregnant women who lacked immunity and protective antibody titers were conferred on both the mothers and their babies (101). Given the extremely high mortality of neonatal tetanus (the World Health Organization estimated 515,000 deaths in 1993), worldwide vaccination strategies are especially targeted at this form of the disease.

Studies also demonstrate that both human immunodeficiency virus (HIV)-infected adults and infants have the ability to develop protective tetanus antibody titers (102,103). In contrast, patients undergoing bone marrow transplantation require reimmunization 9 to 12 months after transplant as they lose their preexisting tetanus immunity (104,105).

After a tetanus-prone injury (punctures, burns, contaminated wounds, frostbite, avulsions, and crush injuries) immunization should be performed if no tetanus booster has been given within the last 5 years (Table 14.4). An injured patient should be given Td vaccine if the

TABLE 14.4. *Tetanus wound management*[a]

Vaccination history	Clean, minor wounds		All other wounds	
	Td	TIG	Td	TIG
Unknown or <3 doses	Yes	No	Yes	Yes
3+ doses	No*	No	No**	No

* Yes, if greater than 10 years since last dose
** Yes, if greater than 5 years since last dose
[a] Based on current US Centers for Disease Control and Advisory Committee on Immunization Practices Guidelines.

patient has not received a dose within the last 10 years. If an immunization history is incomplete or unavailable for the patient, then a series of three monthly Td injections should be performed. HTIG (250 to 500 IU) should be administered concomitantly to patients with an unknown vaccination history, particularly if the wound is tetanus prone.

At the time of this writing, there is a shortage of Td vaccine as a result of Wyeth-Ayerst Laboratories' decision to stop producing the vaccine. The remaining major manufacturer of the vaccine, Aventis Pasteur, subsequently increased production, but there will be a shortage in the United States, and perhaps worldwide, for a while. This appears to be secondary to a ''business decision'' and may reflect the lower profit margin with this vaccine as compared to other patented drugs. Aventis increased the price of the Td vaccine to $6 per dose in 1999, and according to some, this vaccine remains ''grossly underpriced.'' This shortage may be clinically important as there are an estimated 25 million doses of Td vaccine administered in the United States each year.

Current research is aimed at creating improved methods of immunization. A sustained-release preparation of tetanus toxoid may be available in the future, which may allow for a vaccination schedule with fewer doses (106). Oral immunization was possible in mice by genetically engineering a live mutant *Salmonella typhi* strain to carry a fragment of the tetanospasmin gene (fragment C) (107) and oral or nasal administration of liposome-incorporated tetanus toxoid appears possible (108). A recombinant form of tetanus toxin was also shown to be 30 times more potent than the native toxin in preventing tetanus in mice (109).

CONCLUSIONS

Tetanus is a disease that we have thoroughly studied for more than 2,000 years. Despite an inexpensive, widely available vaccine, tetanus continues to remain a significant health concern in developing countries. It is hoped that advances in immunization technology and worldwide immunization programs will reduce future morbidity and mortality and virtually eliminate the disease similar to smallpox.

REFERENCES

1. Breasted JH. *The Edwin Smith surgical papyrus.* Chicago: University of Chicago Press, 1930.
2. Ghalioungui P. *Magic and medical science in ancient Egypt.* London: Hodder & Stoughton, 1963.
3. Adams F. *The extant works of Aretaeus, the Cappadocian.* London: Publications of the Sydenham Society, 1856.
4. Gowers WR. *A manual of diseases of the nervous system.* Philadelphia: Blackiston, 1888:1027–1049.
5. Nicolaier A. Ueber infectiösen tetanus. *Dtsch Med Wochenschr* 1884;10:842–844.
6. Behring E, Kitasato S. Üeber das zustandekommen der diphtherie-immunität und der tetanus-immunität bei thieren. *Dtsch Med Wochenschr* 1890;16:1113–1114.
7. Edsall G. Specific prophylaxis of tetanus. *JAMA* 1959; 171:417–427.
8. Sanford JP. Tetanus forgotten but not gone [Editorial]. *N Engl J Med* 1995;332:812–813.
9. Farrar JJ, Yen LM, Cook T, et al. Tetanus. *J Neurol Neurosurg Psychiatry* 2000;69:292–301.
10. Dietz V, Milstien JB, van Loon F, et al. Performance and potency of tetanus toxoid: implications for eliminating neonatal tetanus. *Bull World Health Organ* 1996;74:619–628.
11. Cvjetanovic B. Public health aspects of tetanus control. In: Veronesi R, ed. *Tetanus: important new concepts.* Amsterdam: Excerpta Medica, 1981:1–7.
12. Health Communications and Public Relations. *Childhood diseases in Africa: neonatal tetanus.* World Health Organization Fact Sheet N 109. March 1996; available at: http://www.who.ch/programmes/inf/facts/fact109.htm.
13. Cvjetanovic B, Grab B, Uemura K, et al. Epidemiological model of tetanus and its use in the planning of immunization programmes. *Int J Epidemiol* 1972;1: 125–137.
14. Schofield F. Selective primary health care: strategies for control of disease in the developing world. XXII. Tetanus: a preventable problem. *Rev Infect Dis* 1986; 8:144–156.
15. Whitman C, Belgharbi L, Gasse F, et al. Progress towards the global elimination of neonatal tetanus. *World Health Stat Q* 1992;45:248–256.
16. Gasse, F. *Elimination of neonatal tetanus will save 1 million newborns annually.* World Health Organization Press Release 1994; available at: http://www.who.ch/press/1994/pr94–07.html.
17. Edmonson RS, Flowers MW. Intensive care in tetanus: management, complications and mortality in 100 cases. *Br Med J* 1979;1:1401–1404.
18. Trujillo MH, Castillo A, Espana JV, et al. Tetanus in the adult: intensive care and management experience with 233 cases. *Crit Care Med* 1980;8:419–423.
19. Harding-Goldson H, Hanna WJ. Tetanus: a recurring intensive care problem. *J Trop Med Hyg* 1995;98: 179–184.
20. Gergen PJ, McQuillan GM, Kiely M, et al. A population-based serologic survey of immunity to tetanus in the United States. *N Engl J Med* 1995;332:761–766.

21. Alagappan K, Rennie W, Kwiatkowski T, et al. Seroprevalence of tetanus antibodies among adults older than 65 years. *Ann Emerg Med* 1996;28:18–21.

22. Bardenheier B, Prevots DR, Khetsuriani N, et al. Tetanus surveillance—United States, 1995–1997. *Mor Mortal Wkly Rep CDC Surveill Sum* 1998;47:1–13.

23. Blumenthal R, Habig WH. Mechanisms of tetanolysin-induced membrane damage: studies with black lipid membranes. *J Bacteriol* 1984;157:321–323.

24. Rottem S, Groover K, Habig WH, et al. Transmembrane diffusion channels in *Mycoplasma gallisepticum* induced by tetanolysin. *Infect Immun* 1990;58:598–602.

25. Craven CJ, Dawson DJ. The chain composition of tetanus toxin. *Biochim Biophys Acta* 1973;317:277–285.

26. Matsuda M, Yoneda M. Dissociation of tetanus neurotoxin into two polypeptide fragments. *Biochem Biophys Res Commun* 1976;57:1257–1262.

27. Bergey GK, Habig WH, Bennett JI, et al. Proteolytic cleavage of tetanus toxin increases activity. *J Neurochem* 1989;53:155–161.

28. Krieglstein K, Henschen A, Weller U, et al. Arrangement of disulfide bridges and positions of sulfhydryl groups in tetanus toxin. *Eur J Biochem* 1990;188:39–45.

29. Bleck TP. Pharmacology of tetanus. *Clin Neuropharmacol* 1986;9:103–120.

30. Middlebrook JL. Cell surface receptors for protein toxins. In: Simpson LL, ed. *Botulinum neurotoxin and tetanus toxin.* San Diego: Academic Press, 1989;95–119.

31. Schmid MF, Robinson JP, DasGupta BR. Direct visualization of botulinum neurotoxin-induced channels in phospholipid vesicles. *Nature* 1993;364:827–830.

32. Williamson LC, Neale EA. Bafilomycin A1 inhibits the action of tetanus toxin in spinal cord neurons in cell culture. *J Neurochem* 1994;63:2342–2345.

33. Schiavo G, Benfenati F, Poulain B, et al. Tetanus and botulinum-B neurotoxins block neurotransmitter release by proteolytic cleavage of synaptobrevin. *Nature* 1992;359:832–835.

34. Manning KA, Erichsen JT, Evinger C. Retrograde transneuronal transport properties of fragment C of tetanus toxin. *Neuroscience* 1990;34:251–263.

35. Bordet T, Castelnau-Ptakhine L, Fauchereau F, et al. Neuronal targeting of cardiotropin-1 by coupling with tetanus C fragment. *Mol Cell Neurosci* 2001;17:842–854.

36. Dobrenis K, Joseph A, Rattazzi MC. Neuronal lysosomal enzyme replacement using fragment C of tetanus toxin. *Proc Natl Acad Sci U S A* 1992;89:2297–2301.

37. Price DL, Griffin JW. Tetanus toxin: retrograde axonal transport of systemically administered toxin. *Neurosci Lett* 1977;4:61–65.

38. Curtis Dr, Felix D, Game CJA, McCulloch RM. Tetanus toxin and the synaptic release of GABA. *Brain Res* 1973;51:358–362.

39. Kerr JH, Corbett JL, Prys-Roberts C, et al. Involvement of the sympathetic nervous system in tetanus. *Lancet* 1968;2:236–241.

40. Parr GH, Wellhoner HH. The action of tetanus toxin in preganglionic sympathetic reflex discharges. *Naunyn Schmiedebergs Arch Pharmacol* 1973;276:437–445.

41. Potgieter PD. Inappropriate ADH secretion in tetanus. *Crit Care Med* 1983;11:417–418.

42. Corbett JL, Harris PJ. Studies on the sympathetic nervous system in tetanus. *Naunyn Schmiedebergs Arch Pharmacol* 1973;276:447–460.

43. Ambache N, Lippold OCH. Bradycardia of central origin produced by injections of tetanus toxin into the vagus nerve. *J Physiol* 1949;108:186–196.

44. Habermann E. Tetanus. In: Vinken PJ, Bruyn GW, eds. *Handbook of clinical neurology.* Amsterdam: North-Holland, 1978;33:491–547.

45. Harvey AM. The peripheral action of tetanus toxin. *J Physiol* 1939;96:348–365.

46. Fernandez JM, Ferrandiz M, Larrea L, et al. Cephalic tetanus studied with single-fibre EMG. *J Neurol Neurosurg Psychiatry* 1983;46:862–866.

47. Duchen LW, Tonge DA. The effects of tetanus toxin on neuromuscular transmission and on the morphology of motor endplates in slow and fast skeletal muscle of the mouse. *J Physiol* 1973;228:157–172.

48. Bleck TP, Brauner JS. Tetanus. In: Scheld WM, Whitley RJ, Durack DT, eds. *Infections of the central nervous system, 2nd ed.* Philadelphia: Lippincott-Raven, 1997:629–653.

49. Udwadia FE. *Tetanus.* New York: Oxford University Press, 1994.

50. Jeffrys JG, Borck C, Mellanby J. Chronic focal epilepsy induced by intracerebral tetanus toxin. *Ital J Neurol Sci* 1995;16:27–32.

51. Luisto M, Iivanainen M. Tetanus of immunized children. *Dev Med Child Neurol* 1993;35:351–355.

52. Spenney JG, Lamb RN, Cobbs CG. Recurrent tetanus. *South Med J* 1971;64:859.

53. Brust JCM, Richter RW. Tetanus in the inner city. *N Y State Med J* 1974;74:1735–1742.

54. Bleck TP. Clincal aspects of tetanus. In: Simpson LL, ed. *Botulinum neurotoxin and tetanus toxin.* San Diego: Academic Press, 1989:379–398.

55. Asa DK, Bertorini TE, Pinals RS. Myositis ossificans circumscripta: a complication of tetanus. *Am J Med Sci* 1986;292:40–43.

56. Dowell VR. Botulism and tetanus: selected epidemiologic and microbiologic aspects. *Rev Infect Dis* 1984;6(Suppl 1):S202–S207.

57. Morbidity and Mortality Weekly Reports. Tetanus—United States, 1982–1984. *MMWR Morb Mortal Wkly Rep* 1985;34:601–611.

58. Patel JC, Kale PA, Mehta BC. Otogenic tetanus: study of 922 cases. In: Patel JC, ed. *Proceedings of an international conference on tetanus, Bombay.* 1965;640–644.

59. deSouza CE, Karnard DR, Tilve GH. Clinical and bacteriologic profile of the ear in otogenic tetanus: a case control study. *J Laryngol Otol* 1992;106:1051–1054.

60. Lathrop DL, Griebel M, Horner J. Dysphagia in tetanus: evaluation and outcome. *Dysphagia* 1989;4:173–175.

61. Saltissi S, Hakin RN, Pearce J. Ophthalmoplegic tetanus. *Br Med J* 1976;1:437.

62. de Ulloa A. *Noticias Americanas: entretenimientos physicohistorios.* Madrid, 1772. Cited in: Mettler CA, Mettler FA. *History of medicine.* Philadelphia: Blakiston, 1947:745–746.

63. Clarke J. An account of a disease which until lately proven fatal to a great number of infants in the Lying-In Hospital of Dublin. *Med Facts Observ* 1792;3:78–104.

Cited in: Mettler CA, Mettler FA. *History of medicine.* Philadelphia: Blakiston, 1947:746.

64. Beumer O. Zur aitologischen Bedeutung der Tetanus-bacillen. *Berl Klin Wochenschr* 1887;00:541–543, 575–577. Cited in: Mettler CA, Mettler FA. *History of medicine.* Philadelphia: Blakiston, 1947.

65. Veronesi R, Focaccia R. The clinical picture. In: Veronesi R, ed. *Tetanus: important new concepts.* Amsterdam: Excerpta Medica, 1981;183–206.

66. Kandeh BS. Causes of infant and early childhood death in Sierra Leone. *Soc Sci Med* 1986;23:297–303.

67. Morbidity and Mortality Weekly Reports. Progress toward the global elimination of neonatal tetanus, 1989–1993. *MMWR Morb Mortal Wkly Rep* 1994;43: 885–894.

68. Schofield FD, Tucker VM, Westbrook GR. Neonatal tetanus in New Guinea: effect of active immunization in pregnancy. *Br Med J* 1961;2:785–789.

69. Gadoth N, Dagan R, Sandbank U, et al. Permanent tetraplegia as a consequence of tetanus neonatorum. *J Neurol Sci* 1981;51:273–278.

70. Anlar B, Yalaz K, Dizmen R. Long-term prognosis after neonatal tetanus. *Dev Med Child Neurol* 1989; 31:76–80.

71. Schon F, O'Dowd L, White J, et al. Tetanus: delay in diagnosis in England and Wales. *J Neurol Neurosurg Psychiatry* 1994;57:1006–1007.

72. Weiss BP, Strasburg MA, Feeley JC. Tetanus and diphtheria immunity in an elderly population in Los Angeles County. *Am J Public Health* 1983;73:802–804.

73. Woo E, Yu YL, Huang CY. Local tetanus revisited. Electrodiagnostic studies in 2 patients. *Electromyogr Clin Neurophysiol* 1988;28:117–122.

74. Boyd RE, Brennan PT, Deng J-F, et al. Strychnine poisoning. *Am J Med* 1983;74:507–512.

75. Moersch FP, Woltman HW. Progressive fluctuating muscular rigidity ("stiff-man syndrome"): report of a case and some observations in 13 other cases. *Mayo Clin Proc* 1956;31:421–427.

76. Band JD, Bennett JV. Tetanus. In: Hoeprich PD, ed. *Infectious diseases, 3rd ed.* Philadelphia: Harper & Row, 1983:1107–1114.

77. Passen EL, Andersen BR. Clinical tetanus despite a protective level of toxin-neutralizing antibody. *JAMA* 1986;255:1171–1173.

78. Gardner P, Schaffner W. Immunization of adults. *N Engl J Med* 1993;328:1252–1258.

79. Trujillo MH, Castillo A, España J, et al. Impact of intensive care management on the prognosis of tetanus. *Chest* 1987;92:63–65.

80. Mukherjee DK. Tetanus and tracheostomy. *Ann Otol Rhinol Laryngol* 1977;86:67–72.

81. Blake PA, Feldman RA, Buchanan TM, et al. Serologic therapy of tetanus in the United States. *JAMA* 1976; 236:42–44.

82. Gupta PS, Kapoor R, Goyal Set al. Intrathecal human tetanus immune globulin in early tetanus. *Lancet* 1980; 2:439–440.

83. Abrutyn E, Berlin JA. Intrathecal therapy in tetanus: a meta-analysis. *JAMA* 1991;266:2262–2267.

84. Begue RE, Lindo-Soriano I. Failure of intrathecal antitoxin in the treatment of neonatal tetanus. *J Infect Dis* 1991;164:619–620.

85. Ahmadsyah I, Salim A. Treatment of tetanus: an open study to compare the efficacy of procaine penicillin and metronidazole. *Br Med J* 1985;291:648–650.

86. Yen LM, Dao LM, Day NPJ, et al. Management of tetanus: a comparison of penicillin and metronidazole. Symposium of antimicrobial resistance in southern Viet Nam. 1997.

87. Müller H, Börner U, Zierski J, et al. Intrathecal baclofen for treatment of tetanus-induced spasticity. *Anesthesiology* 1987;66:76–79.

88. Saissy JM, DemaziPre J, Vitris M, et al. Treatment of severe tetanus by intrathecal injections of baclofen without artificial ventilation. *Intensive Care Med* 1992; 18:241–244.

89. Powles AB, Ganta R. Use of vecuronium in the management of tetanus. *Anaesthesia* 1985;40:879–881.

90. Belmont MR, Moehr RB, Wastilla WB, et al. Pharmacodynamics and pharmacokinetics of benzylisoquinolinium (curare-like) neuromuscular blocking agents. *Anesth Clin North Am* 1993;11:251–283.

91. Anandaciva S, Koay CW. Tetanus and rocuronium in the intensive care unit. *Anaesthesia* 1996;5:505–6.

92. Domenighetti GM, Savary S, Striker H. Hyperadrenergic syndrome in severe tetanus responsive to labetalol. *Br Med J* 1984;288:1483–1484.

93. O'Keefe SJD, Wesley A, Jiala I, et al. The metabolic response and problems with nutritional support in acute tetanus. *Metabolism* 1984;33:482–487.

94. Vieira SRR, Brauner JS. Tetanus: following up 176 patients in the ICU. Proceedings, VI World Congress on Intensive and Critical Care Medicine, Madrid, 1993.

95. Martinelli R, Matos CM, Rocha H. Tetanus as a cause of acute renal failure: possible role of rhabdomyolysis. *Revista Soc Brasileira Med Trop* 1993;26:1–4.

96. Srinivas N, Suresh Kumar Reddy M, Muvagopal S, et al. Dorsal spine compression fracture in tetanus. *J Indian Med Assoc* 1994;92:56–58.

97. Tutuncuoglu S, Demir E, Koprubasi F, et al. The evaluation of late sequelae of tetanus infection. *Indian J Pediatr* 1994;61:263–267.

98. Edwards RA, James B. Tetanus and psychiatry: unexpected bedfellows. *Med J Aust* 1979;1:483–484.

99. Edsall G. The inexcusable disease. *JAMA* 1976;235: 62–63.

100. Bleck TP. Tetanus. *Dis Mon* 1991;37:547–603.

101. Dastur FD, Awatramani VP, Chitre SK, et al. A single-dose vaccine to prevent neonatal tetanus. *J Assoc Phys India* 1993;41:97–99.

102. Kurtzhals JAL, Kjeldsen K, Heron I, et al. Immunity against diphtheria and tetanus in human immunodeficiency virus-infected Danish men born 1950–1959. *APMIS* 1992;100:803–808.

103. Barbi M, Biffi MR, Binda S, et al. Immunization in children with HIV seropositivity at birth: antibody response to polio vaccine and tetanus toxoid. *AIDS* 1992; 6:1465–1469.

104. Prager J, Baumer A, Hermann J, et al. Untersuchungen zur Kinetik der Impfantikörper gegen Tetanustoxoid, Diptherietoxoid, Masern-Virus, Poliomyelitis-Virus and Pneumokokken nach allogener und autologer Knochenmarktransplantation und Widerholungsimpfung. Teil 1: Kinetik der Imfantikörper gegen Tetanustoxoid nach allogener und autologer Knochenmarktransplantation. Kinderätzl. *Praxis* 1992;60:124–130.

105. Prager J, Baumer A, Thilo W, et al. Untersuchungen zur Kinetik der Impfantikörper gegen Tetanustoxoid,

Diptherietoxoid, Masern-Virus, Poliomyelitis-Virus and Pneumokokken nach allogener and autologer Knochenmarktransplantation and Widerholungsimpfung. Teil 3: Kinetik der Impfantikörper gegen Tetanustoxoid und Diptherietoxoid nach allogener and autologer Knochenmarktransplantation kombinierter Wiederholsungsimpfund gegen Diptherie un Tetanus. Kinderätzl. *Praxis* 1992;60:230–238.

106. Chang AC, Gupta RK. Stabilization of the tetanus toxoid in poly (DL-lactic-co-glycolic acid) microspheres for controlled release of the antigen. *J Pharm Sci* 1996; 85:129–132.

107. Fairweather NF, Chatfield SN, Makoff AJ, et al. Oral vaccination of mice against tetanus by use of a live attenuated Salmonella carrier. *Infect Immun* 1990;58: 1323–1326.

108. Alpar HO, Bowen JC, Brown MRW. Effectiveness of liposomes as adjuvants of orally and nasally administered tetanus toxoid. *Int J Pharmaceut* 1992;88: 335–344.

109. Li Y, Foran P, Lawrence G, et al. Recombinant forms of tetanus toxin engineered for examining and exploiting neuronal trafficking pathways. *J Biol Chem* 2001; 276:31394–31401.

NEUROPHYSIOLOGY

Scientific and Therapeutic Aspects of Botulinum Toxin
edited by M.F. Brin, J. Jankovic, and M. Hallett
Lippincott Williams & Wilkins, Philadelphia, © 2002.

15

Effects of Botulinum Toxin at the Neuromuscular Junction

Mark Hallett

It is quite clear that botulinum toxin (BTX) has an effect at the neuromuscular junction. It must also be true that a large part of the clinical efficacy of BTX is a result of the muscle weakness that results from the neuromuscular blockade. On the other hand, there is not always an apparent direct relationship between the amount of weakness and the amount of benefit. Indeed, from initial consideration, it is somewhat surprising that it is possible to block an unwanted spasm, but leave voluntary movement intact. This suggests that there are likely some subtleties that are worth understanding. One such possibility is that BTX has indirect central nervous system effects as well as effects on the neuromuscular junction. That possibility is dealt with in a separate chapter; here, we deal with effects at the neuromuscular junction.

Of course, the benefit of injection depends on the indication. In a trial of BTX for the treatment of hemifacial spasm, we noted that only those parts of the face that were injected and became weak had reduced spasms (1). Indeed, we observed with EMG that the weakened muscles still had electromyographic discharges, but did not produce a spasm because of weakness. In other situations, such as spasticity, where weakness to a certain extent is a goal, it is perhaps easiest to show that weakness correlates with efficacy. For example, in a treatment trial of spastic hyperadduction of the hips in multiple sclerosis, weakness was certainly greater in the treated group than in the placebo group, and there was greater benefit (2). There also was a trend toward greater benefit with higher dose.

Similar findings were observed in the treatment of upper-limb spasticity (3).

For dystonia, the question of efficacy is more difficult because the goal is not weakness as such, but reduced dystonic movements and improved function and motor coordination. Nevertheless, efficacy generally increases with dose, as demonstrated, for example, in the German Dystonia Study group's investigation of multiple doses in the treatment of cervical dystonia (4). It should be noted that side effects also increase with dose, so that the highest dose is not necessarily the best on this account. Another problem is that muscle strength is often difficult to quantify accurately, and the relationship between loss of strength and improvement has not often been shown. EMG methods should help in this regard. One study has clearly demonstrated that increased dose leads to a decline in EMG amplitude in the sternocleidomastoid when treating cervical dystonia (5).

The observation that efficacy does not necessarily correlate with weakness in the treatment of dystonia has been made anecdotally by many investigators (6,7). Either benefit is disproportionate to the weakness produced, or there is marked weakness, but little improvement. In a double-blind trial for treatment of writer's cramp, Tsui et al. looked at objective measures of pen control and subjective improvement in writing (8). Of the 20 patients, 12 had objective improvement, but only 4 claimed subjective improvement.

It can be noted that efficacy can increase with dose, even in the face of minimal weakness (9), so that a positive dose–response relationship does not necessarily mean that more weakness is better.

Botulinum toxin affects the intrafusal neuromuscular junctions as well as the extrafusal neuromuscular junctions (10), and this might be an important aspect of the functional effect. If the gamma-motoneurons cannot activate the intrafusal muscle fibers, muscle spindle output will be diminished, and because muscle activity is supported by afferent feedback, there may be reduced alpha-motoneuron drive. In dystonia, muscle vibration, which strongly activates the spindle afferents, can produce a dystonic spasm. Thus, less sensory input because of the intrafusal effect will lead to less motor output. Such a mechanism was demonstrated by Kaji et al. by using muscle afferent block with lidocaine and alcohol to improve dystonia (11). This treatment effect is described in another chapter.

Another possible reason for benefit to outstrip weakness is that BTX should be more effective in blocking the neuromuscular junctions of the most active muscle fibers (12). For this reason, if only part of the muscle is involved in the involuntary spasm, then that part is more likely to be affected and significant strength could be preserved. The first evidence that BTX preferentially affects active neuromuscular junctions comes from *in vitro* observations of Hughes and Whaler (13). Using a frog diaphragm preparation, they showed that stimulation of the axon

to the diaphragm led to greater uptake of the BTX. This was demonstrated to be relevant in humans by Eleopra et al. (14). In nine patients, they injected both extensor digitorum brevis (EDB) muscles with a low (3 IU) dose of type A BTX (BOTOX). For the first 24 hours after injection, they electrically stimulated only one of the two muscles. Every 4 seconds, there was a 3-second train of stimuli at 4 Hz at an intensity sufficient to cause a muscle contraction. The compound muscle action potential (CMAP) amplitude for each muscle was measured at different intervals over a 30-day period. They found that the effect of the BTX was significantly greater on the stimulated side (Fig. 15.1).

The proposed mechanism of action is supported by the findings of a study on the influence of BTX on ephaptic transmission in ten patients with hemifacial spasm (15). Before the injection, ephaptic transmission in the facial nerve occurred in both directions; that is, stimulation of the zygomatic branch produced a late response in the mentalis muscle and stimulation of the mentalis branch produced a late response in the orbicularis oculi muscle. The orbicularis oculi muscle was then injected, but not the mentalis muscle. After a mean follow-up period of 38 days, with facial nerve stimulation there was a 40% reduction of the CMAP of the injected orbicularis oculi muscle. Ephaptic transmission studied by selective stimulation of facial nerve

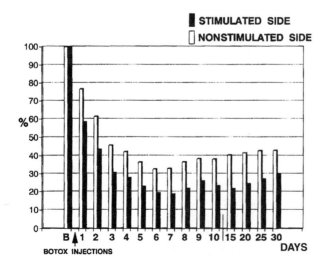

FIG. 15.1. The amplitude of the CMAP of extensor digitorum brevis muscles in nine patients injected on both sides with BTX, but electrically stimulated only on one side. (From Eleopra R, Tugnoli V, De Grandis D. The variability in the clinical effect induced by botulinum toxin type A: the role of muscle activity in humans. *Mov Disord* 1997;12:89–94, with permission.)

branches revealed a preserved delayed response of the affected mentalis muscle. However, no delayed response could be recorded in the injected orbicularis oculi muscle in nine of the patients. The discrepancy between complete loss of the delayed (ephaptic) response and only moderate reduction of the CMAP amplitude of the direct response may be explained by preferential uptake of botulinum toxin type A by hyperactive synapses involved in ephaptic transmission. As those same fibers were likely to be involved in the hemifacial spasm, there was selective blocking of the appropriate muscle fibers. The muscle fibers involved in the spasm tend to be the most active ones and, therefore, should be more affected by the treatment. Thus, botulinum toxin may block the involuntary movement but leave strength relatively intact, because the toxin is preferentially taken up by the most active muscle fibers, those involved in the involuntary movement.

This concept that active synapses after injection should show more blockage has been evaluated in several clinical studies. Hesse et al. tested BTX-A in two groups of hemiparetic patients with lower limb spasticity (16). In the first group ($n = 5$) 2,000 U DYSPORT were injected into the soleus, tibialis posterior and both heads of gastrocnemius muscles; the second group ($n = 5$) received the same injections with additional repetitive alternating electrical stimulation of tibialis anterior and plantar flexors for 30 minutes six times per day during the 3 days following the injection. Muscle tone, rated by the Ashworth spasticity score, and gait analysis were assessed before and 4 weeks after injection. The combined treatment proved to be more effective with respect to reduction of muscle tone, gait velocity, stride length, stance and swing symmetry.

The same group has also investigated whether the combined approach of BTX-A and electrical stimulation is more effective than toxin alone in the treatment of chronic upper-limb spasticity after stroke (17). They performed a randomized, placebo-controlled study with four treatment groups of six patients each: group A: 1,000 units DYSPORT and electrical stimulation; group B: 1,000 units DYSPORT only; group C: placebo

injection and electrical stimulation; and group D: placebo injection only. In groups A and C, the electrical stimulation of the injected muscles was delivered with surface electrodes, three times each day for 30 minutes for 3 days. Muscle tone was rated with the modified Ashworth score, and limb position at rest and difficulties encountered during three upper-limb motor tasks were assessed before and 2, 6, and 12 weeks after injection. The greatest improvements were observed in group A, suggesting that electrical stimulation does enhance the effectiveness of BTX in the treatment of chronic upper-limb flexor spasticity after stroke.

We studied the effects of exercise immediately after BTX-A injection in eight patients with writer's cramp (who were already known to be responders to BTX-A) over two injection cycles in a single-blinded, randomized, crossover design (18). Immediately after the first study injection, they were randomly assigned either to write continuously for 30 minutes or to have their hand and forearm immobilized for 30 minutes. Following the second injection, they had the alternate condition. Patients were assessed just before each injection, and at 2 weeks, 6 weeks, and 3 months postinjection. Assessment included objective strength testing, self-reported rating of benefit and weakness, and blinded evaluation of videotapes and writing samples of the patients writing a standard passage. Strength testing showed that the maximum weakness occurred at 2 weeks postinjection, and the "write" condition resulted in greater reduction in strength than the "rest" condition (Fig. 15.2). Subjective benefit was maximum at 6 weeks postinjection, showing again the dissociation between weakness and benefit. There were improvements in self-reported ratings, writer's cramp rating scale scores by blinded raters, and reduction in writing time, but the differences between the "write" and "rest" conditions were not significant. Thus, while voluntary muscle activity immediately after BTX injection leads to greater reduction in muscle strength, this does not necessarily relate to increased benefit. On the other hand, our findings raise the possibility that voluntary muscle activation may allow reduction of BTX doses and favorably alter the

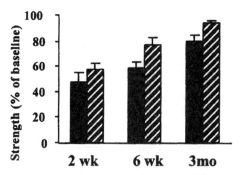

FIG. 15.2. Strength of muscles injected with BTX, comparing the situation when the patients were active (writing) after the injection (*solid bar*) to when they were at rest (*hatched bar*). (From Chen R, Karp BI, Goldstein SR, et al. Effect of muscle activity immediately after botulinum toxin injection for writer's cramp. *Mov Disord* 1999;14: 307–312, with permission.)

balance of benefit and side effects of this type of therapy.

The overall conclusion is that the influence of BTX at the neuromuscular junction is clearly critical in its effect, but that simple weakness is clearly not the whole story. There can be selectivity for the most active synapses, and this will promote a relatively stronger influence on those synapses involved in the involuntary movement. Additionally, the effect on intrafusal synapses will have an influence on sensory feedback, and sensory feedback can be quite important in movement disorders (19,20).

REFERENCES

1. Geller BD, Hallett M, Ravits J. Botulinum toxin therapy in hemifacial spasm: clinical and electrophysiologic studies. *Muscle Nerve* 1989;12:716–722.
2. Hyman N, Barnes M, Bhakta B, et al. Botulinum toxin (DYSPORT) treatment of hip adductor spasticity in multiple sclerosis: A prospective, randomised, double-blind, placebo-controlled, dose-ranging study. *J Neurol Neurosurg Psychiatry* 2000;68:707–712.
3. Simpson DM, Alexander DN, O'Brien CF, et al. Botulinum toxin type A in the treatment of upper extremity spasticity: a randomized, double-blind, placebo-controlled trial. *Neurology* 1996;46:1306–1310.
4. Poewe W, Deuschl G, Nebe A, et al. What is the optimal

dose of botulinum toxin A in the treatment of cervical dystonia? Results of a double-blind, placebo-controlled, dose-ranging study using DYSPORT. German Dystonia Study Group. *J Neurol Neurosurg Psychiatry* 1998;64: 13–17.
5. Dressler D, Rothwell JC. Electromyographic quantification of the paralysing effect of botulinum toxin in the sternocleidomastoid muscle. *Eur Neurol* 2000;43: 13–16.
6. Cohen LG, Hallett M, Geller BD, et al. Treatment of focal dystonias of the hand with botulinum toxin injections. *J Neurol Neurosurg Psychiatry* 1989;52:355–363.
7. Karp BI, Cole RA, Cohen LG, et al. Long-term botulinum toxin treatment of focal hand dystonia. *Neurology* 1994;44:70–76.
8. Tsui JK, Bhatt M, Calne S, et al. Botulinum toxin in the treatment of writer's cramp: a double-blind study. *Neurology* 1993;43:183–185.
9. Brashear A, Lew MF, Dykstra DD, et al. Safety and efficacy of NeuroBloc (botulinum toxin type B) in type A-responsive cervical dystonia. *Neurology* 1999;53: 1439–1446.
10. Rosales RL, Arimura K, Takenaga S, et al. Extrafusal and intrafusal muscle effects in experimental botulinum toxin-A injection. *Muscle Nerve* 1996;19:488–496.
11. Kaji R, Rothwell JC, Katayama M, et al. Tonic vibration reflex and muscle afferent block in writer's cramp: implications for a new therapeutic approach. *Ann Neurol* 1995;38:155–162.
12. Hallett M, Glocker FX, Deuschl G. Mechanism of action of botulinum toxin. *Ann Neurol* 1994;36:449–450.
13. Hughes R, Whaler BC. Influence of nerve-ending activity and of drugs on the rate of paralysis of rat diaphragm preparations by *C. botulinum* type A toxin. *J Physiol* 1962;160:221–233.
14. Eleopra R, Tugnoli V, De Grandis D. The variability in the clinical effect induced by botulinum toxin type A: the role of muscle activity in humans. *Mov Disord* 1997; 12:89–94.
15. Glocker FX, Guschlbauer B, Lucking CH, et al. Effects of local injections of botulinum toxin on electrophysiological parameters in patients with hemifacial spasm: role of synaptic activity and size of motor units. *Neurosci Lett* 1995;187:161–164.
16. Hesse S, Jahnke MT, Luecke D, et al. Short-term electrical stimulation enhances the effectiveness of botulinum toxin in the treatment of lower-limb spasticity in hemiparetic patients. *Neurosci Lett* 1995;201:37–40.
17. Hesse S, Reiter F, Konrad M, et al. Botulinum toxin type A and short-term electrical stimulation in the treatment of upper-limb flexor spasticity after stroke: a randomized, double-blind, placebo-controlled trial. *Clin Rehabil* 1998;12:381–388.
18. Chen R, Karp BI, Goldstein SR, et al. Effect of muscle activity immediately after botulinum toxin injection for writer's cramp. *Mov Disord* 1999;14:307–312.
19. Hallett M. How does botulinum toxin work? *Ann Neurol* 2000;48:7–8.
20. Hallett M. Is dystonia a sensory disorder? *Ann Neurol* 1995;38:139–140.

Scientific and Therapeutic Aspects of Botulinum Toxin
edited by M.F. Brin, J. Jankovic, and M. Hallett
Lippincott Williams & Wilkins, Philadelphia, © 2002.

16

Effects of Botulinum Toxin Type A on Central Nervous System Function

Alfredo Berardelli, Francesca Gilio, and Antonio Currà

Botulinum toxin type A (BoNT-A) has been a major advance in neurologic therapeutics. It is useful in the treatment of focal dystonias, spasticity, and other types of muscular spasms. Patients with focal dystonia can be successfully treated by periodic local injection of BoNT-A into the hyperactive muscles.

Botulinum neurotoxin (BoNT) produces its therapeutic effects by inhibiting acetylcholine (ACh) release from the presynaptic neuromuscular terminals and by weakening the hyperactive muscle fibers involved in the involuntary movement.

Besides acting peripherally, BoNT acts on the central nervous system (CNS) (1,2). Whereas ample research has focused on the peripheral actions of BoNT, its central effects are much less clear. In the following section, we review some of the studies providing clues to the central action of BoNT.

IN VITRO AND IN VIVO ANIMAL EXPERIMENTS

In skeletal muscles, BoNT-A affects the intrafusal as well as the extrafusal neuromuscular junction thereby modifying spindle afferent discharge. Filippi et al. (3) using microelectrode recordings in animal experiments reported that BoNT blocks the gamma motor endings in rat jaw muscles and reduces spindle-afferent discharges without affecting muscle tension. The spindle discharge diminishes within 80 minutes after the injection. In a morphologic and functional study in rats, Rosales et al. (4) compared the effects of BoNT-A on extrafusal and intrafu-

sal muscle fibers. Among its effects, BoNT-A caused fiber atrophy and spread of ACh staining in the endplates, findings indicative of denervation. The toxin's effects on extrafusal and intrafusal fibers over time also paralleled each other. The fusimotor denervation presumably alters the activity of the muscle spindle sensory afferents. Altered spindle afferent input could produce changes in the spinal cord circuitry and central circuitry pathways.

That BoNT can directly or indirectly influence the function of the spinal cord is also supported by findings from retrograde-tracing studies. About 48 hours after injecting radiolabeled BoNT in the cat gastrocnemius, Weigand et al. (5) found a distoproximal gradient of radioactivity in the sciatic nerve, then in the ipsilateral spinal ventral roots, and, finally, in the cord segments innervating the injected muscles. Subsequently, radioactivity also spread to spinal cord segments contralateral to the injection and in smaller amounts to the dorsal roots. These findings suggest that BoNT can be transported on both motor and afferent axons (intrafusal afferents). Studies applying BoNT-A directly into the spinal cord in anesthetized cats demonstrated a decrease in Renshaw cell activity (6). Wiegand and Wellhoner (7) used neurophysiologic techniques to confirm the action of BoNT on the soma membrane of spinal alpha-motoneurons.

Studies in cultured cells show that besides acting on the neuromuscular junction, BoNT acts elsewhere in the CNS (on other types of nerve terminals). In cultured cells of the spinal nerve, BoNT-A inhibited not only the potassium-evoked release of acetylcholine, but also the release of other neurotransmitters (8). In cultured mouse spinal cord neurons, BoNT-A inhibits the release of noncholinergic synaptic transmission blocking both excitatory and inhibitory transmission (9). In addition BoNT-A and BoNT-C partially inhibit the absolute and fractional release evoked by high K^+ concentrations, as well as the fractional basal release of [^{3}H] noradrenaline in primary nerve cell cultures from the brainstem of embryonic mice (10).

Studies of animal brain tissue provide evidence that BoNT-A inhibits the release of acetylcholine in cortical slices and cerebral cortex synaptosomes, with a compensatory decrease in choline uptake and acetylcholine resynthesis (11). When incubated with rat brain homogenate, the radioactive ^{125}I-labeled neurotoxin bound selectively to a large synaptosome fraction (12) and preferentially on both the extrajunctional and junctional areas of the presynaptic membranes that did not exist on the postsynaptic membranes (13). More recently, a protein receptor for BoNT-B was identified in rat brain synaptosomes and its resulting partial amino acid sequence was identical to that of synaptotagmin, a synaptic vesicle membrane protein (14). Studies with electron-microscope autoradiography showed that BoNT neurotoxin binds to synapse-rich areas of rat brain, particularly the hippocampus and cerebellum, with minimal uptake at central nerve terminals (15).

Another important question about the CNS effects of BoNT-A is whether the toxin passes through the blood–brain barrier. Using autoradiography of the toxin marked with ^{125}I and indirect fluorescent labeling, Boroff et al. (16) detected the toxin in the brain parenchyma and blood vessels. Whether BoNT can be diffused through the blood stream and the blood–brain barrier at low doses remains unclear (16).

STUDIES IN HUMANS

Naumann and Reiners (17) investigated the changes in the long latency reflexes elicited by electrical median nerve stimulation in patients with dystonia, and the possible changes induced by BoNT. They found that in writer's cramp, the early part of the long latency reflexes occurring at a latency of about 40 ms was enhanced,

while the late responses at 50 ms were reduced or absent. Treatment with BoNT decreased the size of the later responses on the affected sides. On the basis of these results, Naumann and Reiners concluded that BoNT can induce afferent modifications.

One technique that allows the investigation of spinal cord function is the study of reciprocal inhibition between agonist and antagonist muscles. In normal subjects, reciprocal inhibition consists of an initial phase, which peaks at the conditioning-test intervals of 0 ms and is because of a disynaptic pathway, followed by a second phase, which peaks at the conditioning-test interval of 10 to 20 ms and is a result of presynaptic mechanisms. Patients with upper-limb dystonia have abnormal reciprocal inhibition between flexor and extensor muscles, consisting of a reduced second phase. Priori et al. (18), who investigated reciprocal inhibition before and after BoNT-A injection in forearm flexor muscles in dystonic patients, showed that BoNT injected in the forearm muscles changes reciprocal inhibition between agonist and antagonist muscles. Three weeks after the injection in the dystonic muscles, BoNT increased the second, later phase of reciprocal inhibition but induced no change in the first phase. BoNT also reduced the M wave and the H reflex, but left the H/M ratio unchanged. To explain the toxin's effect on reciprocal inhibition Priori et al. (18) proposed that after injection of BoNT, the presynaptic block of the gamma motoneuron endplate on intrafusal fibers reduces spindle afferent input to the spinal cord, thus increasing presynaptic inhibition of flexor muscle afferents. The effect of BoNT on the second phase of reciprocal inhibition was confirmed in a subsequent study in patients with essential tremor (19). Similarly to patients with dystonia, patients with essential tremor also have a reduced presynaptic phase of reciprocal inhibition. One month after BoNT injection, the second phase of the reciprocal inhibition was restored, whereas the first phase was unaffected. BoNT also reduced the size of the H reflex and the M wave to a similar extent, but left the H/M ratio unaffected. Again after BoNT-A injection, reciprocal inhibition returned to normal. These two studies suggest that BoNT-A injected into the forearm muscles alters the excitability of spinal cord circuitry. On the other hand, in patients with spasticity of the upper limb, BoNT injection fails to reverse the abnormalities of reciprocal inhibition (reduction of both early and late phases) (20). Similar results were reported by Panizza et al. (21), who found no significant changes in the H/M ratio and the H reflex presynaptic inhibition in patients with spasticity performing the vibration test before and after BoNT treatment. The lack of a BoNT-induced effect on reciprocal inhibition in spastic patients suggests that the role of afferent feedback differs in dystonia and spasticity.

In some forms of dystonia, BoNT fails to alter the excitability of central pathways. Blepharospasm is the most common cranial dystonia, a frequent form of focal dystonia. It is characterized by involuntary recurrent spasms of both eyelids. In patients with blepharospasm, the R2 component of the blink reflex has an enhanced recovery cycle (22). The blink reflex is tested by stimulating the supraorbital nerve unilaterally while recording from the orbicularis oculi bilaterally. The stimulation elicits an early response (R1) ipsilateral to the stimulated supraorbital nerve and a late bilateral response (R2). The afferent limb of the reflex loop comprises the sensory trigeminal root and the ophthalmic division. The efferent limb is the facial nerve. The R1 component is relayed centrally through an oligosynaptic arc, the R2 component through a polysynaptic pathway. To determine whether BoNT-A has a central effect on the interneuron circuitry of the brainstem, the excitability of the blink reflex recovery cycle has been studied in patients with blepharospasm before and after BoNT treatment (23). After BoNT injections, the R1 response had reduced amplitude, and the recovery cycle of the R2 response remained enhanced even at the time of maximal BoNT-induced benefit. The same investigation has been replicated in patients with blepharospasm treated with BoNT-A unilaterally, and the R2 response was recorded from the untreated orbicularis oculi after ipsilateral and contralateral supraorbital nerve stimulation (24,25). Also in this study, in recordings before and after BoNT treatment, the R2 component had similar recovery curves, indicating that BoNT-A has no effect on the excitability of the brainstem interneurons mediating the bilateral R2 response.

Studies of Positron Emison Tomography activation in patients with idiopathic dystonia have shown an overactivity of striatum and of nonprimary motor areas and underactivity of the primary motor cortex during voluntary movement. Ceballos-Baumann et al. (26) studied the activation of the motor system in patients with writer's cramp before and after BoNT-A injection. BoNT-A treatment improved writing and increased activation in the parietal cortex and caudal SMA, but it left the pattern of activity in the primary motor cortex and the premotor area unchanged. These results suggest a cortical reorganization secondary to deafferentation of alpha-motoneurons or changes in motor strategy.

In patients presenting with lower-limb spasticity, Pauri et al. (27) investigated the motor-evoked potentials (MEPs) in response to transcranial magnetic stimulation of the leg area at various times after BoNT-A injections in the calf muscles. As shown by the clinical scale records, all patients benefited from the treatment, but 2 weeks later, the MEP latency and central conduction time had lengthened in the injected muscles. This effect has been interpreted as a result of changes in the excitability of spinal motor neurons in response to the descending impulses from the corticospinal tracts.

Evidence for changes in cortical organization after BoNT injection come from studies using transcranial magnetic stimulation (TMS) to map the muscle representation areas in the primary motor cortex. Byrnes et al. (28) studied the topography of the primary motor cortex projections to the upper-limb muscles in patients with writer's cramp by delivering TMS before and after BoNT-A injections into the affected muscles. They found that patients with dystonia had altered corticomotor representation. Cortical maps were distorted in shape, with extensions of the lateral borders. These abnormalities were more evident in patients with long-standing writer's cramp. BoNT-A injection in the dystonic muscles induced a clinical improvement in the hand dystonia and concurrently reversed the cortical changes. After BoNT-A treatment, when the clinical improvement in writer's cramp wore off, the cortical maps returned to their original topography.

EXCITABILITY OF CORTICAL MOTOR AREAS AND BOTULINUM TOXIN

The changes in the cortical representation of hand muscles in the primary motor cortex induced by BoNT and revealed by TMS techniques suggest changes in the balance between inhibition and excitation of the cortical motor neurons.

A sensitive technique for studying cortical excitability is TMS with paired stimuli (conditioning and test shocks) (29). In normal subjects, a conditioning subthreshold transcranial magnetic shock delivered at short interstimulus intervals over the hand motor area suppresses the test response evoked by a suprathreshold transcranial magnetic stimulus. It does so by activating cortical inhibitory interneurons. In normal subjects, experiments with a test response evoked by an anodal electric shock produced no inhibition, and a conditioning transcranial magnetic stimulus produced no inhibitory effect on the forearm flexor H reflex. These results suggest that the inhibition seen with paired stimuli is a consequence of purely cortical mechanisms, probably GABAergic inhibitory interneurons (29).

By using paired TMS, Ridding et al. (30) showed that patients with dystonia had less intracortical inhibition than did normal subjects. Hence, they concluded that a defective cortical inhibitory system probably contributes to the overflow of muscle activity characteristic of dystonic patients. Defective inhibition therefore seems to be of critical importance in the pathophysiology of dystonia (22).

To investigate whether BoNT alters the excitability of cortical motor areas, we used the paired TMS technique to study intracortical inhibition in patients with upper-limb dystonia before, 1 month, and 3 months after the injection of BoNT-A in the affected muscles. We studied 11 normal subjects and 12 patients with dystonia involving the upper limbs (7 with generalized, 2 with segmental, and 3 with focal dystonia). Patients were assessed clinically by using the Dystonia Movement Scale. Paired magnetic stimuli were delivered by two Magstim 200 magnetic stimulators connected through a Bistim module, to a figure-eight coil placed over the forearm muscles motor area. Paired stimulation was given at rest and during voluntary con-

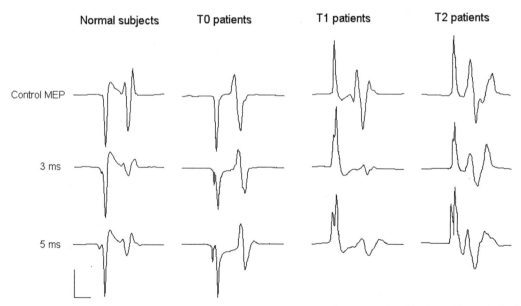

FIG. 16.1. Amplitude of the conditioned MEP in a representative normal subject and in a patient studied before (*T0*), 1 month (*T1*), and 3 months (*T2*) after botulinum toxin injection at rest condition. There is a significant inhibition of the conditioned MEP amplitude in the normal subject and in the patient at T1, but not at T0 or T2. Each trace is the average of 8 single electromyographic trials. Horizontal calibration is 15 ms and vertical calibration is 0.5 mV.

traction. A subthreshold [80% of the motor threshold (Mth) at rest or during contraction] conditioning stimulus was delivered 3 and 5 ms before the suprathreshold (120% Mth) test stimulus. Electromyographic (EMG) signals were recorded over the flexor or the extensor muscles of the forearm on the affected side. We measured the amplitude of the test MEP (expressed as a percentage of the unconditioned MEP).

In all patients, BoNT-A injection (50 to 100 mouse units) reduced dystonic movements in the arm. We found significant inhibition of the test response in normal subjects at rest. Patients with

dystonia had less intracortical inhibition than normal subjects. This finding confirms the results first reported by Ridding et al. (30). One month after BoNT-A injection, intracortical inhibition increased, returning to values seen in normal subjects. When we tested patients again at 3 months, their intracortical inhibition had returned almost to the abnormally low levels seen before botulinum treatment (Figs. 16.1 and 16.2).

During contraction, test responses in normal subjects were significantly inhibited, but the degree of inhibition was less prominent during

CORTICOCORTICAL INHIBITION

AT REST

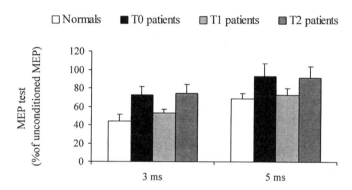

DURING CONTRACTION

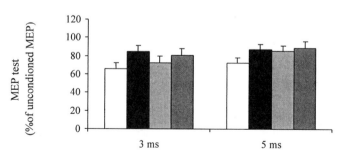

FIG. 16.2. Changes in the amplitude of the conditioned MEP in normal subjects (*open bars*) and T0, T1, and T2 patients (*solid bars*) at rest (*upper panel*) and during voluntary contraction of the target muscle (*lower panel*). At rest, T0 and T2 patients had less intracortical inhibition than normal subjects; T1 patients were similar to normal subjects. During contraction, test responses in normal subjects were significantly inhibited, but less than at rest. At 3-ms interstimulus time interval, at T0 and T2, patients had less cortical inhibition than did normal subjects; at T1, patients and normal subjects had similar intracortical inhibition. Data correspond to means ± SE (standard error).

contraction than in muscles at rest (Fig. 16.2). In patients before BoNT-A treatment, the cortical inhibition was slightly lower than that observed in normal subjects ($p = 0.06$), but 1 month after BoNT-A it was completely normalized. The slight difference in the degree of cortical inhibition already seen between controls and patients before treatment reappeared 3 months after BoNT-A injection. BoNT-A treatment therefore induced clinical benefit and at the same time transiently normalized the dystonic patients' cortical inhibitory abnormalities observed at rest and during voluntary contraction. These findings show that the toxin transiently alters cortical excitability.

BoNT-induced changes in central inhibition could result indirectly from the toxin's peripheral action. BoNT alters the muscle spindle input and the balance between afferent input and motor output. Hence, the abnormal cortical excitability could be an adaptive response in the cortex to the toxin's actions at spinal cord level. Muscle afferent input is tightly coupled to motor cortical output, so that afferents from a stretched muscle go to cortical areas where they can excite neurons capable of contracting the same muscle. BoNT-induced reduction in spindle signals can therefore alter the balance between afferent input and motor output, thereby changing cortical excitability.

The brain is a dynamically changing structure. Support for brain plasticity comes from functional imaging (positron emission tomography) studies and TMS. Reorganization of the human motor system has been demonstrated with motor learning (31), and after lesions of peripheral or central structures. The TMS technique has shown changes in motor cortical topography in patients with upper limb amputations. Transient deafferentation by regional anesthesia or ischemic nerve block also produces changes in the size of MEPs from muscles immediately proximal to the ischemic lesion. Transient deafferentation therefore results in short-term plasticity (32). The phenomenon of cortical plasticity may arise from various mechanisms, including changes in synaptic strength by processes such as long-term potentiation and the alteration of the balance between excitation and inhibition.

Over longer periods of time, anatomic changes may lead to an increase in synaptic density. The toxin-induced changes in motor output presumably reflect a reorganization of the synaptic balance between inhibition and excitation in the pyramidal cells projecting onto the forearm muscles. Cortical plasticity might well explain the intracortical inhibitory changes that we recorded after BoNT injection in patients with dystonia.

In conclusion, our data suggest that BoNT can transiently alter the excitability of the cortical motor areas by reorganizing the inhibitory and excitatory intracortical circuits. The cortical changes probably originate through peripheral mechanisms. Thus, BoNT works not only at the neuromuscular junction but it also alters sensory input, producing secondary changes at central level. BoNT has a complex mechanism of action. Its widening clinical role depends on the multiple direct and indirect effects that the toxin exerts in both the peripheral nervous system and in the CNS.

REFERENCES

1. Simpson LL. The origin, structure, and pharmacological activity of BoNT. *Pharmacol Rev* 1981;33:155–188.
2. Simpson LL. Peripheral actions of the BoNT. In: Simpson LL, ed. *Botulinum neurotoxin and tetanus toxin*. San Diego: Academic Press, 1989:153–178.
3. Filippi GM, Errico P, Santarelli R, et al. Botulinum A toxin effects on rat jaw muscle spindles. *Acta Otolaryngol (Stockh)* 1993;113:400–404.
4. Rosales RL, Arimura K, Takenaga S, et al. Extrafusal and intrafusal muscle effects in experimental BoNT-A injection. *Muscle Nerve* 1996;10:488–496.
5. Wiegand H, Erdmann G, Wellhoner HH. ^{125}I-labeled botulinum A neurotoxin: pharmacokinetics in cats after intramuscular injection. *Naunyn Schmiedebergs Arch Pharmacol* 1976;292:161–165.
6. Hagenah R, Benecke R, Wiegand H. Effects of type A BoNT on the cholinergic transmission at spinal Renshaw cells and on the inhibitory action at Ia inhibitory interneurons. *Naunyn Schmiedebergs Arch Pharmacol* 1977;299:267–272.
7. Wiegand H, Wellhoner HH. The action of botulinum A neurotoxin in the inhibition by antidromic stimulation of the lumbar monosynaptic reflex. *Naunyn Schmiedebergs Arch Pharmacol* 1977;298:235–238.
8. Janicki PK, Haberman E. Tetanus and BoNT inhibit and black widow spider venom stimulates the release of methionine–enkephalin-like material *in vitro*. *J Neurochem* 1983;41:395–402.
9. Bigalke H, Heller I, Bizzini B, et al. Tetanus toxin and botulinum A toxin inhibit release and uptake of various

transmitters, as studied with particulate preparations from rat brain and spinal cord. *Naunyn Schmiedebergs Arch Pharmacol* 1981;316:244–251.

10. Habermann E, Muller H, Hudel M. Tetanus toxin and botulinum A and C neurotoxins inhibit noradrenaline release from cultured mouse brain. *J Neurochem* 1988; 51:522–527.

11. Gundersen CB Jr, Howard BD. The effects of botulinum toxin on acetylcholine metabolism in mouse brain slices and synaptosomes. *J Neurochem* 1978;31:1005–1013.

12. Kitamura M. Binding of botulinum neurotoxin to the synaptosome fraction on rat brain. *Naunyn Schmiedebergs Arch Pharmacol* 1976;295:171–175.

13. Hirokawa N, Kitamura M. Binding of *Clostridium botulinum* neurotoxin to the presynaptic membrane in the central nervous system. *J Cell Biol* 1979;81:43–49.

14. Nishiki T, Kamata Y, Nemoto Y, et al. Identification of protein receptor for *Clostridium botulinum* type B neurotoxin in rat brain synaptosomes. *J Biol Chem* 1994; 269:10498–10503.

15. Black JD, Dolly JO. Selective location of acceptors for botulinum neurotoxin A in the central and peripheral nervous system. *Neuroscience* 1987;23:767–769.

16. Boroff DA, Chen GS. On the question of permeability of the blood–brain barrier to BoNT. *Int Arch Allergy Appl Immunol* 1975;48:495–504.

17. Naumann M, Reiners K. Long-latency reflexes of hand muscles in idiopathic focal dystonia and their modification by BoNT. *Brain* 1997;120:409–416.

18. Priori A, Berardelli A, Mercuri B, et al. Physiological effects produced by BoNT treatment of upper limb dystonia. Changes in reciprocal inhibition between forearm muscles. *Brain* 1995;118:801–807.

19. Modugno N, Priori A, Berardelli A, et al. BoNT restores presynaptic inhibition of group Ia afferents in patients with essential tremor. *Muscle Nerve* 1998;21: 1701–1705.

20. Girlanda P, Quartarone A, Sinicropi S, et al. Botulinum toxin in upper-limb spasticity: study of reciprocal inhibition between forearm muscles. *Neuroreport* 1997;8: 3039–3044.

21. Panizza M, Castagna M, Summa A, et al. Functional and clinical changes in upper-limb spastic patients treated with botulinum toxin. *Funct Neurol* 2000;15: 147–155.

22. Berardelli A, Rothwell JC, Hallett M, et al. The pathophysiology of primary dystonia. *Brain* 1998;121: 1195–1212.

23. Valls-Sole J, Tolosa ES, Ribera G. Neurophysiological observations on the effects of BoNT treatment in patients with dystonic blepharospasm. *J Neurol Neurosurg Psychiatry* 1991;54:310–313.

24. Girlanda P, Quartarone A, Sinicropi S, et al. Unilateral injection of botulinum toxin in blepharospasm: single-fiber electromyography and blink reflex study. *Mov Disord* 1996;11:27–31.

25. Grandas F, Traba A, Alonso F, et al. Blink reflex recovery cycle in patients with blepharospasm unilaterally treated with BoNT. *Clin Neuropharmacol* 1998;21: 307–311.

26. Ceballos-Bauwman AO, Sheean G, Passingham RE, et al. BoNT does not reverse the cortical dysfunction associated with writer's cramp. A PET study. *Brain* 1997; 120:571–582.

27. Pauri F, Boffa L, Cassetta E, et al. BoNT type-A treatment in spastic paraparesis: a neurophysiological study. *J Neurol Sci* 2000;181:89–97.

28. Byrnes ML, Thickbroom GW, Wilson SA, et al. The corticomotor representation of upper-limb muscles in writer's cramp and changes following BoNT injection. *Brain* 1998;121:977–988.

29. Kujirai T, Caramia MD, Rothwell JC, et al. Cortico-cortical inhibition in the human motor cortex. *J Physiol* 1993;471:501–519.

30. Ridding MC, Sheean G, Rothwell JC, et al. Changes in the balance between motor cortical excitation and inhibition in focal, task specific dystonia. *J Neurol Neurosurg Psychiatry* 1995;59:493–498.

31. Pascual-Leone A, Cammarota A, Wassermann EM, et al. Modulation of motor cortical outputs to reading hand of braille readers. *Ann Neurol* 1993;34:33–37.

32. Cohen LG, Ziemann U, Chen R, et al. Studies of neuroplasticity with transcranial magnetic stimulation. *J Clin Neurophysiol* 1998;15:305–324.

Scientific and Therapeutic Aspects of Botulinum Toxin
edited by M.F. Brin, J. Jankovic, and M. Hallett
Lippincott Williams & Wilkins, Philadelphia, © 2002.

17

Impact of Botulinum Toxin on Laryngeal Physiology

Christy L. Ludlow

VOCAL FOLD VIBRATION FOR SPEECH

During speech, a delicate balance must be maintained between the air pressure from the lungs (subglottal pressure) and intrinsic vocal fold tension and length to rapidly initiate and control voice production for vowels. For voice production, the vocal folds must be set into vibration. To begin vibration, the vocal folds are brought together. This increases the subglottal pressure from the lungs, which then moves the closed vocal folds apart, allowing the air from the lungs to flow between the folds producing a negative pressure, which then brings vocal folds again to a close, via the Bernoulli effect. Once closed, the pressure builds up again until the subglottal pressure is adequate to again open the folds. This cycle is repeated at approximately 100 times per second in male voices and approximately 220 times per second in female voices. The length and tension in the folds for closing the folds must be continuously balanced with the subglottal driving pressure (1). This is achieved, in part, by laryngeal muscle contraction on both sides of the larynx and within each of the vocal folds. In general, for voice production, the speaker only activates the laryngeal muscles to a small degree, about 10% to 20% of the maximum activation level and for brief periods of 50 to 100 ms (2). Too low a level of adductor muscle activation will not close the vocal folds; too high a level of activation will override the subglottal pressure, not allowing the vocal folds to be set into vibration. For nonspeech protective functions of the larynx, such as swallow and cough,

between 30% and 70% of the maximum activation levels of the laryngeal muscles are often used. The timing of muscle activation for these functions is also slower and much less precise than for speech (2).

The larynx includes three closing muscles: the thyroarytenoid (TA) muscle, which forms the body of the vocal fold and shortens the fold; the lateral cricoarytenoid, which moves the arytenoid cartilages medially to close the folds; and the interarytenoid, which increases the approximation between the arytenoid cartilages. The cricothyroid muscle lengthens the vocal folds and counteracts the shortening action of the TA. The cricothyroid and TA muscles must be carefully balanced during simultaneous activation to increase the rate of vibration and voice pitch (3). The posterior cricoarytenoid is the only muscle which actively opens the vocal folds.

LARYNGEAL DYSTONIAS

Adductor spasmodic dysphonia (ADSD) is the most common of the dystonic laryngeal motor-control disorders. Voice breaks in adductor spasmodic dysphonia occur during speech in the middle of vowels. As the name denotes, spasmodic bursting of the TA muscle increases the adductory force on the vocal folds, disrupting vibration and producing a voice break (4). In fact, the number of spasmodic muscle bursts corresponds closely with the frequency of voice breaks (5), the major symptom of the disorder. For this disorder, the treatment of choice is now botulinum toxin type A (BTX-A) injections, which is effective in controlling symptoms in well over 90% of persons with ADSD (6). Although only one controlled trial has been published thus far (7), there is little question about the efficacy of this treatment for ADSD. Some controversy still exists, however, over injection technique. Unilateral injections into the TA muscle are effective at large dosages of 15 U which can produce movement reduction on one side (8), while smaller injections of 2.5 U into each vocal fold do not produce observable reduction in vocal fold movement but are similarly effective in controlling symptoms (9–11).

In abductor spasmodic dysphonia (ABSD), patients have difficulties with rapid voice onset following voiceless consonants; that is, moving quickly from the open to the closed position to begin phonation. Persons with voice tremor often have tremor in the laryngeal muscles during the expiratory phase of respiration, affecting voice during speech (12). BTX-A injections are less effective in controlling symptoms in these two disorders than it is in controlling symptoms in ADSD (13).

PATHOPHYSIOLOGY OF SPASMODIC DYSPHONIA

Physiologic studies of ADSD have not found a constant hypertonicity in either the adductor or other laryngeal muscles (14,15). Instead, when muscle activity is examined just before and during speech breaks in ADSD, increases are seen only in the TA muscle (4). The voice breaks in ADSD, then, are caused by spasmodic bursts interfering with continued voicing. The patient is unable to continue voice during these rapid changes in muscle activity resulting in phonatory breaks in vowels.

The results differed when similar muscle comparisons were made in patients with ABSD between muscle activation during speech with and without breaks. Some patients were observed clinically to have bursts of activity in the posterior cricoarytenoid and cricothyroid muscles (16). When quantitative comparisons were made with controls, however, persons with ABSD had increased levels of tone in muscles on one side of the larynx, suggesting a unilateral laryngeal dystonia (17). An asymmetry in tone can interfere with the ability to begin and maintain phonation (18). Patients with vocal tremor, on the other hand, have a variety of laryngeal muscles affected with a 5-Hz tremor both during voice and at rest (12).

CHANGES IN LARYNGEAL FUNCTION FOLLOWING INJECTION WITH BTX-A

Similar changes in laryngeal function occur following either a unilateral or a bilateral injection of the TA muscle with BTX-A in persons with ADSD (Table 17.1).

Phase I

Some persons report changes within the first day, sometimes as early as 6 hours following injection, although no research has been conducted to verify that this is not a result of expectations of a treatment benefit. Such persons report that they sense reduction of tension in the

TABLE 17.1. *Sequence of changes in laryngeal function in persons with adductor spasmodic dysphonia following either a unilateral or bilateral injection with botulinum toxin into the thyroarytenoid muscle(s)*

Time postinjection	Phase	Change in laryngeal function
1 day	I	Sense of reduction in effort
2 to 3 days	II	Reduced volume and breathiness
		Reduction in symptoms
3-7 days	II	Swallowing side effects
1-2 weeks	III	Improvement in swallowing
3 to 4 weeks	IV	Reduction in breathiness
3 weeks to 3 months	V	Normal voice free of symptoms
3 to 5 months	VI	Return of symptoms

larynx, even though reduction in voice loudness has not yet occurred. This Phase I does not occur in all persons and is based only on patient report.

Phase II

Within 3 days, and no later than 5 days, the patient's voice becomes reduced in loudness and the breaks reduce. This can be assumed to be the effect of progressive denervation as the BTX-A is endocytosed and cleaves its substrate, SNAP-25 (synaptosomal-associated protein of 25 kDa). Although a few patients report that they observe a change in laryngeal tension and voice breaks within the first 24 hours, most report the improvement begins and progresses after the second day following an injection. It is during this period, 3 to 5 days postinjection, that patients notice a progressive breathiness as the vocal folds become less adducted. Because breathiness and swallowing difficulties increase over 3 to 5 days after injection, it can be assumed that continued denervation is progressing during this period.

Swallowing difficulties become more pronounced usually between 3 and 5 days postinjection. Most patients report difficulties with liquids and occasional aspiration if they try to drink liquids at a normal speed. They are advised to take liquids in smaller volumes and to drink slower than previously by sipping through a straw.

Phase III

The difficulties with swallowing gradually subside between the first and second week after an injection, normally lasting about 5 days in total (19).

Phase IV

Breathiness resolves, reaching normal loudness levels, usually between 3 to 4 weeks after injection. Improvements in voice volume seem to be independent of recovery from swallowing following injection (19).

Phase V

Between 1 and 3 months postinjection, the patient's voice is close to normal volume and symptoms are controlled. The number of voice breaks is significantly reduced during this period, the patient's speech is more fluent and rapid, and hoarseness is reduced (8). This phase is the period of treatment benefit, and is greater for BTX-A than for treatment with botulinum toxin type F (20). It is also notable that the benefit period differs depending upon the disorder, lasting from 3 to 5 months in ADSD, but is less, on the order of 1 to 2 months, in other disorders following BTX-A injections such as ABSD (13,21,22), tremor, and stuttering (23).

Phase VI

The return of symptoms in ADSD is gradual during Phase VI, beginning about 2 months after injection and usually lasting over 2 months. To maintain symptom control, most patients return for injection around 3 months or slightly later. In our experience, full symptom return does not occur until after 5 or 6 months, but most persons with ADSD seek reinjection before this time period. We have had several patients, however, who have had benefit for more than 1 year following injection, returning 2 or more years later for a repeat injection.

The focus of this review will be to discuss the possible physiologic mechanisms underlying each of these stages in light of some of the recent evidence on the *in vivo* and *in vitro* actions of BTX (24–28). (Table 17.2)

CORRELATION OF CELLULAR EVENTS WITH SYMPTOMATIC CHANGES

Phase I: Sense of Relief Within the First 24 Hours

One usually suspects that expectation plays a role in patients' reports of an early sense of reduction of effort within the first 6 to 24 hours after injection. However, some studies have not only demonstrated denervation of fusimotor endplates (29), but that the denervation effect on

TABLE 17.2. *Physiologic effects of botulinum toxin and proposed corresponding changes in physiologic function*

Action of botulinum toxin	Proposed laryngeal physiologic change	Phase of patient response (time postinjection)
Endocytosis and cleavage of SNAP-25 in muscle spindles (29,30)	Reduced 1a afferent feedback	I. Early report of ease of voice production within 24 hours
Endocytosis and cleavage of SNAP-25 in nerve endings in muscle fibers, loss of function in 50% of neuromuscular junctions (24)	Reduction in muscle tone and movement	II. Breathiness, dysphagia and symptom reduction (1 to 3 days)
	Compensatory slowing of motor pattern to prevent aspiration (33)	III. Reduction in Dysphagia (5 to 10 days)
Collateral sprouting (24)	Innervation of some fibers by collateral sprouts	IV. Reduction in breathiness (2 to 3 weeks) (19)
Retention of cleaved SNAP-25 preventing insertion of renewed SNAP-25 (28)	Continued denervation of both muscle spindles and muscle fibers	V. Normal voice without symptoms (2 to 4 months) (19)
Gradual replacement of cleaved SNAP-25 with renewed SNAP-25 and return of function in neuromuscular junctions (24)	Gradual return of function to original neuromuscular junction	VI. Gradual symptom return (3 to 5 months) (19)
Loss of collaterals (24) (1 year)	Reduction in size of motor units (40)	

muscle spindles occurs much earlier than muscle fiber denervation (30). If feedback from muscle spindles plays a role in ADSD, denervation of muscle spindles might account for patient reports of a sense of relief before significant changes are apparent in the voice. A controversy about the possible role of muscle spindles in laryngeal function has existed for some time. Sanders reported that one portion of the human TA muscle contains muscle spindles (31), but their physiologic significance has not yet been demonstrated. In the cat, laryngeal adductor muscle responses are only elicited by stimulation of the laryngeal mucosa but not by stretch of the TA muscle or joint movement after removal of the mucosa (32). If muscle spindles are not physiologically significant in the human, other mechanisms could be responsible for changes in afferent feedback following laryngeal muscle denervation. Mucosal mechanoreceptor feedback, for example, might reflect reductions in adductory force between the vocal folds following BTX-A injection, independent of changes in muscle spindle feedback.

Phase II: Denervation

As BTX-A is endocytosed and cleaves SNAP-25 beginning between 2 and 5 days postinjection,

denervation progressively affects the voice which sometimes is normalized without symptoms first, then progressively becomes more breathy with swallowing difficulties for drinking water. The speed of laryngeal closure and elevation needed for swallowing liquids is more rapid than for soft or hard foods. Because swallowing difficulties which occur following BTX-A primarily involve liquids, BTX may affect the speed of laryngeal movement for swallowing (33). Such reductions in speed might result from changes in the TA muscles or diffusion to other intrinsic or extrinsic muscles (34). Injections into the posterior cricoarytenoid muscle in ABSD might result in diffusion to the inferior constrictor, which is important for swallowing. Usually the degree of breathiness and the severity of dysphagia correspond during the early denervation period.

The effects of BTX-F during this early denervation period are no different from that occurring following initial injection of BTX-A for blepharospasm (35). We found the time course of symptom reduction and the degree and occurrence of side effects of breathiness and swallowing deficits are similar during the initial denervation period for type A and type F (20). Changes during the denervation period are similar, although the mechanisms by which BTX-A and

BTX-F produce muscle denervation differ: BTX-A cleaves SNAP-25 and BTX-F cleaves VAMP (vesicle-associated membrane protein).

Phase III: Resolution of Swallowing Difficulties

The resolution of the breathiness and swallowing side effects following BTX-A usually follow different and independent time courses (19). The swallowing side effects usually resolve in fewer than 10 days following injection. This would be before reinnervation or significant collateral sprouting is expected to occur (24). Such early improvements in swallowing may be a result of patients learning to compensate within a few days by slowing their swallowing patterns.

We examined the mean number of days of dysphagia following BTX-A with that following BTX-F in a crossover study within the same patients (36). No significant difference was found in the duration of dysphagia following the two types of BTX. Recovery from dysphagia may not be a result of reinnervation, otherwise the resolution of dysphagia would be earlier following BTX-F, which has a shorter duration of action, suggesting a shorter denervation period (20).

Phase IV: Resolution of Breathiness

The resolution of breathiness is later than that for dysphagia, averaging 30 days (1 month) after injection with BTX-A (19). This is the period when collateral sprouting might be at maximum and before the original endplates have again become functionally active (24). The reduction in breathiness usually occurs 1 to 2 months before a return of full function and symptoms and must depend upon a different process than reinnervation.

Comparing the duration of breathiness following BTX-A and BTX-F in a group of spasmodic dysphonia patients showed a nonsignificant trend toward earlier recovery from breathiness following injection with type F than following injection with type A (36). When type A and type F were compared for the treatment of blepharospasm (35), however, no difference

was found in the time of onset of clinical effect, maximum clinical benefit or side effects. It is not known whether the timing of collateral sprouting found following BTX-A differs for BTX-F (24). It may be that restoration of endplate function, which clinically occurs earlier following type F, may contribute to recovery from breathiness following BTX-F, whereas collateral sprouting is responsible for recovery from breathiness following BTX-A.

Phase V: Period of Prolonged Benefit

This prolonged period of normal voice function without symptoms averages 120 days in ADSD (19). There are two explanations offered for the long-term benefit. One is that the catalytically active light chain remains active within the cytosol continuing to cleave SNAP-25 and prevent reinnervation of function (25,26). The other is that the cleaved form of SNAP-25 remains in the nerve ending and is not removed or replaced for a long period preventing the restoration of function (27,28). The possibility of a more rapid turnover and replacement of VAMP following cleavage by type F, than occurs for SNAP-25 following cleavage by type A, might explain the difference in benefit duration for blepharospasm following type A over type F (35).

As was stated earlier there is some evidence that denervation occurs earlier in spindles than in muscle fiber endings (30), but it is not yet known whether the recovery of function differs between muscle spindles and muscle fibers. The duration of the Phase V period of benefit is greater in ADSD than in other laryngeal motor control disorders following injection with BTX-A such as tremor and stuttering (23). In stuttering, for example, the benefit is lost once breathiness reduces and voice production returns (23). This may be a consequence of the differences in the pathophysiology between these disorders.

To examine changes in muscle physiology in persons with ADSD following treatment with BTX-A, we conducted a study injecting the TA muscle on only one side (5). Blinded counts of the numbers of spasmodic muscle bursts before treatment found that there were equal numbers of bursts on the two sides of the larynx in both the TA muscles and the cricothyroid muscles. Following treatment, significant reductions were found in the numbers of muscle spasms in all the muscles on both sides, which corresponded with patients' reductions in voice breaks. Both the overall level of tone (in microvolts) and the percent of maximum activation was reduced in all the muscles. This was interpreted as the possible effect of reductions in muscle spindle feedback from the one muscle that was injected, resulting in reduced level of motor neuron pool drive for all the laryngeal muscles on both sides (5). At least one study has suggested that the physiologic effects of BTX-A might be greater on the fusimotor system and muscle spindle feedback than on muscle fiber innervation (37).

In ADSD, the benefit period continues for a couple of months following recovery from breathiness suggesting that benefit is not directly proportional to the amount of muscle denervation, although this hypothesis awaits experimental confirmation. This phenomenon has been noted in other disorders (38). In bilateral BTX injections for ADSD effective dosages range from 1 to 2.5 U and no movement reduction is seen, although the period of symptom benefit is similar to that found with unilateral injections resulting in unilateral movement reduction (9,10). Other disorders (voice tremor, abductor spasmodic dysphonia, and stuttering) average a 1- to 2-month period of benefit (22,23) in comparison with 3 to 5 months for persons with ADSD. One possibility might be that muscle spindle feedback does not play an important role in the pathophysiology of these other disorders.

Phase VI: Long-Term Changes

BTX-A produces collateral nerve sprouting from the denervated nerve endings (24,39). It has been questioned whether these become physiologically effective and whether they become reduced with restoration of function in the original nerve endings. We examined the effects of BTX-A injection in a group of patients with ADSD between 6 months and up to 3 years following an injection (40). For various reasons, these individuals chose not to have another in-

jection until long after their symptoms had returned. Durations of TA muscle motor units were measured and examined in relation to time since last injection. All of the patients had received their BTX-A injections only on one side. The motor unit durations were increased in the injected muscles relative to noninjected muscles for up to 1 year following injection, demonstrating a possible increase in the numbers of fibers innervated by an axon, which might reflect viable collateral sprouting. Following 1 year postinjection, however, the motor unit durations began to decrease to within the normal range, suggesting that the collateral nerve sprouts were becoming less functional. At the same time, the mean numbers of turns were also measured, to indicate the numbers of motor units (40). Numbers of turns were reduced in the injected muscles prior to 1 year and increased after 1 year.

Finally, some further changes were noted between 1 and 3 years postinjection: the numbers of turns and muscle amplitude increased up to 20 months and then gradually reduced after 20 months. Thus, changes were continuing in the second year postinjection, possibly involving a further refinement in motor unit physiology (40). Therefore, although symptoms return most often around 120 days after injection with BTX-A, physiologic evidence indicates that reinnervation and further changes in muscle physiology continue for at least 1 year in injected muscles. The need for smaller dosages as patients undergo repeated injections every 3 months can be understood in the light of these long-term effects.

Some patients with ADSD have needed increasing dosages over time to achieve benefit (41) in contrast with the usual pattern of decreasing dosages. Such patients may develop antibodies to BTX-A, although these are not always detectable using the mouse assay. To prevent the development of antibodies, caution should be used in reinjecting patients at frequent intervals with increasing dosages, particularly when injections don't result in the usual benefit. We found that a change in the injection technique is often helpful when patients no longer benefit from their previous treatment regimen; for example, changing to a unilateral injection 3 months later when a bilateral injection is no longer beneficial. The converse has also proved effective. The basis for this clinical experience is unknown—perhaps the disorder adapts to a repeated denervation pattern and a change may be needed to alter the pattern of feedback and thus the pathophysiology.

UNEXPLAINED EVENTS

Other unexplainable changes occur in laryngeal motor-control disorders following BTX injection. Clinicians have noted that sometimes when patients have an upper respiratory infection at the time of BTX injection into the laryngeal muscles, there is no noticeable change in the character of the voice and laryngeal motor control. Neither the side effects of dysphagia, breathiness, movement, nor symptom reductions occur. It is not known whether this lack of clinical signs of denervation is caused by destruction of the toxin because of the immune system being up-regulated in response to inflammation in the region. Other possibilities are changes in the gangliosides affecting endocytosis or changes in the cytosol because of the local inflammatory response.

We have noted that about 20% of our patients, particularly those who receive large unilateral injections of BTX-A, do not require injections for long intervals, from 2 to as long as 7 years after an injection. These patients did not always have entirely normal voices during this nontreatment period, but were without the effort or voice breaks. Many of these persons subsequently returned after long periods when their symptoms returned. Although we have seen long-term changes in laryngeal muscle physiology as a result of botulinum toxin, it is highly unlikely that these long-term benefits are solely caused by the injection. Patients may have developed central control strategies or their pathophysiology may have been altered by peripheral denervation. Cortical plasticity following peripheral changes in motor and/or sensory function is well recognized (42). Cortical representation is abnormal in some persons with dystonia (43) and perhaps it can be reversed either when the degree of peripheral denervation is greater or with the use of larger dosages of BTX-A.

CONCLUSIONS

This review of the physiologic changes following BTX-A injection highlights some of the physiologic changes observed following TA muscle treatment in ADSD. Most of the explanations about the physiologic processes that may be involved are hypotheses based on basic research reports in the literature. Much of this is still controversial, however, and *in vitro* findings may not have relevance to the clinical setting. Furthermore, species differences may render some of the *in vivo* findings irrelevant. These interpretations, therefore, should be considered hypotheses concerning the bases for clinical observations and findings following the use of BTX-A for the treatment of laryngeal motor control disorders.

REFERENCES

1. Titze IR. Phonation threshold pressure: a missing link in glottal aerodynamics. *J Acoust Soc Am* 1992;91: 2926–2935.
2. Ludlow CL, Lou G. Observations on human laryngeal muscle control. In: Fletcher N, Davis P, eds. *Controlling complexity and chaos: 9th vocal fold physiology symposium.* San Diego: Singular Press; 1996:201–218.
3. Titze IR, Luschei ES, Hirano M. Role of the thyroarytenoid muscle in regulation of fundamental frequency. *J Voice* 1989;3:213–224.
4. Nash EA, Ludlow CL. Laryngeal muscle activity during speech breaks in adductor spasmodic dysphonia. *Laryngoscope* 1996;106:484–489.
5. Bielamowicz S, Ludlow CL. Effects of botulinum toxin on pathophysiology in spasmodic dysphonia. *Ann Otol Rhinol Laryngol* 2000;109:194–203.
6. Blitzer A, Brin MF, Stewart CF. Botulinum toxin management of spasmodic dysphonia (laryngeal dystonia): a 12-year experience in more than 900 patients. *Laryngoscope* 1998;108:1435–1441.
7. Truong DD, Rontal M, Rolnick M, et al. Double-blind controlled study of botulinum toxin in adductor spasmodic dysphonia. *Laryngoscope* 1991;101:630–634.
8. Ludlow CL, Naunton RF, Sedory SE, et al. Effects of botulinum toxin injections on speech in adductor spasmodic dysphonia. *Neurology* 1988;38:1220–1225.
9. Adams SG, Hunt EJ, Charles DA, et al. Unilateral versus bilateral botulinum toxin injections in spasmodic dysphonia: acoustic and perceptual results. *J Otolaryngol* 1993;22:171–175.
10. Zwirner P, Murry T, Woodson GE. A comparison of bilateral and unilateral botulinum toxin treatments for spasmodic dysphonia. *Eur Arch Otorhinolaryngol* 1993; 250:271–276.
11. Langeveld TP, Drost HA, Baatenburg de Jong RJ. Unilateral versus bilateral botulinum toxin injections in adductor spasmodic dysphonia. *Ann Otol Rhinol Laryngol* 1998;107:280–284.

12. Koda J, Ludlow CL. An evaluation of laryngeal muscle activation in patients with voice tremor. *Otolaryngol Head Neck Surg* 1992;107:684–696.

13. Ludlow CL, Bagley JA, Yin SG, et al. A comparison of different injection techniques in the treatment of spasmodic dysphonia with botulinum toxin. *J Voice* 1992; 6:380–386.

14. Van Pelt F, Ludlow CL, Smith PJ. Comparison of muscle activation patterns in adductor and abductor spasmodic dysphonia. *Ann Otol Rhinol Laryngol* 1994;103: 192–200.

15. Watson BC, Schaefer SD, Freeman FJ, et al. Laryngeal electromyographic activity in adductor and abductor spasmodic dysphonia. *J Speech Hear Res* 1991;34: 473–482.

16. Ludlow CL, Naunton RF, Terada S, Anderson BJ. Successful treatment of selected cases of abductor spasmodic dysphonia using botulinum toxin injection. *Otolaryngol Head Neck Surg* 1991;104:849–855.

17. Cyrus CB, Bielamowicz S, Evans FJ, et al. Adductor muscle activity abnormalities in abductor spasmodic dysphonia. *Otolaryngol Head Neck Surg* 2001;124: 23–30.

18. Titze IR. *Principles of voice production*. Englewood Cliffs, NJ: Prentice Hall, 1994:92–93.

19. Ludlow CL, Rhew K, Nash EA. Botulinum toxin injection for adductor spasmodic dysphonia. In: Jankovic J, Hallett M, eds. *Therapy with botulinum toxin*. New York: Marcel Dekker, 1994:437–450.

20. Ludlow CL, Hallett M, Rhew K, et al. Therapeutic use of type F botulinum toxin. *N Engl J Med* 1992;326: 349–350.

21. Ludlow CL. Treating the spasmodic dysphonias with botulinum toxin: a comparison of results with adductor and abductor spasmodic dysphonia and vocal tremor. In: Tsui J, Calne D, eds. *The dystonias*. New York: Marcel Dekker, 1995:431–446.

22. Bielamowicz S, Squire S, Bidus K, et al. Assessment of posterior cricoarytenoid botulinum toxin injections in patients with abductor spasmodic dysphonia. *Ann Otol Rhinol Laryngol* 2001;110(5 Pt 1):406–412.

23. Stager SV, Ludlow CL. Responses of stutterers and vocal tremor patients to treatment with botulinum toxin. In: Jankovic J, Hallett M, eds. *Therapy with botulinum toxin*. New York: Marcel Dekker; 1994:481–490.

24. de Paiva A, Meunier FA, Molgo J, et al. Functional repair of motor endplates after botulinum neurotoxin type A poisoning: biphasic switch of synaptic activity between nerve sprouts and their parent terminals. *Proc Natl Acad Sci U S A* 1999;96:3200–3205.

25. Keller JE, Neale EA, Oyler G, et al. Persistence of botulinum neurotoxin action in cultured spinal cord cells. *FEBS Lett* 1999;456:137–142.

26. Adler M, Keller JE, Sheridan RE, et al. Persistence of botulinum neurotoxin A demonstrated by sequential administration of serotypes A and E in rat EDL muscle. *Toxicon* 2001;39:233–243.

27. Eleopra R, Tugnoli V, Rossetto O, et al. Different time courses of recovery after poisoning with botulinum neurotoxin serotypes A and E in humans. *Neurosci Lett* 1998;256:135–138.

28. Raciborska DA, Charlton MP. Retention of cleaved synaptosome-associated protein of 25 kDa (SNAP-25) in neuromuscular junctions: A new hypothesis to explain persistence of botulinum A poisoning. *Can J Physiol Pharmacol* 1999;77:679–688.

29. Filippi GM, Errico P, Santarelli R, et al. Botulinum A toxin effects on rat jaw muscle spindles. *Acta Otolaryngol (Stockh)* 1993;113:400–404.

30. Manni E, Bagolini B, Pettorossi VE, et al. Effect of botulinum toxin on extraocular muscle proprioception. *Doc Ophthalmol* 1989;72:189–198.

31. Sanders I, Han Y, Wang J, et al. Muscle spindles are concentrated in the superior vocalis subcompartment of the human thyroarytenoid muscle. *J Voice* 1998;12: 7–16.

32. Andreatta RD, Mann EA, Cyrus CB, et al. Mucosal afferents if the posterior glottis mediate the thyroarytenoid reflex response to low level mechanical displacements in anesthetized cat. *Soc Neurosci Abstracts* 2000;26.

33. Sedory-Holzer SE, Ludlow CL. The swallowing side effects of botulinum toxin type A injection in spasmodic dysphonia. *Laryngoscope* 1996;106:86–92.

34. Shaari CM, George E, Wu BL, et al. Quantifying the spread of botulinum toxin through muscle fascia. *Laryngoscope* 1991;101:960–964.

35. Mezaki T, Kaji R, Kohara N, et al. Comparison of therapeutic efficacies of type A and F botulinum toxins for blepharospasm: a double-blind, controlled study. *Neurology* 1995;45:506–508.

36. Rhew K, Ludlow CL. A randomized cross-over comparison of type A and type F botulinum toxin in patients with adductor spasmodic dysphonia. *(In preparation.)*

37. On AY, Kirazli Y, Kismali B, et al. Mechanisms of action of phenol block and botulinus toxin type A in relieving spasticity: electrophysiologic investigation and follow-up. *Am J Phys Med Rehabil* 1999;78: 344–349.

38. Giladi N. The mechanism of action of botulinum toxin type A in focal dystonia is most probably through its dual effect on efferent (motor) and afferent pathways at the injected site. *J Neurol Sci* 1997;152:132–135.

39. Borodic GE, Ferrante R, Pearce LB, et al. Histologic assessment of dose-related diffusion and muscle-fiber response after therapeutic botulinum-A toxin injections. *Move Dis* 1994;9:31–39.

40. Davidson B, Ludlow CL. Long-term effects of botulinum toxin injections in spasmodic dysphonia. *Otolaryngol Head Neck Surg* 1996;105:33–42.

41. Smith ME, Ford CN. Resistance to botulinum toxin injections for spasmodic dysphonia. *Arch Otolaryngol Head Neck Surg* 2000;126:533–535.

42. Merzenich M, Wright B, Jenkins W, et al. Cortical plasticity underlying perceptual, motor, and cognitive skill development: implications for neurorehabilitation. *Cold Spring Harb Symp Quant Biol* 1996;61:1–8.

43. Bara-Jimenez W, Catalan MJ, Hallett M, et al. Abnormal somatosensory homunculus in dystonia of the hand. *Ann Neurol* 1998;44:828–831.

CLINICAL THERAPEUTICS

Scientific and Therapeutic Aspects of Botulinum Toxin
edited by M.F. Brin, J. Jankovic, and M. Hallett
Lippincott Williams & Wilkins, Philadelphia, © 2002.

18

The Role of Botulinum Toxin Type A in the Management of Strabismus

Alan B. Scott

In his pioneering investigations of botulinum toxin, Justinus Kerner, during the period 1817–1822 (1), made many original observations about causation, diagnosis, prognosis, and treatment of botulism, and noted involvement of eye muscles. He correctly concluded that the toxin paralyzed skeletal muscles and parasympathetic function, and proposed its use as a therapeutic agent in neurologic diseases such as chorea that are characterized by excessive motor movement. But it was a full 160 years after Kerner that the idea of therapy with toxin was implemented. We began in 1970–1971 with injection of various drugs into extraocular muscles as an alternative to surgical treatment for strabismus (2). Among these was botulinum toxin, which immediately stood out for its long paralytic effect of several weeks, specificity for cholinergic terminals, lack of systemic side effects, and controllable dosage/response relationship.

Initially, we thought that toxin treatment of comitant strabismus worked because the extraocular muscles (EOM) were permanently weakened by the induced denervation paralysis. Spencer and McNeer (3) showed changes in the outer (orbital) muscular layer of toxin-treated primate EOM, lasting for 6 months. But active contraction force returns fully to these muscles in most cases. We now believe that the muscles alter alignment of the eyes mostly by adapting their length to the new position of the eye created by toxin-induced paralysis through addition/deletion of sarcomeres. Toxin is just a way of getting the eye into a new position so that the muscles are stretched or shortened (4). The tendency for this internal sarcomere reorganization varies from one individual to another. It also is dependent on the dose response, on creating a large angular change of alignment from the toxin paralysis, and on its persistence for at least 1 month. Therefore, it is not surprising that clinical responses to initial toxin injection for strabismus are variable.

INDICATIONS AND CLINICAL RESULTS

Toxin injection in EOM is most efficient in nonrestrictive strabismus. Scarring and paralysis restrict the inherent ability of the muscle to alter its length/tension characteristics. In general, there is about a 30% to 40% chance that one injection will correct the deviation to 10 prism diopters or less (Table 18.1). Table 18.2 shows that smaller deviations are more frequently corrected to 5 degrees or less by one injection, but that the percentage correction of the deviation is around 60% in most categories. Esotropia and exotropia generally respond similarly to treatment, and children and adults respond alike. Smaller deviations (horizontal or vertical) with minimal sensory changes have a superior prognosis. Large-angle deviations, more common in long-standing adult strabismus, often require repeated injections, resulting in a longer interval from the initiation of therapy to optimal correction. Despite this apparent disadvantage, many adults choose toxin injections to avoid surgery. Use in specific categories of strabismus is de-

TABLE 18.1. *Botulinum toxin correction according to number of injections*

	n	Preinjection deviation (°)	Correction to 5° or less
Children ET 1 injection	146	14	38%
Multiple injections	—	15	68%
Children XT 1 injection	66	13	38%
Multiple injections	—	13	50%
Adults ET 1 injection	225	14	39%
Multiple injections	—	15	68%
Adults XT 1 injection	139	14	28%
Multiple injections	—	16	61%

Follow-up 6 to 83 months (average 20 months).
ET, esotropia; XT, exotropia

tailed below. Unit dosages apply to BOTOX (Table 18.3).

PARALYTIC STRABISMUS

VI Nerve Paralysis

1. *Acute cases* of any age or origin are followed without treatment for 3 to 4 weeks. If healing begins within a month, it typically will be progressive and complete. Adults will be rehabilitated, and children seldom lose binocularity if alignment is restored in a month. After 1 month, if disabling diplopia persists and recovery is not progressing, or if a child remains esotropic in all gaze positions so that binocularity is threatened, then injecting the medial rectus (MR) on the affected side is appropriate. In a randomized trial in ambulatory adults with paresis of diabetic or vascular origin, there was little long-term difference in recovery between a botulinum toxin-treated (86%) and an untreated control group (80%) (5). Thus, for these adults who have a generally good prognosis, the value of botulinum toxin treatment lies in earlier rehabilitation. Small doses of 1.0 to 1.5 units are indicated.

2. *Delayed and partial recovery.* If recovery is delayed several months or takes place very slowly, MR contracture progresses and esotropia increases. Toxin injection of the MR in these non-acute cases allows the lateral rectus (LR) to recover against the treated MR of normal length, rather than against a strong and shortened MR. There is little risk of permanent overcorrection and the patient's alignment is improved, serving both functional and cosmetic goals while waiting healing of the LR. The data from Metz and Mazow (6) indicate that there is a higher per-

TABLE 18.2. *Botulinum toxin correction according to size of deviation*

	Preinjection deviation (°)	Percent correction of deviation	Final 5° or less
Children ET	5 to 12	56%	78%
	12 to 20	63%	63%
	20+	78%	65%
Children XT	5 to 12	59%	67%
	12 to 20	45%	25%
	20+	55%	40%
Adults ET	5 to 20	62%	72%
	20+	62%	35%
Adults XT	5 to 20	53%	67%
	20+	64%	33%

Follow-up 6 to 83 months (average 20 months).

TABLE 18.3. *Botulinum toxin dosage for initial injections*

	Units BOTOX
1. Horizontal strabismus	
a. Under 12°	2.0 to 2.5
b. Over 12°	2.5 to 5.0
c. Further refinements	
1. Smaller doses for medial rectus; larger doses for lateral rectus	
2. Smaller doses for smaller squints; larger doses for larger squints	
2. Medial rectus injection for lateral rectus palsy	
a. Early (1 to 3 months)	1.0 to 2.0
b. Later or in conjunction with transposition surgery	2.5
c. Later for partially or fully healed palsy but with MR contracture	2.5 to 5.0
3. Vertical muscles	
a. Inferior rectus for comitant deviation	2.5
b. Inferior rectus for thyroid	5
c. Inferior oblique	2.5
d. Superior oblique (rare)	2
4. Children with infantile ET or XT (bilateral injections)	2.5
5. Weak muscles: myasthenia, external ophthalmoplegia, aberrant regeneration, cerebral palsy	1.0 to 2.0
6. Retrobulbar injection for nystagmus	25

centage of alignment in treated cases (Table 18.4).

If there is abduction beyond the midline, good abduction saccades, or good LR force (30 g or more), then toxin injection to release the MR contracture will often be fully curative. If LR force is between 10 g and 30 g, then recess–resect surgery is indicated. If LR force is under 10 g, then transposition surgery is indicated, often using toxin to release MR contracture.

3. *Permanent paralysis, with less than 10 g of LR force.* Surgery by lateral transposition of the superior rectus (SR) and the inferior rectus (IR) together with toxin to the MR gives the largest field of single binocular vision. The value of toxin here is primarily to preserve and lengthen the MR so that this muscle, now the only active horizontal mover, has a large range of contraction–relaxation.

In contrast, surgical recession of an already short and contracted MR restores alignment but leads to further shortening of the MR, and a further reduction in range of motion. Also important is that toxin injection leaves the anterior ciliary artery supply of the MR intact, obviating the threat of anterior segment ischemia. The ability of toxin to release MR contracture makes it appropriate to wait a full 6 months after the onset before undertaking transposition surgery. Injection may be done a few weeks before surgery, or deferred until the time of surgery to allow accurate traction testing of the MR. Injection is then easily done under direct visualization. Where MR contracture is mild, injection is best deferred until postoperative alignment can be determined. It may be unnecessary and overcorrection could result. Even several months after surgery, injection can correct undercor-

TABLE 18.4. *Botulinum toxin correction of sixth nerve paresis*

	Number	% Recovered	
		Botulinum toxin treated	Control
Unilateral	34	70%	31%
Bilateral	11	90%	42%

From Metz HS, Mazow M: Botulinum toxin treatment of acute sixth and third nerve palsy. *Graefes Arch Clin Exp Ophthalmol* 1988; 226:141–144, with permission.

rected transposition cases and should be considered before reoperating.

III Nerve Paresis

Saad and Lee (7) corrected three of four cases that had some residual MR function, and Metz and Mazow (6) similarly corrected a majority of their cases using toxin. Toxin is very useful in late aberrant III nerve regeneration, where small deviations interfere with primary-position alignment. The muscles seem to be especially sensitive; small doses should be used.

IV Nerve Paresis

Lozano-Pratt (8) corrected 9 of 9 acute cases with 8 to 15 degrees of vertical deviation. Buonsanti (9) corrected 9 of 15 cases (three others partially improved) by injections of the overacting inferior oblique (IO) muscle. However, I have been disappointed in the long-term effect with consistent recurrence within a year after IO injection in chronic long-standing paresis. Garnham et al. (10) found toxin injection of the yoke IR muscle useful in both acute and chronic IV paresis, and I agree with this observation.

ADULT STRABISMUS

General

Adults must be aware of the intended overcorrection and its cosmetic implications, as well as possible diplopia and spatial disorientation lasting 1 to 2 months. This will require patching in about one-third of adult cases, mostly for the first week or two. Some elderly persons are physically unstable, and many busy adults are unable to drive and work with one eye covered. A trial of patching the eye before injecting can determine this.

The strabismus is often complicated by cicatricial restrictions, excessive muscle recession, poor fusion, or amblyopia. Multiply operated strabismus patients unhappy with the surgical outcome are frequent candidates for injection. In one report of 80 patients, 8 to 20 injections were given as chronic treatment. The intervals

between recurrences gradually increased, and a number of patients became stable (11).

Postretinal Detachment Strabismus

These patients have a past history of normal binocular vision in their favor. In most cases, the strabismic angle is modest. Scott (12) corrected 60% of cases with one injection, and Pettito and Buckley (13), corrected 80% of cases. Scarred extraocular muscles often require larger doses or a repeat injection. Injection of two muscles (e.g., the lateral rectus and inferior rectus simultaneously) is common.

Thyroid Ophthalmopathy

Toxin is useful in acute or active cases to relieve diplopia (14,15). Maintaining alignment to prevent or treat chronic cases is much less secure; surgery is avoided in about 25% to 30% of cases. The medial rectus muscles are frequently affected in thyroid disease and the horizontal deviation is usually modest. Because multiple muscle surgery in thyroid eye disease carries a higher risk of complications, use of toxin for the horizontal muscles while operating on the vertical muscles is very useful. Most late extraocular muscle restrictions are fibrotic. However, the 25% to 30% cure rate and an occasional remarkable loosening of inferior rectus contracture shows that internal muscle shortening plays a role.

Postcataract Strabismus

Immediate diplopia after cataract surgery in previously fusing adults usually presents as hypotropia of the operated eye secondary to IR contracture following retrobulbar anesthesia. When prisms are inadequate and the patient wishes to avoid surgery, toxin injection of the IR will correct over 60% of cases with a single injection. A second useful application is in long-standing unilateral cataract with exotropia and diplopia after cataract removal. Injection of the LR will restore alignment and subsequently maintain fusion in over half of these patients.

Postoperative Adjustment

Avoiding multiple surgical procedures is an integral part of strabismus treatment. Toxin injections are an alternative to additional surgery for strabismus, particularly if the intended goal has not been achieved by recent surgery. Toxin may be used either early or late in the postoperative period (16) or in conjunction with surgery, especially if the planned surgical procedure (e.g., transpositions, additional surgery on rectus muscles) may compromise anterior-segment vascularity.

Intrinsic Muscle Disorders

Unexercised extraocular muscles and other orbital tissues stiffen markedly in some persons but not in others. Strabismus in chronic myasthenia gravis and progressive external ophthalmoplegia is surprisingly responsive to toxin when the eye is stiff on traction testing; the response is less when the eye is readily moved. Caution should be exercised when patients with myasthenia gravis are injected as they may be excessively sensitive to the paralyzing effects of the toxin.

Nystagmus

In acquired nystagmus with oscillopsia and reduced vision, a single retrobulbar injection creates ophthalmoplegia for 6 months to dampen such movements (17). This has dramatically improved vision in several cases from 20/400 to 20/40. Because the induced ophthalmoplegia creates diplopia and marked spatial/balance problems, this works best for wheelchair-bound patients. Only one eye of an ambulatory patient should be injected in this manner. Vision can be improved by two to three lines by intramuscular injection of the horizontal recti in horizontal motor nystagmus, but the effect is transient.

Corneal ulceration caused by lid retraction or poor eyelid closure can be successfully treated by toxin injection (2.5 U) of the levator. The induced ptosis lasts 1 to 3 months and can be repeated.

CHILDHOOD STRABISMUS

Infantile Esotropia

Treatment of infantile esotropia by simultaneous bimedial toxin injection is quite successful. Table 18.5 shows the results of several independent series (18–21). All these reports include 2 years or more of follow-up, and show high correction rates of 60% to 80% with multiple injections. The experience of these investigators suggests the following therapeutic program: (a) simultaneous bimedial injection of 2.5 U of toxin per muscle; (b) inject as early as age 3 months—the good results in the series of Campos et al. were all injected prior to 8 months; (c) Repeat simultaneous bimedial injection with recurrence of esotropia (ET) exceeding 15 prism diopters, increasing the dose to 3 U per eye unless ptosis is a limiting side effect.

Accommodative Esotropia

Bimedial rectus toxin injection has been useful for correcting a high AC/A ratio with residual ET at near (22). Consecutive exotropia has not been seen.

TABLE 18.5. *Infantile esotropia treated by botulinum toxin (no prior surgery)*

Authors	N	Number of injections	% Corrected to 5° or less
McNeer et al.	76	—	89
Scott et al.	61	1.6	66
Gomez de Liano et al.	107	1.6	73
Campos et al.	50	1.0	76

See References 18 through 21.

Acquired Esotropia and the Nonaccommodative Angle in Accommodative Esotropia

Acquired esotropia here refers to strabismus developing after infancy that is neither paretic nor accommodative. Toxin will provide motor alignment, but the best responses are achieved if amblyopia can be improved or reversed prior to injection.

Intermittent Exotropia

As with surgery, full and lasting correction is less common in exotropia (see Table 18.1). An acceptable goal is a lesser exotropic angle with good control. In one investigation of intermittent exotropia (23), 32 patients were treated by one or more simultaneous bilateral toxin lateral rectus injections and followed 3 years from the final injection. Sixty-eight percent of patients developed a stable deviation of 10 prism diopters or less. Seven patients required surgery during the study period when injection failed to prevent recurrent exotropic drift. The response in patients between ages 3 and 5 years was better than the response in younger or older patients. With evidence of exotropia exceeding 10 prism diopters, injection should be repeated.

Cerebral Palsy

Strabismus surgery for neurologically impaired infants and children is less predictable than in normals, has a high rate of overcorrection, and side effects of general anesthesia are more frequent. Toxin injection offers an alternative with an overcorrection rate of about 3%. Low-dose bimedial injections of 1.25 to 2.0 U are preferred with esotropia because the dose-response is less predictable. Exotropia responds normally and the usual beginning dose is 2.5 U. Reinjections are often necessary, increasing the dose as indicated (see Table 18.3). Strabismus in older children with cerebral palsy is treated by unilateral injection to avoid past pointing and balance problems from the induced paralysis.

INJECTION TECHNIQUE

Injection outside the target muscle reduces the treatment effect and increases the likelihood of affecting adjacent muscles. The neuromuscular junctions centered halfway back in the EOM should be the target (24). Injecting horizontal muscles in an alert patient using an electromyogram (EMG) amplifier or by exposing the EOM through a small conjunctival incision are both effective techniques. After age 8 years in an intelligent child, the technique can often be performed as in adults. For children unable to cooperate, sedation is added: (a) Intravenous (IV) ketamine, 0.5 to 1.0 mg/kg, will preserve EMG activity and keep the patient relatively quiet for 2 to 5 minutes. This is 20% of the usual anesthetic dose. The anesthesiologist should be informed that general anesthesia is not desired, but rather some degree of akinesia, amnesia, and light sedation. (b) Inhalation anesthesia is an acceptable alternative, but the EMG signal is much diminished, so the medial rectus is often injected by estimation of its position using no electromyography, or a small conjunctival incision allows injection with the needle tip 10 to 15 mm posterior to the insertion under direct visualization.

TECHNICAL COMPLICATIONS AND DIFFICULTIES

Transient partial ptosis occurs in about 15% of adults and 25% of children because of proximity of the levator muscle and lasts 2 to 4 weeks. Complete ptosis occurs only after injection in the superior orbit. No case of amblyopia as a consequence of ptosis has been documented.

1. Vertical strabismus created by treatment of horizontal rectus muscles occurs in 10% to 25% of cases, depending on dosage. It persists for longer than 6 months in fewer than 1% of patients. This induced vertical strabismus is uncommon in children treated bilaterally, as any vertical effect seems to balance out.

2. The rate of overcorrection of the deviation at 6 months is 1.7%. Cases with muscles that respond strongly to toxin, resulting in overcorrection, are also easily reversed by injecting the antagonist. Smaller doses (1.0 to 1.5 U) should be used.

3. Eye perforation has occurred in unskilled

hands, but even here, no loss of vision has been reported.

CONCLUSIONS

Treatment of strabismus was the first therapeutic application of botulinum toxin. It is indicated in 10% to 15% of cases. Side effects are transient and loss of vision has not occurred in any case in 22 years of use. Toxin injection is simpler than surgery, but the more definitive correction achieved by surgery remains the method of choice in most cases.

REFERENCES

1. Kerner J. Studies published by Gruesser OJ. Die ersten systematischen Beschreibungen und tier experimentellen Untersuchungen des Botulismus. *Sudhoffs Archiv* 1986;70:167.
2. Scott AB, Rosenbaum AL. Pharmacologic weakening of extraocular muscles. *Invest Ophthalmol* 1973;12:924–927.
3. Spencer RF, McNeer KW. Botulinum toxin paralysis of adult monkey extraocular muscle. Structural alterations in orbital, single innervated muscle fibers. *Arch Ophthalmol* 1987;105:1703.
4. Scott AB. Change of eye muscle sarcomeres according to eye position. *J Pediatr Ophthalmol Strabismus* 1994;31:85.
5. Lee J, Harris S, Cohen J, et al. Results of a prospective randomized trial of botulinum toxin therapy in acute unilateral sixth nerve palsy. *J Pediatr Ophthalmol Strabismus* 1994;31:283.
6. Metz HS, Mazow M. Botulinum toxin treatment of acute sixth and third nerve palsy. *Graefes Arch Clin Exp Ophthalmol* 1988;226:141.
7. Saad N, Lee J. The role of botulinum toxin in third nerve palsy. *Aust N Z J Ophthalmol* 1992;20:121.
8. Lozano-Pratt A, Estanol B. Treatment of acute paralysis of the fourth cranial nerve by botulinum toxin A chemodenervation. *Binoc Vis* 1994;9:155.
9. Buonsanti JL, Rivero Sanchez-Covisa ME, Scarfone H, et al. Botulinum toxin chemodenervation of the inferior oblique muscle for chronic and acute IV nerve palsies: results in 15 cases. *Binoc Vis Strabismus Q* 1996;11:119.
10. Garnham L, Lawson J, O'Neill D, et al. Botulinum toxin in chronic superior oblique palsy. In: Spiritus M, ed. *Transactions of the European Strabismological Association.* Buren, The Netherlands: Aeolus Press, 1996:139.
11. Lee JP. Modern management of VI nerve palsy. *Aust N Z J Ophthalmol* 1992;20:41.
12. Scott AB. Botulinum treatment of strabismus following retinal detachment surgery. *Arch Ophthalmol* 1990;108:509.
13. Pettito VB, Buckley EG. Use of botulinum toxin in strabismus after retinal detachment surgery. *Ophthalmology* 1991;98:509.
14. Yons CJ, Vickers SF, Lee JP. Botulinum toxin therapy in dysthyroid strabismus. *Eye* 1990;4:538.
15. Scott AB. Injection treatment of endocrine orbital myopathy. *Doc Ophthalmol* 1984;58:141.
16. McNeer KW. An investigation of the clinical use of botulinum toxin A as a postoperative adjustment procedure in the therapy of strabismus. *J Pediatr Ophthalmol Strabismus* 1990;27:3.
17. Helveston EM, Pogrebniak AE. Treatment of acquired nystagmus with botulinum A toxin. *Am J Ophthalmol* 1988;106:584.
18. McNeer KW, Spencer RF, Tucker MG. Observations on bilateral simultaneous botulinum toxin injection in infantile esotropia. *J Pediatr Ophthalmol Strabismus* 1994;31:214.
19. Scott AB, Magoon EH, McNeer KW, et al. Botulinum treatment of strabismus in children. *Trans Am Ophthalmol Soc* 1989;89:174.
20. Gomez de Liano P, Rodriguez Sanchez JM, Gomez de Liano R, et al. Actitud terapeutica de la POM del VI par craneal: del tratamiento con TBA. In: Prieto-Diaz J, ed. *XII Congreso del Consejo Latinoamericano de Estrabismo.* Buenos Aires: Grafica Lifra, 1996:345.
21. Campos E, Schiavi C, Scorolli L. Botulinum toxin A in essential infantile esotropia. In: Louly M, ed. *Transactions of the VIII International Orthoptic Congress, Kyoto, 1995;* 229–231.
22. McNeer KW, Tucker MG. Botulinum toxin injection into the medial rectus muscle for high accommodative convergence/accommodation esotropia. *Invest Ophthalmol Vis Sci* 1989;30.
23. Spencer RF, Tucker MG, Choi RY, et al. Botulinum toxin management of childhood intermittent exotropia. *Ophthalmology* 1997;104:1762–1767.
24. Kupfer C. Motor innervation of extraocular muscle. *J Physiol* 1960;153:522.

Scientific and Therapeutic Aspects of Botulinum Toxin
edited by M.F. Brin, J. Jankovic, and M. Hallett
Lippincott Williams & Wilkins, Philadelphia, © 2002.

19

The Role of Botulinum Toxin Type A (BOTOX®) in the Management of Blepharospasm and Hemifacial Spasm

Joseph A. Mauriello, Jr.

Local injections of botulinum toxin type A (BTX-A) remain the treatment of choice for blepharospasm and hemifacial spasm (1–24). BTX-A has a local effect on the treated skeletal muscle. The toxin does not appear to affect brainstem interneurons that mediate the bilateral blink reflex recovery cycle in patients with blepharospasm (25). Single-fiber electromyography suggests that new neuromuscular junctions and their functional maturation are responsible for muscle recovery after treatment with BTX-A (26).

TREATMENT OF BLEPHAROSPASM AND CRANIAL DYSTONIA WITH BTX-A

Treatment Outcomes

A study of 239 patients with blepharospasm and cranial dystonia (Meige's syndrome) over an 11-year period demonstrated (a) the long-term acceptance of BTX-A injections by patients and (b) the role of other treatment modalities including oral medications and surgery in treating blepharospasm (26). Of 239 patients evaluated, 228 patients received local injections of BTX-A into the eyelid and facial musculature (16).

Of the 228 patients, 202 (72.1%) were still treated with BTX-A at the end of the 11-year period. Four patients (1.8%) no longer received BTX-A injections because of difficulty in obtaining transportation for medical treatment. Fourteen patients (6.1%) sought no additional treatment of any type. Five patients (2.2%) had apparent remission of their disease after injection. Three patients (1.3%) ultimately obtained relief from orbicularis muscle extirpative surgery and required no additional therapy. Of the 11 patients (4.6%) who chose not to receive BTX-A injections, one patient was successfully managed with psychotherapy and another with oral trihexyphenidyl.

In a study in which BTX types A and F were combined, there was no apparent potentiation of the clinical effectiveness of the two drugs. However, the duration of action with the combined drugs was longer than with type F alone and shorter than with type A alone (27).

Pharmacologic Adjuvant Therapy Combined with BTX Therapy

Of the 228 patients who received BTX-A, 99 patients received adjunctive drug therapy prescribed by their neurologist or primary care physician (16). Drugs used included minor anxiolytics (51 patients) such as alprazolam (25 patients), diazepam (16 patients), and lorazepam (10 patients); anticholinergic medication, trihexyphenidyl (14 patients); antiseizure medications, clonazepam (12 patients) and carbamazepine (6 patients); and a muscle relaxant, baclofen (16 patients). Because antianxiety medications were the most common drugs taken along with botulinum toxin, it was inferred from the data that control of stress by any technique may similarly augment the therapeutic effects of BTX-A.

The authors (16) concluded that BTX-A is the

most highly effective treatment for blepharospasm and Meige's syndrome over a long period of time. In addition, adjunctive oral drug therapy including minor tranquilizers as well as eyelid surgery to excise pretarsal and preseptal orbicularis oculi muscle of the upper eyelid and redundant upper eyelid skin (functional blepharoplasty) may increase the toxin's effectiveness. Any upper eyelid ptosis should be treated by concomitant levator dehiscence repair. It has been the author's impression that after a decade or more of BTX-A injections, eyelid surgery becomes increasingly more likely. In another study, it was found that facial pain and headache may occur with blepharospasm. These symptoms may be similarly relieved by treatment of the blepharospasm with BTX-A (28).

Initial Ophthalmologic Examination

A history and complete ophthalmologic examination are performed. Of particular significance is a history of dry eye. A family history of blepharospasm or other focal dystonia is obtained. A pharmacologic history of neuroleptics, antihistamines, and/or antiepileptic medications including lamotrigine is important as such drugs predispose to blepharospasm. In addition, the role of serotonin reuptake inhibitors is unclear and unsubstantiated to date (29–32). Topical anesthetic is instilled into each eye, and any improvement noted in eyelid spasm may then be attributed to underlying dry eye. Any preexisting ptosis or excess upper eyelid skin should be noted.

Initial Eyelid Treatment with BTX-A

Freeze-dried BTX-A (as BOTOX) is reconstituted by diluting a vial of 100 U with 4 cc of 0.9% saline that is preservative free. The technique involves using a 1-cc tuberculin syringe and a 30-gauge needle.

The toxin is injected into the pretarsal orbicularis muscle of the upper eyelid medially and laterally (2.5 U or 0.1 cc in each location) (Fig. 19.1) (29A). Similarly, the lower eyelids (2.5 U or 0.1 cc in each location) are injected in the same pretarsal location. The lateral canthus (2.5

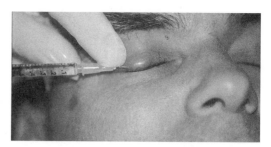

FIG. 19.1. Medial pretarsal injection (0.1 cc of freeze-dried botulinum toxin type A that was reconstituted with 4 cc of saline) of toxin is given as close to eyelid margin as possible.

U) is injected at the initial treatment session (16). A total of 12.5 U is injected into the eyelids on each side.

Injections are performed bilaterally and symmetrically for blepharospasm. Because the orbicularis muscle is located just below the thin skin of the eyelid and there is no intervening subcutaneous fat, electromyographic (EMG) guidance is unnecessary.

In general, treatment of facial areas other than the eyelids is deferred until the effect of the initial eyelid injections is determined 2 weeks after treatment.

Follow-up Evaluation and Treatment

Two weeks after initial injection, patients return for follow-up examinations and are asked to assess their subjective percentage of improvement as compared to pretreatment (16). They are queried about their response relative to the anatomic areas involved: the eyebrow, eyelids, midface (from the cheek to the upper lip), and neck. On examination, the relative weakness on forced closure of the eyelids is objectively graded on a scale from +1 to +4 where +1 is the least-generated forced closure and +4 is the pretreatment level of generated forced closure. The relative weakness of the eyebrow musculature is also assessed.

Patients satisfied with the response and who demonstrate no residual spasm receive no further treatment at that time. Such patients are asked to return for reinjection when the spasms return and become moderate to severe.

Treatment of Residual Eyelid and Eyebrow Spasms

As stated earlier, the physician objectively observes the eyelid and face for evidence of residual spasm. If present, additional drug is given in the upper lid (5 U in each lid). Additional injections are prohibited if upper eyelid ptosis or superior rectus extraocular muscle weakness is present. Generally, the amount of drugs injected into the lower lid and lateral canthal musculature do not need to be increased.

Brow spasms are similarly evaluated. Significant brow spasm is evidenced by marked vertical furrows between the brows medially as well as by downward contraction of the entire brow. Patients who are not satisfied with the result of the first treatment for blepharospasm and have brow spasms receive injections above the medial eyebrows (5 U in two sites above the medial aspect of the brow) (Fig. 19.2). This treatment weakens the corrugator muscle, the depressor supercilii, and the procerus muscles as well as the orbital portion of the orbicularis oculi muscle. These muscles contribute to eyelid closure. Contraction of the corrugator muscle actually raises the head of the brow (medially), but depresses the tail (laterally). More importantly, the depressor supercilii muscle pulls the entire brow downward and contributes to vertical lines between eyebrows. In addition, the procerus muscle contributes to the vertical frown lines between the

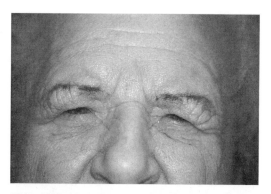

FIG. 19.3. Note descent of entire brow. Vertical lines between brows are mainly a result of corrugator muscle. Patient required eyelid and brow injections for relief.

eyebrows and the horizontal furrows of the radix of the nose (33). The procerus muscle causes descent of the head of the brow (Fig. 19.3). The orbicularis muscle pulls the entire brow downward and creates vertical wrinkles above the medial brow. Residual spasms in the temporal brow area just above the lateral canthus are treated with 2.5 to 5 U depending on the severity of the spasms. Approximately, 20% of patients require brow injections (17).

It is important that the brow injections not weaken the frontalis muscle, which counteracts the brow spasm. In addition, any injections in the frontalis muscle should avoid weakening of the levator muscle. Frontalis muscle activity is evidenced by horizontal furrows across the forehead with concomitant elevation of the eyebrow (Fig. 19.4). The injections should be given just above the medial brow. The middle and upper forehead should be avoided in order to maintain the contractile ability of the frontalis muscle.

Since early 2000, the author has injected BTX-A on each side of the nose 8 mm medial to the medial commissure of the eye. These injections weaken the procerus and the depressor supercilii muscles. The injections are in a plane approximately 5 mm above the level of the medial canthus adjacent to the horizontal nasal wrinkles. These wrinkles are most evident on active contracture, but also tend to be present when the affected muscles are at rest. Treatment includes 2.5 to 5 U injected bilaterally. While

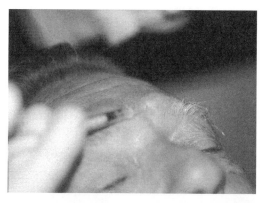

FIG. 19.2. Five units of botulinum toxin type A are injected just above the brow to weaken the procerus, depressor supercilii, and corrugator muscles.

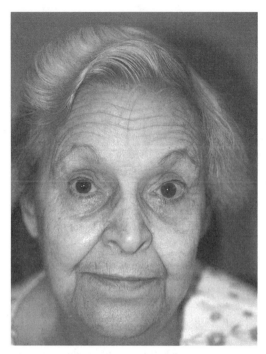

FIG. 19.4. Note use of frontalis muscle to elevate eyebrows to break eyelid spasms. Ten years after successful treatment with botulinum toxin, patient underwent limited myectomy because of decreased duration of toxin effect (less than 2 months). Patient does not have excess dermatochalasis or ptosis.

this treatment is directed specifically at the procerus muscle, diffusion of the toxin also affects the depressor supercilii muscle, which also contracts the eyebrows downward. Such injections effectively control residual blepharospasm that is recalcitrant to the standard protocol outlined above for treatment of the eyelids and medial brow. Marked brow contractures in the medial brow may be treated on the initial visit depending on the overall severity of the eyelid and eyebrow contractures.

Treatment of Residual Facial Spasms

Facial spasms are evaluated 2 weeks after the initial eyelid injections. Eyelid treatment may improve facial spasms and, therefore, treatment of the face may be deferred until the patient is examined 2 weeks after initial eyelid injection.

Residual midfacial and mandibular spasms initially are treated with a total of 5 U injected in two separate locations: (a) in the upper face in the area of the malar eminence and (b) just medial to the mid-aspect of the inferior orbital rim. In patients with spasms of the jaw, 5 U are given at the angle of jaw in the muscle just above the condyle of the jaw (below the zygomatic arch) but not into the joint space. Five to 7.5 U are injected into two to three sites along the ramus of the jaw. Injections may be given in areas where persistent contracture is of concern to the patient (Fig. 19.5). Facial skin, except in the eyelid area, has intervening fat between the dermis and the underlying facial musculature. The target muscle is, therefore, deep to the fat.

Treatment to control spasms in the lower face and mouth should be performed judiciously and incrementally, sometimes in several follow-up treatment sessions as outlined below. Injections adjacent to the corner of the mouth or above the upper lip should be staged in order to avoid excessive muscular weakness with associated drooling, slurred speech, asymmetric facial animation, and biting of the resultant, flaccid buccal mucosa.

Treatment of Subsequent Residual Eyelid and Facial Spasms (4 Weeks After Initial Treatment)

Optimally, patients with significant residual eyelid and facial contractures are reexamined in 2 weeks (4 weeks after the initial injection). At

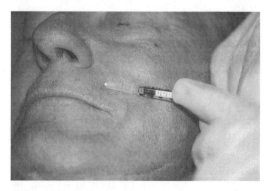

FIG. 19.5. Patient with marked spasm above mouth was treated with 2.5 U and gained relief.

this time, eyelid injections (five additional units in each upper lid) are repeated a third, and even a fourth, time 2 weeks later, if necessary, to obtain a therapeutic effect. The cumulative dose of the previous weeks' injections is given on reinjection several months later after the effect of all the injections dissipates.

In general, patients are requested to return for another treatment session when the effects of the drug are sufficiently dissipated that involuntary eyelid and facial spasms are almost at the pretreatment level. A second treatment session is generally delayed at least 90 days to allow for the production of new receptor sites at the muscle end-plate and for new drug to be effective. As with any drug therapy, the goal of treatment is to control symptoms with the lowest dose and least frequency of injections to minimize complications.

Duration of Action of BTX-A

In our study (16), the mean duration of action was 14.9 weeks for 18 patients with blepharospasm, 16.3 weeks for 7 patients with hemifacial spasm, and 11 weeks for cranial dystonia patients.

Side-Effects of Treatment of Blepharospasm with BTX-A

Acute side-effects include pain on injection. Local bruising resolves within 10 to 14 days. Medications such as coumadin, aspirin, and other anticoagulant medications that predispose to bruising do not need to be discontinued prior to treatment. Garlic, ginseng, and gingko may also cause bleeding.

Resulting lagophthalmos from incomplete involuntary as well as weakened forced eyelid closure may cause symptoms of dry eye. Symptoms include ocular itching, burning, tearing, foreign body sensation, pain in and around the eye, conjunctival injection, photophobia, and blurred vision, and were present in 36% of our patients. Usually, these symptoms are transient and minimal. Dry eye results from an incomplete casual upper eyelid blink. A decreased lacrimal pump from pharmacologic weakening of the orbicu-laris muscle leads to an increased lacrimal lake and tear meniscus present on the lower eyelid margin. Again, transient tearing and blurred vision without other symptoms of dry eye occur. Such symptoms are generally improved by increased forced and complete blinking and topical lubricating eye drops every 2 to 4 hours as needed and usually decrease in intensity 2 to 4 weeks after treatment.

Patients may have an incomplete casual upper eyelid blink that is somewhat counteracted by the increased lacrimal lake inferiorly as a result of a decreased lacrimal pump. These patients should be queried specifically about symptoms of dry eye, including itching, burning, and foreign-body sensation. Corneal epithelial staining with fluorescein may reveal the need for punctal occlusion by silicone plugs or thermal cautery may be necessary. In my experience, only a handful of patients with severe underlying dry eye have required punctal plugs. Rarely, frank recurrent corneal erosion requires prompt ophthalmologic referral.

Mild, transient ptosis lasting for 2 to 4 weeks occurred in 14% of patients (16). Lower-lid ectropion and entropion each occurred in one patient (2%). Such patients may have predisposition of such eyelid malpositions because of preexisting lower-lid laxity.

Tolerance to the drug was not a problem in this series (16). Patients who responded to two or more injections rarely developed tolerance to the drug. Antibodies have not been found in a small number of patients treated for blepharospasm in whom they were sought (12). Theoretically, toxin that is incorrectly formulated, dried, or rehydrated may form inactive, antigenic toxin (toxoid).

In patients with continued blepharospasm after treatment, the poor response is evaluated by assessing forced eyelid closure. In patients with weakened forced closure, the toxin appears to be effective. Such patients should be evaluated for excess dermatochalasis or upper lid ptosis. Other patients in this subgroup have apraxia of eyelid opening that tends to respond to limited myectomy. In my experience, additional BTX-A injections are always necessary.

In patients who continue to show little or no

orbicularis muscle weakness despite repeat botulinum injections, presumed antibodies should be considered as the cause of the failure to respond. No further serum testing is recommended.

Spontaneous Resolution of Blepharospasm After BTX-A Injections

In our study, five patients had spontaneous resolution of the blepharospasm after BTX-A injections (16). While the reason for the resolution is unclear, physicians should probably counsel their patients with blepharospasm and Meige's syndrome that symptoms may rarely abate after treatment with BTX-A. It is impossible to ascertain whether the BTX-A itself influenced the natural history of the disease.

Treatment Choices Other than BTX-A of Patients with Blepharospasm and Meige's Syndrome

Alternative treatments to BTX-A, including radical orbicularis myectomy surgery (three patients), psychotherapy (one patient), and oral medication (one patient), were ultimately chosen as the primary treatment by a small minority of the 239 patient population (16).

Adjunctive treatments included eyelid surgery and oral anxiolytic medications. Six patients underwent excision of excess skin and plication of the levator aponeurosis but continued to receive botulinum treatment. Complications of surgery were minimal and well tolerated.

MANAGEMENT OF HEMIFACIAL SPASM WITH BTX-A

In a retrospective study of patients with hemifacial spasm (HFS), the long-term treatment choices of patients were local BTX-A injections, oral pharmacologic agents, and surgery (neurosurgical decompression of the seventh nerve at the brainstem level and upper eyelid blepharoplasty) (17). Of 119 patients diagnosed with hemifacial spasm, 108 were initially treated with 735 BTX-A injections over an 11-year period

(18). Forty-seven of the 108 patients (43.5%) received 459 injections for a median treatment period of 59 months per patient (17). Eight patients (7.4%) continued treatment elsewhere, and four other patients were injected by the author until their death from other causes. Twenty-two patients (20.4%) were lost to follow-up after receiving 117 injections. Five patients (4.6%) had spontaneous resolution of their condition after BTX-A therapy and nine patients (8.3%) chose not to receive any additional injections or other treatment.

Pharmacologic Adjuvant Therapy Combined with BTX Therapy

In addition to BTX injections, 15 patients required adjunctive minor tranquilizers and/or antiseizure medications. BTX-A is an excellent long-term treatment of hemifacial spasm. As with blepharospasm, patients with hemifacial spasm inexplicably, but only occasionally, experience spontaneous resolution after botulinum therapy (34–36).

Treatment Choices Other than BTX-A in 119 Patients with Hemifacial Spasm

Thirteen patients (12.0%) did not respond adequately to botulinum injections and did not opt for retreatment. Ten of the 13 patients obtained relief from treatments other than BTX: oral pharmacologic agents (two patients), neurosurgical decompression of the seventh nerve (two patients), and upper-eyelid blepharoplasty (one patient).

Duration of Action of BTX-A

The average duration of the therapeutic effect of BTX-A in the treatment of hemifacial spasm is 16 to 18 weeks (8,9,16).

Initial Treatment with BTX-A

In general, 2.5 U are injected into the pretarsal orbicularis oculi muscle in the medial and lateral upper eyelids as well as 12.5 U in the lateral canthus. In patients with only mild disease, 1.25

U rather than 2.5 U are injected into the four pretarsal sites. The lower face is not initially injected.

Follow-up Treatment

When patients are examined 2 weeks after treatment, lower facial spasms are treated with 2.5 to 5 U in the malar eminence region. Lower mouth spasms may be treated with 1.25 to 2.5 U in the corner of the mouth. These injections are given after detailed discussion with the patient about possible asymmetry of smiling and facial weakness with the patient. Occasionally, treatment of the brow protractors including the corrugator muscle and the more central and superficial procerus muscle with 2.5 to 5 U in the medial brow area is helpful.

TREATMENT OF ABERRANT REGENERATION OF THE FACIAL NERVE WITH BTX-A

In a study of six patients with the motor and autonomic effects of aberrant regeneration of facial nerve after a peripheral palsy, BTX-A was found to be an effective treatment. The required dose is similar to or slightly lower than the dose for hemifacial spasm. In two patients with tearing, 20 U were injected into the lacrimal gland area with an almost complete amelioration of tearing (37).

Role of BTX-A Combined with Limited Myectomy and Other Eyelid Surgery

Of 358 patients with focal facial dystonia, 14 underwent (a) upper-eyelid limited myectomy with or without upper-lid blepharoplasty (5 patients), (b) upper-lid blepharoplasty alone (6 patients), or (c) blepharoptosis repair by levator advancement with or without blepharoplasty (3 patients) (38,39). This treatment was reserved for patients who demonstrated orbicularis muscle weakness after BTX injections, but who had a decreased duration of effect or experienced heaviness of the eyelids.

The mean subjective improvement was 68.75% after limited myectomy combined with blepharoplasty, and 58.33% after levator and/or blepharoplasty surgery. Average duration of effect of injections increased from 122.1 days in the patients prior to undergoing eyelid surgery to 210.5 days after surgery. One patient in this series had hemifacial spasm and severe bilateral upper-lid dermatochalasis. Upper-eyelid surgery, including limited myectomy, enhanced the effect of the BTX-A in this small group of patients. In patients who have suboptimal response to injections, or who have moderate to marked dermatochalasis with subjective heaviness of the eyelids, upper-eyelid blepharoplasty and/or limited myectomy should be considered. Function and cosmesis are both improved by such surgery (Fig. 19.6).

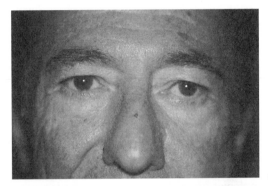

FIG. 19.6. Note patient with left hemifacial spasm and excess skin overhanging the upper eyelid margin (**A**). After bilateral upper-lid blepharoplasty and left-sided upper-lid limited myectomy, the patient enjoyed both an increased duration of botulinum toxin injections and subjective improvement as well. Note improved cosmesis (**B**) several months after surgery. A somewhat higher eyelid crease on the left side as compared to the right side is evident as a result of debulking of orbicularis muscle on the left side.

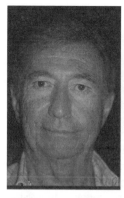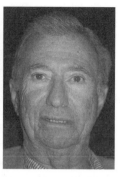

FIG. 19.7. Patient has right upper-eyelid ptosis and dermatochalasis of the upper eyelids with diminished response (decreased duration) to BTX as well as heaviness of the upper eyelids *(left)*. Note patient *(right)* 3 months after bilateral levator advancements, upper-lid blepharoplasty, and limited myectomy. Patient experienced almost immediate improvement in reading and daily visual functions.

Fifteen additional patients have undergone surgical limited myectomy since the original study. Results in this group demonstrate that such surgery has an excellent adjunctive effect to local injections of botulinum for focal facial dystonias (unpublished data). Furthermore, preexisting upper-lid ptosis should be treated in order to improve the effect of the BTX-A injections. In a patient with failure to respond to BTX-A, preexisting should be diagnosed and treated (Fig. 19.7).

CONCLUSION

An analysis of these studies (16,18,38) strongly suggests that BTX-A controls blepharospasm, Meige's syndrome, and hemifacial spasm as well as pharmacologic agents. In patients with eyelid malpositions, including upper-eyelid ptosis, canthal laxity, and upper-lid dermatochalasis, corrective eyelid surgery along with limited myectomy enhances the effectiveness of the injections (16). Because antianxiety medications are the most common drugs taken along with botulinum toxin, control of stress by any other technique may augment the effects of BTX. Pa-

tients with presumed serum antibodies to BTX-A may respond to other types of toxin.

REFERENCES

1. Scott AN, Kennedy RA, Stubbs HA. Botulinum A toxin injections as a treatment for blepharospasm. *Arch Ophthalmol* 1985;103:347–350.
2. Kraft SP, Long AE. Botulinum toxin injections in the treatment of blepharospasm, hemifacial spasm, and eyelid fasciculations. *Can J Neurol Sci* 1988;15:276–280.
3. Frueh BR, Musch DC. Treatment of facial spasm with botulinum toxin: an interim report. *Ophthalmol* 1986; 93:917–923.
4. Shorr N, Seiff RS, Kopelman J. The use of botulinum toxin in blepharospasm. *Am J Ophthalmol* 1985;99: 917–923.
5. Cohen DA, Savino PJ, Stern MB, et al. Botulinum injection therapy for blepharospasm: a review and report of 75 patients. *Clin Neuropharmacol* 1986;9:415–429.
6. Elston JS. Long-term results of treatment of idiopathic blepharospasm with botulinum toxin injections. *Br J Ophthalmol* 1987;71:664–668.
7. Dutton JJ, Buckley EG. Long-term results and complications of botulinum A toxin in the treatment of blepharospasm. *Ophthalmol* 1988;95:1529–1534.
8. Mauriello JA. Blepharospasm, Meige syndrome, and hemifacial spasm: treatment with botulinum toxin. *Neurology* 1985;35:1499–1500.
9. Mauriello JA, Coniaris H, Haupt EJ. Use of botulinum toxin in the treatment of one hundred patients with facial dyskinesias. *Ophthalmol* 1987;94:976–979.
10. Mauriello JA, Aljian J. The natural history of treatment of facial dyskinesias with botulinum toxin: a study of fifty consecutive patients over seven years. *Br J Ophthalmol* 1992;76:349–352.
11. Gonnering RS. Negative antibody response to long term treatment of facial spasm with botulinum toxin. *Am J Ophthalmol* 1988;105:313–315.
12. Barman TA, Prabhakar S. Botulinum toxin treatment of hemifacial spasm and blepharospasm. *Neurol India* 1999;47:206–209.
13. Chang LB, Tsai CP, Liao KK, et al. Use of botulinum toxin A in the treatment of hemifacial spasm and blepharospasm. *Chung Hua I Hsueh Tsa Chih (Taipei)* 1999; 62:1–5.
14. Tan AK. Botulinum toxin for neurological disorders in a movement disorders clinic in Singapore. *Singapore Med J* 1998;39:403–405.
15. Muller-Vahl KR, Kolbe H, Egensperger R, et al. Mitochondriopathy, blepharospasm, and treatment with botulinum toxin. *Muscle Nerve* 2000;23:647–648.
16. Mauriello JA, Dhillon S, Leone T, et al. Treatment profile of 239 patients with blepharospasm and Meige syndrome over 11 years. *Br J Ophthalmol* 1996;80: 1073–1075.
17. Mauriello JA, Leone T, Dhillon S, et al. Treatment choices of 119 patients with hemifacial spasm over 11 years. *Clin Neurol Neurosurg* 1996;98:213–216.
18. Borodic GE, Pearce LB, Johnson E, et al. Clinical and scientific aspects of botulinum A toxin. *Ophthalmol Clin North Am* 1991;4:491–503.
19. Jankovic J, Ford J. Blepharospasm and orofacial-cervi-

cal dystonia: clinical and pharmacologic findings in 100 patients. *Ann Neurol* 1983;13:402–411.
20. Scott AN, Kennedy RA, Stubbs HA. Botulinum A toxin injections as a treatment for blepharospasm. *Arch Ophthalmol* 1985;103:347–350.
21. Deleted in proof.
22. Borodic GE, Cozzolino G. Blepharospasm and its treatment, with emphasis on the use of botulinum toxin. *Plast Reconstr Surg* 1989;83:546–554.
23. American Academy of Ophthalmology. Botulinum toxin therapy of eye muscle disorders: safety and effectiveness. *Ophthalmology* 1989;51:767–772.
24. Marsden C. Blepharospasm-oromandibular dystonia syndrome (Brueghel's syndrome). *J Neurol Neurosurg Psychiatry* 1976;39:1204–1209.
25. Grandas F, Traba A, Alonso F, et al. Blink reflex recovery cycle in patients with blepharospasm unilaterally treated with botulinum toxin. *Clin Neuropharmacol* 1998;21:307–311.
26. Bogucki A. Serial SFEMG studies of orbicularis muscle after the first administration of botulinum toxin. *Eur J Neurol* 1999;6:461–467.
27. Mezaki T, Taki R, Brin MF, et al. Controlled use of type A and F botulinum toxins for blepharospasm: double-blind controlled trial. *Mov Disord* 1999;14:1017–1028.
28. Johnstone SJ, Adler CH. Headache and facial pain responsive to botulinum toxin: an unusual presentation of blepharospasm. *Headache* 1998;38:366–368.
29. Mauriello JA, Carbonaro P, Dhillon S, et al. Drug-associated facial dyskinesias: a study of 238 patients. *J Neuroophthalmol* 1998;18:153–157.
30. Verma A, Miller P, Carwile ST, et al. Lamotrigine-induced blepharospasm. *Pharmacotherapy* 1999;19:877–880.
31. Micheli F, Cersosimo G, Scorticati MC, et al. Blepharospasm and apraxias of eyelid opening in lithium toxicity. *Clin Neuropharmacol* 1999;22:176–179.
32. Salmimen L, Janitti V, Gronross M. Blepharospasm associated with tegafur combination chemotherapy. *Am J Ophthalmol* 1984;97:649–650.
33. Isse N. Endoscopic facial rejuvenation. In: Menick FJ, ed. *Facial anesthetic surgery (clinics in plastic surgery).* Philadelphia: WB Saunders, 1997:213–232.
34. Wang A, Jankovic J. Hemifacial spasm: clinical findings and treatment. *Muscle Nerve* 1998;21:1740–1747.
35. Jitpimolmard S, Tiamkao S, Laopaiboon M. Long-term results of botulinum toxin type A (DYSPORT) in the treatment of hemifacial spasm: a report of 175 cases. *J Neurol Neurosurg Psychiatry* 1998;64:751–757.
36. Karpati S, Desaknai S, Desaknai M, et al. Human herpesvirus type 8-positive facial angiosarcoma developing at the site of botulinum toxin injection for blepharospasm. *Br J Dermatol* 2000;143:660–661.
37. Bojoojerdi B, Ferbert A, Schwarz M, et al. Botulinum toxin treatment of synkinesia and hyperlacrimation after facial palsy. *J Neurol Neurosurg Psychiatry* 1998;65:111–114.
38. Mauriello JA, Keswani R, Franklin MN. Long-term enhancement of botulinum injections by upper eyelid surgery in 14 patients with facial dyskinesias. *Arch Otolaryngol Head Neck Surg* 1999;125:627–631.
39. Mauriello JA. Editorial commentary: causes and treatment of blepharospasm: botulinum toxin, limited myectomy, and pharmacologic therapy. In: Mauriello JA, ed. *Unfavorable results of eyelid and lacrimal surgery prevention and management.* Boston: Butterworth-Heinemann, 2000:197–204.

Scientific and Therapeutic Aspects of Botulinum Toxin
edited by M.F. Brin, J. Jankovic, and M. Hallett
Lippincott Williams & Wilkins, Philadelphia, © 2002.

20

Botulinum Toxin Type A Injections for the Management of the Hyperfunctional Larynx

Andrew Blitzer, Craig Zalvan, Omar Gonzalez-Yanez, and Mitchell F. Brin

Historically, we gave the first laryngeal botulinum toxin injection of the vocal folds in April 1984 (1). The patient was a man who had blepharospasm, and had been successfully treated with botulinum toxin type A (BTX-A). He then developed laryngeal dystonia (spasmodic dysphonia), and was very successfully treated with small amounts of BTX-A, injected under electromyographic (EMG) control. He was initially placed in the intensive care unit for observation. These days, the injections are given during a quick, outpatient visit.

Both the Houston group (39) and the NIH group (40) then began using botulinum toxin for laryngeal dystonia. The Houston and NIH groups continued programs with large doses given unilaterally to simulate the effects of the recurrent nerve section. We observed that bilateral injections permitted the use of smaller doses and produced better voicing. We postulated that if one vocal fold was immobile, the other vocal fold would have to compensate for it and the dystonic symptoms in the functional vocal fold would be exaggerated, leading to poor voicing. Bilateral injections would be expected to address this problem, and should give better voicing results.

SPASMODIC DYSPHONIA

Botulinum toxin injections are performed after a detailed history and head and neck examination are performed. Any neurologic finding is noted, with special attention paid to tremor,

spasm, and tone of the surrounding musculature. Fiberoptic laryngoscopy and stroboscopy is then performed on all patients. In addition to providing videographic documentation, the examination of the larynx is used to confirm the diagnosis, degree of dysfunction, and any relative difference in activity between the two vocal folds.

In adductor dysphonia, vocalization of /i/ and connected speech help to demonstrate which side is more affected by the disease process, from prior BTX injection, and other neurologic conditions that may affect the voice. With abductor dysphonia patients, the vocal fold activity is tested with consonant-based phrases and words such as ''taxi'' or ''Harry's hat.'' The fiberoptic exam is crucial in determining the degree of airway patency, which vocal fold is more affected by the disease, and any residual effect from prior injections. All patients with abductor spasmodic dysphonia undergo a nasopharyngolaryngoscopy prior to any subsequent injection.

The starting dose is based on a large series of patients (1). The starting dose should be adjusted to conform to the needs of the patient. If the patient's profession, or preference, demands a strong voice, the starting dose can be lowered and titrated at subsequent visits. If there is a higher risk for aspiration then the dose can be lowered accordingly.

Lidocaine

The patient is instructed not to cough, talk, or swallow during the injection. Some patients demonstrate increased sensitivity to any airway

---

Mitchell F. Brin is an employee of Allergan, Inc.

manipulation. This can be attenuated by first injecting the subglottic space with 0.4 mL of 1% lidocaine through the cricothyroid membrane. The patient usually coughs after the injection. This helps distribute the anesthetic over the vocal-fold mucosa. This is not routinely performed on all patients because the anesthetic decreases the EMG interference pattern, which pattern helps to identify the most active area of the muscle (2,3).

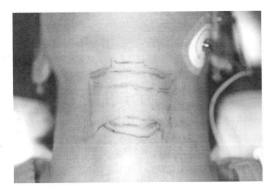

FIG. 20.1. Laryngeal cartilage landmarks drawn on the neck skin.

Botox Titration

We currently use BOTOX (Allergan, Inc.) a brand of BTX-A, to treat our patients. We (Dr. Blitzer) have begun to use Myobloc, a brand of BTX-B, in clinical trials to determine proper dosing, effectiveness, and comparability. All references to botulinum toxin in this chapter refer to BTX-A.

BOTOX is prepackaged with 100 U of toxin that is frozen and lyophilized. This is reconstituted with 4 mL of normal saline (without preservative), giving a final concentration of 2.5 U/0.1 mL. By diluting 0.1 mL of the stock solution with normal saline to a total volume of 0.25 mL, a concentration of 1 U/0.1 mL can be obtained. Similarly, other concentrations are obtained to provide a constant volume of 0.1 mL. Starting dose for adductor dysphonia is typically 1 U in each vocal fold. Starting dose for abductor dysphonia is typically 3.75 U/0.15 mL per one vocal fold.

Positioning

After laryngoscopy has been performed, the patient is positioned comfortably in the examination chair. The chair is raised to an appropriate height. The backrest is lowered until the patient is resting at 30 degrees in the supine position. A pillow is placed behind the back at the level of the shoulders which helps to extend the neck. The EMG leads are placed at and below the angle of the mandible on the side of the EMG machine; one for a skin reference, one a ground,

and the other lead attaches to the injection needle. The neck is palpated and the cricothyroid membrane is located (Fig. 20.1).

The Injection

Adductor

After the skin is cleaned with an alcohol pad, the 27-gauge monopolar, hollow-bore, Teflon-coated EMG needle is connected to the recorder. The right-handed physician then stands to the patient's right side. Prior to insertion, the needle is grasped between the thumb and forefinger and curved gently to provide a slight curvature to the needle. The needle is then inserted through the cricothyroid space with a gentle "pop" as the needle passes the cricothyroid membrane (Fig. 20.2). The tip of the needle is then advanced submucosally superiorly and laterally at approximately 30 degrees in both directions. The audio of the EMG provides feedback guiding the depth of the needle to the most active point of the thyroarytenoid muscle. The patient is asked to phonate a soft /i/ which helps to augment the recruitment signal of the EMG. Once in position, the toxin is injected and the needle is then retracted to the midline. The repeat procedure is performed on the opposite vocal fold when indicated. The procedure is typically well tolerated with rare coughing or gagging noted by the patient. Slight pressure is placed on the

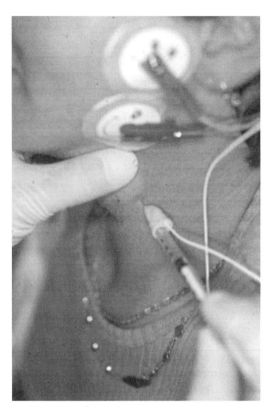

FIG. 20.2. Adductor injection with EMG guidance through the cricothyroid membrane.

needle entrance site to prevent hematoma formation. The patient is then discharged home.

Typically the patient reports back by telephone regarding the effectiveness of the injection at 1 to 2 weeks. Additional injection can be performed as needed. Patients are sent home with a sell return scale. They record any dysphagia, aspiration, breathiness, or any other side effect they encounter. The length and severity of each symptom is recorded. Also recorded are the highest level of function noted on a 0% to 100% scale; 0 being no voice and 100% being a normal voice. We have found this subjective scale to correlate strongly with the degree of function and satisfaction each injection provides the patient. They record a daily report of breathiness and vocal ability for 2 weeks and then on a weekly basis. This sheet is then brought with them on their return visit to help with any adjustment to dosing that may be necessary.

Abductor

The patient is positioned and prepped as stated above. There are two methods that we use to inject the posterior cricoarytenoid muscle (PCA). Both methods use EMG guidance to localize the area of maximum recruitment.

In the first method, the larynx is grasped between the thumb and first two fingers of the left hand (for a right handed-physician). The fingers are positioned lateral and deep to the lateral thyroid ala. With a pulling motion of the fingers and a medial and pushing motion of the thumb, the larynx is gently rotated medially away from the side of the injector. The EMG hollow-bore needle is then advanced medially through the inferior constrictor muscle to the cricoid cartilage, into the PCA muscle (Fig. 20.3). The EMG audible signal is then used to find the area of greatest activity, with increased signal from having the patient sniff, aiding in maximal abduction. Once in position, the botulinum toxin is injected.

An alternative method is used primarily in younger individuals. This is a direct, anterior approach with the EMG needle advanced through the cricothyroid membrane just above the level of the cricoid cartilage. The needle is then directed laterally and forward in the same

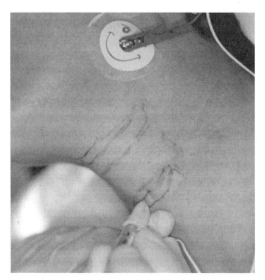

FIG. 20.3. Abductor injection given posterior to the posterior thyroid lamina.

plane until the cricoid cartilage rostrum is encountered. The needle is then advanced through the cartilage until it exits in the PCA muscle lying on the posterior-lateral surface of the cricoid cartilage. The patient is instructed to sniff, confirming placement, and guides the physician to the most active component of the muscle.

As with adductor patients, slight pressure is placed over the entrance site and the patient is sent home with a score sheet to record any post-injection side effects, especially stridor, and degree of vocal ability. With PCA injections, there is an added risk of airway compromise resulting in stridor and potential airway obstruction. In more than 175 patients to date, there has been no need for airway intervention noted by our group. Extreme care must be taken to preserve the airway. There are anecdotal reports of patients who have been intubated or tracheotomized after excessive PCA weakening particularly after bilateral simultaneous insertions.

Adductor Dosing Strategies

After the initial injection, the patient is instructed to record the degree of improvement in their voice as well as any potential side effects. This helps to determine the next dose, usually 3 to 4 months after the first injection. Patients with a heightened sensitivity to botulinum toxin may experience prolonged and debilitating breathiness, hoarseness, or aspiration. If this occurs, the subsequent dose is usually cut in half at the next injection. Also, a patient's profession or preference may require a shorter period of side effects and the dose can be dropped. The patient is instructed that botulinum toxin is used to treat the symptoms produced by spasmodic dysphonia. Therefore the dose is adjusted based on a patient's desire. Some patients prefer a longer interval until the next dose and can tolerate the breathiness in the first few weeks. These patients can have increased dosing resulting with a longer result. In our 13-year report of 901 patients, our range of injection is from 0.005 to 30 U (1). Our average current dose is 1 U per vocal fold. There is an educational curve, and new injectors may need higher doses based upon less

accurate toxin placement. In our series, the average onset of toxin effect was 2.4 days, with the maximum effect at 7 to 10 days. The duration of benefit was 12 to 16 weeks. Patients achieved an average benefit of 89.7% of their normal function.

Some patients have difficulty titrating their dose based on their side-effect profile and time to subsequent injection. With these patients a number of dosing strategies have been devised.

Alternating Vocal Folds

Flexible laryngoscopy is performed to determine which side has more activity and more voicing breaks. This thyroarytenoid (TA) muscle can then be injected (average 2 U). The patient is then contacted by telephone in 2 weeks after the injection to determine efficacy. If the patient desires further symptom relief, a second injection in the opposite vocal fold can be performed any time from 2 weeks up to 4 months after the initial injection. In some patients, this is useful, providing primarily a shorter period of side effects and potentially a longer period of acceptable voicing. The caveat is that the interval between injections may be decreased, depending on the sensitivity to the botulinum toxin. Thus after the initial injection a second injection can be performed on the opposite TA. Alternatively, alternating vocal folds at 4-month intervals provide some patients with minimal side effects and maximal voicing (4).

Another paradigm that we found to be useful in patients who can not tolerate any early side effects is minidosing: 0.1 to 0.2 U per TA per visit. The duration of benefit is usually only 6 to 8 weeks, but there are few side effects. This is very useful for a professional speaker, singer, or teacher, especially if they live nearby the office and can tolerate frequent visits.

In all, it can not be stressed enough that the injections are performed to provide relief from the strained, breaking voice caused by the spasmodic dysphonia. Dosing can be adjusted in a number of ways to provide the patient with the level of control of their symptoms and an adequate interval between injections that supports their lifestyle.

Abductor Dosing Strategies

Prior to any abductor injection, the larynx is examined with a flexible fiberoptic laryngoscope. The vocal folds are examined for symmetry, activity level with voicing tasks, hesitancy, and frank breaks.

For the initial injection of a new patient, the more active vocal fold is chosen for the first injection. The initial dose has been standardized to 3.75 U in 0.15 mL, which is taken from a stock solution of 2.5 U/0.1 mL. Only one PCA is injected at any given treatment. In approximately 20% of our patient population, one PCA injection is sufficient to provide good voicing and control of a patient's abductor spasmodic dysphonia. The patient is usually contacted by phone in 2 to 3 weeks after the initial injection. They are instructed to call sooner if any stridor or respiratory distress develops. If there is no or minimal improvement noted, the patient returns for a second injection. This occurs in the remaining 80% of the abductor population. The patient is then instructed to return for further treatment as symptoms return.

Upon return, the patient's larynx is examined to judge the remaining activity of the vocal folds as well as the patency of the larynx. Any respiratory distress symptoms are also noted. Taken together, the clinical and physical findings help determine which PCA to inject at the followup visit. No further injections are performed if there has been any stridor or extreme narrowing of the posterior glottic chink is noted. The majority of patients have some weakening noted in the vocal fold injected 2 to 3 weeks prior. These patients will receive an injection into the contralateral PCA with doses ranging from 0.625 up to 2.5 U in 0.1 mL. Alternatively, if minimal change is noted from the first injection, the same PCA can be reinjected with a similar dose of 0.625 to 2.5 U/0.1 mL, again based on the physical and clinical findings.

To date none of the abductor patients in our series has required tracheotomy or intubation secondary to respiratory compromise. We strongly suggest that PCA injections be staggered with at least 2 to 3 weeks between injections of each PCA.

Nerve-Section Failure Patients

Patients with adductor SD who have already undergone recurrent laryngeal nerve section have a marked improvement with the BOTOX injections, but to a lesser degree than the nonsurgical patients. When performing the EMG, a decrease in interference pattern is present with few and very small action potentials. In our series, nine patients had failed a recurrent laryngeal nerve section (3). Four of the patients had more than one procedure performed including Teflon injection and laser fold thinning. Most of the recurrent laryngeal nerve section failures were treated unilaterally in the functional vocal fold with an average dose of 2 U. Some of the patients who had activity in the immobile vocal fold did well with the injection in that side. The results showed a functional rating of 81% when the mobile vocal fold was injected, and 60% when the immobile vocal fold was injected. As with nonsurgical cases, follow-up treatment is individualized and the dose may be decreased or increased as needed.

Anterior Commissure Release Failures

We have treated three patients who failed an anterior commissure release procedure. These patients had intense adductor spasms with a postoperative foreshortened appearance of the larynx. These patients required larger doses than the average patient with adductor SD, perhaps because of the barriers to diffusion related to scarring. Although the spasms could be reduced in this group and all experienced some benefit, most noticed a weakened voice with limited pitch range. They also had an extended hypophonia after injection.

Adductor Laryngeal Breathing Dystonia

We attempted to reduce the adductor breathing spasms with doses based on the benefit seen in the adductor group. Patients received between 0.625 and 3.75 U in each thyroarytenoid muscle, depending on the severity of the spasms. The average preinjection function was 27%, based on a rating scale of the percentage of normal function relating to the severity of their breathing. Pulmonary function tests showed abnormal flow volume loops with intermittent interruptions of airflow during inspiration or expiration in 20 of 24 patients. Most of the patients also had diaphragmatic dysfunction on testing. The best postinjection function average was 82% of normal, making the average percentage improvement 55% ($p = .0001$). The mean duration of stridor relief was 14 weeks. A breathy voice lasting 1 to 2 weeks occurred in 50% of patients.

Other Methods of Injection

In our patient experience, we have determined that the EMG-guided transcutaneous method is the most reliable and easiest method of injecting both the TA and PCA muscles. Some groups use the transcutaneous method and augment the localization of the appropriate muscle using flexible endoscopic guidance (5).

Some clinicians have advocated the use of transoral injections using indirect mirror laryngoscopy and a modified injection needle (6). They report an 85% success rate with the transoral injection. They state their method is easy to perform, increases the accuracy of injection, and decreases soft tissue injury. They also report that there was greater patient comfort with most patients indicating the injection was less traumatic than a laryngeal EMG.

Our group does not use the transoral injection technique. Our experience has demonstrated that EMG-guided injections provide access to the most active part of the muscle. The EMG technique requires one transcutaneous puncture that most patients report to be very tolerable. Precise injection into the most active component of the muscle provides for a decreased quantity of toxin and increased efficacy of the procedure. Also, not all laryngologists are as proficient with transoral injection techniques, nor do all patients tolerate oropharyngeal manipulation well.

Green et al. (7) described another approach to the vocal fold injection without the use of EMG guidance. They used a transthyroid cartilage injection through the thyroid cartilage lamina to enter the TA. We also do not use this method for similar reasons.

Rhew et al. (8) reported on vocal fold injections through the operating channel of a flexible fiberoptic laryngoscope. They report satisfactory results with this technique. We feel that not only is placement into the active portion of the muscle not confirmed, dosing may also be difficult because of the long distance of the needle chamber and syringe to the needle.

OTHER USES OF BOTULINUM TOXIN IN THE LARYNX

The use of botulinum toxin in the treatment of spasmodic dysphonia has demonstrated a high degree of success, reliability, and patient satisfaction. Because of its ability to effectively decrease muscular activity, many groups have applied its use to the treatment of a wide range of disorders. In the larynx, the primary role of botulinum toxin has been toward relieving a disabling problem with the voice. Spasmodic dysphonia, tremor, stuttering, vocal tics, ventricular dysphonia, and others are treated primarily by treating the articulatory, phonatory, and respiratory mechanisms which are responsible for the vocal difficulty.

Stuttering

Stuttering is a disorder that affects up to 1% of adults. This disorder presents as an involuntary speech- or action-induced disruption in the fluency of voice. Utterance of words, sounds, or certain syllables can induce audible or silent repetitions in one of the many phonatory mechanisms in voice production including laryngeal, pharyngeal, oral, and lip movements. Botulinum toxin was used to inject the thyroarytenoid muscles of a group of patients with persistent stuttering. Patients noted some improvement in fluency with return of symptoms by 12 weeks. Patients with glottal blocs, laryngeal spasms that obstruct the flow of air, seemed to derive greater benefit (9). Although most stutterers choose behavioral therapy to successfully treat their stutter, botulinum toxin is available to refractory cases.

Vocal Tics

Gilles de la Tourette's syndrome is a devastating psychological and social disorder that is manifested by repetitive dystonic tics of the eyes, mouth, other facial muscles, neck, shoulders, and voice. The vocal tics can range from simple to complex utterances presented as loud screams, grunts, loud talking, repetitive vowel and word utterances, and coprolalia. Psychotropic medications and behavioral therapy remain the mainstay of treatment. Recently, various investigators have focused on the use of botulinum toxin in preventing the multiple dystonic features of the syndrome, including vocal tics (10–13). Although rarely providing a complete cure, botulinum toxin injections into bilateral thyroarytenoid muscles has been shown to decrease the rate of vocal outbreaks, grunts, and coprolalia. The exact mechanism is unknown; however, an effect mediated by the afferent sensory system has been postulated. This suggests that both the disease process and the treatment involve a complex interaction between the central nervous system and the peripheral nervous system, including both afferent and efferent limbs.

Essential Voice Tremor

In an aging population, the prevalence of essential voice tremor has become more noticeable. Generally affecting older individuals, essential voice tremor is defined as an activation-induced tremor with a frequency of 8 to 13 Hz in younger individuals, decreasing to 3 to 7 Hz in older individuals (14). Most noted during utterance of vowels, the voice is characterized by breaks in pitch and fluency marked by vocal arrests secondary to excessive abductive or adductive movements of the vocal folds (15). Voice tremor is commonly seen in association with neurologic disorders including Parkinson's disease, amyotrophic lateral sclerosis, and cerebellar disorders

(16,17). Tremor has also been noted in 25% to 60% of patients with spasmodic dysphonia (9,10,18,19).

Recent attempts to treat essential voice tremor with botulinum toxin injections have demonstrated modest benefit with one-half to two-thirds of patients receiving some subjective improvement of their voice. Objective measures demonstrate significantly less improvement with only one-quarter to one-third of patients showing significant change. However, most patients desire retreatment with botulinum toxin (20,21). Injections are typically performed in bilateral thyroarytenoid muscles. Tremor activity is easily confirmed by electromyographic analysis. Our group and others have confirmed that tremor is not exclusively a glottic phenomenon; other extralaryngeal muscles may contribute (22). Some patients with noted contribution from the cricothyroid and thyrohyoid muscles may need to have these muscles injected in addition to the thyroarytenoid muscles.

Ventricular Dysphonia/Dysphonia Plicae Ventricularis, Supraglottic Spasm

Ventricular dysphonia, known historically as dysphonia plicae ventricularis, presents clinically as a hoarse, ''wet'' voice interrupted by voice breaks, fatigue, and overall poor voice quality. This disorder is thought to be caused by an alteration in the vocal mechanism replacing the false vocal folds as the major vibratory source. This is most commonly secondary to true vocal fold pathology. Long-term hyperfunction of the false vocal folds can result in hypertrophy of the vocal folds. A rating system by Kosokovic demonstrated four stages of ventricular dysphonia based on physical and histologic characteristics. Stages I to III show varying degrees of metaplasia, submucosal edema, and inflammatory infiltrate. Stages I and II are treated primarily with voice therapy. Stage III is unlikely to resolve with voice therapy and is treated surgically (23).

Recently, a number of investigators have used botulinum toxin injected into the false vocal folds to treat this disorder. Transoral injection performed in the operating room and in the office using indirect laryngoscopy resulted in a much higher rate of improvement in conjunction with continued voice therapy. Similar results were observed in patients diagnosed as having supraglottic spasm (24–26).

Puberphonia

Mutational dysphonia, or puberphonia, is the failure of the vocal pitch to descend at puberty. Voice therapy is the mainstay of treatment of this disorder. Injection of each cricothyroid muscle with botulinum toxin in a 47-year-old man resulted in improvement of the voice with normalization of the pitch. In this case, botulinum toxin was hypothesized to help voice therapy achieve a normalization of the voice by temporarily paralyzing, or weakening, certain muscles within the larynx preventing relaxation of the vocal fold. It may be possible to retrain the vocal mechanism to a more functional and acceptable level by manipulating the relative input of muscles responsible for tensing the vocal fold versus relaxing the vocal fold (27).

Arytenoid Rebalancing

Botulinum toxin can be selectively applied to the laryngeal muscles to help create an anatomic change in vocal fold positioning. This can help to change a physical impediment to proper voicing.

One investigator reported the use of ''laryngeal rebalancing,'' referring to the chemodenervation of the interarytenoid muscle, ipsilateral thyroarytenoid muscle, and lateral cricothyroid muscle in the treatment of anteromedial cricoarytenoid dislocation. By weakening the ipsilateral adductory component to the vocal fold position, the relative increase in the abductor strength helped provide traction on the arytenoid. This aided in the repositioning of the arytenoid to a more physiologic position (28).

Another group treated a patient with bilateral vocal fold paralysis by injecting bilateral laryngeal adductor muscles to create a ''rebalancing'' of the abductor and adductor contributions to the vocal fold position. By weakening any residual adductor activity, the airway was increased in patency, and the patient reported significantly less dyspnea (29). Previously, this had only been performed in animal models (30).

Prevention of Posterior Glottic Stenosis; Granuloma

In a similar manner, botulinum toxin has been used to help prevent posterior glottic synechiae in the repair of posterior glottic stenosis. By injecting the adductor muscles, the vocal folds tend to remain more lateralized, allowing faster and more complete healing to occur (31). Botulinum toxin has also been used as an adjunct to the treatment of vocal fold granulomas (32,33). Traditional treatment involves medical therapy consisting of voice therapy and antireflux medication with surgery reserved for treatment failures. By injecting the adductor musculature, there is less local trauma allowing for resolution of the vocal fold granuloma.

Extralaryngeal Uses of Botulinum Toxin in the Laryngopharynx

Dysphagia caused by increased pressure from an inability of the cricopharyngeus muscle to relax may also be treated with botulinum toxin injection. Easily identified by transcutaneous electromyography, the cricopharyngeus can be localized in the office. Alternatively, direct visualization and injection of the cricopharyngeus can be performed in the operating room. In either case, botulinum toxin Type A injection has demonstrated 70% to 100% relief of cricopharyngeal spasm (34–36).

Botulinum toxin injection can also be used as a diagnostic tool. Injections can help to identify those patients who would benefit from a surgical procedure such as cricopharyngeal myotomy. By responding to chemodenervation of the cricopharyngeus with botulinum toxin, a more permanent solution such as surgery can be suggested (27).

Similarly, botulinum toxin Type A has been used to diagnose and treat voice failure in laryngectomy patients using a tracheoesophageal puncture with speech valve. Hypertonicity or spasm of the pharyngoesophageal segment has been postulated as the cause of the voice failure. Botulinum toxin Type A injections into the cricopharyngeus or pharyngoesophageal segment under electromyographic guidance can be used to confirm the diagnosis by providing relief, as well as to treat the problem (37,38).

Botulinum toxin Type A has proven itself as a useful diagnostic and therapeutic tool in the larynx and pharynx. Easy to perform, botulinum toxin Type A injections provide relief of many vocal and pharyngoesophageal disorders. Botulinum toxin Type A allows for a nonsurgical approach to anatomic and neurologic problems encountered in the laryngopharynx.

REFERENCES

1. Blitzer A, Brin MF, Stewart C. Botulinum toxin management of spasmodic dysphonia (laryngeal dystonia): a 12-year experience in more than 900 patients. *Laryngoscope* 1998;108:1435–1441.
2. Brin MF, Fahn S, Blitzer A, et al. Movement disorders of the larynx. In: Blitzer A, Brin MF, Sasaki CT, et al., eds. *Neurological disorders of the larynx.* New York: Thieme, 1992:240–248.
3. Blitzer A, Brin MF. Laryngeal dystonia: a series with botulinum toxin therapy. *Ann Otol Rhinol Laryngol* 1991;100:85–90.
4. Koriwchak MJ, Netterville JL, Snowden T, et al. Alternating unilateral botulinum toxin type A (BOTOX) Injections for spasmodic dysphonia. *Laryngoscope* 1996;106:1476–1481.
5. Truong DD, Rontal M, Rolnick M, et al. Double-blind controlled study of botulinum toxin in adductor spasmodic dysphonia. *Laryngoscope* 1991;101:630–634.
6. Ford CN, Bless DM, Lowery JD. Indirect laryngoscopic approach for injection of botulinum toxin in spasmodic dysphonia. *Otolaryngol Head Neck Surg* 1990;103:752–758.
7. Green DC, Berke GS, Ward PH, et al. Point-touch technique of botulinum toxin injection for the treatment of spasmodic dysphonia. *Ann Otol Rhinol Laryngol* 1992;101:883–887.
8. Rhew K, Fiedlre DA, Ludlow CL. Technique for injection of botulinum toxin through a flexible nasolaryngoscope. *Otolaryngol Head Neck Surg* 1994;111:787–794.
9. Brin MF, Stewart C, Blitzer B, et al. Laryngeal botulinum toxin injections for disabling stuttering in adults. *Neurology* 1994;44;2262–2266.
10. Jankovic J. Botulinum toxin in the treatment of tics. In: Jankovic J, Hallet M, eds. *Therapy with botulinum toxin.* New York: Marcel Dekker, 1994:503–509.
11. Salloway S, Stewart CF, Israeli L, et al. Botulinum toxin for refractory vocal tics. *Mov Disord* 1996;11:746–748.
12. Scott BL, Jankovic J, Donovan DT. Botulinum toxin injection into vocal cord in the treatment of malignant coprolalia associated with Tourette's syndrome. *Mov Disord* 1996; 11:431–433.
13. Trimble MR, Whurr R, Brookes G, et al. Vocal tics in Gilles de la Tourette syndrome treated with botulinum toxin injections. *Mov Disord* 1998;13:617–619.
14. Elble RJ, Higgins C, Leffler K, et al. Factors influencing the amplitude and frequency of essential tremor. *Mov Disord* 1994;9:589–596.
15. Winholtz WS, Ramig LO. Vocal tremor analysis with the vocal demodulator. *J Speech Hear Res* 1992;35:562–573.
16. Smith ME, Ramig LO. Neurological disorders and the voice. In: Rubin JS, Sataloff RT, Korovin GS, et al., eds. *Diagnosis and treatment of voice disorders.* New York: Igaku-Shoin, 1995:203–224.
17. Brin MF, Fahn S, Blitzer A, et al. Movement disorders of the larynx. In: Blitzer A, Brin MF, Sasaki C, et al., eds. *Neurologic disorders of the larynx.* New York: Thieme, 1992:248–278.
18. Blitzer A, Brin MF, Fahn S. Clinical and laboratory characteristics of focal laryngeal dystonia. Study of 110 cases. *Laryngoscope* 1988;98:636–640.
19. Schaefer SD. Neuropathology of spasmodic dysphonia. *Laryngoscope* 1983;93:1183–1204.
20. Warrick P, Dromey C, Irish J, et al. Botulinum toxin for essential tremor of the voice with multiple anatomical sites of tremor: a crossover design study of unilateral versus bilateral injection. *Laryngoscope* 2000;110:1366–1374.
21. Hertegard S, Granqvist S, Lindestad P. Botulinum toxin injections for essential voice tremor. *Ann Otol Rhinol Laryngol* 2000;109:204–209.
22. Blitzer A, Sulica L. Botulinum toxin: basic science and clinical uses in otolaryngology. *Laryngoscope* 2000;111:218–226.
23. Kosokovic F, Vecerina S, Cepelja I, et al. Contribution to therapy of dysphonia plica ventricularis. *Laryngoscope* 1977;87:408–414.
24. Kendall KA, Leonard RJ. Treatment of ventricular dysphonia with botulinum toxin. *Laryngoscope* 1997;107:948–953.
25. Schonweiler R, Wohlfarth K, Dengler R, et al. Supraglottal injection of botulinum toxin type A in adductor type spasmodic dysphonia with both intrinsic and extrinsic hyperfunction. *Laryngoscope* 1998;108:55–63.
26. Rosen CA, Murray T. BOTOX for hyperadduction of the false vocal folds: a case report. *J Voice* 1999;13:234–239.
27. Woodson GE, Murray T. Botulinum toxin in the treatment of recalcitrant mutational dysphonia. *J Voice* 1994;8:347–351.
28. Rontal E, Rontal M. Laryngeal rebalancing for the treatment of arytenoid dislocation. *J Voice* 1998;12:383–388.
29. Ptok M, Schonweiler R. Botulinum toxin type A—induced "rebalancing" in bilateral vocal cord paralysis? *HNO* 2001;49:548–552.
30. Cohen SR, Thompson JW, Camilon FS. Botulinum toxin for relief of bilateral abductor paralysis of the larynx: histologic study in an animal model. *Ann Otol Rhinol Laryngol* 1989;98:213–216.
31. Nathon CO, Yin S, Stucker FJ. Botulinum toxin: adjunctive treatment for posterior glottic synechiae. *Laryngoscope* 1999;109:855–857.
32. Nasri S, Sercarz JA, McAlpin T, et al. Treatment of vocal fold granuloma using botulinum toxin type A. *Laryngoscope* 1995;105:585–588.
33. Orloff LA, Goldman SN. Vocal fold granuloma: suc-

cessful treatment with botulinum toxin. *Otolaryngol Head Neck Surg* 1999;121:410–413.

34. Blitzer A, Brin MF. Use of botulinum toxin for diagnosis and management of cricopharyngeal achalasia. *Otolaryngol Head Neck Surg* 1997;116:328–330.

35. Ashan SF, Meleca RJ, Dworkin JP. Botulinum toxin injection of the cricopharyngeus muscle for the treatment of dysphagia. *Otolaryngol Head Neck Surg* 2000; 122:691–695.

36. Schneider I, Pototschnig C, Thumfart WF, et al. Treatment of dysfunction of the cricopharyngeal muscle with botulinum A toxin: introduction of a new, noninvasive method. *Ann Otol Rhinol Laryngol* 1994;103:31–35.

37. Zormeier MM, Meleca RJ, Simpson ML, et al. Botulinum toxin injection to improve tracheoesophageal speech after total laryngectomy. *Otolaryngol Head Neck Surg* 1999;120:314–319.

38. Blitzer A, Komisar A, Baredes S, et al. Voice failure after tracheoesophageal puncture: management with botulinum toxin. *Otolaryngol Head Neck Surg* 1995; 113:668–670.

39. Miller RH, Woodson, GE, Jankovic J. Botulinum toxin injection of the vocal folds for spasmodic dysphonia. *Arch Otol Head Neck Surg* 1987;113:603–605.

40. Ludlow CL, Naunton RF, Sedory SE, et al. Effects of botulinum toxin injection on speech in adductor spasmodic dysphonia. *Neurology* 1988; 38:1220–1225.

Scientific and Therapeutic Aspects of Botulinum Toxin
edited by M.F. Brin, J. Jankovic, and M. Hallett
Lippincott Williams & Wilkins, Philadelphia, © 2002.

21

The Use of Botulinum Toxin in Juvenile Cerebral Palsy

Mauricio R. Delgado

Cerebral palsy (CP) occurs in 2 to 3 per 1,000 live births and is the most common motor disorder in children (1). CP is actually not a single entity but a group of motor disorders of cerebral origin defined by clinical description. It is not a diagnosis in that its application infers nothing about pathology, etiology, or prognosis. It is an umbrella term covering a wide range of cerebral disorders, which result in a motor disorder manifested from childhood (2). Patients with CP may be affected by other neurologic impairments, including visual and hearing impairments, communication disorders (3), sensory deficits (4), mental retardation (5), epilepsy (6), and behavioral disorders (7). Although the nature of the brain insult is considered static, the effects of the neurologic symptoms may be dynamic and progressive (8).

Most patients with cerebral palsy have hypertonia associated with muscle weakness. Hypertonic signs include spasticity (increased muscle resistance to passive movement of a limb that is velocity dependent), dystonia or rigidity. Rigidity (increased resistance of passive movement of a limb that is not velocity dependent) is rare in children. Many patients with cerebral palsy have a mixed picture with spasticity and dystonia. In 1959, Crothers and Paine proposed to divide cases of CP into three groups: spastic, extrapyramidal, and mixed (9). The anatomic distribution of the weakness has resulted in a classification that includes hemiparesis (one side of the body), diparesis (lower extremities more affected than upper extremities), paraparesis (lower extremities only), triparesis (three extremities), and quadriparesis (four extremities).

The weakness and the hypertonia frequently cause an asymmetric contraction of agonist and antagonist muscles around the joint resulting in a contracture which initially is dynamic (can be overcome by passive manipulation) but with time becomes fixed (cannot be overcome by passive manipulation). Contractures can aggravate already abnormal motor patterns resulting in even more functional impairment and disability. Over time, contractures result in progressive and fixed orthopedic deformities including bone torsions, joint dislocations, and spine deformities. These secondary orthopedic deformities must be distinguished from compensatory or ''coping'' responses, particularly in the ambulatory patient (10).

Unfortunately, many patients with cerebral palsy have also an associated proprioceptive sensory deficit that complicates the motor disorder further (11). In some patients, the poor motor control, weakness, and sensory deficits may contribute more to the disability than the hypertonia itself (12).

In the last 10 to 20 years, several treatments for the management of hypertonia in patients with CP have been developed, including oral medications such as benzodiazepines, baclofen, and tizanidine; surgical procedures such as selective dorsal rhizotomy; and a combination of both, i.e., intrathecal baclofen pump. These methods are mostly used to treat generalized hypertonic symptoms. Chemical denervation, using phenol or alcohol, has been used to treat focal hypertonia or focal aspects of generalized hypertonia. In the last 8 to 9 years, botulinum neurotoxin type A (BTX-A) has been used to produce a reversible neuromuscular blockade and reduce focal hypertonicity.

BTX-A IN CEREBRAL PALSY

Imbalance in muscle tone and weakness across a joint not only can interfere with function but can also lead to fixed contractures, bony torsional abnormalities, and joint instability (13). An attempt to reduce the hypertonic symptoms may help reduce the abnormal muscle imbalance resulting in less contracture and improvement in function. There is experimental evidence that the application of botulinum toxin type A in the spastic mouse reduces the development of contracture (14).

In 1993, the first report of BTX-A for the treatment of children with cerebral palsy appeared in the literature (15). To this date there have been multiple case reports and open-label trials demonstrating the efficacy and safety of this treatment in children with cerebral palsy (16–25). In addition, five randomized placebo-controlled studies demonstrating the efficacy of BTX-A have been published to this date—two of them to evaluate the effect in the upper extremity (26,27), and three others to evaluate the effect of the toxin in the lower extremity (28–30).

It has been demonstrated that BTX-A is more effective to treat dynamic (not fixed) muscle contractures in patients with cerebral palsy (31), and it seems that younger patients respond better than older children. The optimal timing for BTX-A treatment is between 1 and 5 years of age (32), hoping to reduce the incidence of fixed contractures, bone and joint deformity. It is also hoped that early intervention with an effective conservative treatment such as BTX-A could delay and reduce the number of orthopedic interventions in the growing child.

No experience exists with botulinum toxin type B (BTX-B) or any of the other serotypes (BTX-C to -G) in the treatment of patients with CP.

INDICATIONS

CP is a very complex motor disorder that requires a comprehensive and multidisciplinary assessment and management. BTX-A treatment represents only one aspect of what should be an integrated approach rather than a hierarchical approach.

Reasons to use BTX-A in patients with CP include:

1. To improve movement and function: in the upper and lower extremity (i.e., hip adductors and medial hamstrings to reduce leg crossing resulting in less tripping, less falling, longer stride).
2. To improve posture:
   a. To fit better in orthoses [i.e., ankle-foot orthoses (AFO)], hand splints
   b. To facilitate hygiene (i.e., hand and perineal region)
   c. To improve self-care (i.e., dressing, sitting)
   d. To improve cosmesis (i.e., reducing elbow and wrist hyperflexion)
3. To relieve pain associated with hypertonia (i.e., shoulder or hip pain caused by spastic hyperadduction and dislocation), and to improve postoperative recovery (i.e., reduction of pain allows faster recovery).

DOSE

There are two commercially available BTX-A products: BOTOX and DYSPORT. Both have been used to treat patients with CP. Doses for both products are expressed as LD_{50} units. It must be stressed that units of the two preparations are not comparable. The UK Botulinum Toxin and Cerebral Palsy Working Group reported a ratio of BOTOX: DYSPORT of 1:2.5 to 5 units (33).

Recommended Doses for BOTOX

The following are recommendations by a group of practitioners with a combined experience of treating more than 1,000 children with CP treated with BOTOX (32):

1. For the lower limb 3 to 6 U/kg/muscle
2. For the upper limb above the elbow 2 to 3 U/kg/muscle

3. For the upper limb below the elbow and posterior tibialis 0.5 to 2 U/kg/muscle
4. Small muscles of the palm and foot require lower doses (e.g., adductor pollicis requires 5 to 10 U).

The group agreed that a maximum of 12 U/kg/session or 300 U per session was safe. A retrospective study of 270 children with CP, treated with BOTOX between 1996 and 1998 in three major clinical centers in the United States, showed that the average dose per session ranged from 7.7 to 10.8 U/kg (34). However, the upper limit of the dose used, the number of muscles injected and the range of treatment objectives continues to increase, even as we write this chapter. Most experienced injectors use a dilution of 100 U/1 to 2 cc of preservative-free normal saline and do not give more than 50 U per injection site. The optimal number of injection sites per muscle remains undefined. However, most injectors use two to four sites for large muscles (i.e., gastroc-soleus, medial hamstring), two sites for medium size muscles (i.e., hip adductors, biceps brachii), and one site for smaller muscles (i.e., flexor carpi radialis, adductor pollicis).

Recommended Doses for DYSPORT

A wide range of doses of DYSPORT has been used and reported effective, ranging from 0.25 U/kg/injection to 35 U/kg/injection. The Belfast group routinely uses 25 U/kg/session of DYSPORT in the lower limbs, not to exceed 900 U (33). Unfortunately, the report by the UK Botulinum Toxin and Cerebral Palsy Working Group did not provide specific recommendations about how to use this product in children with CP. A recent retrospective multicentered study of 758 children, most with CP (n = 708), aimed to provide dosage guidelines based on risk/benefit assessment. They found that the mean dose of DYSPORT per treatment session was 22.9 U/kg, with the total dose per treatment session ranging from 50 to 2,360 U. Preferred dilutions, number of injection sites and doses per muscle were not specified (25).

DURATION OF EFFECT

The effect of the treatment was usually noticed 24 to 72 hours after the injection and tended to last 3 to 6 months. Rarely, there are patients with a response lasting 12 to 18 months. It seems that children with spasticity show a longer beneficial effect than those with dystonia.

SIDE EFFECTS

With careful use of BTX-A, side effects are uncommon and mild in patients with CP. The two commercially available products that contain BTX-A, BOTOX and DYSPORT, are manufactured in a different way resulting in different bioavailabilities and potencies. Consequently, a separate analysis of their toxicity is warranted.

BOTOX

Experimentation in juvenile primates using BOTOX in the gastrocnemius muscle, dividing the dose into four different injection sites, showed that 12 U/kg marked the onset of systemic toxicity (failure to gain weight) (32). This experiment may indicate that in humans, a dose of 12 U/kg/muscle has the potential to cause systemic side effects, although a dose of more than 6 to 7 U/kg/muscle is rarely used in humans.

In a multicenter, randomized, double-blind, placebo-controlled study involving 145 children with CP, adverse events were reported in 17% of BTX-treated patients. They received a dose of 2 to 4 U/kg muscle of BOTOX in the gastrocnemius-soleus muscles, dividing the dose equally into two different sites. This dose was repeated 4 weeks after the first dose, receiving a total dose of 4 to 8 U/kg/muscle. Only 4% of those receiving placebo reported adverse events. All side effects were rated as mild to moderate and no patients exited the study because of an adverse effect. Leg weakness, leg/calf pain and increased falling were the most common problems (3% of the patients receiving BOTOX vs 0% receiving placebo) (29).

In a retrospective study of 104 children with CP who were injected 257 times over a 2-year period, we found 14 (5.3%) adverse events. The average dose per session of BTX-A was 8 to 9 U/kg, giving 4 to 5 U/kg muscle in the large muscles of the lower extremity. All of the adverse events were mild and included extremity weakness ($n = 9$), low grade fever ($n = 3$) and constipation ($n = 2$) (35).

DYSPORT

A randomized, double-blind, placebo-controlled study of 40 children with CP who were injected in the gastrocnemius muscles, using a 200 U/mL dilution at a dose of 25 U/kg for children with diplegia (12.5 U/kg/muscle) and 15 U/kg/muscle for children with hemiplegia, was performed from 1996 to 1998. Six of 22 (27%) children who received DYSPORT reported adverse events: significant calf pain after injection that required simple analgesia ($n = 2$); increased frequency of falls within the first 2 weeks after the injection ($n = 2$); wheezing ($n = 1$); and increased seizures ($n = 1$). All adverse effects were self-limited (28).

On the other hand, Bakheit et al. (25), found 7% of adverse events in a large multicenter retrospective study of 758 patients who received 1,594 DYSPORT treatments. Focal muscle weakness was the most frequently reported (1%) adverse event. Urinary incontinence was also reported in 1% of the patients. Six patients reported generalized weakness and seven had falls. All other side effects were recorded in less than 1% of the treatments and included pain at the site of the injection, fatigue, somnolence, influenza-like symptoms, fever, and purpuric skin rash. A logistic regression analysis to investigate the effect of the total dose of DYSPORT used per session on the incidence of adverse events found that 22.2% of patients who received a dose in excess of 1,000 U had adverse events as compared to between 5.3% and 9.5% for the other treatment groups.

ADJUNCTIVE TREATMENTS

The complexity of the neurologic and biomechanical abnormalities in the patient with CP demand an integrated approach. Weakening a muscle or muscles with BTX-A should not be used in isolation in this condition. This tempo-

rary weakness actually represents a window of opportunity to work on some of the deficits affecting the patient.

The following are some of the most commonly used adjunctive treatments during BTX-A treatment in CP:

1. *Physical therapy:* A well planned and executed physical therapy program that is tailored for the specific needs of the patient remains central to the management of the child with CP. Clear functional goals need to be established and discussed with the patient and the patient's caregivers. Specific active-assistive, active, and resistive exercises to improve motor control, range of motion, strength, and endurance should be taught to the caregivers so they can carry them out on a daily basis after BTX injections (36). We specifically emphasize the need to strengthen antagonist muscles so that when the effect of BTX wears off, there will be a stronger resistance to the spastic muscle that has been injected.

2. *Orthoses:* Dreannan and Gage (37) recommended the use of orthoses in CP to (a) protect a body segment or joint, (b) prevent deformity, (c) provide stability, and (d) enhance function. Animal experimentation has demonstrated that muscles can adapt to different imposed lengths. This is accomplished by addition or subtraction of sarcomeres (38). A primary reason to use orthoses after BTX injections is to maintain the treated muscle in a stretched position, thereby inducing muscle growth and avoiding the development of a contracture. Tardieu et al. demonstrated in children with CP that progressive contracture of the soleus muscle was avoided when the muscle was stretched for at least 6 hours a day (39). This is the reason why we recommend the use of orthoses for at least 6 hours a day after BTX-A injections to our patients. We also believe this effect has the potential to increase the interval between injections. In our experience, this is true for spastic muscles but not for dystonic muscles.

3. *Casting:* Casting for 2 weeks may be indicated when a mild fixed contracture is present that prevents the joint to get to at least a neutral position. We believe it is important to delay casting for at least 2 weeks after the injection to distinguish between the effects of the toxin and the casting. It is also helpful to wait because there are some patients who have a response to BTX-A that is better than expected and casting may not be necessary (32).

Recommendations for the assessment of the child with CP who is being considered for BTX-A treatment include:

1. Perform a careful neurologic examination to properly identify the motor and sensory deficits of the patient. Increased muscle tone is only one aspect of the motor disorder affecting the patient. Weakness, poor motor control, and proprioceptive sensory deficits may be important factors contributing to the motor impairment, none of which will respond to BTX-A treatment.
2. Measure the passive range of motion (PROM). This will provide an estimate of the passive muscle length (R2) and the presence of fixed joint contractures. The dynamic range of motion can be evaluated using the modified Tardieu Scale, which will identify the angle at which the spastic catch or clonus is identified (R1). R2 minus R1 gives the dynamic range (40). We have noticed that a dynamic range of greater than 15 degrees is associated with a better response to BTX-A treatment.
3. A good understanding of the biomechanics of movement is required to correctly identify the hyperactive muscles responsible for the patient's abnormal movement. Assess the whole child in addition to the multiple levels of the extremity to be treated. We have found that videotaping the patient and reviewing the tape in slow motion is very helpful. Motion analysis in the laboratory is indicated in some patients with very complex movement patterns.
4. Identify one or two levels that are the most critical for the abnormal movement and select the muscles to be treated.
5. Establish very clear functional goals and communicate them to the patient and family.
6. Assess the need for other treatments that will be needed in conjunction with the use of BTX-A (i.e., casting, orthosis, physical therapy).
7. Reassess the patient 2 to 4 weeks after BTX treatment to evaluate effect and decide whether strategy changes need to be made (i.e., need for serial casting, adjustment of orthosis, and so on).

Negative factors against the use of BTX-A in children with cerebral palsy include severe fixed contractures, bony torsion, joint instability, and too many target muscles (32).

CONCLUSIONS

BTX-A is well tolerated, safe, and effective for the treatment of focal or segmental hypertonia in patients with CP. A proper selection of the patient and muscles to be injected is of utmost importance for success. Clear treatment goals need to be identified and communicated to the patient, the patient's family, and the rest of the team working with the patient. An integrated approach with a multidisciplinary team provides the best possible care for children with cerebral palsy.

REFERENCES

1. Anonymous. Surveillance of Cerebral Palsy in Europe (SCPE). *Dev Med Child Neurol* 2000;42:816–824.
2. Badawi N, Watson L, Petterson B, et al. What constitutes cerebral palsy? *Dev Med Child Neurol* 1998;40:520–527.
3. Shapiro BK, Palmer FB, Wachtel RC, et al. Associated dysfunctions. In: Thompson GH, Rubin IL, Bilenker RM, eds. *Comprehensive management of cerebral palsy.* New York: Grune & Stratton, 1983:87–95.
4. Yekutiel M, Jariwala M, Stretch P. Sensory deficit in the hands of children with cerebral palsy: a new look at assessment and prevalence. *Dev Med Child Neurol* 1994;36:619–624.
5. Nicholson A, Alberman E. Cerebral palsy—an increasing contributor to severe mental retardation? *Arch Dis Child* 1992;67:1050–1055.
6. Zafeiriou DI, Kontopoulos EE, Tsikoulas I. Characteris-

tics and prognosis of epilepsy in children with cerebral palsy. *J Child Neurol* 1999;14:289–294.

7. McDermott S, Coker AL, Mani S, et al. A population-based analysis of behavior problems in children with cerebral palsy. *J Pediatr Psychol* 1996;21:447–463.

8. Hoffer MM, Knoebel RT, Roberts R. Contractures in cerebral palsy. *Clin Orthop* 1987;219:70–77.

9. Crothers B, Paine RS. Classification of cerebral palsies. In: Crothers B, Paine RS, eds. *The natural history of cerebral palsy.* Cambridge, MA: Harvard University Press, 1959:34–52.

10. Dabney KW, Lipton GE, Miller F. Cerebral palsy. *Curr Opin Pediatr* 1997;9:81–88.

11. Cooper J, Majnemer A, Rosenblatt B, et al. The determination of sensory deficits in children with hemiplegic cerebral palsy. *J Child Neurol* 1995;10:300–309.

12. Russman BS. Cerebral palsy. Current treatment options. *Neurology* 2000;2:97–108.

13. Boyd R, Graham HK. Botulinum toxin A in the management of children with cerebral palsy: indications and outcome. *Eur J Neurol* 1997;4(Suppl 2):S15–S22.

14. Cosgrove AP, Graham HK. Botulinum toxin A prevents the development of contractures in the hereditary spastic mouse. *Dev Med Child Neurol* 1994;36:379–385.

15. Koman LA, Mooney JF 3rd, Smith B, et al. Management of cerebral palsy with botulinum-A toxin: preliminary investigation. *J Pediatr Orthop* 1993;13:489–495.

16. Cosgrove AP, Corry I, Graham HK. Botulinum toxin in the management of the lower extremity in cerebral palsy. *Dev Med Child Neurol* 1994;36:386–396.

17. Calderon-Gonzalez R, Calderon-Sepulveda R, Rincon-Reyes M, et al. Botulinum toxin A in management of cerebral palsy. *Pediatr Neurol* 1994;10:284–288.

18. Denslic M, Meh D. Botulinum toxin in the treatment of cerebral palsy. *Neuropediatrics* 1995;26:249–252.

19. Garcia Ruiz PJ, Sanchez Bernardos V, Urcelay V, et al. Botulinum A toxins in the treatment of spasticity in cerebral palsy during childhood. *Neurologia* 1996;11: 34–36.

20. Gooch JL, Sandell TV. Botulinum toxin for spasticity and athetosis in children with cerebral palsy. *Arch Phys Med Rehabil* 1996;77:508–511.

21. Arens LJ, Leary PM, Goldschmidt RB. Experience with botulinum toxin in the treatment of cerebral palsy. *S Afr Med J* 1997;87:1001–1003.

22. Sanchez-Carpintero R, Narbona J. Botulinum toxin in spastic infantile cerebral palsy: results in 27 cases during a year. *Rev Neurol* 1997;25:531–535.

23. Wong V. Use of botulinum toxin in 17 children with spastic cerebral palsy. *Pediatr Neurol* 1998;18: 124–131.

24. Friedman A, Diamond M, Johnston MV, et al. Effects of botulinum toxin A on upper limb spasticity in children with cerebral palsy. *Am J Phys Med Rehabil* 2000;79: 53–59.

25. Bakheit AM, Severa S, Cosgrove A, et al. Safety profile of botulinum toxin (DYSPORT) in children with muscle spasticity. *Dev Med Child Neurol* 2001;43:234–238.

26. Corry IS, Cosgrove AP, Walsh EG, et al. Botulinum toxin A in the hemiplegic upper limb: a double-blind trial. *Dev Med Child Neurol* 1997;39:185–193.

27. Fehlings D, Rang M, Glazier J, et al. An evaluation of botulinum-A toxin injections to improve upper extremity function in children with hemiplegic cerebral palsy. *J Pediatr* 2000;137:331–337.

28. Ubhi T, Bhakta BB, Ives HL, et al. Randomised double-blind, placebo-controlled trial of the effect of botulinum toxin on walking in cerebral palsy. *Arch Dis Child* 2000; 83:481–487.

29. Koman LA, Mooney JF 3rd, Smith BP, et al. Botulinum toxin type A neuromuscular blockade in the treatment of lower extremity spasticity in cerebral palsy: a randomized, double-blind, placebo-controlled trial. *J Pediatr Orthop* 2000;20:108–115.

30. Wissel J, Heinen F, Schenkel A, et al. Botulinum toxin A in the management of spastic gait disorders in children and young adults with cerebral palsy: a randomized, double-blind study of "high-dose" versus "low-dose" treatment. *Neuropediatrics* 1999; 30:120–124.

31. Eames NW, Baker R, Hill N, et al. The effect of botulinum toxin A on gastrocnemius length: magnitude and duration of response. *Dev Med Child Neurol* 1999;41: 226–232.

32. Graham HK, Aoki KR, Autti-Ramo I, et al. Recommendations for the use of botulinum toxin type A in the management of cerebral palsy. *Gait Posture* 2000;11: 67–79.

33. Carr LJ, Cosgrove AP, Gringras P, et al. Position paper on the use of botulinum toxin in cerebral palsy. *Arch Dis Child* 1998;79:271–273.

34. Gormley ME, Gaebler-Spira D, Delgado MR. Use of botulinum toxin type A in pediatric patients with cerebral palsy: a three center retrospective chart review. *J Child Neurol* 2001;16:113–118.

35. Delgado MR. The use of botulinum toxin type A in children with cerebral palsy: a retrospective study. *Eur J Neurol* 1999;6(Suppl 4):S11–S18.

36. Leach J. Children undergoing treatment with botulinum toxin: the role of the physical therapist. *Muscle Nerve* 1997;20(Suppl 6):S194–S207.

37. Drennan JC, Gage JR. Orthotics in cerebral palsy. In: Thompson GH, Rubin IL, Bilenker RM, eds. *Comprehensive management of cerebral palsy.* New York: Grune & Stratton, 1983:205–213.

38. Tabary JC, Tabary C, Tardieu C, et al. Physiological and structural changes in the cat's soleus muscle due to immobilization at different lengths by plaster casts. *J Physiol* 1972;224:231–244.

39. Tardieu C, Lespargot A, Tabary C, et al. For how long must the soleus muscle be stretched each day to prevent contracture? *Dev Med Child Neurol* 1988;30:2–10.

40. Boyd RN, Graham HK. Objective measurement of clinical findings in the use of botulinum toxin type A for the management of children with cerebral palsy. *Eur J Neurol* 1999;6(Suppl 4):523–535.

Scientific and Therapeutic Aspects of Botulinum Toxin
edited by M.F. Brin, J. Jankovic, and M. Hallett
Lippincott Williams & Wilkins, Philadelphia, © 2002.

22

Botulinum Toxin Type A in the Treatment of Spasticity

A.P. Moore

Botulinum toxin type A (BTX-A) was first used to treat spasticity in adults by Das and Park (1), who treated six patients with stroke-related spasticity and reported that BTX-A produced both subjective and objective improvement. However, the idea was not new. Justinus Kerner (1786–1862), the German physician and poet who gave us the first accurate and comprehensive description of botulism, deduced that the toxin acts by interrupting signal transmission within the peripheral motor and autonomic nervous systems, and proposed a variety of therapeutic uses for the toxin, including spasticity.

Over the last decade, we have developed considerable anecdotal experience of BTX-A in spasticity through pragmatic clinical practice and open studies, supported recently by randomized controlled trials. This chapter blends these streams of information and emphasizes the importance of using BTX-A for spasticity in the setting of the wider rehabilitation goals. BTX-A should not be used in isolation.

Strictly speaking, a large amount of expert practice with BTX-A remains ''off-license'' and unproven, especially in the field of spasticity. Where relevant, I tell patients and caretakers that BTX-A remains off-license and that they must accept this. I always obtain signed consent before starting any course of BTX-A treatment.

SPASTICITY

Definition of Spasticity

Definitions of spasticity often concentrate on its pathophysiology and stress the velocity-sensi-

tive nature of the involuntary muscle activity, and hyperreflexia. Clinically, spasticity presents as hypertonia, an increased resistance to passive muscle stretch and limb movement caused by disease of the central nervous system, i.e., the brain or spinal cord. It is rarely an isolated problem, and is usually associated with other features such as weakness or poor control of voluntary muscle activation, altered sensation, or sensory inattention. It is often compounded by additional brain disturbance affecting arousal, mood, language, and other functions, and that may profoundly disrupt rehabilitation.

Pathophysiology

The pathophysiology of spasticity is complex, and we do not have a clear understanding of how it develops (2,3). Cerebral and spinal lesions may generate spasticity through different mechanisms releasing monosynaptic or multisynaptic reflexes, respectively (4). Traditionally, spasticity is attributed to disruption of descending corticospinal tract control of reflex activity, causing hyperreflexia and abnormal patterns of reflex activation. In the early stages, this neural component predominates, and as spasticity evolves and becomes more persistent, the muscles remain in a contracted state for long periods. This can lead to soft tissue changes that generate further biomechanical resistance to passive movement, and eventually shortening of the muscle-tendon complex may produce contractures and limb deformity. However, the traditional view is under attack, as the relationship between hypertonia and reflex excitability is weak in many patients with spasticity (5,6). In many "spastic" muscles there is no electromyographic activity, and the resistance to passive movement is due mainly to the biomechanical component. This chapter uses the term spasticity despite its limitations.

The factors that determine whether spasticity progresses or remains a minor problem are not well defined, but the fact that it often does progress reveals an opportunity to influence it.

Importance of Spasticity

Spasticity is common and can significantly impair long-term quality of life in stable patients or recovery of function after new lesions. It does not always need treatment. Patients with a combination of spasticity and voluntary muscle weakness may rely on the spasticity to maintain posture, as when the "spastic prop" of quadriceps spasticity allows patients to stand. However, spasticity is usually detrimental and causes many secondary physical problems with pain and impaired movement, hygiene and self-care, and psychological disturbance with poor self-esteem and body image.

THE PLACE OF BTX-A IN SPASTICITY MANAGEMENT

Spasticity treatment is only part of the wider rehabilitation of patients. Its management requires a multidisciplinary team including the doctor, nurses, physiotherapists, and occupational therapists, as well as orthotists and rehabilitation engineers. The caretakers also play an important role.

There is a wide range of "medical" treatments that the team should deploy in a personalized mix tailored to the spasticity itself, the patient circumstances, and the availability of care and resources. Most clinicians prefer to use reversible, safer, and cheaper treatments first, and begin with prevention of provocative factors such as pain, constipation, infection, and poor postural management. Good physical management is the linchpin of spasticity prevention and treatment, and requires education and considerable staff and caretaker time. There should be a

program of stretching and physical therapies, and regular changes of position to vary pressure points and muscle stretch, together with splints, casts, or orthoses. The aims are to maintain muscle and soft tissue length, and to facilitate function or ease of care.

Widespread or generalized spasticity may respond to oral baclofen, benzodiazepines, tizanidine, or dantrolene. It can be difficult to achieve a satisfactory balance between good suppression of the most spastic segments and weakness or excessive loss of muscle tone elsewhere. If these fail or produce unacceptable drowsiness, weakness, or other side effects, intrathecal baclofen may be valuable. It requires considerable expertise and backup, and thus is not cheap. It carries a significant risk of complications in some units, although this may become less of a problem as experience increases. Rarely, intrathecal phenol may be appropriate, when there is severe leg spasticity with permanent loss of sphincter control.

Focal spasticity, or more widespread spasticity with a prominent focal component, may also respond to some of these measures. Often, however, the adverse effects overshadow the benefits, and more focussed treatments become valuable options. These mainly revolve around medical and surgical techniques for blocking the final common pathway of lower motoneuron activity, and now include BTX-A. Destructive lesions such as phenol injections or nerve, root, or spinal cord surgery can work well, but their effects are not always predictable, and errors or bad luck may result in long-term problems. Phenol nerve or motor point injections are time-consuming, tricky, and uncomfortable, and although they can be very effective, they are not widely used. Cynics argue that this is because they are cheap and not actively promoted by the drug industry. There is a small but significant risk of painful dysesthesia if phenol is used in nerves with a sensory component. Neurosurgical therapies include spinal cord stimulation and selective rhizotomy or more peripheral denervation. Orthopaedic procedures may rescue deforming limbs and return them to more functional postures.

In theory, BTX-A can help at any point in

this range of options. It should not be used in isolation, and clinicians believe that optimum results require combination with physiotherapy and splinting. Patients who need intensive physiotherapy to gain significantly from BTX-A must have access to it arranged before starting. Good use of the window of opportunity starting 1 to 2 weeks after BTX-A injections permits more effective physical therapies and retraining, and may lead to much longer lasting benefit. Physiotherapists can use this time and the impetus of a new treatment to kick-start a stalled patient's progress.

BOTULINUM TOXIN IN SPASTICITY

Mechanism of BTX-A in Spasticity

The most obvious effect of intramuscular BTX-A is the induced muscle weakness and atrophy. The controlled, temporary weakness can logically be expected to reduce the available force of spastic contraction. A more subtle effect was revealed by animal studies showing that muscle spindle afferent activity is reduced even before any detectable weakness (7,8). The γ-motoneurons to the muscle spindles are also cholinergic and probably poisoned by BTX-A in the same way as are the α-motoneurons to somatic muscle fibers. Changes in the sensitivity of the reflex arc may thus help to reduce spasticity. It is possible that remote spread of the toxin to distant muscle spindles contributes to this effect even with no detectable distant weakness. Patients given quite selective injections of BTX-A often gain much more widespread relaxation of spasticity, but this could simply be a result of the removal of a major focus of spasticity with its attendant pain, spasm, and other discomforts that act to provoke the more widespread spasticity.

A "Neuroprotective" Effect?

There is little evidence that BTX-A has a direct effect within the central nervous system. However, it is possible that altering reflex activity and the force of contraction influences the development of central circuitry indirectly. In theory, early treatment of spasticity could break a cycle of spasm, pain, fibrosis, and contracture and influence remodeling of central circuits. It certainly assists physiotherapy by making it easier to manipulate limbs and to retrain antagonists, and allows more-comfortable and better-tolerated splinting.

In early studies using the hereditary spastic rat, Cosgrove et al. injected BTX-A into the gastrocnemius muscle of infant rats, before they developed spasticity. They showed convincingly that BTX-A blocked the development of the expected biomechanical changes of spasticity, of overall shortening of the muscle-tendon unit, and of increase in the tendon:muscle ratio (9). Note that this experiment was in growing rats and perhaps informs human pediatric practice more than adult medicine, but it does suggest the possibility of a therapeutic window early in the development of spasticity, even in adults.

Trial Evidence

Since the first report of Das and Park, many small, uncontrolled or open trials have reported short-term benefit in poststroke spasticity, and in patients with a variety of other disorders causing spasticity, including cerebral palsy, inherited disease, multiple sclerosis, and brain or spinal cord injuries. BTX-A seems to work independently of the cause of the spasticity. The open studies have examined different indications, doses, and techniques, and usually suggested improvement in posture and spasms, and often in function and ease of care. Important adverse events are rare. However, as is clear from the controlled trials with BTX-A that have been performed in spasticity and other disorders, there are many responders in the placebo groups, so we must generate and rely as much as possible on randomized controlled trial evidence. I have confined the rest of this discussion to the randomized controlled trial evidence. Table 22.1 lists the published placebo-controlled randomized controlled trials.

Arm Spasticity

Six randomized controlled trials of BTX-A for arm spasticity all support the use of BTX-A in

TABLE 22.1. *Published placebo-controlled randomized controlled trials*

Authors	Trial type	Spasticity	N	Dose (mu)
Snow et al. 1990 (10)	crossover	adductors	9	BOTOX 400
Grazko et al. 1995 (11)	crossover	leg	12	BOTOX 25 to 290
Simpson et al. 1996 (12)	parallel	arm	37	BOTOX 75/150/300
Burbaud et al. 1996 (13)	crossover	equinovarus	23	DYSPORT 1,000
Hesse et al. 1998 (14)	parallel	arm	24	DYSPORT 1,000 ± electrical stimulation
Bhakta et al. 2000 (15)	parallel	arm	40	DYSPORT 1,000
Bakheit et al. 2000 (16)	parallel	arm	82	DYSPORT 500/1,000/1,500
Smith & Moore 2000 (17)	parallel	arm	24	DYSPORT 500/1,000/1,500
Richardson et al. 2000 (18)	parallel	arm or leg	52	BOTOX various doses
Hyman (19)	parallel	adductors	74	DYSPORT 500/1,000/1,500

a general way (12,14–18,20). Unfortunately, it is extremely difficult to devise outcome measures that are both responsive to change and sufficiently flexible to capture the variety of distinct benefits related in anecdotal reports and less scientifically rigorous formal trials. Functional improvements are especially difficult to demonstrate because the changes permitted by release of spasticity may be swamped by other impairments.

Modified Ashworth scores improve in all trials, and patients usually register "global improvement" on visual analog or Likert scales; but even some of the larger studies can fail to show statistically significant functional improvement (16), especially when the same predefined measure is applied to all subjects. Global measures such as the Barthel index (21) fail to identify benefits reported by patients (14). This reflects the diverse disabilities encountered, none of which is individually present in many patients, so that each measure is rendered statistically unresponsive. However, Bhakta et al. used disability and caretaker burden scales designed to measure the impact of upper limb spasticity. Despite a relatively small sample size, they were able to show statistically significant improvement in disability for at least 6 weeks, and reduction in caretaker burden for at least 12 weeks (15).

Leg Spasticity

Adductor Spasticity

Two placebo-controlled, randomized trials examined adductor spasticity (10,19). The larger

study evaluated 500, 1,000 and 1,500 mouse units (mu) DYSPORT in patients with multiple sclerosis. When 1,500 mu were used, there was statistically significant improvement at week 4 in passive range of movement, with trends to improvement in muscle tone and a hygiene score when 1,000 or 1,500 mu were used. Patients were retreated on request when they felt injections had worn off, and there was a trend towards a dose-response relationship with larger doses lasting longer. However, there was no advantage over placebo in spasm suppression, pain, or global rating. The optimal dose was thought to be 1,000 mu because 1,500 mu was associated with a higher incidence of unwanted muscle weakness (36%).

Spastic Equinovarus

One randomized controlled trial concentrated on spastic equinovarus. Burbaud et al. tested placebo against 1,000 mu DYSPORT distributed between the investigator's choice of gastrocnemius, soleus, and tibialis posterior muscle. At 1 month their patients reported a clear subjective advantage for BTX-A in reducing foot spasticity. Ashworth scores improved significantly. Changes in gait velocity were not significant, possibly because some patients discarded their walking aids and were "walking more cautiously."

OTHER STUDIES

Richardson et al. (18) studied a heterogeneous group of 52 patients with a wide variety of pathologies and types of spasticity. They calculated overall scores at 3, 6, 9, and 12 weeks for a variety of measures. They reported a statistically significant advantage for BTX-A in Ashworth scores, percentage passive range of movement, Rivermead lower-limb scale, and subjective rating of problem severity. The main benefits were concentrated in the first 3 to 6 weeks.

Functional Electrical Stimulation

Two studies suggest that short-term functional electrical stimulation (FES) of the injected muscles, to increase the uptake and therefore toxicity of BTX-A, can enhance the effectiveness of BTX-A in the leg (22) and in the arm (14). These were small studies and a larger study is needed.

BTX-A Versus Phenol

In a randomized controlled trial in 20 stroke patients with spastic equinovarus, Kirazli et al. (23) compared calf muscle injection with BTX-A (BOTOX 400 mu) against tibial nerve injection with 5% phenol, and concluded that BTX-A was generally more effective, with fewer side effects.

PROBLEMS INTERPRETING THE LITERATURE

Trials have generally tested BTX-A in patients receiving inadequate benefit from conventional treatment. BTX-A can retrieve some otherwise difficult situations, yet it may prove better to use it earlier. There are now a few well-controlled studies, but even these have tested only the effects of a single injection session and have followed relatively small numbers of patients for 3 to 4 months. All the patients have had established spasticity, often present for many years. We are still at the stage of optimizing technical details of patient, dose, and distribution of BTX-A. Even so, most trials use a rigidly defined protocol specifying BTX-A dose and muscles to be injected. Outcome measures showing benefit tend to be impairment rating scales such as the

modified Ashworth scale (MAS), and it is more difficult to show improvement in function.

Most experienced BTX-A users believe that BTX-A is more effective in the early stages of spasticity, and that flexibility of dose and muscle selection improves results because they allow personalized patterns of injection. Many of the indications and benefits are specific to the patient (Table 22.2). They relate to factors other than improvement in function, such as reduced pain, spasm, and difficulty caring for the patient, and are more difficult to measure. Most available trial outcome measures struggle to cope with such variety, and are thus insensitive to change. The few responsive measures are poorly validated.

There is a tension between designing smaller, cheaper trials with homogeneous problems more likely to respond to rigid protocols, and larger, expensive studies using more heterogeneous patients and flexible protocols. Pharmaceutical companies have generally aimed to gain a license for "spasticity" as represented by a limited disorder such as spastic drop foot, and hope that, once licensed, BTX-A will creep into more general use.

Although these beliefs remain untested, they do have a ring of logic and do highlight the problems of designing studies and assessing the available trial data. In addition, if clinicians think that BTX-A is helping, in practice, they will give regular treatments over many sessions, yet there are no formal studies in adults of long-

TABLE 22.2. *Indications for BTX-A in spasticity*

Reduce pain or spasm
Aid hygiene (e.g., perineal, axillary, palmar)
Improve fit and comfort of orthoses (wrist, ankle)
Ease dressing and mobility for caretakers
Increase range of movement
Improve wheelchair posture
Improve function
Cosmesis (e.g., natural arm posture)
Treat/prevent pressure sores (e.g., medial knees)
Reduce need for systemic drugs
Optimize physiotherapy
Prevent injury from involuntary movements
Postpone or avoid orthopaedic surgery
Predict results of orthopaedic surgery
Reduce pain and aid postoperative healing

term safety and efficacy, of the role of BTX-A relative to other treatments for spasticity, or of cost-effectiveness. There are no guidelines on when to stop BTX-A injections.

PRINCIPLES OF CLINICAL USE

Spasticity Service

It seems clear from experience (but is not proven in any study) that it is better to use BTX-A to treat spasticity in the setting of a wider rehabilitation service, with a range of staff and facilities as described above. BTX-A should only be injected by clinicians with appropriate knowledge of functional anatomy, general experience in diagnosis and management of spasticity, and specific training in the use of BTX-A. Guidelines to development of a botulinum toxin service for spasticity were recently published (24).

Selection of Patients

It is easier to define the principles of selection than to issue a precise menu of indications. The underlying cause of the spasticity probably does not matter. Patients should have clinically important spasticity that is causing or is about to cause a problem: the presence of spasticity is not in itself currently an indication for treatment. Appropriate alternative treatments should have been tried or at least considered. There should be a significant focal element to the spasticity, and the muscles to be treated should not be severely contracted and fixed. The clinician must understand the dynamic anatomy of the spasticity and be aware of the risks of undue weakness of the target or nearby muscles. The goals of treatment should be clearly defined; Table 22.2 sets out the more common indications.

SPASTICITY SYNDROMES COMMONLY TREATED WITH BTX-A

Spastic Arm

Common patterns include shoulder abduction, flexion at the elbow, wrist and fingers, plus pronation of the forearm, thumb-in-palm, and fist-

1. Pectoralis
2. Biceps; Brachialis; Brachioradialis
3. Flexor carpi ulnaris; Flexor carpi radialis; Pronator teres/quadratus
4. Flexor digitorum profundus/superficialis
5. Flexor pollicis longus; Thenar muscles

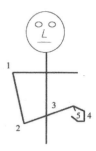

FIG. 22.1. Common injection patterns for the arm

ing (Fig. 22.1). Occasional variants may occur, such as shoulder adduction or wrist supination. All of these can be treated with BTX-A injections into the appropriate muscles. The total dose required is likely to be between 500 and 1,500 mu DYSPORT or its equivalent, depending on the number and bulk of muscles needing injection.

Control of muscle spasm pain is a common indication for injections around the shoulder, and reducing resistance to passive extension at any level can make dressing easier. Functional improvements can occur, for instance when release of elbow flexion permits a patient to control a wheelchair or to use the hand to brace an object. In ambulant patients an arm swinging more naturally at the patient's side can help walking and is a great cosmetic bonus, restoring confidence and social activity. It is very difficult to restore fine dexterity, which is often due more to loss of motor control than to spasticity, but even fractional release of severe fisting can transform caretakers' problems in maintaining palmar skin hygiene. The combination of BTX-A with physiotherapy, regular muscle stretch by the patient and all attendants, and progressive splinting can open flexed postures for longer than the usual duration of BTX-A-induced weakness.

Spastic Leg

The simplest situations are dynamic spastic equinus (13) and adductor spasticity (10,19)

1. Hip flexors
2. Adductors
3. Hamstrings
4. Gastrocnemius;
   Soleus;
   Tibialis posterior
Occasional:
   Quadriceps;
   Extensor hallucis
   longus

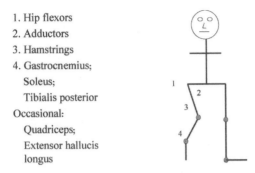

FIG. 22.2. Common injection patterns for the leg

(Fig. 22.2). It is straightforward to identify the muscles clinically and inject freehand, though I use the EMG for adductor injections in obese patients. Proximal flexor spasms can arise from hamstrings or hip flexors and require more careful analysis. In practice, there is often a mixture, and injections into the hamstrings are technically easier and often work. Other less-common injections include BTX-A into quadriceps to block extensor spasms, tibialis posterior for foot inversion or toe flexors or extensors, especially to suppress an intrusive extensor toe. Injections into the deeper muscles, such as tibialis posterior or the smaller long toe muscles, may need EMG control.

Benefits of adductor injections include easier perineal hygiene and sexual intercourse. Anecdotally, weakening hamstrings may block spasms, improve wheelchair posture, and sometimes help with walking. Injections into gastrocnemius and soleus can make splints more comfortable to wear, and may sometimes improve walking. As spastic equinus can be a fairly simple pattern of spasticity several investigators have chosen it for initial trials of the concept of BTX-A use in spasticity. Drug manufacturers may be hoping that the award of a licensed indication in this limited spasticity syndrome will promote wider use of BTX-A for spasticity in adults, as seems likely to happen in cerebral palsy.

Spastic Neck

Occasional patients develop a torticollis after a stroke or head injury. If injected before muscle contracture sets in, BTX-A may straighten the neck. Recurrent treatments may be needed, as for dystonic torticollis. There are no randomized controlled trials relevant to spastic torticollis (as opposed to spasmodic or dystonic torticollis).

SITUATIONS TO AVOID

Patients with spasticity are less likely to benefit if they have severe muscle contractures. There must be a dynamic component to the spasticity. I help patients understand this by comparing a dynamic contracture with a piece of elastic, a contracture with string. Weakening elastic allows it to stretch, weakening string does not. It is sometimes difficult to know whether a fixed posture is caused by contracture. Assessment during sleep or sedation can help. If the patient is to have surgery for any reason, take the chance to examine joint range of movement (ROM) while the patient is anesthetized. Sometimes temporary motor point blocks with lidocaine will clarify the pattern of muscle involvement, and reveal whether there is severe contracture.

It is important to be realistic. There may be little value in abolishing modest spasticity in patients whose main disability is weakness or loss of higher functions such as in sensory inattention. There is unlikely to be much improvement in function, and BTX-A will only help if the spasticity is causing other problems.

Muscle Selection

The history will reveal some candidate muscles that are clearly responsible for spasms, abnormal posturing, or other disability. Clarify whether the problem is progressing, and consider other treatment options for each muscle. Observation of static posture and the effects of orthoses, and examination of passive and active movement, muscle hypertrophy, and tenderness will pick out most other muscles. It is rarely necessary to resort to laboratory evaluation with tests such as gait analysis or electromyography. It is often not possible to treat all the candidate muscles, and then clinicians must judge which would be the most useful ones to weaken within the dose allowed for the injection session.

When Should Electromyography Be Used?

Some units use EMG to help in muscle selection, employing multichannel recordings to study the patterns and amplitudes of muscle activation and to decide whether particular muscles are triggering symptoms, being recruited (cocontraction), or antagonizing the primary involuntary contraction. In spasticity, EMG may help to distinguish actively contracting muscles from those resisting stretch because of passive biomechanical changes in muscle viscosity, or even contracture. Muscles without a clear EMG burst when stretched may not respond usefully to BTX-A. The pattern of activation is often unhelpful because any stimulus tends to produce widespread cocontraction.

After muscles have been selected, either clinically or by EMG, it can be helpful to use EMG with special hollow combination EMG/injection needles. EMG can confirm needle placement in the chosen muscle using various activation procedures, or simply prove that the needle is in muscle and not other tissue when BTX-A is injected. This can be essential in obese patients. Portable EMG equipment is available, either as a full system giving visual and sound confirmation of needle placement, or as a simpler, more portable, less-expensive audio-only system. The latter can be very helpful but must be used with caution for reinjections. To an inexperienced electromyographer the sound from an EMG needle in a previously treated muscle is similar to that from a distant untreated muscle. This is not just a theoretical problem because previously treated muscles may remain atrophic at the time of retreatment and can be more difficult to locate.

INJECTION TECHNIQUE

The best sites for injection are theoretically the nerve endplate zones deep in the muscle bulk. Note that these are different from the motor point, which is the point at which the nerve enters the muscle and is the target for some phenol injections. The patterns of endplate zones are not clearly mapped, and it is impractical to make multiple passes with an EMG/injection needle

looking for their subtle but characteristic electrical signature. Fortunately, small- and moderate-size muscles will usually respond to BTX-A injected simply into the belly of the muscle. Although there is some diffusion through muscle fascia (25), muscles with well-delineated separate components, such as quadriceps, will need separate injections for each major section. Some authorities recommend multiple scattered smaller injections to spread the toxin. Muscles with fibers arrayed in parallel may be more effectively weakened by multiple injections transversely across the muscle belly, whereas muscles with fibers arranged longitudinally may require a spread of injections along their length. The clinician should consider the discomfort of multiple injections, and remember that patients may let an unpleasant experience persuade them not to undergo repeat injections. The psychology can be important, especially in frail or confused patients, and trying to get an extra few percent benefit may be counterproductive in the long run.

Although EMG can be very helpful, a simpler technique will suffice in many cases. If the needle is placed in the belly of the muscle and the muscle then gently activated or stretched passively, the differential movement of muscle and skin tilts the needle and syringe and confirms its position inside the muscle fascia (26). This is most helpful in long-limb muscles such as hamstrings, gastrocnemius, long finger flexors, and the like, and much less useful in adductors, wrist pronators, and neck muscles.

DOSES

In some situations, I use a cautious strategy with modest doses on the first injection session, titrating upwards if the effect is inadequate. This works well when there is a risk of inconvenient weakness, such as in occupational dystonias, e.g., writer's cramp or musician's cramp. The disadvantage is that it may take several sessions over 3 to 6 months to find the optimum compromise. In most patients with spasticity, I prefer to give a fuller dose and reduce it if there are problems. This is appropriate when a more rapid effective response is needed and where undue collateral weakness is unlikely to matter, as commonly occurs in spasticity in a limb unlikely to be functionally useful even if the spasticity is abolished. Recommended doses for particular muscles are given elsewhere (27).

FOLLOW UP

Monitoring the Response

Clinicians should establish a clear and objective baseline description of the nature and severity of any condition being treated. Only then can the response be monitored. Unfortunately, the huge variety of clinical problems makes it difficult to devise satisfactory scales for clinical trials. Ranges of movement and modified Ashworth scores may be useful, but can only rate the impairment crudely. They may not reflect clinically important benefit, for instance when severe poststroke fisting relaxes enough to prevent palmar trauma and skin infection, but the modified Ashworth scores category is unchanged. It can be very helpful to agree on treatment goals specific to the patient in advance and concentrate on monitoring those goals.

Spasticity is an excellent example of a complex situation where progress must be monitored in a broader sense. I use a generic diary showing a visual analog score tailored to the patient's own goals. The patient, caretakers, or therapists can fill it in once a week. Regular reports from therapists are extremely useful. Until the pattern of response is clear, clinicians may need to see the patient at 3 to 6 weeks after each injection, at the time of anticipated maximal response. Once everyone is satisfied of benefit, such intensive monitoring becomes unnecessary, and if a pattern is established after a few sessions, I rely on patients, caretakers, or therapists to tell me when a repeat injection is needed. I keep any diary forms completed early on because they give an excellent and personalized measure of baseline severity and responsiveness to BTX injections.

Retreatment

Occasional patients derive enough improvement from a single cycle of injection, with attendant splinting and physiotherapy, to manage with no further injections. The duration of benefit is usually about 3 months. Avoid reinjection before 3 months to minimize the risk of antibody formation and secondary nonresponse. Many patients do need to have repeat injection cycles, and do need reevaluation at each visit. If BTX-A is thought to be helping and there is still a clear indication to treat, consider whether to adjust the dose or the pattern of muscles injected. It is sometimes possible to "chase" residual spasticity or spasticity elsewhere. Other treatments may be preferable or worth adding. There are no clear rules for stopping treatment with BTX-A.

CONCLUSIONS

BTX-A is an emerging treatment for spasticity. It has many advantages and some disadvantages (Table 22.3). There is a great deal of experience and anecdotal evidence to support its use, but we need more good-quality trials before we can be sure of its value and its place in spasticity management. Even if the doctors and patients become convinced, health care purchasers are increasingly demanding incontrovertible evidence of clinical benefit and value for money before they dispense funding.

TABLE 22.3. *Potential advantages and disadvantages of BTX-A in spasticity*

Advantages	Disadvantages
Simple, given in outpatients, focused	Can be complex, requiring experience
Side effects few and short-lived	Wears off, has to be repeated
Flexible; can "chase" spasticity	Potentially expensive
Reduces need for systemic drugs	Logistical; organizing a clinic
Easily integrated with other treatment	Long-term commitment
Independent of cause of spasticity	Inadequate for widespread spasticity
Possible prevention of contractures	Discomfort of multiple injections

REFERENCES

1. Das TK, Park DM. Effect of treatment with botulinum toxin on spasticity. *Postgrad Med J* 1989;65:208–210.

2. Brown P. Pathophysiology of spasticity. *J Neurol Neurosurg Psychiatry* 1994;57:773–777.

3. O'Dwyer NJ, Ada L. Reflex hyperexcitability and muscle contracture in relation to spastic hypertonia. *Curr Opin Neurol* 1996;9:451–455.

4. Herman R, Freedman W, Meeks S. Physiological aspects of hemiplegic and paraplegic spasticity. In: Desmedt J, ed. *New developments in electromyography and clinical neurophysiology: human reflexes, pathophysiology of motor systems, methodology of human reflexes.* Basel: Karger, 1973:579–589.

5. O'Dwyer NJ, Ada L, Neilson PD. Spasticity and muscle contracture following stroke. *Brain* 1996;119: 1737–1749.

6. Powers R, Campbell D, Rymer W. Stretch reflex dynamics in spastic elbow flexor muscles. *Ann Neurol* 1989;25:32–42.

7. Filippi GM, Errico P, Santarelli R, et al. Botulinum A toxin effects on rat jaw muscle spindles. *Acta Otolaryngol* 1993;113:400–404.

8. Manni E, Bagolini B, Pettorossi VE, et al. Effect of botulinum toxin on extraocular muscle proprioception. *Doc Ophthalmol* 1989;72:189–198.

9. Cosgrove AP GH. Botulinum toxin A prevents the development of contractures in the hereditary spastic mouse. *Dev Med Child Neurol* 1994;36:379–385.

10. Snow BJ, Tsui JK, Bhatt MH, et al. Treatment of spasticity with botulinum toxin: a double-blind study. *Ann Neurol* 1990;28:512–515.

11. Grazko MA, Polo KB, Jabbari B. Botulinum toxin A for spasticity, muscle spasms, and rigidity. *Neurology* 1995;45:712–717.

12. Simpson DM, Alexander DN, O'Brien CF, et al. Botulinum toxin type A in the treatment of upper extremity spasticity: a randomized, double-blind, placebo-controlled trial. *Neurology* 1996;46:1306–1310.

13. Burbaud P, Wiart L, Dubos JL, et al. A randomised, double-blind, placebo-controlled trial of botulinum toxin in the treatment of spastic foot in hemiparetic patients. *J Neurol Neurosurg Psychiatry* 1996;61: 265–269.

14. Hesse S, Reiter F, Konrad M, Jahnke MT. Botulinum toxin type A and short-term electrical stimulation in the treatment of upper-limb flexor spasticity after stroke: a randomized, double-blind, placebo-controlled trial. *Clin Rehabil* 1998;12:381–388.

15. Bhakta B, Cozens J, Chamberlain M, et al. Impact of botulinum toxin type A on disability and carer burden due to arm spasticity after stroke: A randomised double-blind placebo-controlled trial. *J Neurol Neurosurg Psychiatry* 2000;68:217–222.

16. Bakheit A, Thilmann A, Ward A, et al. A randomized, double-blind placebo-controlled, dose-ranging study to compare the efficacy and safety of three doses of botulinum toxin type A (DYSPORT) with placebo in upper-limb spasticity after stroke. *Stroke* 2000;31:2402–2406.

17. Smith S, Ellis E, White S, et al. A double-blind placebo-controlled study of botulinum toxin in upper-limb spasticity after stroke or head injury. *Clin Rehabil* 2000;14: 5–13.

18. Richardson D, Sheean G, Werring D, et al. Evaluating the role of botulinum toxin in the management of focal hypertonia in adults. *J Neurol Neurosurg Psychiatry* 2000;69:499–506.

19. Hyman N, Barnes M, Bhakta B, et al. Botulinum toxin (DYSPORT) treatment of hip adductor spasticity in multiple sclerosis: a prospective, randomised, double-blind, placebo-controlled, dose-ranging study. *J Neurol Neurosurg Psychiatry* 2000;68:707–712.

20. Childers M, Brashear A, Jozefczyk P, et al. A multicenter, double-blind, placebo-controlled dose response trial of botulinum toxin type A (BOTOX) in upper-limb spasticity post-stroke. *Neurology* 1999;52(suppl 2): A295 (abstract).

21. Mahoney F, Barthel D. Functional evaluation: the Barthel index. *MD Med J* 1965;14:61–65.

22. Hesse S, Jahnke MT, Luecke D, et al. Short-term electrical stimulation enhances the effectiveness of Botulinum toxin in the treatment of lower-limb spasticity in hemiparetic patients. *Neurosci Lett* 1995;201:37–40.

23. Kirazli Y, Yagiz A, Kismali B, et al. Comparison of phenol block and botulinus toxin type A in the treatment of spastic foot after stroke. A randomized, double-blind trial. *Am J Phys Med Rehabil* 1998;77:510–515.

24. Barnes M, Bhakta B, Moore P, et al. *The management of adults with spasticity using botulinum toxin: a guide to clinical practice.* Radius Healthcare, Byfleet, Surrey 2001.

25. Shaari CM, George E, Wu BL, et al. Quantifying the spread of botulinum toxin through muscle fascia. *Laryngoscope* 1991;101:960–964.

26. Cosgrove AP, Graham HK. Cerebral palsy. In: Moore A, ed. *Handbook of botulinum toxin treatment.* Oxford: Blackwells Scientific, 1995;222–247.

27. Brin M, the Spasticity Study Group. Dosing, administration and a treatment algorithm for use of botulinum toxin A for adult-onset spasticity. *Muscle Nerve* 1997; 20(Suppl 6):S208–S220.

23

Botulinum Toxin Type A BOTOX® for Pain and Headache

Mitchell F. Brin, William Binder, Andrew Blitzer, Lawrence Schenrock, and Janice M. Pogoda

INITIAL OBSERVATIONS OF THE ANALGESIC EFFECTS OF BOTULINUM TOXIN A

Botulinum toxin type A (BTX-A; commercial preparations BOTOX®, manufactured by Allergan Inc., Irvine, California, USA; and DYSPORT, manufactured by Ipsen Pharmaceuticals, France) is one of seven distinct serotypes (A to G) of neurotoxin produced by the bacterium *Clostridium botulinum.* When injected directly into contracting muscles, BTX-A binds to the presynaptic nerve terminal, becomes internalized, and interferes with the docking of the neurotransmitter acetylcholine (ACh) with the presynaptic membrane at the neuromuscular juncture by cleaving the synaptosomal-associated protein of 25 kDa (SNAP-25) protein. This action creates chemical denervation so that muscle contraction is inhibited, thereby producing muscle weakness or relaxation. The effects of BTX-A are dose dependent. In addition, the effects are temporary because the presynaptic terminal sprouts new accessory terminals and the main terminal recovers its ability to release ACh. The recovery process takes about 3 months (1).

Therapeutic use of BTX-A in humans was first reported in 1980 for pediatric strabismus (2), and later for other ophthalmologic disorders (3,4), blepharospasm (5), and other dystonias, such as hemifacial spasm (6). Its analgesic effects were first reported in 1985 in a pilot study

of BTX-A treatment for cervical dystonia, characterized by abnormal, involuntary neck and shoulder muscle contractions and often resulting in significant, disabling musculoskeletal pain. Tsui et al. described that the most marked benefit of BTX-A injections was pain relief in all six patients who reported severe neck pain caused by muscle spasm (7). In a small, double-blind, placebo-controlled extension of this pilot study, 16 patients treated with BTX-A experienced significantly reduced pain compared to placebo (8). In subsequent open-label, prospective studies involving larger numbers of patients, we reported pain relief in 74% to 84% of cervical dystonia patients following BTX-A injections (9–12). Additional double-blind, placebo-controlled studies confirmed the observed effects on pain of BTX-A in cervical dystonia patients (13–16).

In 1992, Memin et al. reported results from a pilot study conducted in Paris, France, of BTX-A as treatment for spasticity following upper motor neuron lesion; five of six patients with pain experienced significant pain relief (17). Also in 1992, Dengler et al. reported analgesic effects of BTX-A among 10 patients treated for spastic drop foot (18). Later, a larger prospective study of patients with chronic limb spasticity as a result of various causes observed that 28 (90%) of 31 patients with painful flexor spasm or passive stretching experienced at least moderate pain relief and 8 (26%) patients experienced complete pain resolution after BTX-A injections (19). Another prospective study in Thailand observed joint pain relief in 22 poststroke spasticity patients (20). Double-blind, placebo-controlled

Mitchell F. Brin became an employee of Allergan, Inc. in January 2001, subsequent to the international meeting in 1999.

studies provided further support for the effect of BTX-A on pain relief in spasticity patients (21,22).

Early in its use as a therapeutic agent, BTX-A was observed to provide pain relief in disorders other than dystonia and spasticity. Published case reports detail analgesic effects of BTX-A injections for muscle hypertrophy associated with complex repetitive discharges (23) and for stiff-person syndrome (24). In a prospective study of 60 achalasia patients, BTX-A improved chest pain associated with this disease of the esophagus (25). Among 100 patients treated for anal fissure, 78 (78%) reported pain resolution within 3 days after initial injection (26).

USES OF BTX-A SPECIFICALLY FOR PAIN RELIEF

The earliest published reports of therapeutic uses of BTX-A focused primarily on relief of muscle spasm and secondarily on pain relief. By the mid-1990s, BTX-A was recognized as a viable therapeutic approach specifically for pain-associated disorders that were otherwise difficult to treat. Acquadro and Borodic reported the successful treatment of chronic myofascial pain in two patients who had been nonresponsive to conventional therapies (27). Girdler presented a case report of a patient with a 6-year history of temporomandibular joint dysfunction in whom BTX-A injections produced functional denervation of specific masticatory muscles that led to temporary weakness but ongoing pain relief (28). Polo and Jabbari successfully used BTX-A injections in a case of painful limb myoclonus that had been nonresponsive to a wide range of therapies (29). Diaz and Gould reported the successful treatment of a case with a 10-year history of postthoracotomy myofascial pain in the left upper-thorax and arm (30). In a double-blind, placebo-controlled study, cerebral palsy patients given BTX-A for postoperative pain following adductor-release surgery had significantly reduced pain scores, analgesic requirements, and hospital stays as compared to placebo (31). In a prospective study of 11 patients with severe, chronic prostatic pain, 9 (82%) patients experienced pain relief after BTX-A injections (32).

A double-blind, placebo-controlled study of patients suffering from chronic low-back pain showed statistically and clinically significant pain reduction in BTX-A treated subjects, as compared to placebo (33).

Johnstone and Adler reported on an unusual case of blepharospasm that presented with severe headaches and periorbital pain (34). After treatment with BTX-A injections, blepharospasm improved and complete pain resolution was achieved. They noted that blepharospasm usually does not present with pain as the primary complaint, and thus speculated whether this patient's pain was blepharospasm-induced or whether her blepharospasm was pain-induced. Therefore, this case offered possible evidence that not only muscle relaxation but also sympathetic mechanisms may be involved in pain relief as a result of BTX-A treatment.

STUDIES OF BTX-A FOR BRUXISM AND TEMPOROMANDIBULAR DISORDER

Historically, bruxism has had various definitions but it is generally characterized as grinding, clenching, or gnashing of the teeth. If left untreated, it results in masseter hypertrophy, headache, temporomandibular joint destruction, and complete edentulousness. There are two distinct manifestations of bruxism: that which occurs, usually diurnally, in patients with idiopathic, tardive, and/or posttraumatic cranial dystonia; and that which occurs nocturnally and is commonly seen in dental practice. Population prevalence of the latter, more common form has been estimated at 21% (35). The etiology is unclear and is somewhat controversial. At one time, it was thought that occlusal disorders and/or orofacial anatomy might be contributory, but more recently, the focus has been on pathophysiologic and psychological factors, such as sleep arousal response, disturbances in the central dopaminergic system, and stress (36). There is no consensus as to the best treatment; treatments typically prescribed include occlusal appliance, medication, counseling (37) and, for symptom relief, massage and stretching exercises (38).

In 1990, Van Zandijcke and Marchau presented a case report of successful treatment of bruxism with BTX-A injections in a patient who was comatose as a consequence of a car accident (39). In 1997, Ivanhoe et al. similarly reported cessation of bruxism after BTX-A injections in a patient who sustained an anoxic brain injury secondary to cardiac arrest (35). In 1998, a report from the Netherlands reported successful treatment of masseteric hypertrophy in two bruxism patients using BTX-A; pain relief was also achieved in one of the patients (40).

While pain relief was addressed and/or achieved in only one of the above cases, these reports provided evidence that bruxism, which often results in orofacial muscle pain, was responsive to BTX-A. It has been hypothesized that pain results when bruxism intensity exceeds the adaptation capacity of the musculoskeletal structures (38).

A relationship between bruxism and temporomandibular disorder (TMD) exists, but the nature of the relationship is not entirely clear. One line of thought is that bruxism predisposes to, and in fact plays a role in, the initiation of TMD (41). However, another belief is that bruxism itself should be classified as TMD (42).

TMD is defined as a group of conditions affecting the temporomandibular joint, masticatory muscles, and related structures that typically presents as jaw pain; other symptoms can include earache, headache, neck pain, and facial swelling (43). TMD-related pain is usually articular, from inflammation of associated tissues, as well as myofacial (43). The source of myofacial pain is unclear, although it has been suggested that both peripheral and central mechanisms are involved (44).

The prevalence of TMD in adults has been estimated at 10% (45). Typical treatments include analgesics, antiinflammatory medications, muscle relaxants, massage, acupuncture, and orthotic devices, none of which are known to be unusually effective (43).

Open-Label, Prospective Study of BTX-A for Severe Bruxism

An open-label, prospective study of BTX-A injections for the treatment of severe bruxism was conducted with patients from the Baylor College of Medicine Parkinson's Disease Center and Movement Disorders Clinic in Houston, Texas (46). Over an 8-year period, patients who satisfied the following diagnostic criteria were recruited and followed: tooth-grinding sounds that could be corroborated by family members or caregivers; impaired chewing, swallowing, or speech; tooth wear; nonresponsiveness to conventional therapies; and tender or hypertrophied masseter muscles. Eighteen patients (17 female) participated; mean duration of bruxism was 15 years. Most had predominantly diurnal symptoms and nine (50%) had associated dystonia. At each treatment visit, masseter muscles were injected with 25 to 100 U of BTX-A (BOTOX) per side. The primary outcome was "peak effect," defined as the maximum benefit observed after treatment and scored as follows: 0, no effect; 1, mild improvement; 2, moderate improvement but no change in function; 3, moderate improvement in severity and function; and 4, marked improvement in severity and function. Peak effect was determined by personal diaries and perception as well as interviews with family and friends. Two measures of duration of response were obtained: (a) maximum, defined as the duration of peak effect, and (b) total, defined as the duration of observance of any improvement.

The study included 123 treatment visits, or an average of 6.8 treatment visits per patient. Time between treatment visits ranged from 3.2 to 9.7 months (mean, 5.0 ± 1.8 months). Mean peak effect was 3.4 ± 0.9 (range, 0 to 4), which equates to moderate improvement in severity and function. Sixteen patients (89%) reported marked improvement after at least one treatment visit. Time to response ranged from 12 hours to 5 days (mean, 2.7 ± 1.7 days). Maximum duration ranged from 2.5 to 17 weeks (mean, 11.7 ± 4.1 weeks), and total duration ranged from 6 to 78 weeks (mean, 19.1 ± 17 weeks). One subject reported dysphagia at six treatment visits with duration ranging from 21 to 40 days (mean, 34.7 ± 7 days).

Based on the theory of a "central bruxism generator," defined as phasic jaw activity that is dependent on interaction among motor, limbic, and autonomic systems (47), the authors speculated that jaw muscle relaxation induced by BTX-A disrupts the feedback loop from the trigeminal motor nucleus and inhibits the central bruxism generator. They also proposed that BTX-A may deactivate periodontal mechanoreceptors that are thought to facilitate jaw closure motoneurons (48).

Open-Label, Prospective Study of BTX-A for TMD

An open-label, prospective Canadian study of BTX-A injections for the treatment of TMD was conducted with patients with one of three diagnoses: myofascial symptoms alone, myofascial symptoms with internal joint derangement or arthralgia, or myofascial symptoms with internal joint derangement and arthralgia (43). Patients who had never failed to respond to conventional treatment were excluded. Forty-six patients, predominantly female, participated; median duration of TMD was 8 years. Both masseter and temporalis muscles of each patient were injected with BTX-A (BOTOX): masseter with 50 U and temporalis with 25 U, each divided evenly over five sites. Five outcome measures were used: subjective facial pain measured by a visual analog scale (VAS); VAS-measured orofacial function (a series of ten different functions); interincisal opening; bite force; and objective masticatory muscle tenderness (scored by a clinician). Assessments were made before treatment and every other week after treatment for 8 weeks. Table 23.1 shows the results.

Reduction of both subjective and objective

pain occurred in most patients (87% and 96%, respectively). In all cases, pain reduction coincided with muscle weakening. For all outcomes except bite force, baseline measurements were significantly different from all posttreatment measurements. For bite force, posttreatment measurements returned to baseline values by week 8. Age was inversely correlated with improvement. Median time to subjective bite weakness was 9 days. No adverse events were reported.

The authors postulated that pain relief occurred because of reduction of mechanical stimulation of sensitized peripheral nociceptive afferent pathways via one or both of the following events, based on experimental evidence (49): BTX-A inhibition of α motor neurons resulting in reduced maximum contractile force of the injected muscles, or BTX-A inhibition of γ efferents resulting in reduced resting muscle tone. They further speculated that the reduction in muscle activity indirectly altered the release of neuropeptides and modulators of local inflammation peripherally such that stimulation of central wide dynamic range neurons and nociceptive specific neurons was reduced.

STUDIES OF BTX-A FOR MYOFASCIAL PAIN SYNDROME

Myofascial pain syndrome (MPS) is a very common pain disorder. It is estimated that 14% of the US population suffers from chronic musculoskeletal pain and that 21% to 93% of patients with regional pain complaints have MPS (50).

TABLE 23.1. *Median (range) outcome measurements by time posttreatment in a prospective, open-label study of BTX-A for temporomandibular disorder, Ontario, Canada, 2000 (43)*

Outcome	Baseline	2 weeks	4 weeks	6 weeks	8 weeks
Pain[a]	8.0 (3–10)	6.0 (1–9)	5.0 (0–9)	5.0 (0–10)	5.0 (0–9)
Function[b]	5.3 (1–9)	4.4 (0.6–9)	4.1 (1–9)	4.1 (0.5–9)	3.9 (0.6–9.5)
Jaw opening (mm)	29.5 (12–54)	33.5 (12–55)	33.0 (14–50)	33.0 (16–50)	34.5 (18–53)
Bite force (lb)	12.0 (1–37)	9.0 (1–27)	11.0 (1–28)	11.0 (0–30)	14.0 (1–37)
Tenderness[c]	15.0 (5–30)	8.0 (1–30)	6.0 (0–24)	4.5 (0–26)	6.0 (0–30)

[a] Measured by VAS on a 0 to 10 scale (0, no pain).
[b] Median score of ten functions, each measured by VAS on a 0 to 10 scale (0, no limitation).
[c] Sum of scores from five muscles measured bilaterally by a clinician on a 0 to 3 scale (0, no discomfort upon palpation).

Unfortunately, MPS does not have a uniformly accepted definition or a well-understood pathology; it is underdiagnosed and lacks a satisfactory treatment regimen (51). The clinical hallmark of MPS is the "trigger point," a region of focal tenderness in a taut band of muscle fibers (52) that, upon compression, produces referred pain in characteristic areas for specific muscles. Current research supports a relationship between trigger points and integrative mechanisms in the spinal cord in response to sensitized nerve fibers associated with abnormal endplates (53). Most conventional treatments emphasize muscle relaxation; e.g., massage, heat application, therapeutic stretching, relaxant medications, and biofeedback.

Double-Blind, Placebo-Controlled Crossover Study of BTX-A for MPS

A double-blind, placebo-controlled crossover study of BTX-A injections for the treatment of MPS was conducted in 1994 with patients from the University of North Carolina Pain Clinic (54). Six subjects (four female, two male) with chronic myofascial pain (mean duration, 3 years) were injected with BTX-A (BOTOX) and placebo, in random order, 8 weeks apart. Trigger points were injected with a total of 50 U of BTX-A. At weekly intervals during the first 4 weeks after each injection and at 8 weeks after the final injection, four pain outcome measurements were obtained: (a) VAS for pain; (b) muscle tenderness; (c) patient verbal descriptions of current pain intensity (from a predetermined list of terms); and (d) patient verbal descriptions of current pain unpleasantness. For the latter two, numerical values were assigned to correspond to the verbal descriptions. Positive response was defined as a reduction from baseline of more than 30% on at least two occasions. Table 23.2 summarizes the results.

Numbers of subjects who responded positively after BTX-A but not placebo per VAS, tenderness, pain intensity, and pain unpleasantness were 4, 5, 3, and 2, respectively. Onset of benefit occurred within the first week of injection but not within 30 minutes. Mean duration of benefit was 5 to 6 weeks, with a significant difference between BTX-A and placebo from 2 to 4 weeks per VAS, tenderness, and pain intensity. BTX-A had no effect on trigger point locations or their ability to produce radiating pain. No adverse events were reported. The authors concluded that BTX-A exerts its effect on MPS by interrupting sustained muscle contraction of intrafusal muscle fibers surrounding the trigger point.

Randomized, Comparative Study of BTX-A Versus Methylprednisolone for MPS

A randomized study to compare BTX-A to methylprednisolone for the treatment of MPS was conducted in Italy (51). Forty MPS patients (predominantly female) with chronic muscle spasm in the piriformis, iliopsoas, or scalenus anterior muscles of duration greater than 6

TABLE 23.2. *Positive response[a] by outcome measurement in a double-blind, placebo-controlled study of BTX-A for myofascial pain syndrome, University of North Carolina Pain Clinic, 1994 (54)*

Patient	Visual analog scale	Pain tenderness	Pain intensity	Pain unpleasantness	Spasm
1	B	B	B	B/P	B
2	N	N	N	N	N
3	B/P	B	B/P	B/P	B/P
4	B	B	N	B	B
5	B	B	B	B/P	N
6	B	B	B	B	B

[a] Positive response means greater than 30% reduction from baseline on at least two occasions.
B, responded after botulinum injection; N, responded after neither botulinum nor placebo injection; P, responded after placebo injection.

months but less than 2 years were injected with either BTX-A (BOTOX) or methylprednisolone (20 patients each) into the affected muscle(s). BTX-A dose was muscle-dependent: 100 U for piriformis, 150 U for iliopsoas, and 80 U for scalenus anterior. The pain outcome measurement, VAS, was obtained at baseline and at 30 and 60 days postinjection. Patients were given a stringent program of physiotherapy to follow over the course of the study.

Table 23.3 shows the changes from baseline VAS. BTX-A patients had significantly higher VAS at baseline than did methylprednisolone patients; however, no adjustments were made for this in the analyses. Nonetheless, BTX-A patients experienced significantly greater reductions in pain at 60 days postinjection as compared to methylprednisolone patients and, unlike methylprednisolone patients, experienced further pain reduction between 30 and 60 days postinjection. Also, at 60 days postinjection, VAS was significantly lower in BTX-A patients as compared to VAS in methylprednisolone patients ($p < 0.0001$). Seven patients were noncompliant with the physiotherapy program, all of whom were in the methylprednisolone group. The author surmised that noncompliance was because of more painful stretching in methylprednisolone patients as compared to BTX-A patients. Data on time to benefit, duration of benefit, and adverse events were not provided. The author suggested that, in addition to inducing muscle relaxation, BTX-A might also provide pain relief by affecting afferent pathways that relate to pain perception and posture.

STUDIES OF BTX-A FOR HEADACHE

Three types of headache—tension, cluster, and migraine—account for 80% of all headaches (55). Another type, cervicogenic headache, similar to migraine, was defined in 1983 by Sjaastad et al. (56) as unilateral headache triggered by forceful neck movement and/or sustained awkward position. Because of the inconsistency of headache definitions and the resulting difficulty in epidemiologic and pathophysiologic study of headache, the International Headache Society (IHS) published guidelines, in 1988, for discriminating among 13 major types (57). Although the pathophysiology of headache is not entirely clear, there is evidence that BTX-A has potential as an effective treatment for this debilitating and often underdiagnosed disease.

Cervicogenic Headache

Cervicogenic headache is characterized by unilateral pain originating in the neck and shoulders and radiating to the occiput and frontal regions. It is associated with decreased range of motion (ROM), tenderness, and abnormal neck muscle tone. Some theories of pathophysiology suggest involvement of myofascial pain (58,59) or muscular activity (60,61). Very few epidemiologic studies of cervicogenic headache exist. There are reports suggesting that it comprises 15% of headache patients visiting a headache clinic and has a population prevalence of less than 1% to 18%, depending on the criteria used to define it (62). In 1997, Hobson and Gladish reported successful treatment with BTX-A of cervicogenic headache resulting from a whiplash injury

TABLE 23.3. *Mean (standard deviation) change from baseline in pain score[a] in a randomized, placebo-controlled comparative study of BTX-A and methylprednisolone for myofascial pain syndrome, Policinico San Marco Pain Center, Zingonia/Bergamo, Italy, 2000 (51)*

Time postinjection	BTX-A ($n = 20$)	Methylprednisolone ($n = 20$)	p value[b]
30 days	−3.9 (0.2)	−3.5 (0.9)	0.06
60 days	−5.5 (0.3)	−2.5 (0.7)	<0.0001

[a] Visual analog scale from 0 (no pain) to 9 (unbearable pain).
[b] Two-tailed t-test.

from a car accident (63). A double-blind, placebo-controlled pilot study of BTX-A for cervicogenic headache is detailed below.

Double-Blind, Placebo-Controlled Pilot Study of BTX-A for Chronic Cervical-Associated Headache

A double-blind, placebo-controlled pilot study of BTX-A treatment for chronic cervical-associated headache was conducted in Canada (64). Twenty-six subjects with chronic headache secondary to cervical whiplash injury at least 2 years prior to study entry participated. Confirmation by anesthetic block, one of the IHS criteria for cervicogenic headache, was not done because it was felt that this would unacceptably confound the study results. Therefore, the term "cervical-associated headache" was chosen to describe the condition of the study subjects. Patients were injected with either 100 U of BTX-A (BOTOX) (14 patients) or placebo (saline; 12 patients) into the patient-specific five most tender cervical muscle trigger points. Muscles treated included the splenius capitis, rectus capitis, semispinalis capitis, and trapezius. Outcome measurements were pain, self-measured by VAS, and clinician-rated ROM based on rotation, flexion, extension, and lateral bending. Measurements were made at baseline and at 2 and 4 weeks postinjection. Table 23.4 shows the results.

BTX-A patients had significantly higher pain at baseline than placebo; however, no adjustments were made for this in the analyses. Nonetheless, BTX-A patients experienced improving pain and ROM scores over the course of the study and, at 4 weeks postinjection, had significantly improved scores compared to baseline. No such trends were observed for placebo. No adverse events were reported. The authors suggested that the effect of BTX-A on cervicogenic headache may result from mechanisms similar to those that produce BTX-A effects in disorders such as temporomandibular dysfunction and dystonias.

Tension Headache

Tension headache is the most common headache type and can be either episodic or chronic. It is the least distinctive type of headache, but is generally characterized by aching, tenderness, or sensations of pressure or constriction. The role of pericranial muscles or whether they are even a factor in the pathophysiology of tension headache has been debated. Other theories postulate that pain originates from myofascial tissue or from central mechanisms in the brain (65). One hypothesis of pathophysiology proposes vascular, myofascial, and supraspinal involvement (66). It suggests that minor myofascial stimuli trigger tension headache as a result of increased sensitization of the trigeminal nuclear complex and possibly the dorsolateral C2 segment of the spinal cord and thalamus. Stress is considered the most common precipitating factor in episodic tension headache (67), while depression, anxiety, and possibly heredity are associated with the chronic form (68–71).

One-year population prevalence of tension headache is estimated at 38%, with higher preva-

TABLE 23.4. *Median (range) outcome measurements by time posttreatment in a double-blind, placebo-controlled study of BTX-A for chronic cervical-associated headache, Ontario, Canada, 2000 (64)*

Outcome	Baseline		2 Weeks		4 Weeks	
	BTX-A	Placebo	BTX-A	Placebo	BTX-A	Placebo
Pain[a]	6.5 (2–9)	3.0 (0–8)	5.0 (1–10)	3.0 (0–6)	3.5 (1–8)	4.5 (1–9)
Range of motion[b]	312 (80–400)	337 (225–380)	317 (145–435)	347 (250–395)	343 (285–420)	325 (225–370)

[a] Measured by VAS on a 0 to 10 scale (0, no pain).
[b] Measured by rotation, flexion, extension, and lateral bending; increasing scores indicate improvement.

lence among women, and racially among whites (72). By age, prevalence peaks in 30- to 39-year olds and declines thereafter. It is estimated that an average of 9 work days per year per patient are lost because of tension headache and that half of all sufferers experience reduced effectiveness an average of 5 work days per year (72). Treatments for acute episodes include simple analgesics, nonsteroidal anti-inflammatories, and muscle relaxants. About 2% of tension headache patients suffer from chronic tension headache, which is defined as at least 15 attacks per month (72); 12% of these patients miss an average of 27 work days per year and 47% suffer reduced effectiveness an average of 20 days per year. Females are twice as likely as males to have chronic tension headache. Successful treatment usually depends on treating underlying depression or chronic states of anxiety (73).

The earliest reported study of BTX-A treatment for tension headache, specifically for chronic tension headache, was in 1994, by Zwart et al. (73a). In an open-label study of six patients, they observed no effect of BTX-A on either pain or pressure pain threshold, and concluded that temporal muscle tension is not a major direct factor in the pathophysiology of the chronic stage of chronic tension headache. Subsequent studies followed with mixed results. In Relja's open-label study of ten patients with individualized treatment regimens, BTX-A was associated with reduced headache duration, pain intensity, and pain sensitivity (74). Using the same methods, the same investigator observed similar effects in a second, larger open-label study (75). In a pilot study of eight patients injected with BTX-A into frontal, temporal, occipital, and sternocleidomastoid muscles, 25 U per injection, mean area-under-the-curve was significantly reduced at 4 weeks postinjection as compared to baseline (76). A study comparing BTX-A to methylprednisolone injections into the tender points of cranial muscles of tension headache patients observed significantly decreased VAS pain scores at 60 days postinjection (77). In an open-label, individualized-treatment study of 50 patients, 30 (60%) responded positively to BTX-A (78). None of three double-blind, placebo-controlled studies, two from Germany and one

from Switzerland, found a BTX-A effect on tension headache, although quality of life improvement was demonstrated in some (79–81). However, Carruthers et al. found efficacy in cosmetic patients who also suffered from tension headache, as detailed below (82).

Retrospective, Open-Label Study of BTX-A for Tension Headache

Patients who experienced tension headache relief as an unexpected consequence of BTX-A treatment for hyperfunctional facial lines were studied retrospectively at the Vancouver Hospital and Health Sciences Center in Canada (82). The study included eight patients (seven female, one male) treated over 39 sessions with 10 to 40 U of BTX-A (BOTOX) injected into the glabella and adjacent forehead areas. Table 23.5 summarizes the findings. Responses ranged from "mildly better" to "cleared." No adverse events were reported. The authors suggested as possible mechanisms of BTX-A effect on tension headache a direct effect on paralyzed muscles reducing nociceptive stimulation, loss of biofeedback as a result of paralyzed muscles, and perhaps a secondary central effect.

In view of the efficacy observed in some of the above studies, additional investigation is warranted to assess the key patient population characteristics and treatment paradigm for these chronic tension-type headache patients.

Cluster Headache

Arguably, the most painful type of headache is the cluster headache, which is characterized by recurrent unilateral attacks occurring over a "cluster period" (usually weeks) of severe pain lasting 15 minutes to 3 hours untreated. Cluster headache can be chronic, but usually is episodic, with attacks occurring once per day with an average cluster period of 6 to 12 weeks and a remission period of 1 year (83,84). It is not uncommon for individual attacks to occur at the same time each day and for the cluster of attacks to occur at the same time each year (85).

Some conclusions about the pathophysiology of cluster headache can be drawn from its clini-

TABLE 23.5. *Characteristics of patients who experienced tension headache relief after BTX-A treatment for hyperfunctional facial lines, Vancouver Hospital and Health Sciences Center, Vancouver, Canada, 1999 (82)*

Patient	Headache severity	No. treatments	BOTOX units per treatment	Subjective postinjection response	Time to response	Response duration
1	mild	21	10–37	mildly better	3 days	2 months
2	moderate	4	25–28	much better	4 days	2 months
3	moderate	4	20–21	cleared	2 weeks	4 months
4	severe	2	35–40	much better	few minutes	2 months
5	mild	2	23–26	much better	2 weeks	several months
6	moderate	2	14–35	much better	3 weeks	4 months
7	moderate	2	12–15	cleared	1 week	3 months
8	moderate	2	23–26	mildly better	2 days	2 weeks

cal presentation: (a) ipsilateral trigeminal nociceptive pathways are likely involved because of pain centered around the eye and forehead; (b) activation of the cranial parasympathetic system and dysfunction of the ipsilateral sympathetic nerves probably occur because of the ipsilateral autonomic features; and (c) consistency in timing of attacks and clusters suggests the involvement of a central pacemaker or biologic clock, i.e., the suprachiasmatic nucleus (85).

Cluster headache is strongly associated with heavy smoking and drinking (85); there may also be a heredity factor (86–91). Very few epidemiologic studies have been performed to estimate cluster headache prevalence, but it is extremely rare; in large male cohort studies, rates ranged from 0.13% to 0.45% (84,92–94). Cluster headache is about three times more prevalent in males than in females; however, the gender ratio appears to be decreasing over time, possibly because of the association with certain lifestyle factors that are not as gender-discrepant as they once were. In men, peak age of onset is in the third decade. In women, there are two peak ages of onset: the second and sixth decades (85).

Treatment of cluster headache often begins with patient education as to their personal etiologic factors so that future attacks can be reduced or altogether prevented. Treatments aimed at quick relief of symptoms include oxygen inhalation, triptans such as sumatriptan and zolmitriptan, dihydroergotamine, and lidocaine. Short-term or "transitional" prophylactic agents to be used during cluster periods to rapidly suppress attacks include ergot derivatives

and corticosteroids. Maintenance prophylactics that can be used throughout the cluster period include verapamil, lithium carbonate, methysergide, valproic acid, topiramate, and melatonin. Surgery, typically directed toward the sensory trigeminal nerve, is an option for patients unresponsive to other treatments (85).

Probably because of the rarity of the disease, no formal studies of effects of BTX-A on cluster headache have been published. Ginies et al. were the first to provide case reports detailing the use of BTX-A in cluster headache patients; they found that BTX-A ended current cluster periods in three of five patients (95). Subsequently, Freund and Schwartz reported that BTX-A ended current cluster periods in two of two patients treated (96), and Smuts and Barnard reported positive response in two of four cluster headache patients treated (78).

Migraine

Migraine is characterized by unilateral, pulsating pain associated with nausea, vomiting, photophobia, and phonophobia (97). An IHS diagnosis of migraine without aura requires at least five attacks over a lifetime of duration 4 to 72 hours. About 15% of migraine cases include a visual or sensory phenomenon called "aura" (98). IHS diagnosis of migraine with aura requires two lifetime attacks of migraine headache, either with or following aura of duration 4 to 60 minutes. Time between aura and headache is less than 1 hour.

Many models of migraine pathophysiology

have been proposed (99). The earliest modern theory on the pathophysiology of migraine was the "vascular" theory, conceived by H. Wolff in the 1940s and 1950s, which proposes that migraine aura is caused by cerebral vasoconstriction and that migraine pain is caused by subsequent vasodilation. However, current opinion on the pathophysiology of migraine is that it involves more than what the vascular theory alone proposes. The "spreading depression" theory hypothesizes that migraine results from vasodilation but that vasodilation is caused by a prolonged period of neuronal depression that follows a brief wave of excitation. The "neurovascular" theory proposes that either spreading depression or other migraine triggers (e.g., stress, glare, noise, carotid artery dilation) activate trigeminal nerve axons which results in a series of pain-inducing events: (a) vasodilation and inflammation of areas surrounding innervated vessels through the release of neuropeptides (e.g., substance P); (b) sensitization of nerve endings, also through the release of neuropeptides; and (c) transmission of pain impulses to the trigeminal nucleus caudalis and, in turn, to higher brain centers. According to the "serotonin abnormalities" theory, a surge in plasma serotonin levels causes vasoconstriction and reduced blood flow, leading to migraine aura and to a subsequent drop in serotonin levels, which, in turn, leads to vasodilation and migraine pain. The "integrated" theory attempts to combine all of these theories into a complex mechanism by which migraine occurs and is sustained.

Several migraine etiologic factors have been proposed and studied. Heredity appears to play a role in 70% to 80% of all migraine cases (100). In females, migraine has been correlated with events that produce cyclical changes in hormone levels, such as use of oral contraception, pregnancy, menopause, and estrogen replacement therapy (101). Various lifestyle and dietary factors have also been implicated: physical activity; smoking; caffeine; alcohol; chocolate; food additives; and sleep pattern, quality, and duration (67,102–104). Psychosocial factors are also believed to play an important role in migraine etiology. It has been reported that up to 54% of all migraine attacks are stress-related (104). Major

depression is also a correlate of migraine (105). Certain medications are hypothesized to initiate or increase the frequency of migraine attacks: nitroglycerin, certain calcium channel-blockers, tetracycline, and sildenafil citrate (104).

Worldwide prevalence of migraine is estimated to be 13% to 17% in women and 8% to 14% in men, based on meta-analyses of international data collected from 1962 to 1992 (106–108). In the United States, prevalence is estimated at 18% in women, 7% in men, and 13% overall, with higher prevalence among 35- to 45-year olds, lower-income populations, and whites (109). The gender ratio is equal before puberty, then increases in favor of women until 40 to 45 years of age (103,110,111). Overall, migraine is twice as prevalent in women as in men. Among female migraineurs, 60% experience at least one severe attack per month; 42% of this subgroup experience at least four severe attacks per month (112).

The effect of migraine on quality of life is profound. Nearly all migraine patients experience functional impairment as a result of their condition, and more than half report severe impairment or required bedrest (109). It is estimated that migraine results in 112 million bedridden days in the United States per year, and results in an annual cost to employers of $13 billion (113). Given the prevalence pattern by age, most of these days occur during the most productive employment and most important childrearing years (114). The effect of migraine extends beyond the attacks themselves in terms of quality of life, productivity, and comorbidities such as depression, anxiety disorders, epilepsy, and stroke (115). Direct costs of migraine—i.e., medical costs—are estimated at $1 billion per year, far less than the indirect costs; about 60% of direct costs are from physician visits and 30% from prescription medications (113). Most migraineurs do not seek medical treatment; instead, they rely on over-the-counter medications (109) because they believe that effective prescribed treatments do not exist (114).

As with cluster headache, treatment of migraine often begins with patient education so that future attacks can be reduced or prevented. Pharmacologic therapy falls into two categories:

acute and prophylactic (116). Acute medication typically consists of simple analgesics for mild to moderate attacks. For moderate to severe attacks, medication used to be prescribed in the form of ergot derivatives. However, the advent of triptans, with greater receptor specificity than ergot derivatives, revolutionized acute migraine therapy for more severe attacks. Opioids are reserved for rescue therapy when other medications cannot be used. Prophylactic medications commonly prescribed include propranolol, timolol, sodium divalproex, and amitriptyline.

William Binder, an otolaryngologist and facial plastic surgeon, observed that BTX-A provided relief to migraine sufferers whom he was treating for hyperfunctional facial lines (117). Subsequently, Binder et al. conducted an open-label study to further investigate the possibility of a BTX-A effect on migraine (detailed below). Various open-label (78,118) as well as double-blind studies followed and reported promising results. Representative studies are detailed below.

Open-Label, Prospective Study of BTX-A for Migraine

We conducted an open-label study of BTX-A for migraine that included a sample of 106 patients (95 female, 11 male) recruited from private practice cosmetic surgery clinics in Los Angeles and San Francisco, and from otolaryngology and neurology clinics in New York City (119). Patients either sought BTX-A (BOTOX) treatment for hyperfunctional facial lines or other dystonias with concomitant headache disorders, or were candidates for BTX-A treatment specifically for headaches. Based on IHS criteria, patients were classified as true migraineurs (75%), possible migraineurs (17%), or nonmigraineurs (9%), and received prospective BTX-A treatments either prophylactically (93 patients) or for acute migraine episodes (4 patients); a small subgroup (9 patients) received both types of treatments. Injections were administered to the glabellar, temporal, frontal, and, in two subjects, the suboccipital regions of the head and neck. Average dose per injection was 31 U. True migraineurs received higher doses, and patients treated specifically for headache

tended to receive larger doses as the study progressed. Length of follow-up ranged from 3 weeks to 6 months. Treatment benefit was evaluated by self-reported degree and duration of response. Degree of response was defined as (a) complete response (elimination of headache symptoms), (b) partial response (at least 50% reduction in frequency or severity of headaches), and (c) nonresponse (less than 50% reduction in frequency or severity of headaches). Patients lost to follow-up were considered nonresponders.

Among true migraineurs treated prophylactically, 51% (95% CI = 39% to 62%) were complete responders with mean (SD) duration of benefit of 4.1 (2.6) months. Complete response was related to lower baseline migraine frequency ($p = 0.06$) and severity ($p = 0.07$). Figure 23.1 shows the response by baseline severity. "Improvement," defined as complete or partial response, was unrelated to baseline frequency and severity. Mean (SD) duration of benefit among improvers was 3.2 (2.3) months. Complete responders with severe baseline headaches had somewhat longer duration of benefit [mean (SD), 4.6 (3.1) months] compared to those with less severe headaches at baseline [mean (SD) 3.7 (2.3) months]. Although there was no evidence of dose-response, injection site appeared to be related to response; 87% of complete responders received glabellar injections versus 66% of non- or partial responders ($p = 0.01$). Of 13 subjects treated for acute migraine, 10 were complete responders, and all responded within 1 to 2 hours postinjection. Two patients reported transient brow ptosis; other adverse effects were limited to transient local pain and ecchymosis at the injection site.

Based on observations from this study, we proposed that the effect of BTX-A on migraine may not be limited to muscle relaxation. Among these patients, dose-duration curve did not necessarily directly correlate with the duration of action associated with muscle relaxation. Also, in some patients, relief of migraine symptoms persisted beyond the time that muscle function returned (after 3 months). We suggested that BTX-A for migraine acts by inhibiting the sensory trigeminal nerve endings, the vesicular re-

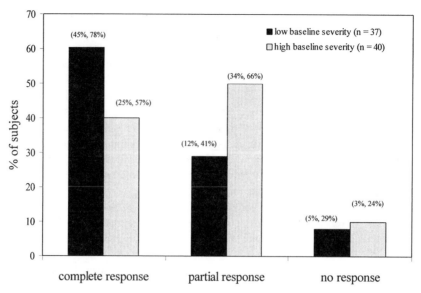

FIG. 23.1. Proportion (95% confidence intervals) of self-reported complete, partial, and nonresponders among 77 true migraineurs treated prophylactically by baseline headache frequency (high frequency, at least three times per month) and severity (high severity, "severe"); open-label, prospective study of BTX-A for migraine (119).

lease of pain-associated neurotransmitters, or the vasculature and extracranial inflammatory process believed to be involved in the vicious trigeminal-neurovascular cycle of migraine pathophysiology. Specifically, we hypothesized that (a) BTX-A injected into the temple or forehead muscles recognizes the parasympathetic neurons innervating the extracranial vasculature and causes a disruptive effect on the vesicular release of ACh as well as other ACh-like neuropeptides; (b) blockade of these neuropeptides may also inhibit neurogenic inflammation, thought to play a role in migraine, that may result from the release of neuropeptides from trigeminal nerves innervating both the intracranial and extracranial vasculature; and (c) parasympathetic neurons may be a likely site of action for BTX-A because of their known cholinergic component and possible colocalization of the other vasodilatory neuropeptides within these nerves.

Double-Blind, Placebo-Controlled Study of BTX-A for Migraine

A double-blind, placebo-controlled study of BTX-A (BOTOX) for migraine was conducted with 123 (105 female, 18 male) patients from 12 headache centers across the United States (120). Patients were randomized to one of three groups: (a) placebo (41 patients); (b) 25 U BTX-A (42 patients); or (c) 75 U BTX-A (40 patients). Symmetrical injections were administered to the frontal, temporal, and glabellar regions of the head. The primary outcome in intent-to-treat analysis was change from baseline in number of moderate-to-severe migraines per month. Other outcome measurements were the occurrence of migraines, severity of migraines, migraine-associated symptoms, use of acute migraine medications, and Subject Global Assessment. Outcome data were collected at three monthly postinjection visits.

Twenty-five units BTX-A resulted in significantly greater reduction in moderate-to-severe migraine frequency than did placebo at month 2 (-1.57 vs -0.37, $p = 0.008$) and at month 3 (-1.88 vs -0.98, $p = 0.04$) postinjection. Twenty-five units BTX-A also resulted in a significantly greater reduction in frequency of migraines of any severity than did placebo at month 3 (-2.12 vs -0.90, $p = 0.01$) and a tendency toward fewer migraines at month 2 (-1.55 vs

−0.37, $p = 0.07$). At month 3, when compared to placebo, significantly more subjects who received 25 U BTX-A reported at least two fewer migraines of any severity ($p = 0.01$) and a decrease in migraine frequency of at least 50% ($p = 0.046$). When compared to placebo, 25 U BTX-A resulted in a significantly greater reduction in migraine severity at months 1 and 2 ($p < 0.03$) and in use of migraine medications at month 2 ($p = 0.03$). At month 3, significantly fewer subjects who received 25 U BTX-A experienced migraine-associated vomiting compared to placebo ($p = 0.01$). Regardless of dose, BTX-A-treated patients had significantly better Subject Global Assessment scores than did placebo-treated patients at month 2 (75 U BTX-A = 1.25, 25 U BTX-A = 1.19, vehicle = 0.46; $p = 0.041$).

Seventy-five units BTX-A resulted in higher incidence of treatment-related adverse events as compared to placebo (50% vs 24%, $p = 0.02$), whereas 25 U BTX-A and placebo were similar in adverse event incidence. All adverse events were transient and included blepharoptosis, diplopia, and injection-site weakness.

The authors surmised that 75 U BTX-A did not perform as well as 25 U because patients randomized to the higher-dose group had lower baseline migraine frequency than did the lower-dose group. However, they reported adjusting for this in the analyses. Their explanation of BTX-A effect on migraine was that pericranial muscle contractions are part of the trigger process for migraine and that BTX-A reduces such contractions. They also acknowledged the possibility of a central secondary effect through inhibition of pain pathways.

Double-Blind, Placebo-Controlled Study of BTX-A for Migraine

We conducted a double-blind, placebo-controlled study of BTX-A (BOTOX) for migraine with 53 patients (50 female, 3 male) recruited from three headache centers in New York City, Loma Linda, California, and Englewood, Colorado (121). Patients were randomized to one of four treatment groups: group 1, BTX-A to the frontal and temporal regions (45 and 30 U, re-

spectively; 14 patients); group 2, BTX-A to the frontal region (45 U), placebo to the temporal region (12 patients); group 3, BTX-A to the temporal region (30 U), placebo to the frontal region (14 patients); and group 4, placebo to the frontal and temporal regions (13 patients). Primary outcome measurements in intent-to-treat analyses were change from baseline in frequency, duration, and pain intensity (0 to 10 scale) of migraine headaches. Outcome data were collected at baseline and at 2, 4, 8, 12, and 16 weeks postinjection. Group 1 versus group 4 at week 12 was defined as the key comparison.

Maximum pain decrease for group 1 occurred by week 12 and was significantly greater than for group 4 [median (range) = −4.0 (−7.5, −0.1) for group 1 and −0.2 (−5.1, 3.5) for Group 4; $p = 0.01$]. At week 12, when compared to placebo (group 4), BTX-A (groups 1 to 3) produced a greater decrease in the number of migraines per month [median (range) = −1.7 (−7.2, 20.6) for BTX-A; −0.5 (−8.5, 10.7) for placebo] and had the largest difference in maximum duration (hours) decrease [least-squares mean (SE) adjusted for baseline = −19.2 (3.7) for BTX-A and −8.0 (6.5) for placebo; $p = 0.15$]. Only group 1 experienced a significant increase in proportion of participants with a two-migraine decrease in frequency since baseline ($p = 0.006$) and a significant decline in medication use ($p < 0.0001$) over the course of follow-up.

CONCLUSIONS

BTX-A has emerged as a promising option for patients suffering from chronic pain disorders. A primary benefit of BTX-A is its duration of effect, which typically begins within 1 to 14 days, peaks within 2 to 6 weeks, and may require retreatment 12 to 16 weeks subsequently. These time frames coincide with known properties of BTX-A. Another benefit is its established safety and tolerability. In headache, therapeutic doses of BTX-A range from 25 to 250 U (116). Adverse effects associated with BTX-A for pain are generally mild and reversible; the most common are excessive weakness in the treated muscle and unwanted weakness in adjacent muscles. Examples include ptosis after injection to the levator muscle for treatment of blepharospasm, hyperfunctional facial lines, or headache, and dysphagia after treatment for cervical dystonia (122).

An uncommon complication of BTX-A therapy is the formation of neutralizing antibodies that render it ineffective (for review, see reference 123). Estimated prevalence of BTX-A resistance is less than 5% (124) and appears to be correlated with dose and frequency rather than with duration of exposure (125,126). In 1997, Allergan released the current BOTOX with a lower protein exposure per unit than the original BOTOX. Current BOTOX is thought to have a lower potential for antibody formation because of the lower protein exposure. Cervical dystonia patients who develop BTX-A immunoresistance can benefit from different preparations of BTX-A or from other botulinum toxin serotypes (127–131). However, there is laboratory evidence that cross-reactivity and cross-neutralization among different botulinum toxin serotypes may occur (132).

The association between BTX-A and pain relief was originally thought to relate only to its effect on muscle contraction. However, some studies of BTX-A for various conditions suggest that muscle relaxation may not directly coincide with pain relief, suggesting alternative mechanisms for analgesic effects of BTX-A. There is experimental evidence that BTX-A affects afferent transmission (49,133), which may be a factor in pain relief, and that BTX-A inhibits the release of substance P (134) and potentially other neuromodulators. Substance P is a neuropeptide that plays a role in pain perception, vasodilation, and neurogenic inflammation. Also, it has been shown experimentally that BTX-A relieves formalin-induced pain in laboratory animals (135). This is an important observation in understanding the action of BTX-A on pain because formalin causes pain not through muscle tension, but by first directly stimulating nociceptors and then through inflammation. It seems likely that the analgesic effects of BTX-A relate not only to its well-established effect at the neuromuscular juncture, but also to an effect on the nociceptor system (122).

Unanswered questions include optimum treatment regimen (i.e., dose and injection sites), as well as specific headache and patient characteristics that are associated with the maximum clinical response. However, it should be emphasized that an ''optimum treatment regimen'' for a generalized patient population may not exist; i.e., ''optimum treatment'' might be highly individualized for reasons such as the dose-dependency on targeted muscles and injection regions. Furthermore, pain clinical trials are challenged to manage the ''placebo effect,'' particularly when an injectable therapy is evaluated. These factors undoubtedly contribute to the findings from some studies that failed to show a consistent BTX-A effect on pain. In medical practice, the appropriate dose for a given patient is determined through controlled and systematic observations after each treatment, beginning at low doses and adjusting dose and injection sites until maximum effect is achieved.

BTX-A as BOTOX is currently FDA-approved for use in strabismus, blepharospasm, and cervical dystonia. It is approved in other countries for hyperhidrosis, poststroke spasticity, juvenile cerebral palsy, and cosmetic conditions. It is used clinically for numerous other disorders in patients for whom conventional therapies are ineffective or poorly tolerated, and it is likely that additional applications will continue to be discovered. Further research is warranted to fully understand the potential and limitations of such a widely applicable therapeutic agent as botulinum toxin type A.

ACKNOWLEDGMENTS

This work was supported by the Bachmann-Strauss Dystonia and Parkinson Foundation.

REFERENCES

1. de Paiva A, Meunier FA, Molgo J, et al. Functional repair of motor endplates after botulinum neurotoxin type A poisoning: biphasic switch of synaptic activity between nerve sprouts and their parent terminals. *Proc Natl Acad Sci U S A* 1999;96:3200–3205.
2. Scott AB. Botulinum toxin injection into extraocular muscles as an alternative to strabismus surgery. *J Pediatr Ophthalmol Strabismus* 1980;17:21–25.
3. Scott AB. Injection treatment of endocrine orbital myopathy. *Doc Ophthalmol* 1984;58:141–145.
4. Scott AB. Botulinum toxin treatment of strabismus. *Am Orthopt J* 1985;35:28–29.
5. Frueh BR, Felt DP, Wojno TH, et al. Treatment of

blepharospasm with botulinum toxin. A preliminary report. *Arch Ophthalmol* 1984;102:1464–1468.

6. Mauriello JA Jr. Blepharospasm, Meige syndrome, and hemifacial spasm: treatment with botulinum toxin. *Neurology* 1985;35:1499–1500.

7. Tsui JK, Eisen A, Mak E, et al. A pilot study on the use of botulinum toxin in spasmodic torticollis. *Can J Neurol Sci* 1985;12:314–316.

8. Tsui JKC, Eisen A, Stoessl AJ, et al. Double-blind study of botulinum toxin in spasmodic torticollis. *Lancet* 1986;2:245–247.

9. Brin MF, Fahn S, Moskowitz C, et al. Localized injections of botulinum toxin for the treatment of focal dystonia and hemifacial spasm. *Mov Disord* 1987;2:237–254.

10. Tsui JKC, Fross RD, Calne S, et al. Local treatment of spasmodic torticollis with botulinum toxin. *Can J Neurol Sci* 1987;14:533–535.

11. Jankovic J, Schwartz K. Botulinum toxin injections for cervical dystonia. *Neurology* 1990;40:277–280.

12. Poewe W, Schelosky L, Kleedorfer B, et al. Treatment of spasmodic torticollis with local injections of botulinum toxin. One-year follow-up in 37 patients. *J Neurol* 1992;239:21–25.

13. Greene P, Kang U, Fahn S, et al. Double-blind, placebo-controlled trial of botulinum toxin injections for the treatment of spasmodic torticollis. *Neurology* 1990;40:1213–1218.

14. Blackie JD, Lees AJ. Botulinum toxin treatment in spasmodic torticollis. *J Neurol Neurosurg Psychiatry* 1990;53:640–643.

15. Lorentz IT, Subramaniam SS, Yiannikas C. Treatment of idiopathic spasmodic torticollis with botulinum toxin A: a double-blind study on twenty-three patients. *Mov Disord* 1991;6:145–150.

16. Lu CS, Chen RS, Tsai CH. Double-blind, placebo-controlled study of botulinum toxin injections in the treatment of cervical dystonia. *J Formos Med Assoc* 1995;94:189–192.

17. Memin B, Pollack P, Hommel M, et al. Effects of botulinum toxin on spasticity. *Rev Neurol (Paris)* 1992;148:212–214.

18. Dengler R, Neyer U, Wohlfarth K, et al. Local botulinum toxin in the treatment of spastic foot drop. *J Neurol* 1992;239:375–378.

19. Dunne JW, Heye N, Dunne SL. Treatment of chronic limb spasticity with botulinum toxin A. *J Neurol Neurosurg Psychiatry* 1995;58:232–235.

20. Viriyavejakul A, Vachalathiti R, Poungvarin N. Botulinum treatment for post-stroke spasticity: low-dose regime. *J Med Assoc Thai* 1998;81:413–422.

21. Grazko MA, Polo KB, Jabbari B. Botulinum toxin A for spasticity, muscle spasms, and rigidity. *Neurology* 1995;45:712–717.

22. Hyman N, Barnes M, Bhakta B, et al. Botulinum toxin (DYSPORT) treatment of hip adductor spasticity in multiple sclerosis: a prospective, randomised, double blind, placebo controlled, dose ranging study. *J Neurol Neurosurg Psychiatry* 2000;68:707–712.

23. Nix WA, Butler IJ, Roontga S, et al. Persistent unilateral tibialis anterior muscle hypertrophy with complex repetitive discharges and myalgia: report of two unique cases and response to botulinum toxin. *Neurology* 1992;42:602–606.

24. Davis D, Jabbari B. Significant improvement of stiff-

25. person syndrome after paraspinal injection of botulinum toxin-A. *Mov Disord* 1993;8:371–373.

25. Fishman VM, Parkman HP, Schiano TD, et al. Symptomatic improvement in achalasia after botulinum toxin injection of the lower esophageal sphincter. *Am J Gastroenterol* 1996;91:1724–1730.

26. Jost WH. One hundred cases of anal fissure treated with botulin toxin: early and long-term results. *Dis Colon Rectum* 1997;40:1029–1032.

27. Acquadro MA, Borodic GE. Treatment of myofascial pain with botulinum A toxin [Letter]. *Anesthesiology* 1994;80:705–706.

28. Girdler NM. Use of botulinum toxin to alleviate facial pain. *Br J Hosp Med* 1994;52:363

29. Polo KB, Jabbari B. Effectiveness of botulinum toxin type A against painful limb myoclonus of spinal cord origin. *Mov Disord* 1994;9:233–235.

30. Diaz JH, Gould HJ. Management of post-thoracotomy pseudoangina and myofascial pain with botulinum toxin. *Anesthesiology* 1999;91:877–879.

31. Barwood S, Baillieu C, Boyd R, et al. Analgesic effects of botulinum toxin A: a randomized, placebo-controlled clinical trial. *Dev Med Child Neurol* 2000;42:116–121.

32. Zermann D, Ishigooka M, Schubert J, Schmidt RA. Perisphincteric injection of botulinum toxin type A. A treatment option for patients with chronic prostatic pain? *Eur Urol* 2000;38:393–399.

33. Foster L, Clapp L, Erickson M, et al. Botulinum toxin A and chronic low back pain: a randomized, double-blind study. *Neurology* 2001;56:1290–1293.

34. Johnstone SJ, Adler CH. Headache and facial pain responsive to botulinum toxin: an unusual presentation of blepharospasm. *Headache* 1998;38:366–368.

35. Ivanhoe CB, Lai JM, Francisco GE. Bruxism after brain injury: successful treatment with botulinum toxin-A. *Arch Phys Med Rehabil* 1997;78:1272–1273.

36. Lobbezoo F, Naeije M. [Etiology of bruxism: morphological, pathophysiological and psychological factors]. *Ned Tijdschr Tandheelkd* 2000;107:275–280.

37. van der Zaag J, Lobbezoo F, Naeije M. [Dental and pharmacological treatment options for bruxism]. *Ned Tijdschr Tandheelkd* 2000;107:289–292.

38. Visscher CM, Lobbezoo F, Naeije M. [Treatment of bruxism: physiotherapeutic approach]. *Ned Tijdschr Tandheelkd* 2000;107:293–296.

39. Van Zandijcke M, Marchau MM. Treatment of bruxism with botulinum toxin injections [Letter]. *J Neurol Neurosurg Psychiatry* 1990;53:530.

40. Rijsdijk BA, van ES RJ, Zonneveld FW, et al. [Botulinum toxin type A treatment of cosmetically disturbing masseteric hypertrophy]. *Ned Tijdschr Geneeskd* 1998;142:529–532.

41. Stegenga B, Lobbezoo F. [Bruxism and temporomandibular disorders]. *Ned Tijdschr Tandheelkd* 2000;107:285–288.

42. Lobbezoo F, Lavigne GJ. Do bruxism and temporomandibular disorders have a cause-and-effect relationship? *J Orofac Pain* 1997;11:15–23.

43. Freund B, Schwartz M, Symington JM. Botulinum toxin: new treatment for temporomandibular disorders. *Br J Oral Maxillofac Surg* 2000;38:466–471.

44. Sessle BJ. Biological and psychological aspects of orofacial pain. In: Stohler CS, Carlson DS, eds. *Craniofacial growth series 29, Center for Human Growth &*

Development. Ann Arbor, MI: University of Michigan, 1994:1–33.

45. LeResche, L. Epidemiology of temporomandibular disorders: implications for the investigation of etiologic factors. *Crit Rev Oral Biol Med* 1997;8:291–305.

46. Tan EK, Jankovic J. Treating severe bruxism with botulinum toxin. *J Am Dent Assoc* 2000;131:211–216.

47. Hartmann E. Bruxism. In: Kryger MH, Roth T, Dement WC, eds. *Principles and practice of sleep medicine, 2nd ed.* Philadelphia, PA: WB Saunders, 1994: 598–601.

48. Lavigne G, Kim JS, Valiquette C, et al. Evidence that periodontal pressoreceptors provide positive feedback to jaw closing muscles during mastication. *J Neurophysiol* 1987;58:342–358.

49. Filippi GM, Errico P, Santarelli R, et al. Botulinum A toxin effects on rat jaw muscle spindles. *Acta Otolaryngol* 1993;113:400–404.

50. Finley JE. Myofascial pain. *eMed J* 2 (Oct. 2, 2001) (http://www.emedicine.com/PMR/topic84.htm).

51. Porta M. A comparative trial of botulinum toxin type A and methylprednisolone for the treatment of myofascial pain syndrome and pain from chronic muscle spasm. *Pain* 2000;85:101–105.

52. Travell JG, Simons DG. Myofascial pain and its trigger points. In: Travell JG, Simons DG, eds. *Myofascial pain and dysfunction.* Baltimore, MD: Williams and Wilkins, 1983:5–164.

53. Hong CZ, Simons DG. Pathophysiologic and electrophysiologic mechanisms of myofascial trigger points. *Arch Phys Med Rehabil* 1998;79:863–872.

54. Cheshire WP, Abashian SW, Mann JD. Botulinum toxin in the treatment of myofascial pain syndrome. *Pain* 1994;59:65–69.

55. Winner PK. Migraine: diagnosis and rational treatment. *Int J Fertil Womens Med* 1998;43:104–110.

56. Sjaastad O, Saunte C, Hovdahl H, et al. "Cervicogenic" headache. An hypothesis. *Cephalalgia* 1983;3: 249–256.

57. Headache Classification Committee of the International Headache Society. Classification and diagnostic criteria for headache disorders, cranial neuralgias and facial pain. *Cephalalgia* 1988;8:19–28.

58. Pfaffenrath V, Dandekar R, Pollmann W. Cervicogenic headache—the clinical picture, radiological findings and hypotheses on its pathophysiology. *Headache* 1987;27:495–499.

59. Jaeger B. Are "cervicogenic" headaches due to myofascial pain and cervical spine dysfunction? *Cephalalgia* 1989;9:157–164.

60. Pikoff H. Is the muscular model of headache still viable? A review of conflicting data. *Headache* 1984;24: 186–198.

61. Bansevicius D, Sjaastad O. Cervicogenic headache: the influence of mental load on pain level and EMG of shoulder-neck and facial muscles. *Headache* 1996;36: 372–378.

62. Sjaastad O, Fredriksen TA. Cervicogenic headache: criteria, classification and epidemiology. *Clin Exp Rheumatol* 2000;18:S3–S6.

63. Hobson DE, Gladish DF. Botulinum toxin injection for cervicogenic headache. *Headache* 1997;37:253–255.

64. Freund BJ, Schwartz M. Treatment of chronic cervical-associated headache with botulinum toxin A: a pilot study. *Headache* 2000;40:231–236.

65. Jensen R. Pathophysiological mechanisms of tension-type headache: a review of epidemiological and experimental studies. *Cephalalgia* 1999;19:602–621.

66. Olesen J. Clinical and pathophysiological observations in migraine and tension-type headache explained by integration of vascular, supraspinal and myofascial inputs. *Pain* 1991;46:125–132.

67. Rasmussen BK. Migraine and tension-type headache in a general population: precipitating factors, female hormones, sleep pattern and relation to lifestyle. *Pain* 1993;53:65–72.

68. Rasmussen BK. Migraine and tension-type headache in a general population: psychosocial factors. *Int J Epidemiol* 1992;21:1138–1143.

69. Holroyd KA, France JL, Nash JM, et al. Pain state as artifact in the psychological assessment of recurrent headache sufferers. *Pain* 1993;53:229–235.

70. Mitsikostas DD, Thomas AM. Comorbidity of headache and depressive disorders. *Cephalalgia* 1999;19: 211–217.

71. Russell MB, Ostergaard S, Bendtsen L, et al. Familial occurrence of chronic tension-type headache. *Cephalalgia* 1999;19:207–210.

72. Schwartz BS, Stewart WF, Simon D, et al. Epidemiology of tension-type headache. *JAMA* 1998;279: 381–383.

73. Diamond S. Tension-type headache. *Clin Cornerstone* 1999;1:33–44.

73a. Zwart JA, Bovim G, Sand T, et al. Tension headache: botulinum toxin paralysis of temporal muscles. *Headache* 1994;34:458–462.

74. Relja M. Treatment of tension-type headache by local injection of botulinum toxin. *Eur J Neurol* 1997; 4(Suppl 2):S71–S74.

75. Relja MA. Treatment of tension-type headache by local injection of botulinum toxin: 1-year followup. *Cephalalgia* 2000;20:336.

76. Schulte-Mattler WJ, Wieser T, Zierz S. Treatment of tension-type headache with botulinum toxin: a pilot study. *Eur J Med Res* 1999;4:183–186.

77. Porta M. A comparative trial of botulinum toxin type A and methylprednisolone for the treatment of tension-type headache. *Curr Rev Pain* 2000;4:31–35.

78. Smuts JA, Barnard PWA. Botulinum toxin type A in the treatment of headache syndromes: a clinical report of 79 patients. *Cephalalgia* 2000;20:332.

79. Gobel H, Lindner V, Krack P, et al. Treatment of chronic tension-type headache with botulinum toxin. *Cephalalgia* 1999;19:455.

80. Rollnik JD, Tanneberger O, Schubert M, et al. Treatment of tension-type headache with botulinum toxin type A: a double-blind, placebo-controlled study. *Headache* 2000;40:300–305.

81. Schmitt WJ, Slowey E, Fravi N, et al. Effect of botulinum toxin A injections in the treatment of chronic tension-type headache: a double-blind, placebo-controlled trial. *Headache* 2001;41:658–664.

82. Carruthers A, Langtry JA, Carruthers J, et al. Improvement of tension-type headache when treating wrinkles with botulinum toxin A injections. *Headache* 1999;39: 662–665.

83. Ekbom K. A clinical comparison of cluster headache and migraine. *Acta Neurol Scand* 1970;Suppl 41:11.

84. Kudrow L. Cluster headache mechanisms and management. New York: Oxford University Press, 1980.

85. Dodick DW, Rozen TD, Goadsby PJ, et al. Cluster headache. *Cephalalgia* 2000;20:787–803.

86. Kudrow L, Kudrow DB. Inheritance of cluster headache and its possible link to migraine. *Headache* 1994; 34:400–407.

87. Russell MB. Genetic epidemiology of migraine and cluster headache. *Cephalalgia* 1997;17:683–701.

88. Eadie MJ, Sutherland JM. Migrainous neuralgia. *Med J Aust* 1966;1:1053–1057.

89. Couturier EG, Hering R, Steiner TJ. The first report of cluster headache in identical twins [see Comments]. *Neurology* 1991;41:761.

90. Roberge C, Bouchard JP, Simard D, et al. Cluster headache in twins [Letter; Comment]. *Neurology* 1992;42: 1255–1256.

91. Sjaastad O, Shen JM, Stovner LJ, et al. Cluster headache in identical twins. *Headache* 1993;33:214–217.

92. Ekbom K, Ahlborg B, Schele R. Prevalence of migraine and cluster headache in Swedish men of 18. *Headache* 1978;18:9–19.

93. D'Alessandro R, Gamberini G, Benassi G, et al. Cluster headache in the Republic of San Marino. *Cephalalgia* 1986;6:159–162.

94. Swanson JW, Yanagihara T, Stang PE, et al. Incidence of cluster headaches: a population-based study in Olmsted County, Minnesota. *Neurology* 1994;44: 433–437.

95. Ginies PR, Fraimount JL, Siou DK, et al. Treatment of cluster headache by subcutaneous injection of botulinum toxin (abst). In: Jensen TS, editor. *Progress in Pain Research and Management.* Seattle: IASP Press, 1996:501.

96. Freund BJ, Schwartz M. The use of botulinum toxin A in the treatment of refractory cluster headache: case reports. *Cephalalgia* 2000;20:329–330.

97. Olesen J, Lipton RB. Migraine classification and diagnosis. International Headache Society criteria. *Neurology* 1994;44(Suppl 4):S6–S10.

98. Cady RK. Diagnosis and treatment of migraine. *Clin Cornerstone* 1999;1:21–32.

99. Silberstein SD, Lipton RB, Dalessio D, eds. *Wolff's Headache.* 7th ed. South Melbourne, NZ: Oxford University Press, 2001.

100. Hickey JV. The clinical practice of neurological and neurosurgical nursing, 4th ed. New York: Lippincott, 1997.

101. Edelson RN. Menstrual migraine and other hormonal aspects of migraine. *Headache* 1985;25:376–379.

102. Spierings EL, Sorbi M, Haimowitz BR, et al. Changes in daily hassles, mood, and sleep in the 2 days before a migraine headache. *Clin J Pain* 1996;12:38–42.

103. Stang P, Sternfeld B, Sidney S. Migraine headache in a prepaid health plan: ascertainment, demographics, physiological, and behavioral factors. *Headache* 1996; 36:69–76.

104. Rapoport AM. Pharmacological prevention of migraine. *Clin Neurosci* 1998;5:55–59.

105. Breslau N, Davis GC, Schultz LR, et al. Joint 1994 Wolff Award Presentation. Migraine and major depression: a longitudinal study. *Headache* 1994;34: 387–393.

106. Lipton RB, Silberstein SD, Stewart WF. An update on the epidemiology of migraine. *Headache* 1994;34: 319–328.

107. Stewart WF, Shechter A, Rasmussen BK. Migraine prevalence. A review of population-based studies. *Neurology* 1994;44(Suppl 4):S17–S23.

108. Stewart WF, Simon D, Shechter A, et al. Population variation in migraine prevalence: a meta-analysis. *J Clin Epidemiol* 1995;48:269–280.

109. Lipton RB, Stewart WF, Diamond S, et al. Prevalence and burden of migraine in the United States: data from the American Migraine Study II. *Headache* 2001;41: 646–657.

110. Stewart WF, Linet MS, Celentano DD, et al. Age- and sex-specific incidence rates of migraine with and without visual aura. *Am J Epidemiol* 1991;134:1111–1120.

111. Stewart WF, Lipton RB, Celentano DD, et al. Prevalence of migraine headache in the United States. Relation to age, income, race, and other sociodemographic factors. *JAMA* 1992;267:64–69.

112. Lipton RB, Stewart WF. Prevalence and impact of migraine. *Neurol Clin* 1997;15:1–13.

113. Hu XH, Markson LE, Lipton RB, et al. Burden of migraine in the United States: disability and economic costs. *Arch Intern Med* 1999;159:813–818.

114. Mannix LK. Epidemiology and impact of primary headache disorders. *Med Clin North Am* 2001;85: 887–895.

115. Lipton RB, Stewart WF, Vonkorff M. Burden of migraine: societal costs and therapeutic opportunities. *Neurology* 1997;48(Suppl 3):S4–S9.

116. Silberstein SD. Review of botulinum toxin type A and its clinical applications in migraine headache. *Expert Opin Pharmacother* 2001;2:1649–1654.

117. Binder W, Brin MF, Blitzer A, et al. Botulinum toxin type A (BOTOX) for treatment of migraine headaches: An open-label study. *Otolaryngol Head Neck Surg* 2000;123:669–676.

118. Mauskop A, Basedo R. Botulinum toxin A is an effect prophylactic therapy of migraines. *Cephalalgia* 2000; 20:422.

119. Binder WJ, Brin MF, Blitzer A, et al. Botulinum toxin type A (BOTOX) for treatment of migraine headaches: An open-label study. *Otolaryngol Head Neck Surg* 2000;123:669–676.

120. Silberstein S, Mathew N, Saper J, et al. Botulinum toxin type A as a migraine preventive treatment. *Headache* 2000;40:445–450.

121. Brin MF, Swope DM, Abassi S, et al. BOTOX for migraine: double-blind, placebo-controlled, region-specific evaluation. *Cephalalgia* 2000;20:421–422.

122. Aoki KR. Pharmacology and immunology of botulinum toxin serotypes. *J Neurol* 2001;248(Suppl 1): 3–10.

123. Brin MF. Botulinum toxin therapy: basic science and overview of other therapeutic applications. In: Blitzer A, Binder WJ, Boyd JB, et al, eds. *Management of facial lines and wrinkles.* New York: Lippincott Williams & Wilkins, 2000:279–302.

124. Jankovic J, Schwartz K. Response and immunoresistance to botulinum toxin injections. *Neurology* 1995; 45:1743–1746.

125. Gonnering RS. Negative antibody response to long-term treatment of facial spasm with botulinum toxin. *Am J Ophthalmol* 1988;105:313–315.

126. Tsui JK. Botulinum toxin as a therapeutic he agent. *Pharmacol Ther* 1996;72:13–24.

127. Ludlow CL, Hallett M, Rhew K, et al. Therapeutic use of type F botulinum toxin [Letter]. *N Engl J Med* 1992; 326:349–350.

128. Greene PE, Fahn S. Use of botulinum toxin type F injections to treat torticollis in patients with immunity to botulinum toxin type A. *Mov Disord* 1993;8: 479–483.

129. Mezaki T, Kaji R, Kohara N, et al. Comparison of therapeutic efficacies of type A and F botulinum toxins for blepharospasm: a double-blind, controlled study. *Neurology* 1995;45:506–508.

130. Sheean GL, Lees AJ. Botulinum toxin F in the treatment of torticollis clinically resistant to botulinum toxin A. *J Neurol Neurosurg Psychiatry* 1995;59: 601–607.

131. Sankhla C, Jankovic J, Duane D. Variability of the immunologic and clinical response in dystonic patients immunoresistant to botulinum toxin injections. *Mov Disord* 1998;13:150–154.

132. Halpern JL, Smith LA, Seamon KB, et al. Sequence homology between tetanus and botulinum toxins detected by an antipeptide antibody. *Infect Immun* 1989; 57:18–22.

133. Rosales RL, Arimura K, Takenaga S, et al. Extrafusal and intrafusal muscle effects in experimental botulinum toxin-a injection. *Muscle Nerve* 1996;19: 488–496.

134. Ishikawa H, Mitsui Y, Yoshitomi T, et al. Presynaptic effects of botulinum toxin type A on the neuronally evoked response of albino and pigmented rabbit iris sphincter and dilator muscles. *Jpn J Ophthalmol* 2000; 44:106–109.

135. Cui M, Aoki KR. Botulinum toxin type A (BTX-A) reduces inflammatory pain in the rat formalin model. *Cephalalgia* 2000;20:414(abstr).

Scientific and Therapeutic Aspects of Botulinum Toxin
edited by M.F. Brin, J. Jankovic, and M. Hallett
Lippincott Williams & Wilkins, Philadelphia, © 2002.

24

The Role of Botulinum Toxin Type A in the Management of Occupational Dystonia and Writer's Cramp

Barbara Illowsky Karp

The term "focal hand dystonia" encompasses the most common form, writer's cramp, as well as occupational cramp in which dystonia arises during tasks needed to perform a particular job. Because many professions and activities rely on precise hand control, the unwanted contractions and motor-control deficits associated with hand dystonia can be particularly debilitating.

HISTORY

Descriptions of writer's cramp first appeared in the eighteenth century. Ramazzini, in a section on "Disease of Scribes and Notaries" in his 1713 publication of *De Morbis Artificum* (*Diseases of Workers*), described selective failure of writing caused by intense fatigue and strain on the muscles and tendons (1). In *The Lancet* in 1864, Solly reported "scrivener's palsy or paralysis of writers," a disease that "...shows itself outwardly in a palsy of the writing powers. The muscles cease to obey the mandates of the will. It comes on very insidiously, the first indication often being only a painful feeling in the thumb or forefinger of the writing hand, accompanied by some stiffness; these unnatural sensations subside during the hours of rest and sleep, to return with the writer's work on the next day" (2). W.C. Gowers' 1890 *A Manual of Diseases of the Nervous System* discussed "occupational neuroses" in writers (3). Although writer's cramp was the most common form of occupational dystonia, similar abnormalities were described in shoemakers, milkers, musicians, seamstresses, cobblers, and others whose work had involved frequent repetitive hand movements (3,4).

EPIDEMIOLOGY AND PHYSIOLOGY

The Epidemiological Study of Dystonia in Europe Collaborative Group found the incidence of writer's cramp to be 14 per 10^6 population in eight countries in Europe (5). Nutt et al. reported an incidence of 2.7 per 10^6 population and a prevalence of 69 per 10^6 population in Rochester, Minnesota, in 1988, similar to the prevalence of Huntington's disease or amyotrophic lateral sclerosis (6). While most other focal dystonias are more common in women, hand dystonia affects men and women equally. Men, however, may have an earlier age of onset (7).

Writer's cramp usually presents in middle age (8). Spontaneous remission is rare, occurring in less than 5% of patients. Although symptoms can progress over months or years, few patients cease writing entirely (8). When hand dystonia does spread, it next involves more proximal muscles in the same arm or corresponding muscles in the opposite limb (9).

Hand dystonia may be precipitated by prolonged, repetitive hand use. It can also occur with overt hand trauma (10,11), peripheral nerve injury (8,12,13), or cerebral lesions, especially of the contralateral basal ganglia. The hands and arms are involved in hemidystonia and many symptomatic secondary dystonias (14).

Up to 20% of patients with writer's cramp

have family members with dystonia (15,16), however, no genetic mutations specific for focal hand dystonia have yet been identified. The DYT1 mutation is rarely present in patients with idiopathic writer's cramp or musician's cramp (17–19), although the arms are frequently affected in patients with DYT1-positive early onset dystonia (20).

Electromyography during writing with a dystonic hand shows a variety of abnormalities, including a loss of the normal alternating pattern of agonist/antagonist contraction, cocontraction of agonist and antagonist muscles, prolonged muscle bursts and abnormally decreased reciprocal inhibition. Overflow activity is present in muscles not normally involved in the task being performed (21–23). Other physiologic abnormalities in focal hand dystonia include distorted finger and hand representations on cortical sensory mapping (24–27), abnormal long-latency reflexes (28,29), loss of reciprocal inhibition (30–32), abnormal regulation of grip force (33), cortical hyperexcitability (34,35), defects in sensorimotor integration (36), and defects in intracortical inhibition (21,37,38).

SIGNS AND SYMPTOMS

The initial symptoms of writer's cramp are often feelings of arm tightness and hand fatigue during writing that worsen with continued effort. Severe pain is unusual. Over time, there is increasing difficulty with motor control including loss of speed, motor fluency and accuracy. Abnormal muscle contraction causes a distortion of normal posture. Undesired, excessive flexion of the wrist and fingers lead to a tendency to grip the pen too tightly. Less commonly, the fingers or wrist extend and pull away so that pen grip cannot be maintained. The process of writing becomes labored and the patients stop frequently to rest and shake out their hands. Although brief periods of rest help, dystonia quickly reappears once writing resumes. In "simple" writer's cramp, the dystonia remains limited to writing; in "dystonic" writer's cramp, the dystonia is present during other tasks as well. In severe cases, dystonic posture may be apparent at rest.

Involved hand and forearm muscles may hypertrophy over time.

Muscle strength, reflexes and sensation are normal in patients with focal hand dystonia. Tremor, myoclonic jerks, decreased arm swing, or a slight increase in tone of the affected arm may be present (15,39).

DIFFERENTIAL DIAGNOSIS

Repetitive stress injury (RSI; overuse syndrome) is an increasingly recognized cause of hand disability (40,41). Similar to focal hand dystonia, RSI is associated with repetitive hand use. Unlike dystonia, hand function is retained; the predominant symptom of this disorder is pain persisting despite rest. RSI is usually caused by tenosynovitis and can be treated with analgesics, antiinflammatories and rest.

Ulnar neuropathy can produce symptoms similar to focal hand dystonia, especially excessive flexion of the fourth and fifth fingers (42). In addition to dystonia, these patients frequently have sensory signs and symptoms or weakness in an ulnar distribution. Ross et al. demonstrated that patients with ulnar neuropathy may have prolonged muscle bursts and defects on agonist/antagonist activation similar to those in writer's cramp, suggesting that ulnar neuropathy leads to central remodeling (13). In the uncommon case of dystonia associated with ulnar neuropathy, the dystonic symptoms may resolve when the ulnar neuropathy is treated.

The forearm and hand discomfort of focal hand dystonia may be mistaken for carpal tunnel syndrome. However, median nerve sensory and motor signs are absent, as are Tinel's and Phalen's signs. Patients with reflex sympathetic dystrophy (complex regional pain syndrome) may have dystonia in the affected limb along with the more typical symptoms of pain, autonomic dysfunction and trophic skin changes (43,44). Psychogenic hand dystonia is a diagnosis of exclusion, but should be suspected if symptom onset was abrupt and if there are other somatizations or psychogenic neurologic symptoms (45).

TREATMENT

Before seeking medical attention, many patients try adaptive measures to cope with the dystonia. Musicians refinger passages, adjust their instruments, or alter hand position. Those with writer's cramp try thicker pens, different grips, or switch to writing with the nondominant hand. Unfortunately, about 25% of those who switch hands will develop dystonia in the second hand (8).

Nonpharmacologic approaches to treating focal hand dystonia include the use of splints or braces, which may occasionally be helpful. Acupuncture, psychotherapy, chiropractic manipulation, relaxation therapy, hypnosis, and transcutaneous nerve stimulation have not proven useful. Biofeedback (46,47), physical therapy, sensory discrimination retraining (48), and constraint-induced movement therapy (49,50) may be helpful, but it is not clear if they produce sustained relief.

Peripheral surgical approaches to hand dystonia have included tendon and nerve surgery. As noted above, ulnar nerve transposition may help the occasional patient whose dystonia is associated with ulnar neuropathy. Carpal tunnel release may improve carpal tunnel symptoms if present, but has no impact on the dystonia. Tenotomy and thoracic rib removal are similarly of little use. There is presently only limited experience with stereotactic neurosurgical procedures for focal hand dystonia. Iacono found improvement in a single patient with arm dystonia and tremor following ventroposterior Vim thalamotomy (51), as did Goto in a single writer's cramp patient who underwent Vo-complex thalamotomy (52).

Oral medications including dopamine agonists, dopamine antagonists, baclofen, benzodiazepines, muscle relaxants, herbal preparations, and anticholinergics generally produce little benefit in patients with focal hand dystonia and their use is often complicated by significant adverse effects. Botulinum toxin injection avoids systemic effects and is now the treatment of choice for focal hand dystonia. It is safe and effective and can be combined with surgery, oral medications, or ancillary therapies.

Botulinum Toxin Type A Treatment of Focal Hand Dystonia

For occupational and writer's cramp, botulinum toxin is injected into the dystonic arm and hand muscles. Determining which muscles are involved and selecting injection sites may not be straightforward as many dystonic limb movements are accompanied by voluntary or involuntary compensatory movements. The patient should be observed during the dystonia-provoking activities for abnormal posture, disruption of movement, and the presence of tremor. The patient should also be examined at rest and with other actions that might elicit the dystonia without compensatory movements. Patients may be asked to tap their fingers sequentially on a desk with the wrist unsupported or to draw a spiral with outstretched fingers (Fig. 24.1A). Writing with the nondominant hand may elicit mirror dystonia in the resting dominant hand (Fig. 24.1B).

Some patients experience tightness, fatigue, or aching in the forearm without an observable change in posture. In this circumstance, injections can be targeted to areas of specific discomfort. Wire electromyography recorded during dystonic activation may also be helpful in detecting the involvement of deep or nonobvious muscles. The selection of muscles for injection therefore depends on clinical evaluation, patient report of local discomfort or tightness, and/or electromyographic (EMG) evidence of excessive muscle activation.

EMG also aids proper needle placement during botulinum toxin injection. Forearm muscle bellies are thin and overlapping. At times it is necessary to place the needle in a specific part of a larger muscle, such as the fascicle for single finger in the flexor digitorum superficialis or profundus. Without EMG it is not possible to be certain whether the needle is in the targeted muscle or fascicle, or even if it is in muscle at all (53). With EMG, needle localization can be verified by observing an interference pattern with activation of the selected muscle. In patients with cocontraction who cannot isolate a single muscle voluntarily, needle position can be determined by passing a small current through the tip to evoke muscle contraction.

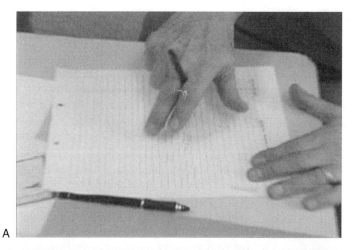

A

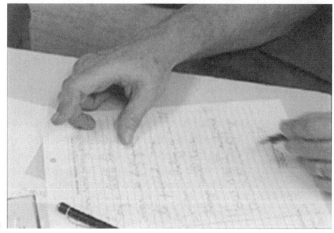

B

FIG. 24.1. A: Flexion dystonia of the fourth and fifth fingers while trying to write with all fingers outstretched. **B:** Flexion dystonia of the fourth and fifth fingers while writing with the nondominant hand.

A detailed knowledge of forearm anatomy is necessary for accurate injection. The flexor digitorum superficialis fascicles for digits 2 and 5 are deep and distal to those for digits 3 and 4 (54). In flexor digitorum profundus, the fascicles for digits 2 and 3 are proximal to those for digits 4 and 5.

For focal hand dystonia, injection is needed into the forearm muscles mediating wrist and finger movement (Table 24.1). Injection of hand intrinsics or proximal arm muscle may also be necessary. As a guide, the initial dose of BOTOX (type A toxin) is in the range of 5 to 25 U for muscles in the forearm and 2.5 to 10 U for hand intrinsics. To accurately inject such small doses, BOTOX should be reconstituted in a low concentration such as 2.5 to 5 U/0.1 cc,

TABLE 24.1. *Muscles injected for writer's cramp in descending order of frequency*

Flexor digitorum sublimis
Flexor digitorum profundus
Flexor pollicis longus
Flexor carpi ulnaris
Extensor digitorum communis
Flexor carpi radialis
Extensor carpi ulnaris
Extensor pollicis longus
Extensor carpi radialis
Extensor indicis proprius
Flexor pollicis brevis
Extensor pollicis brevis
Adductor pollicis
Pronator teres
Supinator
Interossei
Lumbricals
Pronator quadratus

rather than to 10 to 20 U/0.1 cc as used in torticollis. Large doses into a single muscle may best be divided into multiple sites to aid delivery of the toxin to a wide area of the selected muscle while limiting diffusion to adjacent muscles. At a given injection session, patients require a mean total dose of 25 to 50 U divided among two to four muscles.

The doses should be adjusted according to muscle and body size. We have observed that extensor muscles become weaker at lower doses than flexors and that women are more sensitive to a given botulinum toxin dose than are men. Therefore, lower doses should be used in women and in extensor muscles.

Patients with symptomatic dystonia associated with basal ganglia disorders or following stroke may develop tightly clenched fists. Botulinum toxin can be used to open the hand for patient comfort and improved palmar hygiene. This use requires higher doses of botulinum toxin than those for idiopathic focal hand dystonia. Doses greater than 150 U of BOTOX for each hand are often needed.

The dose of botulinum toxin is titrated over the initial several injection sessions to that which maximizes relief from the dystonia while minimizing muscle weakness. As with botulinum toxin use for other dystonias, injection sessions should be no more frequent than every 3 months. "Booster" injections 2 weeks after the initial injection should be avoided as they may increase the likelihood of antibody formation.

When the patient returns for evaluation of response or for reinjection, the patient should be examined for weakness that might postpone injection or require a change in dose. The dystonia should also be reevaluated at each session because the pattern of muscle contraction can change (55). Variation in the pattern of muscle contraction may be caused by a change in the hand dystonia, alteration because of botulinum toxin treatment, or unmasking of muscles not previously thought to be involved. After three or four injection sessions, many patients have a relatively stable response to injection so that the same muscles and doses can be used each time. In others, the muscles or doses fluctuate (Fig. 24.2). Goals of hand dystonia treatment include improvement in abnormal posture, relief of dis-

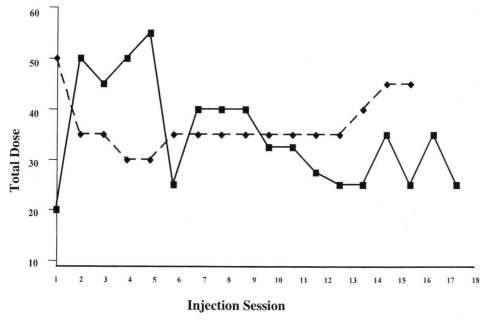

FIG. 24.2. Dose fluctuation in two patients receiving long-term botulinum toxin injections for focal hand dystonia. Injection sessions were at least 3 months apart.

TABLE 24.2. Rating scales

Five-point rating scale for dystonia
benefit and weakness

Benefit
0 =   No improvement
1 =   Minimal improvement (<25%)
2 =   Mild improvement (25%–49%)
3 =   Moderate improvement (50%–74%)
4 =   Major improvement (>75%)

Weakness
0 =   No weakness
1 =   Minimal weakness
2 =   Mild weakness
3 =   Moderate weakness
4 =   Severe weakness

Visual analog scales for benefit and weakness

Draw an x on the line below indicating the extent of
improvement:

No improvement 0%_____100% (normal use)

Draw an x on the line below indicating the extent of
weakness:

No weakness 0% _____ 100% (inability to move)

comfort, and restoration of function. Functional improvement can be assessed by observing the ease and smoothness of writing, musical performance, or task activity. Subjective scales, such as a five-point dystonia rating scale and a visual analog scale (Table 24.2), are frequently used. Benefit is difficult to quantify objectively. Wissel et al. devised a standardized writer's cramp rating scale that generates a composite score reflecting pathologic flexion and extension, tremor, and writing speed (56). Timed writing of a standardized passage allows objective assessment of changes in writing speed and comparison of writing samples (Fig. 24.3). Video-

tapes made before and after injection allow for direct comparison of actions at different times.

Adverse effects of limb botulinum toxin injection include mild malaise, pain or bruising at the injection site and greater weakness than intended in the injected or nearby muscles. Unlike injections for torticollis, botulinum toxin injection for hand dystonia is almost always accompanied by some loss of strength. The weakness, if severe, can be as functionally disabling as the dystonia itself (57,58). The degree of weakness cannot be predicted accurately from patient size, severity of dystonia, or botulinum toxin dose. Nor can the balance between weakness and benefit: Some patients have dramatic improvement with minimal change in strength; others have severe weakness and with little relief of the dystonia.

Efficacy of Injection

The efficacy of botulinum toxin for focal hand dystonia has been studied in both open-label and double-blind trials (56,58–66). In some studies, set botulinum toxin doses were used. In most studies, doses were based on clinical judgment resulting in a range of doses from 10 to 120 U per muscle and 10 to 300 U per treatment session. Reinjection intervals ranged from 2 weeks to 9 months.

Although the studies varied in injection technique and doses, they produced similar results. On at least one occasion, 67% to 93% of focal hand dystonia patients benefited from injection. The latency to response was 5 to 28 days and benefit lasted 60 to 77 days. Approximately 15% of patients did not respond to botulinum toxin injection, although the presence of weakness demonstrated that the lack of response was not because of the presence of blocking antibodies. Almost all patients with benefit had weak-

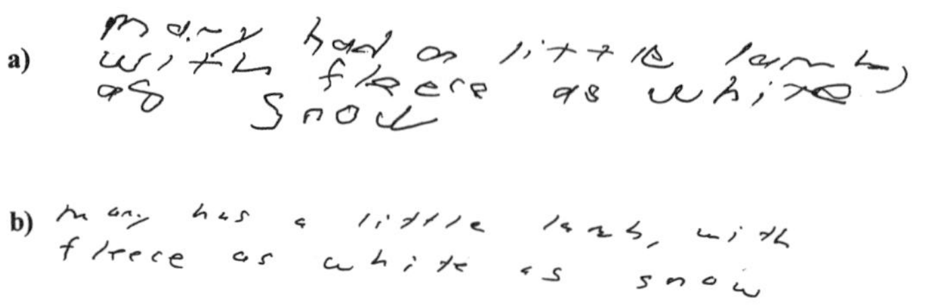

FIG. 24.3. A: Writing sample before botulinum toxin injection. **B:** Writing sample after botulinum toxin injection.

ness, which was severe in approximately 5% of sessions (58). Weakness was rarely a reason for discontinuation of treatment (55). The duration of overt weakness was 6 to 8 weeks, shorter than the period of benefit.

Botulinum toxin injections for focal hand dystonia can continue on a quarterly basis for years with a stable response in many patients (55,67). About 10% of patients discontinue injections because of antibody formation and loss of response. Many patients who maintain response eventually discontinue injections, largely because the treatment fails to meet their expectations or needs. This is especially so in musicians, for whom even marked improvement in the dystonia is inadequate if the ability to play professionally is not restored.

CONCLUSIONS

The clinical use of botulinum toxin for neurologic disorders was reviewed in 1990 at an NIH Consensus Development Conference and by the American Academy of Neurology (68,69). At that time, limited information was available on botulinum toxin efficacy in focal hand dystonia. Experience over the past 15 years shows that most patients with hand cramp improve when given botulinum toxin injections. The safety and efficacy are also now well-established. Botulinum toxin injection should be considered first-line therapy for focal hand dystonia.

REFERENCES

1. Ramazzini B. Diseases of scribes and notaries. In: *Diseases of workers*. New York: Hafner Publishing Company, 1713:421–425.
2. Solly S. Scrivener's palsy, or the paralysis of writers. *Lancet* 1864;2:709–711.
3. Gowers WR. *A manual of diseases of the nervous system*. Philadelphia, PA: P. Blakiston, Son & Co., 1888.
4. Hunter D. *The diseases of occupations*. London: Hodder & Stoughton, 1978.
5. The Epidemiological Study of Dystonia in Europe (ESDE) Collaborative Group. A prevalence study of primary dystonia in eight European countries. *J Neurol* 2000;247:787–792.
6. Nutt JG, Muenter MD, Aronson A, et al. Epidemiology of focal and generalized dystonia in Rochester, Minn. *Mov Disord* 1988;3:188–194.
7. The Epidemiological Study of Dystonia in Europe (ESDE) Collaborative Group. Sex-related influences on the frequency and age of onset of primary dystonia. *Neurology* 1999;53:1871–1873.
8. Marsden CD, Sheehy MP. Writer's cramp. *Trends Neurosci* 1990;13:148–153.
9. Greene P, Kang UJ, Fahn S. Spread of symptoms in idiopathic torsion dystonia. *Mov Disord* 1995;10:143–152.
10. Frucht S, Fahn S, Ford B. Focal task-specific dystonia induced by peripheral trauma. *Mov Disord* 2000;15:348–349.
11. Jankovic J, Van Der Linden C. Dystonia and tremor induced by peripheral trauma: Predisposing factors. *J Neurol Neurosurg Psychiatry* 1988;51:1512–1519.
12. Scherokman B, Husain F, Cuetter A, et al. Peripheral dystonia. *Arch Neurol* 1986;43:830–832.
13. Ross MH, Charness ME, Lee D, et al. Does ulnar neuropathy predispose to focal dystonia? *Muscle Nerve* 1995;18:606–611.
14. Marsden CD, Obeso JA, Zarranz JJ, et al. The anatomical basis of symptomatic hemidystonia. *Brain* 1985;108:463–483.
15. Sheehy MP, Marsden CD. Writer's cramp—a focal dystonia. *Brain* 1982;105:461–480.
16. Waddy HM, Fletcher NA, Harding AE, et al. A genetic study of idiopathic focal dystonias. *Ann Neurol* 1991;29:320–324.
17. Kamm C, Naumann M, Mueller J, et al. The DYT1 GAG deletion is infrequent in sporadic and familial writer's cramp. *Mov Disord* 2000;15:1238–1241.
18. Kamm C, Castelon-Konkiewitz E, Naumann M, et al. GAG deletion in the DYT1 gene in early limb-onset idiopathic torsion dystonia in Germany. *Mov Disord* 1999;14:681–683.
19. Friedman JR, Klein C, Leung J, et al. The GAG deletion of the DYT1 gene is infrequent in musicians with focal dystonia. *Neurology* 2000;55:1417–1418.
20. Bressman SB, Sabatti C, Raymond D, et al. The DYT1 phenotype and guidelines for diagnostic testing. *Neurology* 2000;54:1746–1752.
21. Berardelli A, Rothwell JC, Hallett M, et al. The pathophysiology of primary dystonia. *Brain* 1998;121:1195–1212.
22. Cohen LG, Hallett M. Hand cramps: clinical features and electromyographic patterns in a focal dystonia. *Neurology* 1988;38:1005–1012.
23. Farmer SF, Sheehan GL, Mayston MJ, et al. Abnormal motor unit synchronization of antagonist muscles underlies pathological cocontraction in upper limb dystonia. *Brain* 1998;121:801–814.
24. Bara-Jimenez W, Catalan MJ, Hallett M, et al. Abnormal somatosensory homunculus in dystonia of the hand. *Neurology* 1998;44:828–831.
25. Bara-Jimenez W, Shelton P, Sanger TD, et al. Sensory discrimination capabilities in patients with focal hand dystonia. *Ann Neurol* 2000;47:377–380.
26. Elbert T, Candia V, Altenmuller E, et al. Alteration of digital representations in somatosensory cortex in focal hand dystonia. *Neuroreport* 1998;9:3571–3575.
27. Byl NN, McKenzie A, Nagarajan SS. Differences in somatosensory hand organization in a healthy flutist and a flutist with focal hand dystonia: a case report. *J Hand Ther* 2000;13:302–309.
28. Panizza M, Lelli S, Nilsson J, et al. H-reflex recovery curve and reciprocal inhibition of H-reflex in different kinds of dystonia. *Neurology* 1990;40:824–828.

29. Naumann M, Reiners K. Long-latency reflexes of hand muscles in idiopathic focal dystonia and their modification by botulinum toxin. *Brain* 1997;120:109–116.
30. Chen RS, Tsai CH, Lu CS. Reciprocal inhibition in writer's cramp. *Mov Disord* 1995;10:556–561.
31. Chen R, Wassermann EM, Canos M, et al. Impaired inhibition in writer's cramp during voluntary muscle activation. *Neurology* 1997;49:1054–1059.
32. Panizza M, Hallett M, Nilsson J. Reciprocal inhibition in patients with hand cramps. *Neurology* 1989;39:85–89.
33. Serrien DJ, Burgunder JM, Wiesendanger M. Disturbed sensorimotor processing during control of precision grip in patients with writer's cramp. *Mov Disord* 2000;15: 965–972.
34. Curra A, Berardelli A, Rona S, et al. Excitability of the motor cortex in patients with dystonia. In: Fahn S, Marsden CD, DeLong M, eds. *Dystonia 3: advances in neurology.* Philadelphia, PA: Lippincott-Raven, 1998: 33–40.
35. Ikoma K, Samii A, Mercuri B, et al. Abnormal cortical motor excitability in dystonia. *Neurology* 1996;46: 1371–1376.
36. Murase N, Kaji R, Shimazu H, et al. Abnormal premovement gating of somatosensory input in writer's cramp. *Brain* 2000;123:1813–1829.
37. Ibanez V, Sadato N, Karp B, et al. Deficient activation of the premotor cortical network in patients with writer's cramp. *Neurology* 1999;53:96–105.
38. Ridding MC, Sheean G, Rothwell JC, et al. Changes in the balance between motor cortical excitation and inhibition in focal, task specific dystonia. *J Neurol Neurosurg Psychiatry* 1995;59:493–498.
39. Jedynak CP, Bonnet AM, Agid Y. Tremor and idiopathic dystonia. *Mov Disord* 1991;6:230–236.
40. Pitner MA. Pathophysiology of overuse injuries in the hand and wrist. *Hand Clin* 1990;6:355–364.
41. Ranney D. Work-related chronic injuries of the forearm and hand: their specific diagnosis and management. *Ergonomics* 1993;36:871–880.
42. Charness ME, Ross MH, Shefner JM. Ulnar neuropathy and dystonic flexion of the fourth and fifth digits: clinical correlation in musicians. *Muscle Nerve* 1996;19: 431–437.
43. Schwartzman R, Kerrigan J. The movement disorder of reflex sympathetic dystrophy. *Neurology* 1990;40: 57–61.
44. Birklein F, Riedl B, Sieweke N, et al. Neurological findings in complex regional pain syndromes—analysis of 145 cases. *Acta Neurol Scand* 2000;101:262–269.
45. Lang AE. Psychogenic dystonia: a review of 18 cases. *Can J Neurol Sci* 1995;22:136–143.
46. Deepak KK, Behari M. Specific muscle EMG biofeedback for hand dystonia. *Appl Psychophysiol Biofeedback* 1999;24:267–280.
47. O'Neill MA, Gwinn KA, Adler CH. Biofeedback for writer's cramp. *Am J Occup Ther* 1997;51:605–607.
48. Byl NN, McKenzie A. Treatment effectiveness for patients with a history of repetitive hand use and focal hand dystonia: a planned, prospective follow-up study. *J Hand Ther* 2000;13:289–301.
49. Taub E, Uswatte G, Pidikiti R. Constraint-induced movement therapy: a new family of techniques with broad application to physical rehabilitation—a clinical review. *J Rehabil Res Dev* 1999;36:237–251.
50. Candia V, Elbert T, Altenmuller E, et al. Constraint-induced movement therapy for focal hand dystonia in musicians [Letter]. *Lancet* 1999;353:42.
51. Iacono RP, Kuniyoshi SM, Schoonenberg T. Experience with stereotactics for dystonia: case examples. *Adv Neurol* 1998;78:221–226.
52. Goto S, Tsuiki H, Soyama N, et al. Stereotactic selective Vo-complex thalamotomy in a patient with dystonic writer's cramp. *Neurology* 1997;49:1173–1174.
53. Comella CL, Buchman AS, Tanner CM, et al. Botulinum toxin injection for spasmodic torticollis: increased magnitude of benefit with electromyographic assistance. *Neurology* 1992;42:878–882.
54. Bickerton LE, Agur AMR, Ashby P. Flexor digitorum superficialis: locations of individual muscle bellies for botulinum toxin injections. *Muscle Nerve* 1997;20: 1041–1043.
55. Karp BI, Cohen LG, Cole R, et al. Long-term botulinum toxin treatment of focal hand dystonia. *Neurology* 1994; 44:70–76.
56. Wissel J, Kabus C, Wenzel R, et al. Botulinum toxin in writer's cramp: objective response evaluation in 31 patients. *J Neurol Neurosurg Psychiatry* 1996;61: 172–175.
57. Ross MH, Charness ME, Sudarsky L, et al. Treatment of occupational cramp with botulinum toxin: diffusion of toxin to adjacent noninjected muscles. *Muscle Nerve* 1997;20:593–598.
58. Jankovic J, Schwartz K, Donovan DT. Botulinum toxin treatment of cranial-cervical dystonia, spasmodic dysphonia, other focal dystonias and hemifacial spasm. *J Neurol Neurosurg Psychiatry* 1990;53:633–639.
59. Cohen LG, Hallett M, Geller BD, et al. Treatment of focal dystonias of the hand with botulinum toxin injections. *J Neurol Neurosurg Psychiatry* 1989;52:355–363.
60. Yoshimura DM, Aminoff MJ, Olney RK. Botulinum toxin therapy for limb dystonias. *Neurology* 1992;42: 627–630.
61. Rivest J, Lees AJ, Marsden CD. Writer's cramp: treatment with botulinum toxin injections. *Mov Disord* 1991; 6:55–59.
62. Poungvarin N. Writer's cramp: the experience with botulinum toxin injections in 25 patients. *J Med Assoc Thai* 1991;74:239–247.
63. Cole R, Hallett M, Cohen LG. Double-blind trial of botulinum toxin for treatment of focal hand dystonia. *Mov Disord* 1995;10:466–471.
64. Cole RA, Cohen LG, Hallett M. Treatment of musician's cramp with botulinum toxin. *Med Prob Perf Art* 1991;6:137–143.
65. Lees AJ, Turjanski N, Rivest J, et al. Treatment of cervical dystonia, hand spasms and laryngeal dystonia with botulinum toxin. *J Neurol* 1992;239:1–4.
66. Behari M. Botulinum toxin in the treatment of writer's cramp. *J Assoc Physicians India* 1999;47:694–698.
67. Chen R, Karp BI, Hallett M. Botulinum toxin type F for treatment of dystonia: long-term experience. *Neurology* 1998;51:1494–1496.
68. National Institutes of Health Consensus Development Conference Statement. Clinical use of botulinum toxin. *Arch Neurol* 1991;48:1294–1298.
69. National Institutes of Health Consensus Development Conference Statement. Assessment: the clinical usefulness of botulinum toxin-A in treating neurologic disorders. *Neurology* 1990;40:1332–1336.

Scientific and Therapeutic Aspects of Botulinum Toxin
edited by M.F. Brin, J. Jankovic, and M. Hallett
Lippincott Williams & Wilkins, Philadelphia, © 2002.

25

Botulinum Toxin A Therapy for Temporomandibular Disorders

Marvin Schwartz and Brian Freund

DEFINING TEMPOROMANDIBULAR DISORDER

Temporomandibular disorder (TMD) is a collective term used to describe a group of pathologic conditions involving the temporomandibular joint (TMJ), masticatory muscles, and/or associated structures. As such, the TMDs encompass a wide variety of medical disorders of orthopedic and myofascial origin that closely resemble those described for other joint and muscular conditions. The unique nature of TMD resides in the proximate anatomy of numerous other facial and cranial structures, thereby complicating, interacting with, and mimicking other sources of head and neck pain (Figs. 25.1 and 25.2).

Symptoms commonly associated with TMDs include:

- Difficulty speaking
- Difficulty eating
- Difficulty sleeping
- Chronic headaches
- Earaches, hearing impairment
- Jaw dysfunction including hyper- and hypomobility
- General orofacial pain

The differential diagnosis for TMD is a gallery of conditions applicable to almost all head and neck pain. Table 25.1 provides an incomplete list (1).

An historical review by Kaplan (2) reveals that TMD was described as early as 1920 in the guise of ''abnormalities of mandibular articulation'' (Wright, 1920; Goodfriend, 1933). Subsequent nomenclatures for TMD and its subtypes reinforce the observations, vanities and biases of the investigators, including:

- Costen's syndrome (Costen, 1956)
- TMJ dysfunction syndrome (Schore, 1959)
- TM pain syndrome (Schwartz, 1959)
- Pain dysfunction syndrome (Voss, 1964)
- Myofacial pain dysfunction syndrome or MPDS (Laskin, 1969)
- Myoarthropathy of the TMJ (Graber, 1971)
- Occlusomandibular disturbance (Gerber, 1971)
- Internal joint derangement (Farrar, 1971)

Statistics from epidemiologic studies are difficult to compare as a universally accepted classification system for TMD does not exist (see below). De Kanter and coworkers published the results of their meta-analysis of 51 studies in 1993 (3). The results were confounded by some limitations, including a lack of uniformity in classification. However, more than 15,000 subjects in 23 studies reported a dysfunction rate of 30%. Professionally assessed dysfunction was identified in 44% of subjects. While the statistics may be difficult to pin down, it is clear that TMDs are common in nonpatient populations (4).

Thorough reviews of data from large studies reveal that 20% to 25% of a population (5,6) sought professional care for their TMD at some point in their life. Significantly, advanced care requiring the expertise of specialists was required in 5% to 10% of the population (7–10). The economic and societal costs are substantial (11).

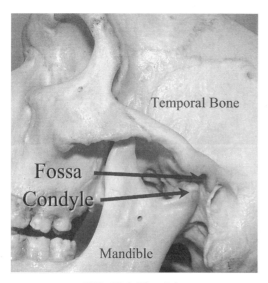

FIG. 25.1. The Joint

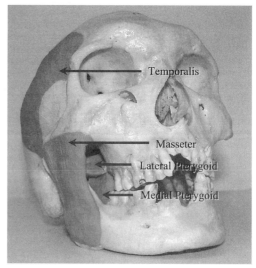

FIG. 25.2. The Musculature

CLASSIFICATION OF TMD

At this writing, there exists no unanimity in the TMD community regarding a single universally acceptable taxonomy. A comprehensive, historical overview and analysis by Ohrbach and Stohler (12) of proposed systems include Bell, 1960, 1982, 1986; American Academy of Craniomandibular Disorders, 1980, 1990; Block, 1980; President's Conference on the Examination, Diagnosis and Management of TMJ Disorders, 1982; Farrar, 1982; Eversole and Machado, 1985; Fricton, 1988; International Headache Society (fits ICD system), 1988; Stegenga et al. (based on system of American Rheumatism As-

sociation), 1989; and Research Diagnostic Criteria (RDC), 1992. Currently, the RDC and ICD systems appear to be used more commonly than any of the others.

Despite the differences, a practical review of these classification systems yields several common underlying themes. First, while most of the schemes attempt to provide comprehensive coverage of all possible pathologic conditions, the most prevalent clinical TMDs are primary craniomandibular pains. These are usually divided, based upon anatomic etiology, among pain originating in the TMJ proper or intracapsular (i.e., arthrogenic) and pain originating in the muscula-

TABLE 25.1. *Differential diagnosis of TMD*

Source of pathology	Common examples
Systemic diseases	Multiple myeloma; diabetes mellitus; systemic lupus erythematosus (SLE); giant-cell arteritis
Myofascial pain	Masticatory muscles; cervical muscles; frontalis-occipitalis and other facial muscles involved in tension headaches, cervicogenic headaches, myofascial pain dysfunction (MPD), fibromyalgia
Skeletal pain	Osteomyelitis; neoplasia; fibrous dysplasia; gout; osteomalacia; Paget's disease
Proximate anatomic structure pain	Odontogenic; ophthalmic; otic; nasal; sinus; salivary; Eagle's syndrome
Intracranial pathology	Neoplasm; aneurysm; abscess; hemorrhage; hematoma; edema
Neurologic disorders	Migraine variants; cluster headaches; neuralgias; paroxysmal hemicrania; cranial arteritis; carotidynia
Psychogenic pain disorders	Psychotic syndromes; mood disturbances; anxiety disorders; organic disorders; somatoform disorders

ture (i.e., myogenic). Second, there is a notable overlap between TMD taxonomy and those of other disciplines caring for patients with primary head and neck pain (below). Third, stress, psychologic factors, and chronicity are common and significant factors in TMD, as with most complicated head and neck pain. The contribution of central input and neuroplasticity is significant and must be considered in the successful diagnosis and management of TMD.

INTERDISCIPLINARY MANIFESTATIONS OF TMD

A studied approach transcending medical and dental disciplines yields numerous instances of overlap that have historically resulted in the artificial segmentation of TMDs. Three poignant examples are presented.

Tension headaches (TH): The majority of TH anatomically originate or involve the temporalis and/or masseter muscles. As such, there is no distinction between the classification of this clinical phenomenon as a myogenous TMD versus a TH. It is of little coincidence that some TH researchers use temporalis muscle pain induced by tooth clenching as a valuable experimental model (13).

Oromandibular dystonia: Belonging to the group of movement disorders characterized by involuntary spasms and muscle contractions that induce abnormal movements and postures, this particular subset constitutes a focal form that involves the musculature of the masticatory apparatus and lower face. It manifests as distorted oral position and function resulting in difficulty in speaking, eating, swallowing, and facial appearance. Although it is a neurologic disorder, there is no doubt of its inclusion as a subset of TMDs owing to the involvement of the masticatory apparatus.

Bruxism: This clinical entity may occur as a solitary form of TMD involving only the musculature or as an initiating and/or perpetuating factor in more involved forms of TMD involving joint damage. Taking a wider view of the literature brings an interesting correlation. Bruxism manifests many of the characteristics of dystonia including similar epidemiology, as well as the features of pain and exacerbation by external factors such as fatigue, stress, and emotional extremes. Wooten-Watts, Tan, and Jankovic (14) postulated the possibility that bruxism may be a form of dystonia. With this knowledge, it is entirely possible to view the current treatment of bruxism with intraoral appliances or occlusal adjustments as "sensory tricks" that relieve the dystonia. Perhaps this explains the success of a myriad of splint designs and occlusal therapies despite the lack of fundamental understanding of their basis of action. It may also explain the common failure of splint and occlusal therapies in some TMD cases. After all, the sensory trick is not the same for all patients with dystonias.

PATHOPHYSIOLOGY OF TMD

The masticatory system is a dynamic one involving joint, musculature and supporting structures. A simple etiology for TMD is not usually found. Rather, it is a combination of factors that lead to overuse or abuse of the apparatus and resultant pain (15–18). These factors include:

- Parafunctional muscle activity (e.g., bruxing, clenching)
- Trauma (e.g. whiplash, subluxation)
- Psychological factors
- Occlusion
- Systemic diseases (e.g., arthritis)

In the majority of cases, TMD may be considered to be a multifactorial disease.

TREATMENT OF TMD

The range of treatment modalities available for the treatment of TMD is as extensive as the presentations of the different disorders found under this umbrella. It is not surprising, therefore, that there is no consistently effective method of treatment. However, directed treatment of the arthrogenic and myogenic components often yields success, as these are the most common cause for patient presentation (19).

Treatment of joint pathology includes supportive care, indirect joint care and direct intervention. Supportive care includes pharmacotherapy, rest, physical therapies, and psychotherapy

(20–23). Indirect joint care techniques take advantage of the fact that the dentition is an appendage of the mandible as are the TMJs. Manipulation of the teeth and mandible can affect the TMJ. Therefore, orthotics such as oral splints and alterations of the dentition and its alignment can be used to change joint function (24,25). Finally, surgical intervention in the form of arthrocentesis, arthroscopy, and open arthrotomy are available for the advanced correction of arthrogenic pathology (26–29).

The care of the myogenic component of TMD has been limited largely to supportive care. Physical therapies, oral pharmacotherapy, biofeedback, and other modalities usually provide short-term and inadequate relief in more severe cases. However, the importance of muscle therapy is significant because the majority of TMD cases include a myogenous component as an etiologic and/or perpetuating factor. Relaxation of the appropriate muscles yields significant therapeutic gains due to direct muscle effects and indirect joint effects (30–32). Therefore, an ideal agent would provide enduring and specific muscular therapy with an acceptable side effect profile. Botulinum toxin type A (BTX-A) would appear to fulfill these criteria better than any other currently available modality.

Because most patients present with simultaneous arthrogenic and myogenic aspects to their TMD, best results are obtained when providing care for both the concurrently.

EVOLUTION OF BTX-A THERAPY FOR TMD

The long history of BTX-A treatment of movement disorders led to the early treatment of the oromandibular dystonia subset of TMD by pioneers in the field [Blitzer et al. (33), Brin and Blitzer (34), and Tan and Jankovic (35)]. Success in the form of improved function and amelioration of cosmetic disability was demonstrated. Even more significantly, early evidence of pain relief was reported. In light of the similarities between bruxism and dystonias, an attempt to treat bruxism with BTX-A followed. The innovators have reported early successes with this therapy for bruxism (36,37).

Concurrent basic scientific evidence of BTX-A effects beyond the neuromuscular junction supports the unfolding picture of a therapy that has broad-reaching significance for the treatment of pain.

Muscle spindle: Sensory motor transmission is affected by BTX-A (38). Afferent muscle spindle discharge is modified and intrafusal muscle spindles atrophy in response to BTX-A (39). These studies support an afferent mechanism of BTX-A that may play a role in pain modulation.

Antinociceptive effects: Cui and Aoki (40) observed that subcutaneous BTX-A prophylaxis effectively relieved pain associated with formalin-induced inflammation in rats. This report further supports the hypothesis that BTX-A possesses an antinociceptive effect that is independent of its effects on neuromuscular transmission.

CNS effects: Aoki (41) demonstrated a retrograde neuronal uptake of radioactively labeled BTX-A into the central nervous system (CNS). Ishikawa and colleagues (42) observed that BTX-A inhibits the release of substance P from trigeminal nerves. BTX-A may also act via a central mechanism after retrograde transport into the CNS.

The association of pain relief with BTX-A therapy for movement disorders and bruxism provided an early glimpse into the potential for this therapy for complicated TMDs. Fundamental principles of myofascial pain overlay on the joint pathology, chronic myofascial pain, reduction of joint loading by diminution of the activity of the major jaw-closing muscles, and enhancement of postsurgical physical rehabilitation were daily, unresolved clinical challenges that resulted in failures of treatment. The promise of a comprehensive, long-lasting therapy was worthy of investigation.

To date, the only published TMD clinical work has been produced at The Crown Institute and its predecessor. Three studies were undertaken in the past few years.

Feasibility Study

Using the past experience from the dystonia field and dosages used in the masticatory muscles in oromandibular dystonias, a handful of patients were recruited for a proof-of-concept trial (unpublished). Despite the fact that these patients had the most severe forms of TMD that were resistant to other treatments, the early findings were encouraging. All of the patients experienced a clinical effect ranging from weakened chewing muscles to profound and prolonged pain relief.

Two unexpected findings were identified. The multiple injections into already aching muscles were very painful for some patients, to the extent that they refused follow-up BOTOX injections without some form of sedation/anesthesia. Second, injection of BOTOX only into the clinically symptomatic muscle(s) resulted in a compensatory overactivity and pain in the agonist muscles. This mirroring effect, also seen in cervicogenic headaches, compelled bilateral injection of the musculature subsequently. Finally, particular note was made of the importance of chronicity and complexity of the pain. The more chronic pain sufferers obtained less relief qualitatively. Furthermore, few of the subjects experienced pure myogenic pain. Most had concomitant arthrogenic pain and experienced chronic headaches, including tension and migraine headaches. This observation would consistently repeat in future work in this field and is consistent with findings in the headache field where chronic sufferers rarely present with pure headache forms.

Preliminary Study

This first clinical trial (43) was undertaken to objectively demonstrate the effectiveness of BOTOX in providing relief of symptomatology associated with TMD and to begin to establish a dose response curve (Table 25.2).

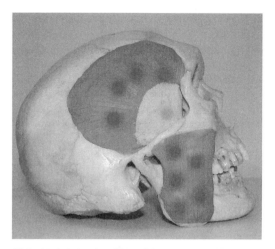

FIG. 25.3. Injection Sites: Masseter and Temporalis

Nineteen patients (mean age, 31 years) were recruited for this randomized study that was neither controlled nor blinded. Eight patients received a total of 100 U of BOTOX distributed equally to the two masseter and two temporalis muscles (Fig. 25.3). Each muscle received five injections of 5 U BOTOX (diluted to 5 U/0.1 cc) delivered via percutaneous injection under EMG guidance. The remaining 11 patients received the same dose to the temporalis muscles and double the dose (50 U) to each masseter muscle in the form of five injections of 10 U BOTOX (diluted to 10 U/0.1 cc) for a total of 150 U BOTOX per patient. All patients were followed for 3 months using numerous objective and subjective criteria.

This preliminary study demonstrated several significant findings:

- No toxicity or side effects were encountered by any patient despite the use of doses up to 3 times the amounts previously reported for the treatment of dystonias involving these muscles.
- There was a dose-dependent, statistically significant difference in clinical improvement indices between the two groups. Despite the small sample size, statistical significance was most likely attainable as a result of the profound difference between the group responses.

TABLE 25.2. *Outcomes for 150 patients randomized to 100 U or 150 U BOTOX*

	Low dose group (*n* = 8)	High dose group (*n* = 11)
Improvement	25%	91%
No change	75%	9%
Worse	0%	0%
Mean onset (weeks)	2.0	1.2
Mean duration (weeks)	3.0	6.2

The dosage for the two groups differed by a full 50%.

• The speed of onset and duration of action trended toward dose dependence.

The details of this study were published in 1998 (43). The encouraging results prompted three important sequelae. First, BTX-A treatment became an important, albeit experimental, adjunct in the treatment of TMD for patients with chronic pain with a myogenic source. Its utility for nonsurgical patients, as well as pre- and postsurgical patients, proved clinically significant. Second, addressing patient needs became more achievable, but accurate diagnosis became more important. BTX-A seemed to have only an indirect effect on arthrogenic pathology, perhaps by unloading the joint as a result of a reduction in jaw-closing muscle strength, but a more direct effect on myogenic pain and chronic pain. Treatment exclusively with BTX-A for a combined (arthrogenic and myogenic) TMD could not yield relief as good as BTX-A combined with directed joint care. Third, a need for a follow-up study with refinements and a larger sample size was indicated.

Coincidentally and importantly, many of these patients who reported a prior medical history of headaches described profound improvement or prevention during the course of the study.

Pilot Study

This follow-up clinical trial (44,45) was designed to correlate treatment effect to different TMD diagnostic subcategories, to assess clinical correlates such as psychological and demographic profiles, and to establish a temporal relationship between follow-up measures (objective pain, subjective pain, maximum contraction, range of motion) and muscle relaxation.

Fifty subjects with TMD were recruited and 46 completed the study. The design was prospective with no controls as the very effective dose of 150 U of BOTOX (high-dose group above) established previously was used for all patients. The mean age was 40.5 years (range, 16 to 75 years). Each patient was followed at 2-week intervals for a total of 8 weeks. Outcome measures included pain by visual analog scale (VAS), tenderness to palpation, functional index based on multiple VAS, interincisal oral opening, and mean maximum voluntary contraction (MVC) as measured with a custom strain gauge device.

Preliminary results were published in 1999 in the *Journal of Oral and Maxillofacial Surgery* (44), and final results were reported in 2000 in the *British Journal of Oral and Maxillofacial Surgery* (45). In summary, the following significant findings are enumerated:

• Statistically significant improvement from pretreatment levels in pain experience, tenderness to palpation, functional index, and mouth opening were observed.
• These outcome measures remained significantly different from the pretreatment findings at 8 weeks.
• No significant difference was found between diagnostic categories, and between demographic and psychological profiles.
• MVC initially diminished but then returned to pretreatment values.

This study strongly demonstrates that BTX-A therapy produces a reduction in symptoms and an improvement in functional abilities for patients with TMD. The prospects for this new modality of TMD care were clearly positive. An advanced study was indicated and a Phase II multicenter clinical trial began in 2001 with support from Allergan Inc. of Irvine, California (makers of BOTOX).

An apparently paradoxical finding of this study was that all measured patient improvements extended temporally beyond the muscle-relaxing effects as measured objectively by the bite meter. This fact belies the simplistic notion of BTX-A having purely a muscle-relaxing effect, and, along with other recent, disparate observations regarding BTX-A use in treating migraines and its effect on locations other than the neuromuscular junction (e.g., nociceptive afferents), leads one to search for broader understanding of the observed phenomena. A unifying hypothesis is presented below.

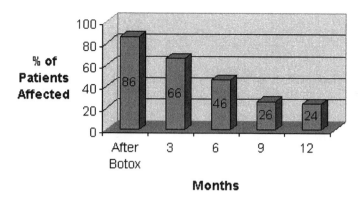

FIG. 25.4. Patients affected by BOTOX vs. time.

Long-term Follow-up

Seventeen patients have now been followed for more than 1 year. While this is not a part of any official study, the observations are presented in chart form (Fig. 25.4). Improvement within 2 weeks following BOTOX injections in almost 90% of patients is a consistent finding in practice. The effect lasts from 1 to 3 months, usually dependent on severity of the TMD. The plateau at approximately 25% beyond 9 months is interesting and may be significant. This is either demonstrative of the natural extinction of the disease or a truly profound long-term effect of BTX-A therapy. Further studies are warranted.

FINAL THOUGHTS: MAKING SENSE OF IT ALL

On cursory examination, it is easy to view BTX-A therapy as a simple muscular agent that has found utility in another orthopedic application, i.e., relating to the TMJ. TMD, however, is not a simple orthopedic problem. It is often associated with headaches and cervicogenic pain. BTX-A's effectiveness extends beyond the muscle-relaxing effect. BTX-A is also useful in treating other head and neck primary pains such as migraine. There is a commonality between TMD, headaches, and neck pain in presentation and response to treatment. These cannot all be coincidental. Furthermore, there is pain relief and functionality that outlasts the muscle relaxant effect of BTX-A. A unifying model based upon known neuroanatomy, neurophysiology, and current understanding of TMD, headaches, and cervicogenic pain is presented.

The trigeminal nucleus (TN), with emphasis on subnucleus caudalis and interpolaris, receives almost all primary afferent input from all of the craniofacial structures, including the intracranial vasculature and dura. It also receives input from the cervical region and cranial nerves VII, IX, X, and XII. Unique to the TN, as compared to spinal nerves, is this extensive convergence pattern of cranial and cervical nerves. Further input to the nucleus is provided from higher centers, many times in the form of inhibitory and regulatory influences.

Second-order afferent neurons synapse within the nucleus and project extensively to other parts of the brainstem and higher centers. Some of these neurons are involved in multisynaptic brainstem paths that function in craniofacial and cervical muscle reflex pathways, as well as autonomic reflex responses. The filtered afferent nociceptive signals ultimately project to the cortex for interpretation as pain. An excellent review with extensive and thorough referencing is provided by Sessle (46). In summary, the TN is the first gateway for afferent head and neck input with wide-ranging integrative function and significant output activity directly through the brainstem and indirectly through higher centers.

The modulation of nociceptive transmission in the TN bears significance in clinical practice as numerous pain phenomena can be explained at the cellular level. Peripheral sensitization, ex-

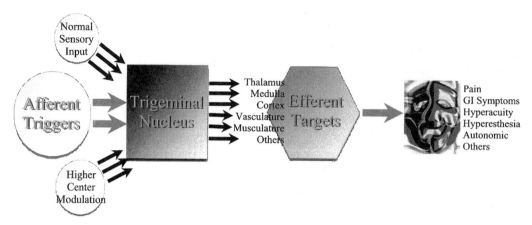

FIG. 25.5. A model of trigeminal nucleus functional trigeminopathy

pansion of receptor fields, recruitment of A-beta fibers and wind-up are all understood in the context of the function of the TN and its constituent parts.

TRIGEMINOPATHY: DEFINITION

The term "trigeminopathy" is intended to unify current understanding of primary head and neck pain. It builds on the knowledge base that exists and is therefore consistent with current thoughts on the diagnosis, classification and treatment of these pains. It is defined as a diverse group of primary head and neck pains that share these features:

- Afferent trigger(s) stimulation
- TN stimulation
- Receptive efferent target(s) activation

The afferent triggers may be peripheral or central and are usually a combination of both. In a state of homeostasis, the TN continuously receives numerous inputs, both excitatory and inhibitory in nature, that result in an output which signals normalcy. There is a sense of balance. In a headache sufferer, this balance is upset beginning with an afferent barrage. This afferent overdrive is triggered only in susceptible individuals. In migraine sufferers the result of a stimulus (often peripheral such as food) is an intracranial vascular response mediated, in sus-

ceptible individuals, by a channelopathy that results in an excitatory neural message barrage to the TN. This results in a stimulation of the TN. The TN performs an integrative function that results in selective efferent output, both central and peripheral. In people who have receptive efferent targets, their activation manifests as a clinical sign or symptom. The susceptibility of efferent targets is variable within and between individuals. In the case of migraine, centers in the hypothalamus, the periaqueductal gray, raphe nuclei, red nucleus, and others have been identified with positron emission tomography (PET) scans and magnetic resonance imaging (MRI) to be responsible for symptoms such as aura, nausea and vomiting, photophobia, phonophobia, and more [reviewed recently by Hargreaves and Shepheard (47)]. This same schema may be used to understand TMD and cervicogenic pain.

The philosophic significance of trigeminopathy lies in the fundamental shift from the current practice of diagnosis of head and neck pains based on symptomatology, especially difficult because of efferent variability, to a mechanistic diagnosis based on the underlying physiologic disturbance. The core commonality is the TN and its integrative function. Almost all afferent input is funneled into the TN, and almost all efferent outcomes commence at the TN.

Just as the medical community now understands the term "coagulopathies" to be a group of related abnormalities pertaining to our hemostatic system, so trigeminopathies refers to a group of related abnormalities pertaining to pain mechanisms of the head and neck. Perhaps this new understanding will be one of the more significant legacies of BTX-A treatment of primary head and neck pain.

REFERENCES

1. Block SL. Differential diagnosis of masticatory muscle pain and dysfunction. *Oral Maxillofac Clin North Am* 1995;7:29–49.
2. Kaplan, AS. Classification. In: Kaplan AS, Assael LA, eds. *Temporomandibular disorders; diagnosis and treatment, 1st ed.* Philadelphia, PA: WB Saunders, 1991:106–117.
3. De Kanter RJ, Truin GJ, Burgersdijk RC, et al. Prevalence in the Dutch population and a meta-analysis of signs and symptoms of temporomandibular disorder. *J Dent Res* 1993;72:1509–1518.
4. Carlsson GE, LeResche L. Epidemiology of temporomandibular disorders in temporomandibular disorders and related pain conditions. In: Sessle BJ, Bryant PS, Dionne RA, eds. *Progress in pain research and management, Vol. 4.* Seattle, WA: IASP Press, 1995:211–226.
5. Carlsson GE. Epidemiology and treatment need for temporomandibular disorders. *J Orofac Pain* 1999;13:232–237.
6. Carlsson GE, Helkimo M. Epidemiologic studies of mandibular function. *J Prosthet Dent* 1983;50:134–135.
7. Rugh JD, Solberg WK. Oral health status in the United States: temporomandibular disorders. *J Dent Educ* 1985;49:398–406.
8. Locker D, Slade G. Prevalence of symptoms associated with temporomandibular disorders in a Canadian population. *Community Dent Oral Epidemiol* 1988;16:310–313.
9. Schiffman EL, Fricton JR, Haley DP, et al. The prevalence and treatments needs of subjects with temporomandibular disorders. *J Am Dent Assoc* 1990;120:295–303.
10. Magnusson T, Carlsson GE, Egermark-Eriksson I. An evaluation of the need and demand for treatment of craniomandibular disorders in a young Swedish population. *J Craniomandib Disord* 1991;5:57–63.
11. Von Korff M. Health services research and temporomandibular disorders. In: Sessle BJ, Bryant PS, Dionne RA, eds. *Progress in pain research and management, Vol. 4.* Seattle, WA: IASP Press, 1995:227–236.
12. Ohrbach R, Stohler C. Research diagnostic criteria for temporomandibular disorders: current diagnostic systems. *J Craniomandib Disord Facial Oral Pain* 1992;6:307–317.
13. Jensen R, Olesen J. Initiating mechanisms of experimentally induced tension-type headache. *Cephalalgia* 1996;16:175–182.
14. Wooten-Watts M, Tan E-K, Jankovic J. Bruxism and cranial-cervical dystonia: is there a relationship? *Cranio* 1999;17:1–6.
15. Steed PA, Wexler GB. Temporomandibular disorders—traumatic etiology vs. nontraumatic etiology: a clinical and methodological inquiry into symptomatology and treatment outcomes. *Cranio* 2001;19:188–194.
16. Greene CS. The etiology of temporomandibular disorders: implications for treatment. *J Orofac Pain* 2001;15:93–105.
17. Kamisaka M, Yatani H, Kuboki T, et al. Four-year longitudinal course of TMD symptoms in an adult population and the estimation of risk factors in relation to symptoms. *J Orofac Pain* 2000;14:224–232.
18. Molin C. From bite to mind: TMD—a personal and literature review. *Int J Prosthodont* 1999;12:279–288.
19. Clark GT, Kim YY. A logical approach to the treatment of temporomandibular disorders. *Oral Maxillofac Clin North Am* 1995;7:149–166.
20. Stohler CS, Zarb GA. On the management of temporomandibular disorders: a plea for a low-tech, high-prudence therapeutic approach. *J Orofac Pain* 1999;13:255–261.
21. Dionne RA. Pharmacologic treatments for temporomandibular disorders. *Oral Surg Oral Med Oral Pathol Oral Radiol Endod* 1997;83:134–142.
22. Murphy GJ. Physical medicine modalities and trigger point injections in the management of temporomandibular disorders and assessing outcome. *Oral Surg Oral Med Oral Pathol Oral Radiol Endod* 1997;83:118–122.
23. Dahlstrom L. Psychometrics in temporomandibular disorders. An overview. *Acta Odontol Scand* 1993;51:339–352.
24. Dao TT, Lavigne GJ. Oral splints: the crutches for temporomandibular disorders and bruxism? *Crit Rev Oral Biol Med* 1998;9:345–361.
25. Major PW, Nebbe B. Use and effectiveness of splint appliance therapy: review of the literature. *Cranio* 1997;15:159–166.
26. Dolwick MF. The role of temporomandibular joint surgery in the treatment of patients with internal derangement. *Oral Surg Oral Med Oral Pathol Oral Radiol Endod* 1997;83:150–155.
27. Foster ME, Gray RJ, Davies SJ, Macfarlane TV. Therapeutic manipulation of the temporomandibular joint. *Br J Oral Maxillofac Surg* 2000;38:641–644.
28. Kropmans TJ, Dijkstra PU, Stegenga B, et al. Therapeutic outcome assessment in permanent temporomandibular joint disc displacement. *J Oral Rehabil* 1999;26:357–363.
29. Mercuri LG. Considering total temporomandibular joint replacement. *Cranio* 1999;17:44–48.
30. Svensson P, Graven-Nielsen T. Craniofacial muscle pain: review of mechanisms and clinical manifestations. *J Orofac Pain* 2001;15:117–145.
31. Rauhala K, Oikarinen KS, Raustia AM. Role of temporomandibular disorders (TMD) in facial pain: occlusion, muscle and TMJ pain. *Cranio* 1999;17:254–261.
32. Stohler CS. Muscle-related temporomandibular disorders. *J Orofac Pain* 1999;13:273–284.
33. Blitzer A, Brin MF, Greene PE, et al. Botulinum toxin injection for the treatment of oromandibular dystonia. *Ann Oto Rhinol Laryngol* 1989;98:93–97.
34. Brin M, Blitzer A, Herman S, et al. Oromandibular dystonia: treatment of 96 cases with botulinum A. In: Jankovic J, Hallett M, eds. Therapy with botulinum toxin. New York: Marcel Dekker, 1994:429–435.
35. Tan E-K, Jankovic J. Botulinum toxin A in patients with

oromandibular dystonia: long-term follow-up. *Neurology* 1999;53:2102–2105.

36. Tan E-K, Jankovic J. Treating severe bruxism with botulinum toxin. *J Am Dent Assoc* 2000;131:211–216.

37. Tan E-K, Jankovic J. Bruxism in Huntington's disease. *Mov Disord* 2000;15:171–173.

38. Fillippi GM, Errico P, Santarelli R, et al. Botulinum A toxin effects on rat jaw muscle spindles. *Acta Otolaryngol* 1993;113:400–404.

39. Rosales RL, Arimura K, Takenaga S, et al. Extrafusal and intrafusal muscle effects in experimental botulinum toxin-A injection. *Muscle Nerve* 1996;19:488–496.

40. Cui M, Aoki KR. Botulinum toxin type A (BTX-A) reduces inflammatory pain in the rat formalin model. *Cephalagia* 2000;20:414.

41. Aoki R. The development of BOTOX—its history and pharmacology. *Pain Dig* 1998;8:337–341.

42. Ishikawa H, Mitsui Y, Yoshitomi T, et al. Presynaptic effects of botulinum toxin type A on the neuronally evoked response of albino and pigmented rabbit iris sphincter and dilator muscles. *Jpn J Ophthalmol* 2000; 44:106–109.

43. Freund B, Schwartz M. The use of botulinum toxin for the treatment of temporomandibular disorder. *Oral Health* 1998;88:32–37.

44. Freund B, Schwartz M, Symington JM. The use of botulinum toxin for the treatment of temporomandibular disorders: preliminary findings. *J Oral Maxillofac Surg* 1999;57:916–920; discussion 920–921.

45. Freund B, Schwartz M, Symington JM. Botulinum toxin: new treatment for temporomandibular disorders. *Br J Oral Maxillofac Surg* 2000;38:466–471.

46. Sessle BJ. Acute and chronic craniofacial pain: brainstem mechanisms of nociceptive transmission and neuroplasticity, and their clinical correlates. *Crit Rev Oral Biol Med* 2000;11:57–91.

47. Hargreaves RJ, Shepheard SL. Pathophysiology of migraine—new insights. *Can J Neurol Sci* 1999;26(Suppl 3):S12–S19.

Scientific and Therapeutic Aspects of Botulinum Toxin
edited by M.F. Brin, J. Jankovic, and M. Hallett
Lippincott Williams & Wilkins, Philadelphia, © 2002.

26

The Role of Botulinum Toxin in Gastrointestinal Disorders

Giuseppe Brisinda, Giorgio Maria, Anna Rita Bentivoglio,
and Alberto Albanese

Following the discovery that botulinum neurotoxins (BTX) inhibit neuromuscular transmission (1), these powerful poisons have become drugs with many indications. First used to treat strabismus (2), local injections of BTX are now considered a safe and efficacious treatment for neurologic and nonneurologic conditions (3). A recent achievement in the field is the observation that BTX is a treatment for disorders of the gastrointestinal tract (GIT). BTX is not only potent in blocking skeletal neuromuscular transmission, but it is also active on cholinergic nerve endings in the autonomic nervous system (4). The capability to inhibit contraction of GIT smooth muscles was first suggested based on *in vitro* observations and was later demonstrated *in vivo* (5). In addition, BTX does not block nonadrenergic noncholinergic (NANC) responses mediated by nitric oxide (NO). This has further promoted interest in using BTX as a treatment for overactive smooth muscles and sphincters, such as the anal sphincters to treat anal fissure, and the puborectalis muscle to treat outlet-type constipation and anterior rectocele.

Information on the anatomy of the pelvic floor and the anal canal, and functional organization of GIT innervation is a prerequisite to understanding many features of BTX action on the GIT and the effects of injections placed into specific sphincters. This review presents current data on the use of BTX to treat GIT diseases and summarizes recent knowledge on the pathogenesis of GIT disorders caused by a dysfunction of the enteric nervous system (ENS).

ANATOMY AND PHYSIOLOGY OF THE PELVIC FLOOR

The complex anatomy and physiology of the anal canal and the rectum account for their important role in continence and for their susceptibility to diseases (6,7). There is an intrinsic relationship between the anal canal, the rectum, and pelvic floor musculature. The main component of the pelvic floor is the levator ani muscle, composed of a pair of broad, symmetric sheets encompassing three striated muscles: the iliococcygeus, the pubococcygeus, and the puborectalis (Fig. 26.1). The puborectalis is a U-shaped strong loop of striated muscle that pulls the anorectum junction to the back of the pubis. It represents the most medial portion of the levator ani and is situated immediately cephalad to the deep component of the external anal sphincter (EAS) (Fig. 26.2). The junction between these two muscles is indistinct and they have a similar innervation; therefore, the puborectalis has been regarded by some authors as a part of the EAS and not of the levator ani complex (6–8). The anorectal angle indicates bending of the rectum by the sling-shaped fibers of the puborectalis muscle at the level of the anorectal junction; it is important to maintain gross fecal continence (Fig. 26.3).

At the anal level, the sphincter complex consists of two overlapping sphincters (Fig. 26.4) (6,9). The EAS, which forms the outer layer, is composed of voluntary, striated, skeletal muscle. It has been described as a single continuous sheet, a double compartment, or a triple-loop

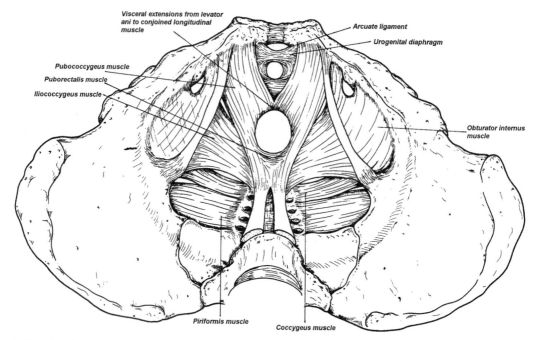

FIG. 26.1. Drawing of the pelvic floor musculature and its connections to the skeleton as seen from inside the abdomen.

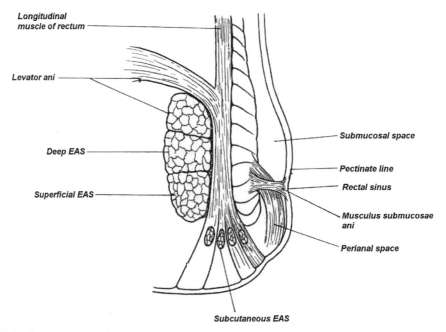

FIG. 26.2. Connections of the levator ani muscle and of the external anal sphincter to the rectum and the perineum.

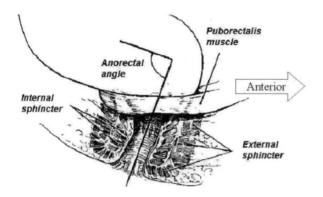

FIG. 26.3. Drawing of the muscles surrounding the anal canal. The anorectal angle is reduced when the puborectalis muscle pulls the rectum anteriorly.

system. In this latter view, the deep EAS and the puborectalis make the loop on the top, which arises from and inserts on the pubis. The middle loop attaches to the coccyx (superficial EAS) and the lower loop inserts on the anterior perianal skin (subcutaneous EAS) (6). Each U-shaped loop is a separate sphincter with distinct attachments and directions of muscle bundles and innervation, and that complements with the others to maintain continence (6,7). The internal anal sphincter (IAS) is the involuntary, smooth, muscle component of the sphincter complex. Being in a state of continuous maximal contraction, the IAS is a natural barrier to the involuntary loss of stool and gas. This is a result of a combination of intrinsic myogenic and extrinsic autonomic neurogenic properties (7,8,10). The IAS is responsible for 50% to 85% of resting anal tone. Being of visceral origin, it is supplied both by sympathetic and parasympathetic nerves; in addition, the ENS modulates its tonic activity. Noradrenergic sympathetic nerves are considered excitatory and the parasympathetic inhibitory to the IAS. Vagal neurons do not act directly, but rather form synaptic connections with neurons whose cell bodies are in the intrinsic GIT ganglia. This transmission is principally mediated by acetylcholine (ACh) acting on nicotinic receptors (10).

Recently, it was shown that the longitudinal layer and the circular smooth muscle in the human rectum receive an intrinsic NO-mediated inhibitory innervation (11,12). The exact site of involvement remains to be determined, but recent data suggest that the carbon monoxide and heme oxygenase pathway may have a role in neurally mediated relaxation of the IAS (13).

In vitro studies on strips of human IAS revealed excitatory α-adrenergic receptors, inhibitory β-adrenergic receptors, excitatory or biphasic cholinergic receptors, and inhibitory NANC receptors. Experimental evidence suggests that norepinephrine induces contraction of isolated IAS strips, whereas adrenaline has a variable response and isoprenaline induces relaxation (14). Furthermore, blockade of α_1-adrenoceptors by a single oral dose of indoramin causes a long-lasting reduction in resting pressure along the length of the anal canal either in patients with fissure or in healthy subjects (15).

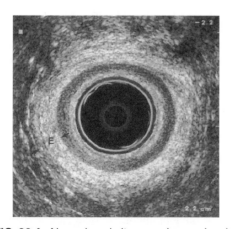

FIG. 26.4. Normal anal ultrasound scan showing the anal sphincter muscles in cross-section. The darker homogeneous ring is the internal anal sphincter *(I)*. The white heterogeneous ring surrounding this is the external anal sphincter *(E; arrows)*. The top of the figure is anterior.

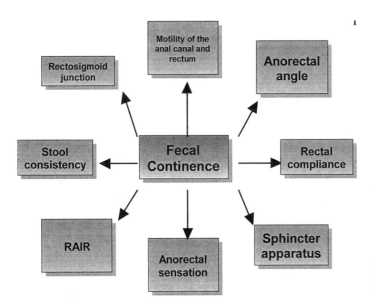

FIG. 26.5. Factors contributing to the maintenance of fecal continence.

The mechanisms responsible for both fecal continence and defecation are complex and interrelated (15). Continence is maintained by the interaction of multiple mechanisms (Fig. 26.5). To achieve defecation, descending commands from the brain are transmitted to the sacral parasympathetic neurons that initiate a motor program in the colon. The ENS in the colon is responsible for coordinating contractions of the smooth muscles and of some striated pelvic floor muscles. Motor neurons located in the anterior column of the sacral spinal cord innervate, via the pudendal nerve, the EAS, and the pelvic floor musculature. Tonic discharges of these neurons cause contraction of the EAS and of pelvic floor musculature, which maintain continence (15). Inhibition of such tonic discharge is necessary for defecation. A fecal bolus in the rectum results in reflex relaxation of the IAS, the so-called rectoanal inhibitory reflex (RAIR). There is agreement on the local intramural nature of the reflex, and morphologic data provide compelling anatomic evidence that NO mediates RAIR (15).

Neuromyogenic Properties of the GIT Smooth Muscles

GIT motility depends on its extrinsic and intrinsic innervation. The autonomic nervous system, because of preganglionic parasympathetic nerves and postganglionic sympathetic nerves, provides extrinsic innervation (10,16); the ENS provides the intrinsic innervation. It is a highly complex system, responsible for the coordination of motility, secretion, and microcirculation in the GIT and for the regulation of the local response to immune inflammatory processes (10,16,17). ENS has been described as the "brain of the gut," because the neurons can function independently of the central nervous system (CNS); however, the CNS maintains an important role in coordinating the diverse functions of enteric neurons via sympathetic and parasympathetic motor and sensory pathways. A deficiency of enteric neurons causes obstruction because of a lack of intestinal propulsion and relaxation of GIT sphincters.

Functional Organization of the ENS

The two main ganglionated plexuses are Auerbach's myenteric plexus and Meissner's submucous plexus. Other nonganglionated plexuses, such as the longitudinal muscle plexus, the circular muscle plexus, the plexus of the muscularis mucosae, and the mucosal plexus, supply GIT layers. In addition, perivascular plexuses are found around arteries and arterioles in the gut wall (10,16,17).

Intraparietal neurons encompass motor neurons (excitatory and inhibitory), interneurons, and intrinsic sensory neurons. Sympathetic and parasympathetic neurons also innervate the GIT.

Excitatory motor neurons innervate longitudinal and circular muscles and the muscularis mucosae. Their primary transmitter is ACh, but they also release tachykinins, substance P, neurokinin A, neuropeptide K, and neuropeptide Y (10,16–18). Inhibitory motor neurons relax smooth muscles and are involved in reflexes that facilitate the passage of food along the GIT (Fig. 26.6). Inhibitory neurons release a combination of at least three transmitters: NO, adenosine triphosphate (ATP), and vasoactive intestinal polypeptide (VIP) (10,14,16,17).

Sympathetic pathways to the GIT are noradrenergic; they inhibit motility, constrict the sphincters, and, in general, inhibit contractile activity by means of a presynaptic action on the myenteric plexus. The vagus nerve includes the axons of neurons located in the brainstem. Vagal neurons form synaptic connections with neurons whose cell bodies are in the intrinsic ganglia of the GIT. ACh principally mediates this transmission (10).

Smooth Muscle Contraction

This function is regulated by changes in cytosol calcium levels. Calcium regulation is affected by a variety of regulatory proteins, including myosin light chains, calmodulin, and calponin. Contraction is dependent on an increase in cellular calcium. The activation of myosin may induce relaxation or allow cross bridges to enter a state of prolonged contraction, the so-called ''latch state.'' The precise mechanisms responsible for the maintenance of smooth-muscle tone are still not entirely known. Relaxation of smooth muscles occurs when there is a resulting decrease in cytosolic calcium. These functions

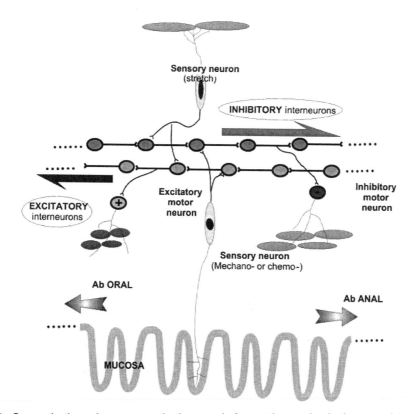

FIG. 26.6. Sympathetic and parasympathetic control of smooth muscles in the gastrointestinal tract.

depend on the intrinsic electrical and mechanical properties of GIT smooth muscles and are regulated by the ENS and by sympathetic and parasympathetic influences (16). An increase in cellular calcium can be produced by the influx of calcium through membrane channels or by stimulation of α_1 adrenoceptors, resulting in a release of calcium from the sarcoplasmic reticulum mediated by inositol triphosphate. Stimulation of β_2 adrenoceptors brings about cAMP-mediated return of calcium to the sarcoplasmic reticulum. Stimulation of NO induces cGMP-mediated decrease in cellular calcium (14).

Interstitial cells of Cajal act as local pacemakers to generate the rhythmic activity of the circular muscle layer throughout the GIT. Motor neurons act on Cajal's cells that are innervated by the myenteric and the submuscular plexuses (19). Hormones and autocoids, such as histamine, serotonin, adenosine, and eicosanoids, produced by nonneural cells in the gut wall, also regulate muscle activity and influence GIT motility during meals and in between (10,16,17).

CHRONIC ANAL FISSURE

A chronic fissure is a cut or crack in the anal canal or anal verge that may extend from the mucocutaneous junction to the dentate line (6,7,20). It is a common complaint in young adults with a roughly equal incidence in both sexes, and shows great reluctance to heal without intervention. Classic symptoms are pain on or after defecation that is often severe and may last from minutes to several hours. Often there is bright blood on the toilet paper. The patient may report that constipation is the antecedent event, but once pain develops, the fear of the act of defecation and a refusal of the call to stool can exacerbate this problem (6). However, a history of constipation is obtained only in one of four cases and diarrhea is seen to be a predisposing factor in about 6% of patients (20).

Fissure is associated with childbirth in 3% to 11% of patients, and commonly occurs in the anterior midline (6,20). Shearing forces from the fetal head on the anal mucosa or mucosal tethering after childbirth rendering it more susceptible to trauma have both been incriminated; post-

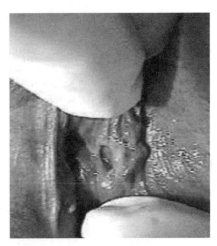

FIG. 26.7. Direct observation of a chronic anal fissure; the sharp borders and the exposure of fibers of the internal anal sphincter are evident.

partum anal fissure is associated with reduced anal canal pressures (21).

The majority of fissures occur in the posterior midline of the anal canal; fissures are located in the anterior midline in 10% of women and 1% of men. Multiple fissures, or fissures occurring in the lateral position, raise suspicion of other diseases, including Crohn's disease, ulcerative colitis, tuberculosis, human immunodeficiency virus, or syphilis (6,20).

The fissure can be seen as the buttocks are parted (Fig. 26.7). It is often suspected because there is marked spasm of the anus making examination difficult. Digital or proctoscopic examination is often impossible because of pain experienced by the patient. Spasm of the IAS has been noted in association with chronic fissure and for many years treatment has focused on alleviating IAS hypertonia.

Pathophysiology of Chronic Fissure

The cause of chronic fissures and the reasons for their failure to heal remain unclear. Also unexplained are the main characteristics of this painful condition, including the predilection for posterior midline and the lack of granulation tissue at the fissure site. Several theories have been advanced to unravel the underlying cause of anal fissure. Most of them are conflicting and none gives a satisfactory explanation for the characteristic features of chronic fissure. Recognized features common to most chronic fissure are a high resting anal pressure caused by hypertonicity of the IAS, reduced vascular perfusion index at the site of the anal fissure, and the presence of "ultraslow" pressure wave activity in the IAS (14). It is generally believed that small traumatic tears in the lining of the anal canal fail to heal because of a reduced blood supply, producing anal fissure.

In addition, the IAS of patients with anal fissure is fibrotic, when compared with that of controls (22), leading to the hypothesis that a myositis might occur early in the course of a fissure and that this is the underlying cause of both spasm and fibrosis. Furthermore, in patients healed by a conservative treatment, resting pressure tends to increase to pretreatment level while the patient remains symptom free. This means that sphincter hypertonus does not necessarily cause pain.

It has been postulated that the increased incidence of fissure in the anterior and posterior midline positions is related to the distribution of vessels supplying blood to the anal canal. Relief of symptoms and healing induced by treatment could be attributed to a decrease in anal pressure that would increase the mucosal blood flow and relieve ischemia. The inferior rectal arteries branching from the internal pudendal artery provide blood supply to the distal anal canal. These vessels cross the ischiorectal fossa; their divisions pass through the anal sphincters to reach the mucosa. Postmortem angiography of the inferior rectal artery has revealed a paucity of inferior rectal artery branches at the posterior commissure in 85% of 41 subjects (23). A morphologic study of the capillaries revealed a reduced density in the subanodermal space and within the IAS in the posterior midline in the majority of subjects. The predilection of anal fissures for the posterior midline and the lack of granulation tissue seen in the base of a chronic fissure may be explained by ischemia (23,24).

Decreased anodermal blood flow may be promoted by endothelial cell dysfunction associated with reduced NO synthesis, which is known to be involved in the regulation of local blood flow. Interruption of the endothelial continuity not only removes the anticoagulant and vasodilator functions of the endothelium, but also exposes the subendothelium, which has several procoagulant functions. In addition, even in the absence of detectable microscopic changes, endothelial function can change from vasodilator to vasoconstrictor and from anticoagulant to procoagulant. These changes may be induced by inflammatory or immune cytokines. Activation of the endothelium may express antigens as the endothelial cells can act as antigen-presenting cells. Antiendothelial cell antibodies have been found in many patients with anal fissure, but not in healthy controls (25). In antibody-positive patients, higher resting anal tone, with no change of maximum voluntary contraction, has been observed (25). This supports a role of the endothelium in the pathogenesis of anal ischemia. Circulating antibodies may activate the endothelium to produce vasoactive autacoids, which could contribute to the increased basal tone and aggravate the ischemia at the level of the posterior anal commissure. The observation that the topical application of glyceryl trinitrate (GTN) may induce healing of anal fissure in up to 60% of cases supports a pathogenic role of endothelial NO synthesis (26).

A primary IAS disturbance may be a contributing etiologic factor. IAS supersensitivity to β_2-agonists has been observed in the patients with chronic fissure (27). This may be induced by a prolonged absence of the neurotransmitter, by abnormalities at neurotransmitter or metabolic level, or by a modification of cholinergic and adrenergic receptors. The efficacy of BTX in inducing fissure healing and reduction of resting tone suggests that increased IAS adrenergic or cholinergic activity is likely to occur in patients with chronic fissure (28–36).

Conservative Therapies

Because the passage of a hard stool is thought to contribute to the development of anal fissure, the control of constipation has been considered the main treatment for years. Patients with a history suggestive of fissure of recent onset are often treated successfully by conservative measures, such as stool softeners, bulking agents, a high-fiber diet, and sitz bath (6,20). To prevent recurrence, a patient should be encouraged to continue with the diet and to use bulked laxative agent, if required, even after symptoms have resolved.

Anal dilators have been employed in the treatment of anal fissure for many years. However, it has been shown that the addition of a dilator is not more useful than stool softeners or topical anesthesia alone. It has been reported that more than half of the patients were initially cured using this technique, but that half of those cured relapsed (20).

Surgical Treatment

If symptoms fail to resolve or have been present for a long period of time, resolution without surgery becomes increasingly less likely. Lateral internal sphincterotomy (LIS) has been the most commonly used treatment for chronic fissure since the 1950s (37). It may be performed under local or general anesthesia, through a radial or circumferential incision, or using a subcutaneous approach. Open or subcutaneous methods produce adequate and equivalent falls in anal pressure. The IAS may be divided from medial to lateral or vice versa. LIS results have been reported from many centers. Surgery is associated with several complications, most of which can be prevented by the use of a judicious technique and, of course, by familiarity with anorectal anatomy. Although LIS heals and relieves symptoms of chronic fissure in nearly all patients (96%) (38,39), the incidence of incontinence varies. The largest studies report impairment of continence in up to 30% of patients. Although most episodes of incontinence are minor and transient, incontinence is permanent in a subset of patients (40).

An incision of the IAS throughout its whole length is inadvisable, but it is uncertain how much of the sphincter should be divided. A common practice is to divide the sphincter for the length of the fissure. It has been suggested that the length of LIS does not affect the incidence of recurrence and the alterations of continence,

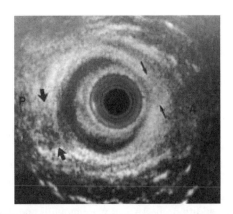

FIG. 26.8. Ultrasound scan of a woman with anterior *(A, thin arrows)* damage to both the internal and the external anal sphincters as a result of childbirth, and posterior *(P, thick arrows)* damage to both the internal and the external anal sphincters related to hemorrhoidectomy.

but there is some disagreement on this point (41). A prospective study with endoanal sonography has revealed that more of the IAS than intended was divided by LIS, particularly in multiparous women, who may have an unrecognized obstetric-related sphincter injury (Fig. 26.8) (42).

Treatment with NO Donors

NO donors may promote healing of anal fissure by increasing local blood flow in two ways: they reduce intraanal pressure and are vasodilators of the anal vessels. The indication for the use of NO donors has been documented. Local application of nitro derivates reduces anal pressures, improves anodermal blood flow, and significantly reduces pain within 5 minutes of application, as assessed by a linear analog pain score (26). Many patients (from 19% to 44%) experience transient headache when using topical GTN preparations and report a burning sensation in the anus (26,43–49). Benefit from GTN is not always permanent. A review of 23 patients with chronic anal fissure showed that 3 months after successful healing with GTN ointment eight patients (35%) recurred, six healed spontaneously, and two healed with a further course of treatment (48). Recently, it was stated that the treatment with topical GTN is less efficacious than previously reported (47). This study highlighted issues related to poor patients' compliance, and reckoned that 62% of the patients had relevant side effects that interfered with their quality of life. High doses of GTN are not more efficacious in inducing healing (49). An important issue is the development of drug tolerance, which is well documented when the same drugs are used to treat cardiovascular diseases. Nitrates have a short duration of action; thus, their frequent application is necessary. Side effects, such as headaches and tachyphylaxis, greatly limit their utility (49). Recent studies suggest that GTN is labor intensive for patients and that it is not superior to LIS (50).

Alternative nitrates, such as isosorbide dinitrate (ISDN), have been investigated. ISDN (1 g of 1% ointment applied every 3 hours throughout the day) achieved healing in 30 (88%) of 34 patients (51). Similarly, its healing has been demonstrated in 34 (83%) of 41 patients following use of topical ISDN in a dose of 1.25 mg or 2.5 mg applied three times a day (52).

Calcium Channel Antagonists

Calcium channel antagonists, such as nifedipine, which has been used in the management of achalasia, decrease anal sphincter tone if given sublingually or orally. In the first clinical study, 30 minutes after 20 mg of sublingual nifedipine there was a 32% and 24% reduction in anal canal pressure in patients with anal fissures and in normal volunteers, respectively, but no significant effect on blood pressure or heart rate (53). An oral dose of 20 mg twice daily was used to treat 15 patients with a chronic fissure (54). The initial dose of nifedipine caused a 36% fall in anal mean resting pressure and healing was achieved in 60% by 8 weeks. The principal side effect was flushing of the face and limbs, which was usually short-lived. The effectiveness of time-released nifedipine (40 mg) daily was assessed over a 5-day period in healing chronic anal fissure (55). Healing was complete in nine patients and symptomatic improvement was documented in a further three patients. In addition, a 93% incidence of side effects has been reported.

The effectiveness of topical diltiazem in decreasing anal canal pressure was recently demonstrated (56,57). In a pilot study, 67% of patients healed using a 2% gel without any reported side effects (56). There was also a significant reduction in the pain score and in resting anal pressure after treatment with diltiazem as compared with pretreatment values. Preliminary results suggest that this therapy does not have significant side effects, as with the oral preparation (57); this may aid compliance to treatment.

Muscarinic Agonists

Few studies have involved topical muscarinic agonists (14). These agents promote the NO synthesis in NANC neurones. Bethanecol, used as a 0.1% topical cream, decreased anal sphincter pressure and healed fissures without side effects (56). Rates of healing may be similar to those with GTN and diltiazem.

Sympathetic Neuromodulators

Both oral indoramin (an α_1-antagonist) and salbutamol (a β_2-agonist) reduce anal canal pressure by relaxing the IAS in healthy volunteers and in patients with anal fissure (15). The effectiveness of these drugs in the treatment of anal fissures has yet to be evaluated.

BTX Treatment

BTX can be used to treat anal fissure (Table 26.1), particularly when a patient is at high risk of incontinence. With the patient lying on a side (usually the left side when the operator is right-handed), the IAS can be easily palpated and injected. The lower rounded edge of the IAS can be felt on physical examination about 1 to 1.5 cm to the dentate line.

In an open-label study (28), we have observed that six (60%) of ten patients healed following a single infiltration of 15 BOTOX units into the IAS. In a subsequent double blind study, a success rate of 76% was achieved following a single treatment with 20 U (32). A prospective comparison between two-dose regimens (15 and 20 U) showed negligible side effects and no complica-

TABLE 26.1. *Comparison of published results on the treatment of patients with chronic anal fissure using botulinum toxin*

No. of patients	Dose of toxin (units)	Healing rate at 6 weeks %	Temporary incontinence %	Recurrence %	Complications %	Reference
10	15 BOTOX	70	10	20	10	28
12	5 BOTOX	83	0	8	0	29
54	5 BOTOX	78	6	6	11	59
5	Nr DYSPORT	60	0	0	0	82
100	5 BOTOX	82	7	6	0	31
36	10/15 BOTOX	65/81	0	0	0	83
25	20 BOTOX	88	4	0	0	32
57	15/20 BOTOX	44/68	0	0	0	33
69	10-21 BOTOX	48–70	0	37–52	0	35
50	20/40 DYSPORT	76/80	4/12	4/8	0	60
25	20 BOTOX	96	0	0	0	34
50	20 BOTOX	74	0	0	0	36

tions; symptomatic improvement was achieved in both groups of patients, but the healing rate was higher in the 20 U group (33). We have also been able to demonstrate that fissure healing is induced more effectively by BTX treatment than by GTN, and that IAS hypertonia is also alleviated more effectively (34). When compared to baseline values 1 month after treatment, resting pressure was reduced by 26.2% in BTX-treated patients and by 16.6% in GTN-treated patients. Two months after treatment resting anal pressure was reduced by 28.4% in the BTX group and by 13.7% in the GTN group. Recently, it was noted that topical ISDN potentiates the effect of BTX in patients with refractory chronic fissure (58).

The therapeutic efficacy of different BTX doses in chronic fissure was recently reported (35). It was found that the healing rate does not differ significantly when the total dose and the number of injection sites are varied. The healing rate was 83% in the patients treated with 10 BOTOX units, 78% in those treated with 15 U and 90% in the group treated with 21 U. A between-group comparison did not reveal significant differences. The injections were administered through the intersphincteric groove in the direction of the IAS; however, 1 month after treatment, the mean squeeze pressure was reduced more than resting pressure, suggesting diffusion of the toxin to the EAS (35).

Based on the theory that low anodermal perfusion at the base of the fissure contributes to the

pathophysiology, additional applications of BTX have been performed at this point (35). In our experience, patients with a posterior chronic fissure have better results, represented by a lowering of resting anal tone and the early development of a healing scar, when BTX is injected anteriorly into the IAS (34,36). Anteriorly placed injections induce a higher fall in resting pressure and improve clinical outcome. Fibrosis of the IAS that is more prominent in the site of the fissure than elsewhere in the smooth muscle may reduce IAS compliance and limit BTX diffusion. It is known that the myenteric plexus and myenteric ganglia are located between the circular and longitudinal smooth-muscle layers along the entire extent of the IAS. A chronic reduction of perfusion in the posterior part of the anus may affect the myenteric nervous fibers at this location and make them less sensitive to the action of BTX.

BTX injections into the EAS are also effective for treating fissures (31,59). The mechanism is probably mediated by diffusion to the IAS, as shown by the observation that maximum squeeze pressure and resting pressure are both reduced with this procedure. Because the fundamental pathogenic event in chronic fissure is the IAS spasm, the injection into the EAS is not the first choice for treatment. In addition, the IAS is readily visible and easier to inject than the EAS. In a series of 50 patients, who received 10 or 20 DYSPORT units into the EAS adjacent to the fissure margins, 78% of patients healed by

TABLE 26.2. *Variables affecting the outcome of treatment with botulinum toxin for chronic anal fissure*

	Influence of dose regimens (33)		Influence of site of injections (36)	
	15 units	20 units	Posterior	Anterior
Number of patients	23	34	25	25
Baseline characteristics				
Age (years)	45±17	41±13	40±13	46±15
M/F ratio	10/13	18/16	14/11	11/14
Duration of symptoms (months)	11±8	13±12	17±16	16±15
Baseline anal pressures				
Resting tone (mm Hg)	94±35	111±30	109±30	101±27
Voluntary contraction (mm Hg)	66±34	84±40	83±38	84±31
1 month evaluation				
Fissure healing	5	17	12	22
Symptomatic improvement	12	24	–	–
Resting tone (mm Hg)	68±26	80±23	84±24	69±18
Voluntary contraction (mm Hg)	54±28	72±36	79±43	83±40
2 months evaluation				
Fissure healing	10	23	15	22
Symptomatic improvement	13	24	–	–
Resting tone (mm Hg)	80±34	79±28	84±29	69±14
Voluntary contraction (mm Hg)	58±30	74±35	79±37	83±39
Rescue treatment	5 (20 U)	7 (25 U)	6 (posterior injections)	3 (anterior injections)
Healing	13	30	20	25

3 months (60). There was no significant difference in healing rates between the two treatment groups, but the patients treated with the higher dosage had a greater reduction in sphincter tone of the puborectalis muscle and a higher incidence of transient incontinence and other complications.

In conclusion, BTX appears to be a safe treatment for patients with anal fissure. It is less expensive and easier to perform than surgical treatment and does not require anesthesia. It is also more efficacious than nitrate therapy. In the patients with a posterior chronic fissure, better results are achieved when BTX is injected anteriorly into the IAS (Table 26.2). No adverse effects or permanent IAS damage have resulted from BTX injection.

CHRONIC CONSTIPATION CAUSED BY PELVIC FLOOR DYSFUNCTION

Constipation is a common primary presenting symptom and a common chronic complaint. A diagnosis of constipation is made when there are fewer than three bowel movements per week and at least one of the following occurs on a mini-mum of 25% of occasions: hard bowel movements, difficulty passing the bowel movement, or sense of inadequate defecation (6). Patients with chronic idiopathic constipation can be classified into two pathophysiologic groups: slow transit constipation and pelvic floor dysfunction.

Pelvic floor dysfunction is characterized by a failure of the puborectalis muscle to relax during efforts to defecate, or by its paradoxical contraction. With an effort to evacuate the rectum, the puborectalis and the EAS normally relax to straighten the anorectal angle and open the anal canal. The diagnosis is suggested by the demonstration of a persistent impression of the puborectalis on the posterior surface of the anal canal during attempted evacuation of barium paste and, more reliably, by EMG evidence of increased electrical activity in the puborectalis muscle during straining.

The etiology of pelvic floor dysfunction is unclear. As in other forms of constipation, the patients are commonly females, who developed constipation as adolescents or young adults. Prolonged efforts to empty the rectum may aggravate the condition. It has been suggested that paradoxical puborectalis contraction during straining represents a focal dystonia, characterized by excessive recruitment of synergistic and antagonistic muscle groups during voluntary activity and lack of reciprocal inhibition (61). Signs of anismus have been noted in normal subjects, in patients with anorectal pain, and even in patients with fecal incontinence (62,63).

BTX has been used to selectively weaken the EAS and puborectalis muscle in constipated patients. It has been observed that BTX relaxes the puborectalis muscle (64); as a consequence, the anorectal angle increases during straining and evacuation becomes possible. However, despite good results, the effect of BTX injections is fairly short term. From 6 to 15 BOTOX units were injected, under electromyography guidance, into the EAS or the puborectalis muscle (65). This brought about short-term improvement of all four treated patients who had failed to respond to conventional biofeedback treatment, but in the long-term, only half of the patients remained successful. In a recent study, symptomatic improvement was noted in 13 of 15 patients after injections of 25 BOTOX units into the EAS (66). Improvement was maintained for a mean of 5 months, and reinjection was thereafter necessary. In a group of 50 patients with chronic outlet obstruction constipation, four patients with a puborectalis syndrome were studied using anorectal manometry, defecography, and electromyography. They were then treated with a total of 30 BOTOX units injected into two sites on either side of the puborectalis muscle under ultrasonographic guidance (67). One patient was lost to follow up; in the remaining three, the frequency of natural bowel movements increased from 0 to 6 per week and only one patient needed laxatives. Anorectal manometry demonstrated decreased tone during straining from 96 ± 12 mm Hg to 42 ± 13 mm Hg at 4 weeks ($p = 0.003$) and 63 ± 22 mm Hg at 8 weeks ($p = 0.009$). Defecography performed 8 weeks after treatment showed improvement in the anorectal angle (increased from $94° \pm 11°$ to $114° \pm 13°$, $p = 0.01$) and evacuation of barium paste. EMG demonstrated that the puborectalis muscle was still capable of producing a mild paradoxical contraction. Still, one patient suffered from symptomatic recurrence 16 weeks

after treatment. He was retreated with 50 U; 8 months later he received a further 60 U. Seven months after the last injection he had normal daily bowel movements with no use of laxatives.

Outlet-type constipation may also occur in Parkinson's disease (PD). Following the observation of the dramatic improvement of a PD patient with outlet-type constipation treated with BTX injections into the puborectalis muscle (68), we performed a prospective study to identify the prevalence of this condition among PD outpatients. Patients with a diagnosis of PD filled an inventory of gastrointestinal function (evaluating the number of bowel movements and defecatory function) and received a proctologic evaluation. Of 120 patients who met the inclusion criteria for chronic constipation, 13 (11%) had isolated or combined outlet-type constipation. Ten of the 13 patients (1 female, mean age 70 ± 8 years) were enrolled in the prospective study. They were evaluated by means of manometry, defecography, and electromyography, and received BTX injections into the puborectalis, the total dose per session being 30 (3 patients), 60 (1 patient), or 100 BOTOX units (6 patients). The results indicate a reduction of tone during straining and an improvement of the anorectal angle (Fig. 26.9). In these patients, anal tone during straining was reduced from 95 ± 42 mm Hg at baseline to 38 ± 11 mm Hg at 1 month ($p < 0.05$) and 38 ± 9 mm Hg ($p < 0.05$) at 2 months evaluation. Resting anal tone and maximum voluntary contraction were unchanged as compared with baseline values. At defecography, the anorectal angle measured during straining increased from a mean of $98° \pm 8°$ before treatment to a mean of $124° \pm 15°$ ($p < 0.05$) after treatment.

ANTERIOR RECTOCELE

Rectocele is a hernia of the anterior rectal wall into the lumen of the vagina. It is a frequent finding in women and its clinical relevance is questionable: from 20% to 81% of nonsymptomatic women and of constipated people may present a rectocele (69,70). If less than 2 cm in diameter, rectocele is considered a normal finding in constipated or healthy subjects. When the diam-

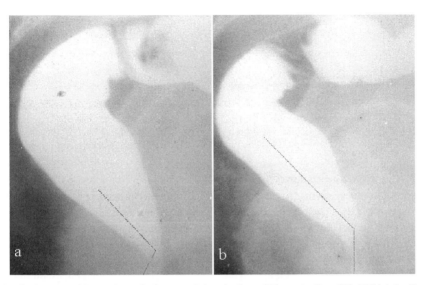

FIG. 26.9. Defecographies taken during straining before (**A**) and after (**B**) BTX injections in the puborectalis muscle. This parkinsonian patient had severe constipation as a result of puborectalis syndrome. Following treatment, during straining, the pelvic floor descends about 3 cm and the anorectal angle becomes obtuse (compare **A** and **B**).

eter increases beyond 2 cm, the rectocele can cause outlet obstruction and rectal emptying difficulties (69–71).

It has been suggested that in some instances, the rectocele is caused by failure of relaxation or paradoxical contraction of the puborectalis muscle occurring during attempted evacuation, but the reason for its establishment is not clear. It is important to identify a rectocele when it is the primary cause of intractable obstructed evacuation. A rectocele may cause mild to severe anorectal symptoms, which are usually associated with severe constipation. It is conceivable that straining aggravates the rectocele, enlarges it, and makes evacuation even more difficult. When there is a rectocele or a paradoxical sphincter reaction, defecation has to occur through the nonrelaxed pelvic floor (69–71).

Although simple to diagnose, the rectocele is difficult to treat. The initial phase of management usually involves a high-residue diet and the use of increasing doses of laxatives and enemas to try to elicit rectal voiding. Neither procedure is effective in solving the problem. A wide variety of surgical approaches has been proposed with the aim of assuring rectal emptying by reducing the dimension of the rectocele.

However, the results of surgery are often disappointing with regard to emptying difficulties. Surgical repair, either vaginal, transperineal, or transanal, does not always alleviate symptoms, and in some patients causes impaired fecal continence. Furthermore, transanal repair may compromise anal sphincter pressures and an alternative approach should be considered when the anal sphincter is lax. From 30% to 72% of patients still had difficulties with evacuation in the postoperative period: 54% of patients still complained of constipation, often severe, after the surgical procedure; 17% of them noted persistent anorectal pain; and 34% had impaired fecal continence. Six months after successful transanal repair of rectoceles, a significant impairment in resting and squeezing anal pressures, probably correlated to stretch of the anal sphincters, were still found (72). Moreover, increased incidences of rectovaginal fistulas and vaginal narrowing and significant postoperative pain have been reported when the transvaginal approach is used.

Recently, 14 women (mean age of 55 ± 11 years) were treated with a total of 30 BOTOX units evenly divided into three sites, two on either side of the puborectalis muscle and the third anteriorly in the EAS (73). At 1 month, inspection revealed a symptomatic improvement in seven patients. Incomplete evacuation had disappeared in seven patients and was reduced in two patients. Blood and/or mucus discharge had disappeared in all seven patients who had previously reported it. The pressure during straining was reduced by 41%, as compared with the baseline value, and was significantly lower than the resting pressure value at the same time. At 2-month evaluation, a symptomatic improvement was found in nine patients. At defecography, the rectocele depth was reduced from 4.3 ± 0.6 cm to 1.8 ± 0.5 cm ($p < 0.001$) and the rectocele area was reduced from 9.2 ± 1.3 cm^2 to 2.8 ± 1.6 cm^2 ($p < 0.001$). The anorectal angle measured during straining increased from a mean of $98° \pm 15°$ before treatment to a mean of $121° \pm 19°$ ($p = 0.001$). At 1-year evaluation, there was no report of digitally assisted rectal voiding and rectocele was not found at physical examination.

OTHER APPLICATIONS IN THE GIT

Recently, interest has focused on the use of BTX to treat motility disorders of the upper GIT other than achalasia. BTX may have a potential for treating these disorders.

Obesity

BTX injection into the gastric antrum may be used to transiently decrease gastric emptying as a treatment for obesity. Preliminary data in rats have shown a loss of body weight ($14 \pm 8\%$ BTX group, $4 \pm 3\%$ saline group, $p < 0.001$) and a reduction of dietary intake ($38 \pm 22\%$ of the basal value in BTX group vs $65 \pm 32\%$ in saline group, $p < 0.05$) in the BTX-treated group (74). Experiments in humans are now being considered.

Delayed Gastric Emptying

BTX has been used to facilitate gastric emptying in patients who underwent pylorus-preserving duodenopancreatectomy (75). Six patients were treated with 80 BOTOX units injected into the pylorus at the end of the surgical procedure. In the postoperative period, only one patient reported symptoms related to delayed gastric emptying.

Infantile Hypertrophic Pyloric Stenosis

This is a congenital hereditary disorder characterized by a functional gastric outlet obstruction that occurs in 1 per 750 births. Pyloric obstruction is the result of a gradual hypertrophy of the circular smooth muscle of the pylorus. Although myenteric neurons have a normal appearance, neurons that innervate the circular-muscle layer of the pyloric sphincter lack NO synthase. Recently, a failure of response to BTX injection was reported in two patients with pyloric stenosis (76).

Sphincter of Oddi Dysfunction

Recurrent upper abdominal pain is a common clinical problem that affects 10% or more of patients undergoing cholecystectomy. Sphincter of Oddi dysfunction has been implicated in the etiology of 10% to 20% of these cases. Unfortunately, it is difficult to diagnose this disorder without performing a manometry of the sphincter, a procedure with a potential risk of pancreatitis. Sphincterotomy is considered the most effective treatment because response to medical therapy is poor (77); however, it is not easy to establish a direct relationship between Oddi dysfunction and pain before sphincterotomy.

Experimental studies have demonstrated that local injections of BTX significantly reduce wave amplitude and phasic contractile activity in the sphincter of Oddi, by means of a selective inhibition of cholinergic influences. At least two potential uses of BTX can be hypothesized: first, an intrasphincteric injection may serve as a handy test to select patients whose pain is directly related to Oddi dysfunction (78); second, repeated BTX treatments may provide a treatment modality alternative to sphincterotomy (79,80). Further prospective studies are needed to investigate the potential use of BTX in these patients.

Recently, 15 consecutive patients with frequent attacks of acute pancreatitis during 6 months and manometrically proven pancreatic sphincter of Oddi dysfunction were treated by endoscopy with 100 BOTOX units into the major papilla (81). No side effects occurred. Twelve patients (80%) remained asymptomatic for 3 months after BTX treatment. One of the three patients who had no symptomatic benefit suffered from continued elevated pancreatic sphincter pressure and benefited from pancreatic sphincterotomy later on. Eleven of the 12 patients who initially responded to BTX had a symptomatic relapse on average 6 months after BTX treatment and then achieved long-term clinical remission when treated with pancreatic or combined sphincterotomy.

REFERENCES

1. Burgen ASV, Dickens F, Zatman LJ. The action of botulinum toxin on the neuromuscular junction. *J Physiol* 1949;109:10–24.
2. Scott AB. Botulinum toxin injection into extraocular muscles as an alternative to strabismus surgery. *Ophthalmology* 1980;87:1044–1049.
3. Munchau A, Bhatia KP. Uses of botulinum toxin injection in medicine today. *BMJ* 2000;320:161–165.
4. Bhutani MS. Gastrointestinal uses of botulinum toxin. *Am J Gastroenterol* 1997;92:929–933.
5. MacKenzie I, Burnstock G, Dolly JO. The effects of purified botulinum neurotoxin type A on cholinergic, adrenergic and nonadrenergic, atropine-resistant autonomic neuromuscular transmission. *Neuroscience* 1982; 7:997–1006.
6. Corman ML. *Colon and rectal surgery, 4th ed.* Philadelphia, PA: Lippincott, 1998.
7. Beck DE, Wexner SD. *Fundamentals of anorectal surgery, 2nd ed.* London: WB Saunders, 1998.
8. Jorge JM, Wexner SD. Anatomy and physiology of the rectum and anus. *Eur J Surg* 1997;163:723–731.
9. Sangwan YP, Solla JA. Internal anal sphincter: advances and insights. *Dis Colon Rectum* 1998;41:1297–1311.
10. Albanese A, Brisinda G, Mathias CJ. The autonomic nervous system and gastrointestinal disorders. In: Appenzeller O, ed. *The autonomic nervous system. Part II. Dysfunctions.* Amsterdam: Elsevier, 2001:613–663.
11. Stebbing JF, Brading AF, Mortensen NJ. Nitrergic innervation and relaxant response of rectal circular smooth muscle. *Dis Colon Rectum* 1996;39:294–299.
12. Stebbing JF, Brading AF, Mortensen NJ. Role of nitric oxide in relaxation of the longitudinal layer of rectal smooth muscle. *Dis Colon Rectum* 1997;40:706–710.
13. Chakder S, Cao GY, Lynn RB, et al. Heme oxygenase activity in the internal anal sphincter: effects of nonadrenergic, noncholinergic nerve stimulation. *Gastroenterology* 2000;118:477–486.
14. Bhardwaj R, Vaizey CJ, Boulos PB, et al. Neuromyogenic properties of the internal anal sphincter: therapeutic rationale for anal fissures. *Gut* 2000;46:861–868.
15. Pitt J, Craggs MM, Henry MM, et al. Alpha-1 adrenoceptor blockade: potential new treatment for anal fissures. *Dis Colon Rectum* 2000;43:800–803.
16. Goyal RK, Hirano I. The enteric nervous system. *N Engl J Med* 1996;334:1106–1115.
17. Furness JB, Bornstein JC. The enteric nervous system and its extrinsic connections. In: Yamada T, ed. *Textbook of gastroenterology.* Philadelphia, PA: Lippincott, 1995:2–24.
18. Brookes SJ, Steele PA, Costa M. Identification and immunohistochemistry of cholinergic and noncholinergic circular muscle motor neurons in the guinea-pig small intestine. *Neuroscience* 1991;42:863–878.
19. Der-Silaphet T, Malysz J, Hagel S, et al. Interstitial cells of Cajal direct normal propulsive contractile activity in the mouse small intestine. *Gastroenterology* 1998;114: 724–736.
20. Lund JN, Scholefield JH. Aetiology and treatment of anal fissure. *Br J Surg* 1996;83:1335–1344.
21. Corby H, Donnelly VS, O'Herlihy C, et al. Anal canal pressures are low in women with postpartum anal fissure. *Br J Surg* 1997;84:86–88.
22. Brown AC, Sumfest JM, Rozwadowski JV. Histopathology of the internal anal sphincter in chronic anal fissure. *Dis Colon Rectum* 1989;32:680–683.
23. Klosterhalfen B, Vogel P, Rixen H, et al. Topography of the inferior rectal artery: a possible cause of chronic, primary anal fissure. *Dis Colon Rectum* 1989;32:43–52.
24. Schouten WR, Briel JW, Auwerda JJ, et al. Ischaemic nature of anal fissure. *Br J Surg* 1996;83:63–65.
25. Maria G, Brisinda D, Ruggieri MP, et al. Identification of anti-endothelial cell antibodies in patients with chronic anal fissure. *Surgery* 1999;126:535–540.
26. Lund JN, Scholefield JH. A randomised, prospective, double-blind, placebo-controlled trial of glyceryl trinitrate ointment in treatment of anal fissure. *Lancet* 1997; 349:11–14.
27. Regadas FS, Batista LK, Albuquerque JL, et al. Pharmacological study of the internal and sphincter in patients with chronic anal fissure. *Br J Surg* 1993;80:799–801.
28. Gui D, Cassetta E, Anastasio G, et al. Botulinum toxin for chronic anal fissure. *Lancet* 1994;344:1127–1128.
29. Jost WH, Schimrigk K. Therapy of anal fissure using botulin toxin. *Dis Colon Rectum* 1994;37:1321–1324.
30. Mason PF, Watkins MJ, Hall HS, et al. The management of chronic fissure in-ano with botulinum toxin. *J R Coll Surg Edinb* 1996;41:235–238.
31. Jost WH. hundred cases of anal fissure treated with botulin toxin: early and long-term results. *Dis Colon Rectum* 1997;40:1029–1032.
32. Maria G, Cassetta E, Gui D, et al. A comparison of botulinum toxin and saline for the treatment of chronic anal fissure. *N Engl J Med* 1998;338:217–220.
33. Maria G, Brisinda G, Bentivoglio AR, et al. Botulinum toxin injections in the internal anal sphincter for the treatment of chronic anal fissure: long-term results after two different dosage regimens. *Ann Surg* 1998;228: 664–669.
34. Brisinda G, Maria G, Bentivoglio AR, et al. A comparison of injections of botulinum toxin and nitroglycerin ointment for the treatment of chronic anal fissure. *N Engl J Med* 1999;341:65–69.
35. Minguez M, Melo F, Espi A, et al. Therapeutic effects of different doses of botulinum toxin in chronic anal fissure. *Dis Colon Rectum* 1999;42:1016–1021.

36. Maria G, Brisinda G, Bentivoglio AR, et al. Influence of botulinum toxin site of injections on healing rate in patients with chronic anal fissure. *Am J Surg* 2000;179: 46–50.

37. Eisenhammer S. Surgical correction of chronic internal anal sphincter contracture. *S Afr Med J* 1951;25: 486–489.

38. Hananel N, Gordon PH. Lateral internal sphincterotomy for fissure-in-ano—revisited. *Dis Colon Rectum* 1997; 40:597–602.

39. Argov S, Levandovsky O. Open lateral sphincterotomy is still the best treatment for chronic anal fissure. *Am J Surg* 2000;179:201–202.

40. Nyam DC, Pemberton JH. Long-term results of lateral internal sphincterotomy for chronic anal fissure with particular reference to incidence of fecal incontinence. *Dis Colon Rectum* 1999;42:1306–1310.

41. Garcia-Aguilar J, Belmonte MC, Perez JJ, et al. Incontinence after lateral internal sphincterotomy: anatomic and functional evaluation. *Dis Colon Rectum* 1998;41: 423–427.

42. Sultan AH, Kamm MA, Nicholls RJ, et al. Prospective study of the extent of internal anal sphincter division during lateral sphincterotomy. *Dis Colon Rectum* 1994; 37:1031–1033.

43. Watson SJ, Kamm MA, Nicholls RJ, et al. Topical glyceryl trinitrate in the treatment of chronic anal fissure. *Br J Surg* 1996;83:771–775.

44. Bacher H, Mischinger HJ, Werkgartner G, et al. Local nitroglycerin for treatment of anal fissures: an alternative to lateral sphincterotomy? *Dis Colon Rectum* 1997; 40:840–845.

45. Oettle GJ. Glyceryl trinitrate vs. sphincterotomy for treatment of chronic fissure-in-ano: a randomized, controlled trial. *Dis Colon Rectum* 1997;40:1318–1320.

46. Kennedy ML, Sowter S, Nguyen H, et al. Glyceryl trinitrate ointment for the treatment of chronic anal fissure: results of a placebo-controlled trial and long-term follow-up. *Dis Colon Rectum* 1999;42:1000–1006.

47. Dorfman G, Levitt M, Platell C. Treatment of chronic anal fissure with topical glyceryl trinitrate [see Comments]. *Dis Colon Rectum* 1999;42:1007–1010.

48. Lund JN, Armitage NC, Scholefield JH. Use of glyceryl trinitrate ointment in the treatment of anal fissure. *Br J Surg* 1996;83:776–777.

49. Carapeti EA, Kamm MA, McDonald PJ, et al. Randomised controlled trial shows that glyceryl trinitrate heals anal fissures, higher doses are not more effective, and there is a high recurrence rate. *Gut* 1999;44:727–730.

50. Richard CS, Gregoire R, Plewes EA, et al. Internal sphincterotomy is superior to topical nitroglycerin in the treatment of chronic anal fissure: results of a randomized, controlled trial by the Canadian Colorectal Surgical Trials Group. *Dis Colon Rectum* 2000;43: 1048–1057.

51. Schouten WR, Briel JW, Boerma MO, et al. Pathophysiological aspects and clinical outcome of intra-anal application of isosorbide dinitrate in patients with chronic anal fissure. *Gut* 1996;39:465–469.

52. Lysy J, Israelit-Yatzkan Y, Sestiery-Ittah M, et al. Treatment of chronic anal fissure with isosorbide dinitrate: long-term results and dose determination. *Dis Colon Rectum* 1998;41:1406–1410.

53. Chrysos E, Xynos E, Tzovaras G, et al. Effect of nifedi-pine on rectoanal motility. *Dis Colon Rectum* 1996;39: 212–216.

54. Cook TA, Smilgin Humphreys MM, Mortensen NJMcC. Oral nifedipine reduces resting anal pressure and heals chronic anal fissure. *Br J Surg* 1999;86: 1269–1273.

55. Cook TA, Mortensen NJ. Nifedipine for treatment of anal fissures. *Dis Colon Rectum* 2000;43:430–431.

56. Carapeti EA, Kamm MA, Evans BK, et al. Topical diltiazem and bethanechol decrease anal sphincter pressure without side effects. *Gut* 1999;45:719–722.

57. Knight JS, Birks M, Farouk R. Topical diltiazem ointment in the treatment of chronic anal fissure. *Br J Surg* 2001;88:553–556.

58. Lysy J, Israelit-Yatzkan Y, Sestiery-Ittah M, et al. Topical nitrates potentiate the effect of botulinum toxin in the treatment of patients with refractory anal fissure. *Gut* 2001;48:221–224.

59. Jost WH, Schanne S, Mlitz H, et al. Perianal thrombosis following injection therapy into the external anal sphincter using botulin toxin. *Dis Colon Rectum* 1995;38:781.

60. Jost WH, Schrank B. Repeat botulin toxin injections in anal fissure: in patients with relapse and after insufficient effect of first treatment. *Dig Dis Sci* 1999;44: 1588–1589.

61. Mathers SE, Kempster PA, Swash M, et al. Constipation and paradoxical puborectalis contraction in anismus and Parkinson's disease: a dystonic phenomenon? *J Neurol Neurosurg Psychiatry* 1988;1:1503–1507.

62. Wexner SD, Marchetti F, Salanga VD, et al. Neurophysiologic assessment of the anal sphincter. *Dis Colon Rectum* 1991;34:606–612.

63. Voderholzer WA, Neuhaus DA, Klauser AG, et al. Paradoxical sphincter contraction is rarely indicative of anismus. *Gut* 1997;41:258–262.

64. Hallan RI, Williams NS, Melling J, et al. Treatment of anismus in intractable constipation with botulinum A toxin. *Lancet* 1988;2:714–717.

65. Joo JS, Agachan F, Wolff B, et al. Initial North American experience with botulinum toxin type A for treatment of anismus. *Dis Colon Rectum* 1996;39: 1107–1111.

66. Shafik A, El Sibai O. Botulin toxin in the treatment of nonrelaxing puborectalis syndrome. *Dig Surg* 1998;15: 347–351.

67. Maria G, Brisinda G, Bentivoglio AR, et al. Botulinum toxin in the treatment of outlet obstruction constipation caused by puborectalis syndrome. *Dis Colon Rectum* 2000;43:376–380.

68. Albanese A, Maria G, Bentivoglio AR, et al. Severe constipation in Parkinson's disease relieved by botulinum toxin. *Mov Disord* 1997;12:764–766.

69. Siproudhis L, Dautreme S, Ropert A, et al. Dyschezia and rectocele—a marriage of convenience? Physiologic evaluation of the rectocele in a group of 52 women complaining of difficulty in evacuation. *Dis Colon Rectum* 1993;36:1030–1036.

70. Van Laarhoven CJ, Kamm MA, Bartram CI, et al. Relationship between anatomic and symptomatic long-term results after rectocele repair for impaired defecation. *Dis Colon Rectum* 1999;42:204–210.

71. Karlbom U, Graf W, Nilsson S, et al. Does surgical repair of a rectocele improve rectal emptying? *Dis Colon Rectum* 1996;39:1296–1302.

72. Ho YH, Ang M, Nyam D, et al. Transanal approach to

rectocele repair may compromise anal sphincter pressures. *Dis Colon Rectum* 1998;41:354–358.

73. Maria G, Brisinda G, Bentivoglio AR, et al. Anterior rectocele due to obstructed defecation relieved by botulinum toxin. *Surgery* 2001;129:524–529.

74. Gui D, De Gaetano A, Spada PL, et al. Botulinum toxin injected in the gastric wall reduces body weight and food intake in rats. *Aliment Pharmacol Ther* 2000;14: 829–834.

75. Wiesel PH, Bettschart V, Suter M, et al. Prevention of delayed gastric emptying after pylorus-preserving pancreatoduodenectomy with intrapyloric injection of botulinum toxin. *Gastrointest Endosc* 1997;45:44(abstr).

76. Heinen F, Mall V, Ruckauer KD, et al. Lack of response to botulinum toxin A in patients with hypertrophic pyloric stenosis. *Eur J Pediatr* 1999;158:436.

77. Geenen JE, Hogan WJ, Dodds WJ, et al. The efficacy of endoscopic sphincterotomy after cholecystectomy in patients with sphincter-of-Oddi dysfunction. *N Engl J Med* 1989;320:82–87.

78. Pasricha PJ, Miskovsky EP, Kalloo AN. Intrasphincteric injection of botulinum toxin for suspected sphincter of Oddi dysfunction. *Gut* 1994;35:1319–1321.

79. Sand J, Nordback I, Arvola P, et al. Effects of botulinum toxin A on the sphincter of Oddi: an *in vivo* and *in vitro* study. *Gut* 1998;42:507–510.

80. Muehldorfer SM, Hahn EG, Ell C. Botulinum toxin injection as a diagnostic tool for verification of sphincter of Oddi dysfunction causing recurrent pancreatitis. *Endoscopy* 1997;29:120–124.

81. Wehrmann T, Schmitt TH, Arndt A, et al. Endoscopic injection of botulinum toxin in patients with recurrent acute pancreatitis due to pancreatic sphincter of Oddi dysfunction. *Aliment Pharmacol Ther* 2000;14: 1469–1477.

Scientific and Therapeutic Aspects of Botulinum Toxin
edited by M.F. Brin, J. Jankovic, and M. Hallett
Lippincott Williams & Wilkins, Philadelphia, © 2002.

27

Botulinum Toxin Type A in the Treatment of Hyperfunctional Facial Lines and Cosmetic Disorders

Alastair Carruthers and Jean Carruthers

One of the more common uses of botulinum toxin type A (BTX-A) is in the treatment of cosmetic concerns. Similarly, botulinum toxin injections are the most common cosmetic procedures performed today in North America. The use of this powerful therapeutic for aesthetic purposes is the result of its ease of use, excellent safety profile, striking efficacy, and the fact that it treats the underlying musculature responsible for the formation of hyperfunctional facial lines rather than just treating the lines themselves.

As far as we know, Dr. Alan Scott, who pioneered the development of BTX-A for clinical use (1), was the first to use BTX-A to treat hyperfunctional facial lines in the mid-1980s. We published the first systematic study of the use of BTX-A for hyperfunctional facial lines in 1992 (2), but this was quickly followed by reports by many other investigators.

At this time, numerous studies have been published that demonstrate the efficacy and safety of BTX-A injections for cosmetic purposes in close to 900 patients (2–18). In addition, two large (total N = 535), double-blind, placebo-controlled studies of the efficacy of BTX-A in the treatment of glabellar lines were recently completed. The results of these studies were presented at the American Academy of Dermatology annual meetings (in 2000 and 2001) and the European Academy of Dermatology and Venereology meeting (2000) and are expected to be published in 2002. These well-controlled studies demonstrated peak responder rates of 70% to 90% for all efficacy variables and a very low rate of adverse events.

Most studies on the cosmetic use of BTX-A describe a time course of response that is similar to what has been reported for BTX-A use in other indications. Typically, the beneficial effects of BTX-A first begin to appear within 2 days, peak in 1 to 4 weeks, and gradually decline after 3 to 4 months. However, several physicians report seeing a much longer duration of effect (up to 6 to 12 months) in some patients. This seems to be most common in patients that have been treated several times with BTX-A for the same condition over a period of a year or so. As the number of repeat injection increases, the duration of effect tends to become more prolonged (2,19).

At this time, there are two different BTX-A products on the market in different parts of the world: BOTOX, available in 100-U vials, and DYSPORT, which is sold in 500-U vials. However, the appropriate doses of the two commercial products are very different. Consequently, it is important to always indicate the specific BTX-A product used when reporting the results of a clinical study or providing practical guidelines for clinical use. Because the majority of the published information on the cosmetic use of BTX-A refers specifically to the BOTOX formulation, all doses and injection procedures described in this review are for BOTOX unless otherwise indicated.

More recently, a BTX-B formulation (MYOBLOC) was approved by the United States Food and Drug Administration (FDA) for use in cervical dystonia. Cosmetic experience with this product is limited. However, it has obvious differences from the BTX-A products discussed above and dosing and injection technique will need to be modified accordingly.

GENERAL CONSIDERATIONS WHEN USING BTX-A FOR COSMETIC PURPOSES

Dilution and Handling

The effect of BTX-A treatment can be controlled by varying not only the dose, but the dilution. Studies show that higher doses in smaller volumes tend to keep the toxin and the area of muscle weakening confined to a more localized area, while smaller doses in larger volumes tend to cause more widespread effects (20,21).

A 1998 review of BTX-A dilution and storage practices among physicians using BTX-A for cosmetic purposes found that most are using a volume of 2.5 to 3 mL of preservative-free saline to dilute one 100-U vial of BTX-A, resulting in a concentration of 33 to 40 U/mL (22). However, a few investigators are using very low concentrations (5 to 10 U/mL) in higher volumes to deliberately spread the toxin over a wider area (6,17,23), while we prefer to use a very high concentration (100 U/mL) in our clinical practices in order to tightly control BTX-A placement. A dilution study by Fulton in 1998 (23) suggested that going below 6.7 U/mL produced inferior results, but no thorough systematic study of the effect of dilution volume and concentration on duration, efficacy, or the incidence of adverse effects has been done. At this time, dilution volume appears to be mostly a matter of personal preference. However, if adverse effects due to spread of the toxin to unintended targets is a problem, increasing BTX-A concentration and decreasing injection volume may be beneficial.

There seems to be less variability in the dilution of DYSPORT. Three studies that used this formulation of BTX-A for cosmetic purposes used 2.5 mL of preservative-free saline to dilute each 500-U vial (200 U/mL) (24–26).

The manufacturers recommend that reconstituted BTX-A be stored at 2°C (35.6°F) to 8°C (46.4°F) and used within 4 hours of reconstitution. However, many clinicians have stored reconstituted BTX-A (BOTOX) for as long as 1 week without any noticeable loss of potency or increase in adverse events (9,22,27).

Injection Technique

In many of the early studies of the cosmetic uses of BTX-A, the use of electromyographic (EMG) guidance to place the toxin in the most active part or the muscle was common. This technique can be useful to the beginner, but after a thorough understanding of the relevant facial anatomy is attained, EMG guidance provides little benefit. When not using EMG recording, a 30-gauge needle is commonly used in order to minimize discomfort to the patient.

COMMON COSMETIC USES

Glabellar Frown Lines

In the treatment of glabellar frown lines, the goal is to produce a significant weakening, or even complete paralysis, of corrugator and orbicularis, which move the brow medially, as well as procerus and depressor supercilii, which pull the brow inferiorly. Because the location, size, and use of these muscles vary greatly between individuals, the best outcomes will come from individualizing the treatment sites and doses to match each patient's needs.

Injection sites and dosing. In the medical literature, procedures for softening glabellar frown lines with BTX-A range from placing a single injection of 10 U into the belly of each corrugator (16) to total doses of 20 to 50 U spread over seven sites (28).

Pribitkin and colleagues, in 1997 (16), demonstrated that 10 U per side was a good starting dose when using a single injection to each corrugator. They found that starting at lower doses and titrating upward as needed at 2-week intervals did not work well for most patients. They observed that the best outcomes were seen in patients with thin skin and fine wrinkles or shallow folds that were amplified by scowling but that could still be spread out with the fingers.

Patients with deep dermal scarring and exceptionally deep glabellar crevices that could not be pulled apart with the fingers tended to not respond as well.

A very systematic dose-ranging study was conducted by Hankins and colleagues in 1998 (29). Forty-six patients were injected in five sites (one in the midline glabellar area 4 mm below brow line; and two more on each side, one just above and one just below the medial brow in line with the medial canthus of the eye) with total doses that ranged from 1 to 10 U per site. The volume was held constant at either 0.05 or 0.1 mL per site. They determined that the minimum effective dose was 2.5 to 4 U per site and that increasing the dose above that level did not produce any significant increase in efficacy. Both injection volumes used were equally effective. One problem with this study was that the treatment groups were small (five subjects per group) and so statistical significance was difficult to achieve.

In the two, large, placebo-controlled studies mentioned earlier, 4 U BTX-A were injected in each of five sites (one in the procerus and two in each corrugator). This treatment paradigm gave good results in the overwhelming majority of patients, while producing only a few, transient, adverse effects. The dilution used in these studies was 40 U/mL which kept the volume of each injection at 0.1 mL.

In our clinics, we currently use seven injection sites when treating glabellar frown lines, and vary the dosage depending on the individual brow. In an average female brow without a great deal of muscle mass, we use a total of 25 U BTX-A. When there is a greater muscle mass, a total dose of 35 U or even higher is used. Typically, 5 to 10 U are injected into the procerus at the midline, another 4 to 7 U just above each eyebrow, directly above the caruncle of the inner canthus and above the bony supraorbital ridge, and another 3 to 7 U at least 1 cm superior to the previous injection site on each side. In most individuals, especially those with horizontal brows, 3 to 5 U is injected 1 cm above the supraorbital rim in the mid-pupillary line on each side. Patients are advised that they should be reinjected every 3 to 4 months during the first year,

but that after that time they should return for reinjection when they feel in need of retreatment.

The most undesirable adverse event reported with BTX-A treatment of glabellar frown lines is blepharoptosis. This happens when the injected toxin diffuses to the eyelid muscles. Our injection technique is designed to keep the risk of this complication as low as possible. To minimize the risk of ptosis (which is less than 1% in our clinic), we recommend keeping the injected volume at the minimum needed for efficacy, accurately placing the injection (no closer than 1 cm above the central eyebrow), and advising the patient to stay vertical and not to manipulate the injected area for several hours after injection.

The doses of DYSPORT that have been reported in the literature for glabellar lines range from a total of 16 U (30) to 80 U (24,26).

Crow's-Feet

In the treatment of crow's-feet with BTX-A, the goal of treatment is to produce a selective weakening of the orbicularis oculi just in the area of the crow's-feet lines.

Injection sites and dosing. The total doses of BTX-A that have been reported for the treatment of crow's-feet range from 4 to 5 U/side (9,17) to 5 to 15 U/side (7,12), distributed over two or three injection sites. Some physicians use EMG guidance (7,12,13) to locate the most active part of the muscle while the patient grimaces, whereas other physicians (17) inject the "hills" formed between the crow's-feet lines when the patient grimaces. The reported duration of effect for these injections range from 3 to 6 months (12) to 5 to 6 months (13).

According to the results reported in the literature, this appears to be a particularly successful and safe procedure. Most studies report few, if any, adverse effects. In an early study (7), a few cases of temporary lower eyelid droop were seen in some of the first patients enrolled. However, this complication was eliminated by moving the injection site farther from the lateral canthus.

In our clinic, we start with 12 to 15 U per side, distributed in equal parts between two and four injection sites. We keep the injections intradermal in order to minimize the risk of bruising. We have not noted any other adverse effects following this procedure.

The doses of DYSPORT that have been reported in the literature for the orbicularis oculi range from a total of 8 U (30) to 60 U (26).

Horizontal Forehead Lines

The challenge in treating horizontal forehead lines with BTX-A is to soften the undesirable lines without causing brow ptosis or a complete elimination of expressiveness. This can be difficult because the frontalis muscle that produces these forehead lines also helps keep the brow elevated.

Injection sites and dosing. The most important thing to remember when treating forehead lines with BTX-A is that the injections must be kept well above the brow in order to reduce the risk of ptosis. Guerrissi and Sarkissian (14) recommend keeping injections 2.5 cm or more above the brow, while Goodman (17) describes his injection sites as being at least two finger breadths above the brow. It seems that 2.5 cm may not be far enough away from the brow in some patients as 2 of 17 patients in the study by Guerrissi and Sarkissian (14) developed brow ptosis lasting 55 to 70 days.

The specific descriptions of dosing and technique in the literature vary significantly. Guerrissi and Sarkissian (14) describe using a total dose of 14 to 20 U BTX-A (in a 25 U/mL dilution), depending on the number of lines and their lateral extension, but do not specify the number or location of the injection sites. Goodman (17) injects the ridges appearing between the forehead lines when the patient raises his or her eyebrows. Two sites per wrinkle per side are injected with 1 to 2 U (in a 10 U/mL dilution).

In our clinic, patients are treated with a total of 10 to 20 U BTX-A distributed over four to five injection sites horizontally across the midbrow and 2 to 3 cm above the eyebrows. In individuals with a narrow brow (less than 12 cm between the temporal fusion lines at the midbrow level), we use four injection sites. For broader-browed individuals (greater than 12 cm) we use five injection sites and a slightly higher

total dose. It is our belief that the brow depressors should always be treated at the same time as frontalis. The technique is described under ''Brow Lift'' below. Even with this cautious approach, we still see a minor degree of brow ptosis or swelling of the upper eyelids in a few patients. The beneficial effects typically last from 4 to 6 months.

The doses of DYSPORT that have been reported in the literature for the frontalis muscle range from a total of 40 U (26) to 70 U (30).

Brow Lift

Injections of BTX-A can be used either alone or in combination with surgical procedures to lift the brow and give patients a more open and friendly look. However, as is true for the treatment of forehead lines, it is important to use BTX-A to selectively weaken the brow depressors without weakening that portion of the frontalis responsible for keeping the brow elevated. Failure to do so will result in brow ptosis. This can be a challenge because the lower portion of the frontalis interdigitates with the brow depressors (corrugator supercilii, procerus, and the medial and lateral portions of orbicularis oculi) and may be affected by toxin injections in those locations. However, the bulk of frontalis is superior to the brow depressors, so keeping the injection sites low should prevent significant brow ptosis.

Injection sites and dosing. Early reports of the use of BTX-A to produce brow elevation describe using moderate doses (20 to 30 U total) distributed over a total of one (32) to three sites (33). This approach produces a modest brow elevation of 1 mm or so with no ptosis. More recent reports describe achieving slightly greater brow elevations by distributing the BTX-A over three to four sites along the underside of each brow (34,35). Ahn and colleagues (34) injected 7 to 10 U into the superolateral orbicularis oculi at three sites below the lateral third of the brow (but superior and lateral to the orbital rim). Huang and colleagues (35), injected a total dose of 10 U (in a 50 U/mL dilution), distributed in 2.5 U increments between four sites along the underside of the lateral half of the brow. An additional 5 U was injected into each corrugator muscle just above and medial to the brow.

In our clinics, we currently use the same approach as described in the paper by Huilgol, Carruthers, and Carruthers (33). One injection of 7 to 10 U BTX-A is made in the glabellar area at the midline, immediately below the line joining the eyebrows, followed by 1 injection on each side into the supralateral eyebrow where orbicularis is curving inferolaterally, outside the bony orbital rim.

Initial approaches to produce brow elevation relied on the suppression of brow depression by injecting the depressor muscles. We now understand that the brow elevation seen with glabella injection is actually lateral brow elevation caused by overaction of lateral frontalis resulting from minor weakness of medial frontalis. An extreme form of this is seen with the ''Mr. Spock'' eyebrow, which can be a complication of brow injections but which can also be a desirable result in some individuals. Understanding which individuals will get brow elevation and which will get central brow ptosis is a major challenge.

Other

Facial asymmetry. The correction of facial asymmetry should be considered just as much of a therapeutic treatment as it is a cosmetic one. Facial asymmetries typically result from trauma or pathology and their correction can be of great psychological as well as physical benefit to the patient. There have been several reports of the successful use of BTX-A in the treatment of facial asymmetries caused by a variety of facial nerve palsies (36–39), facial dystonia (3,40), surgery (39,41), or trauma (39). In cases of hemiparesis, BTX-A is used to decrease expressivity on the unaffected side. In cases of hyperkinesia, the affected muscles are treated.

Neck lines. Injections of BTX-A can reduce vertical neck bands resulting from the action of the platysma muscle (12,42). There have also been reports of its usefulness in the treatment of horizontal neck lines.

Melolabial folds. The use of BTX-A to treat melolabial folds is complicated by the fact that much of the fold is formed by excess skin that will be unaffected by BTX-A. In addition, sufficient tone in the muscles in that area (e.g., levator labii superioris alaeque) is necessary to maintain normal appearance and expressiveness. Some clinicians have treated this area successfully (3), but we do so only rarely and with very small doses (2 U).

ADJUNCTIVE USE

Although BTX-A treatment can produce impressive results when used alone, it is reasonable to expect that much of its cosmetic use will be in combination with other procedures. The simplicity, safety, and versatility of BTX-A treatment make it well suited for use with a variety of surgical procedures and skin resurfacing techniques. The use of BTX-A to weaken certain muscles before surgery can make it easier to manipulate the tissues during surgical procedures, allowing for a greater surgical correction or for better concealment and healing of the surgical incision. In addition, the use of BTX-A during or after a procedure can prevent or slow the return of wrinkles by reducing the action of the muscles that created the wrinkles in the first place.

With laser resurfacing. The adjunctive use of BTX-A gives a superior and longer-lasting outcome by preventing the underlying muscles from recreating the glabellar furrows and crows feet removed by the laser. Regular postoperative injections (every 6 to 12 months) can prolong the effects of this procedure. The ability of BTX-A injections to improve and prolong the effects of laser resurfacing has been documented in a recent study by West and Alster (43). We first described the use of BTX-A injections in combination with laser resurfacing in 1998 (44), but today, it is a common component of the standard laser resurfacing protocol used by many clinicians (45).

With surgical brow lift. As mentioned above, BTX-A can be used on its own to create a mild brow elevation. However, surgery is often required when brow ptosis is moderate to severe and a greater elevation is desired. Preoperative relaxation of the brow depressors with BTX-A may allow for a greater brow elevation. Postoperatively, BTX-A treatment may help prolong the benefits of surgery by relaxing the muscles that are working to reestablish the depressed brow.

With upper- and lower-lid blepharoplasty. We have found that pretreatment of the crow's-feet area with BTX-A allows the muscles to relax, leading to a more accurate estimation of the amount of skin to be resected during surgery and better placement of the incision so that it is concealed within the orbital margin. The crow's-feet area can also be treated intraoperatively by directly injecting the lateral area of the exposed orbicularis oculi (31).

With lower eyelid ectropion and "round-eye" repair. Following these procedures, the quality of the surgical result can be damaged by dehiscence of the temporal incision. The use of BTX-A to transiently weaken the lateral fibers of the orbicularis (the muscles that are pulling on the medial side of the incision) can prevent this. First briefly reported in an article in *Ophthalmology Times* (46), this is now our standard procedure, and dehiscence has been eliminated.

With repair of facial wounds. The constant action of underlying musculature can slow the healing of skin wounds and promote scar formation. Immobilization of underlying musculature with BTX-A has been shown to promote the healing of experimentally induced facial wounds in monkeys (47). As mentioned above, we have seen similar improvements in the healing of surgical incisions when BTX-A is used with eyelid surgery. However, this technique may prove particularly beneficial in the repair of traumatic injury.

CONCLUSIONS

Botulinum toxin type A is one of the most common cosmetic procedures performed today. It is effective in a wide range of applications, as well as safe, easy to use, and easy to combine with other procedures. It provides a valuable alternative for those patients for whom surgery is inappropriate, and can also be a valuable adjunctive treatment for patients receiving surgical or skin resurfacing procedures.

REFERENCES

1. Scott AB. Clostridial toxins as therapeutic agents. In: Simpson LL, ed. *Botulinum neurotoxin and tetanus toxin.* New York: Academic Press, 1989:399–412.
2. Carruthers JDA, Carruthers JA. Treatment of glabellar frown lines with *C. botulinum*-A exotoxin. *J Derm Surg Oncol* 1992;18:17–21.
3. Blitzer A, Brin MF, Keen MS, et al. Botulinum toxin for the treatment of hyperfunctional lines of the face. *Arch Otolaryngol Head Neck Surg* 1993;119: 1018–1022.
4. Carruthers A, Carruthers JDA. The use of botulinum toxin to treat glabellar frown lines and other facial wrinkles. *Cosmet Dermatol* 1994;7:11–15.
5. Guyuron B and Huddleston SW. Aesthetic indications for botulinum toxin injection. *Plast Reconstr Surg* 1994; 93:913–918.
6. Keen M, Blitzer A, Aviv J, et al. Botulinum toxin A for hyperkinetic facial lines: results of a double-blind, vehicle-controlled study. *Plast Reconstr Surg* 1994;94: 94–99.
7. Keen M, Kopelman J, Avia J, et al. Botulinum toxin A: a novel method to remove periorbital wrinkles. *Facial Plast Surg* 1994;10:141–146.
8. Foster JA, Barnhorst D, Papay F, et al. The use of botulinum A toxin to ameliorate facial kinetic frown lines. *Ophthalmology* 1996;103:618–622.
9. Garcia A, Fulton JE Jr. Cosmetic denervation of the muscles of facial expression with botulinum toxin: a dose-response study. *Dermatol Surg* 1996;22:39–43.
10. Lowe NJ, Maxwell A, Harper H. Botulinum A exotoxin for glabellar folds: a double-blind, vehicle-controlled study with an electromyographic injection technique. *J Am Acad Dermatol* 1996;35:569–572.
11. Matsudo PK. Botulinum toxin for correction of frontoglabella wrinkles: preliminary evaluation. *Aesth Plast Surg* 1996;20:439–441.
12. Blitzer A, Binder WJ, Aviv JE, et al. The management of hyperfunctional facial lines with botulinum toxin: a collaborative study of 210 injection sites in 162 patients. *Arch Otolaryngol Head Neck Surg* 1997;123:389–392.
13. Ellis DAF, Tan AKW. Cosmetic upper-facial rejuvenation with botulinum. *J Otolaryngol* 1997;26:92–96.
14. Guerrissi J, Sarkissian P. Local injection into mimetic muscles of botulinum toxin A for the treatment of facial lines. *Ann Plast Surg* 1997;39:447–453.
15. Koch JR, Troell RJ, Goode RL. Contemporary management of the aging brow and forehead. *Laryngoscope* 1997;107:710–715.
16. Pribitkin EA, Greco TM, Goode RL, et al. Patient selection in the treatment of glabellar wrinkles with botulinum toxin type A injection. *Arch Otolaryngol Head Neck Surg* 1997;123:321–326.
17. Goodman G. Botulinum toxin for the correction of hyperkinetic facial lines. *Aust J Dermatol* 1998;39: 158–163.
18. Oliver JM. Botulinum toxin A treatment of overactive corrugator supercilii in thyroid eye disease. *Br J Ophthalmol* 1998;82:528–533.
19. Ahn K-Y, Park M-Y, Park D-H, et al. Botulinum toxin A for the treatment of facial hyperkinetic wrinkle lines in Koreans. *Plast Reconstr Surg* 2000;105:778–784.
20. Shaari CM, Sanders I. Quantifying how location and

dose of botulinum toxin injection affect muscle paralysis. *Muscle Nerve* 1993;16:964–969.

21. Borodic GE, Ferrante R, Pearce B, et al. Histologic assessment of dose-related diffusion and muscle fiber response after therapeutic botulinum A toxin injection. *Mov Disord* 1994;9:31–39.

22. Klein AW. Dilution and storage of botulinum toxin. *Dermatol Surg* 1998;24:1179–1180.

23. Fulton JE. Botulinum toxin: The Newport Beach experience. *Dermatol Surg* 1998;24:1219–1224.

24. Ascher B, Klap P, Marion M-H, et al. La toxine botulique dans le treatment de rides fronto-glabellaires et de la region orbitaire. *Ann Chir Plast Esthet* 1995;4:69–75.

25. Le Louarn C. [Botulinum toxin and facial wrinkles: a new injection procedure.] *Ann Chir Plast Estet* 1998; 43:526–533.

26. Lowe NJ. Botulinum Toxin type A for facial rejuvenation: United States and United Kingdom perspectives. *Dematol Surg* 1998;24:1216–1218.

27. Sloop RR, Cole BA, Escutin RO. Reconstituted botulinum toxin type A does not lose potency in humans if it is refrozen or refrigerated for 2 weeks before use. *Neurology* 1997;48:249–253.

28. Carruthers A, Carruthers J. Cosmetic uses of botulinum A exotoxin. In: Klein AW, ed. *Tissue augmentation in clinical practice.* New York: Marcel Dekker, 1998: 207–236.

29. Hankins CL, Strimling R, Rogers GS. Botulinum A toxin for glabellar wrinkles: dose and response. *Dermatol Surg* 1998;24:1181–1183.

30. Tambasco N, Lalli F, Mancini ML, et al. [Botulinum toxin in the treatment of facial expression wrinkles.] *Riv Ital Chir Plast* 1997;29:197–200.

31. Guerrissi JO. Intraoperative injection of botulinum toxin A into orbicularis oculi muscle for the treatment of crow's-feet. *Plast Reconstr Surg* 2000:105:2219–2228.

32. Frankel AS, Kamer FM. Chemical brow lift. *Arch Otolaryngol Head Neck Surg* 1998;124:321–323.

33. Huilgol SC, Carruthers A, Carruthers JDA. Raising eyebrows with botulinum toxin. *Dermatol Surg* 1999;25: 373–376.

34. Ahn MS, Catten M, Maas CS. Temporal brow lift using botulinum toxin A. *Plast Reconstr Surg* 2000;105: 1129–1135.

35. Huang W, Rogachefsky AS, Foster JA. Brow lift with botulinum toxin. *Dermatol Surg* 2000;26:55–60.

36. May M, Croxon GR, Klein SR. Bells palsy, management and sequelae using EMG rehabilitation, botulinum toxin and surgery. *Am J Otology* 1989;220–229.

37. Clark RP, Berris CE. Botulinum toxin: a treatment for facial asymmetry caused by facial nerve paralysis. *Plast Reconstr Surg* 1989;84:535–555.

38. Smet-Dielman H, Van de Heyrung PH, Tassigrin MJ. Botulinum toxin A injection in patients with facial nerve palsy. *Acta Otorhinolaryngol Belg* 1993;47:2359–2363.

39. Armstrong MWJ, Mountain RE, Murray JAM. Treatment of facial synkinesis and facial asymmetry with botulinum toxin type A following facial nerve palsy. *Clin Otolaryngol* 1996;21:15–20.

40. Carruthers J, Stubbs HA. Botulinum toxin for benign essential blepharospasm, hemifacial spasm and age-related lower eyelid entropion. *Can J Neurol Sci* 1987; 14:42–45.

41. Borodic GE. Botulinum A toxin for (expressionistic) ptosis overcorrection after frontalis sling. *Ophthal Plast Reconstr Surg* 1992;8:137–142.

42. Carruthers A, Carruthers JDA. Botulinum toxin in the treatment of glabellar frown lines and other facial wrinkles. In: Jankovic J, Hallett M, eds. *Therapy with botulinum toxin.* New York: Marcel Dekker, 1994;577–595.

43. West TB, Alster TS. Effect of botulinum toxin type A on movement-associated rhytides following CO_2 laser resurfacing. *Dermatol Surg* 1999;25:259–261.

44. Carruthers J, Carruthers A. Combining botulinum toxin injection and laser for facial rhytides. In: Coleman WP, Lawrence N, eds. *Skin resurfacing.* Baltimore, MD: Williams & Wilkins, 1998:235–243.

45. Carruthers J, Carruthers A, Zelichowska A. The power of combined therapies: BOTOX and ablative facial laser resurfacing. *Am J Cos Surg* 2000;17:129–131.

46. Fagien S. Botulinum toxin can eradicate rhytides, improve overall results. *Ophthalmology Times International* 1998;Jan/Feb:20–22.

47. Gassner HG, Sherris DA, Otley CC. Treatment of facial wounds with botulinum toxin A improves cosmetic outcome in primates. *Plast Reconstr Surg* 2000;105: 1948–1955.

Scientific and Therapeutic Aspects of Botulinum Toxin
edited by M.F. Brin, J. Jankovic, and M. Hallett
Lippincott Williams & Wilkins, Philadelphia, © 2002.

28

Botulinum Toxin for Achalasia and Related Disorders

Willemijntje A. Hoogerwerf, Dennis D. Dykstra, and Pankaj J. Pasricha

In addition to its potent skeletal neuromuscular blockade, botulinum neurotoxin type A (BTX-A) inhibits smooth muscle activity (1). This inhibition was first suggested *in vitro,* when the toxin interfered with cholinergic signaling in the myenteric nervous system (2). Based on these *in vitro* studies, it was later demonstrated *in vivo* that BTX-A could inhibit contraction of the gastrointestinal smooth muscle (3).

ACHALASIA

Achalasia is a gastrointestinal motility disorder characterized by dysphagia for solids and liquids, regurgitation of undigested food, chest pain, and weight loss. Achalasia occurs in one to two patients per 200,000 population per year. The diagnosis is confirmed by manometric characteristics including an elevated lower esophageal sphincter (LES) resting pressure, aperistalsis of the esophagus, and incomplete sphincter relaxation after swallowing. Failure of LES relaxation (Fig. 28.1) may occur because of selective degeneration of nitrinergic inhibitory neurons in the surrounding myenteric plexus (4–6). As a result, the smooth-muscle tone is mainly under control of excitatory cholinergic nerves leading to a functional obstruction of the esophagus. The current methods of treatment for achalasia have focused on reducing the LES pressure to enable the patient to eat without the disabling symptoms of this disorder. These methods include mechanical disruption of the LES fibers either by pneumatic dilatation (PD) or by surgical myotomy.

Speculating that botulinum toxin (BTX) could restore the muscle tone by inhibition of acetylcholine (ACh) release from excitatory cholinergic nerves, Pasricha et al. first investigated the effect of BTX type A in piglets (3). BTX injections into the LES of piglets significantly decreased LES pressure as compared to both baseline and saline-injected controls. Pasricha et al. were also the first to demonstrate that BTX-A can be effective for the treatment of achalasia in a double-blind, placebo-controlled study (7). The efficacy of BTX-A injections ranged from 65% to 90% following a single injection. Associated clinical obstructive symptoms such as dysphagia and regurgitation were markedly improved.

Eighty to 100 U of BTX-A is injected endoscopically approximately 1 cm above the Z line into the LES in four aliquots of 1.0 mL, using a standard sclerotherapy needle (7). Higher doses of toxin and better localization by use of endoscopic ultrasound have not improved results (8). Patients are discharged from the endoscopy unit after postsedation requirements have been met and are allowed to eat later in the day. Improvement in symptoms is usually observed only after 24 hours; peak effects occur even later in some patients.

Several formulations of BTX-A are available. A comparison between BOTOX 100 U and DYSPORT 250 U showed a similar efficacy for up to 6 months of follow-up (9).

Injection of BTX-A is considered safe. Transient chest pain and heartburn are the most commonly reported complications of injections. Paraesophageal tissue inflammation and esophageal wall injury has been reported (10). Re-

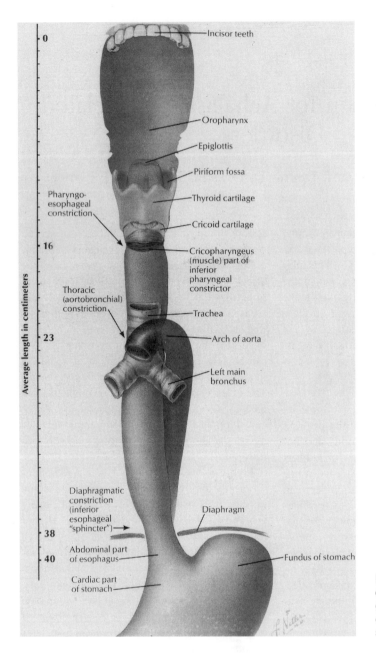

FIG. 28.1. The common types of dysfunction of the esophagus are shown, including those of the lower and upper sphincter.

cently, reports from the surgical literature have suggested that identification of tissue planes is technically more difficult in patients who require laparoscopic Heller myotomy after previous BTX injections (11). This has not translated, however, into a worse postsurgical outcome. Caution needs to be exercised to potential late side effects such as antibody development against the toxin, although this has never been reported in this indication. One case report described fatal heart block following treatment with BTX, but there was little to suggest that two events were causally related (12). Overall, the treatment appears to be remarkably safe, and is therefore of particular value in the elderly and in high-risk patients.

A variety of studies have been published in recent years on the effect of BTX-A injections in achalasia. In a study of the long-term efficacy of BTX-A treatment, Annese studied 57 patients with achalasia (13). Patients had a mean age of 51 years, 30 were male, and 27 were female. All patients had a baseline evaluation consisting of clinical assessment and esophageal manometry. They received an injection of 100 U of BTX-A (BOTOX) through a 2.3-mm sclerotherapy needle during an upper gastrointestinal endoscopy. Eight aliquots of 0.5 cc each (25 U/cc) were injected at two different levels of each quadrant of the LES. One month after treatment, 50 patients (88%) improved. After a mean follow-up of 24 (± 15) months (range, 6 to 48), 43 patients (75%) continued to do well, although repeat injections were required to avoid relapse. The authors speculate that the higher proportion of patients maintaining remission may be attributed to the use of a higher dose of toxin (100 U) over a wider area of the LES and earlier retreatment as compared to previous studies.

Kolbasnik et al. examined the long-term efficacy of intrasphincteric BTX-A in a prospective cohort study of 30 patients with achalasia (14). Follow-up consisted of clinical assessment, symptom scoring, and postinjection manometry. A good initial clinical response was seen in 23 of 30 patients (77%). Of these 23 responders, 7 (30%) had a sustained symptomatic response after a single injection (mean follow-up of 21 months). The remaining 16 initial responders (70%) eventually relapsed (mean initial response time of 11 months). Of these 16 patients, 9 have maintained good symptomatic relief with further BTX-A injections. The remaining seven patients opted for pneumatic dilatation or surgical myotomy. Five of the seven patients who had no initial response received a second injection, but again did not respond. Neither initial nor sustained response to BTX-A could be predicted based on gender, age, duration of illness, or previous pneumatic dilatation or esophageal motility before treatment. The authors concluded that 77% of patients with classical achalasia experienced a good symptomatic response after BTX-A injection and 30% of initial responders achieved symptomatic relief after a single injection. The initial responders who relapsed did well with subsequent injections.

A multicenter randomized study of intrasphincteric BTX-A compared the effect of different doses of BTX-A and identified predictors of response in achalasia patients (15). A total of 118 achalasia patients were randomized to receive one of three doses of BTX-A (BOTOX) in a single injection: 50 U, 100 U, and 200 U. Of those who received 100 U, responsive patients were reinjected with an identical dose after 30 days. Clinical and manometric assessments were performed at baseline, 30 days after the initial injection and at the end of follow-up (mean 12 months). Patients with a mean esophageal body contraction amplitude greater than 40 mm Hg in the distal two leads measured by manometry were diagnosed as having vigorous achalasia. Thirty days after the initial injection, 97 (82%) of the patients were considered responders without a clear dose-related effect. At the end of follow-up, relapse of symptoms were evident in 6 of 32 patients (19%) who received two injections of 100 U as compared with 14 of 30 (47%) and 15 of 35 (43%) in the 50 U and 200 U groups, respectively. Side effects reported by nine patients were mild and transient retrosternal or epigastric pain. These side effects did not appear to be dose dependent. The authors concluded that two injections of 100 U of BTX-A 30 days apart appeared to be the most effective therapeutic schedule. The presence of vigorous achalasia was the principal determinant of the response to BTX-A.

Vaezi and Richter reviewed several studies using BTX-A in the treatment of achalasia (16,17). They found that out of a total of 244 patients in 9 separate studies, BTX-A is effective in relieving symptoms initially in about 207 (85%) of the patients. However, this is a short-term response, with symptom recurrence reported in more than 50% of the initial responders by 6 months. In those responding to the first BTX-A injection, 76% will respond to a second injection with decreasing response to further injections. An overall initial resistance of BTX-A is present in up to 26% of patients who never show any clinical response. There was a time-dependent decline in clinical remission, with only 42% of the patients still in remission by 12 months (50 of 118 patients in 4 studies). Older patients (older than 60 years of age) and those with vigorous achalasia are more likely to have a sustained response (up to 1.5 years) to BTX-A. One author found the long-term symptom improvements in patients treated with BTX-A were not associated with a sustained decrease in LES pressure or esophageal barium column height, suggesting that BTX-A may be preferentially affecting esophageal sensory neurons (18).

Comparing BTX Injections to Pneumatic Dilatation

The common limitation with PD and BTX-A injection in the treatment of achalasia is the need for repeat intervention (20). A recent randomized controlled, double-blind study compared PD with BTX-A injections (18). The authors found that one to two BTX-A injections were as effective as PD in short-term (less than 12 months) relief of dysphagia. Other studies found that there is a higher long-term efficacy (more than 12 months) with PD as compared to BTX-A (21,22). The calculated mean duration of the effect of BTX-A for dysphagia and regurgitation on the basis of an intention to treat analysis was 7.3 and 8.5 months, respectively. Another study found that although the treatment efficacy of both techniques was similar, the initial treatment failure was higher with BTX-A injections (23). Patients fearful of perforation or those felt to be at high risk for more aggressive therapy may be the best candidates for BTX-A injections at this time (19). Both PD and intrasphincteric BTX-A injection can provide effective symptom relief for patients with achalasia. However, in general, pharmacologic therapy will have a temporizing effect only. It is therefore to be expected that a single injection of BTX-A, given its pharmacologic nature, will not reach similar efficacy when compared to PD. However, repeat injections given on an "as needed" basis will reach efficacy rates that are comparable to PD.

Cost-effectiveness

The incidence of achalasia is low and it is therefore unlikely that a study will be undertaken di-

rectly comparing the different treatment options. Several studies have addressed the issue of cost-effectiveness comparing surgery, PD, and BTX-A injections based on currently available data (24–26). Laparoscopic Heller myotomy is the most costly intervention despite higher short- and long-term efficacy (24). The calculated costs were $10,792, $3,111, and $3,723 for surgical myotomy, PD, and BTX-A, respectively. PD was less costly than BTX-A so long as the rates of PD efficacy and perforation were greater than 70% and less than 10%, respectively, and the cost of BTX-A, including endoscopy, was more than $450. A Canadian cost minimization analysis comparing BTX-A to PD suggested that BTX-A injections were less costly only if the life expectancy was less than 2 years (25).

BTX for High-risk Patients

While evaluating the effects of BTX-A on elderly patients with achalasia, Wehrmann found that the mean remission period for their patients after a single injection of 100 U (BOTOX) to be 5 months (range, 2 to 9 months) (27). The authors note that the duration of BTX-A reported in the literature for patients with achalasia is in the range of 2 to 12 months. Gordon et al. studied the effects of BTX-A in achalasia patients at high surgical risk because of age or concomitant medical problems such as severe coronary artery disease, diabetes, and obstructive lung disease (28). Sixteen patients underwent an upper endoscopy with four-quadrant BTX-A injections. All patients tolerated the procedure well. Seventy-five percent of patients (12/16) demonstrated clinical improvement at 1 month; however, five patients did develop recurrent symptoms within 6 months.

Because older patients are more likely to respond to BTX and the procedure is relatively safe, BTX may be a good alternative for those elderly patients who are considered to be at high risk for more invasive procedures such as pneumatic dilatation or surgical myotomy. Symptomatic relief will allow for optimization of the physical and nutritional status in a subgroup of high-risk patients, so that a more invasive procedure, if necessary at all, can be scheduled electively under optimal circumstances.

Botulinum Toxin as a Diagnostic Tool

Katzka et al. used the response to BTX-A as a means to support a diagnosis of achalasia in patients with achalasia-like symptoms but with atypical manometric findings (29). Response to BTX-A injections can therefore be used as a guide that may justify the use of more invasive therapy.

BTX-A After Failure of Myotomy or Pneumatic Dilatation

Only one study has reported the use of BTX-A injection in patients that failed prior therapy with surgical myotomy or pneumatic dilatation (30). Five patients were included; two patients underwent a surgical Heller myotomy and three patients underwent PD. Four patients responded favorably and were asymptomatic at the 6-month follow-up; three patients required a second injection after the first 3 months for recurrence of dysphagia (with an equally good response).

Achalasia in the Pediatric Population

Achalasia is rare in children. Injection of BTX-A into the lower esophageal sphincter has been studied as an alternative to esophageal pneumatic dilatation or surgical myotomy in 23 pediatric patients (31). Nineteen patients initially responded to BTX-A. The mean duration of effect was 4.2 months ±4.0 (SD). At the end of the study period (3.5 years), three patients were repeat responders, three experienced dysphagia but did not receive pneumatic dilatation or surgery, three underwent pneumatic dilatation, eight underwent surgery, three underwent pneumatic dilatation with subsequent surgery, and three awaited surgery. The authors concluded that BTX-A effectively initiated the resolution of symptoms associated with achalasia in children. However, one-half of patients are expected to need an additional procedure approximately 7 months after one injection session.

OTHER GASTROINTESTINAL SMOOTH-MUSCLE DISORDERS

Diffuse Esophageal Spasms

BTX-A has also been tried in esophageal motility disorders other than achalasia. Cassidy et al. treated 10 patients with manometrically proven diffuse esophageal spasm by BTX-A injection into the LES (32). Sixty days after injection, 80% of the patients had responded by a 50% or more decrease in pre- and posttreatment symptom scores for dysphagia, chest pain, and regurgitation.

Upper Esophageal Sphincter Dysfunction

BTX-A has been used for treatment of upper esophageal sphincter (UES) dysfunction (33). UES dysfunction is characterized by either incomplete or poorly coordinated opening of the UES during the pharyngeal phase of swallowing (Fig. 28.1). This may lead to hypopharyngeal retention and sometimes to laryngeal penetration or tracheal aspiration of swallowed food. Neuromuscular diseases or postoperative changes can cause UES dysfunction. In most cases, however, the cause is unknown. Treatments are aimed at lowering the resting pressure of the cricopharyngeal muscle. These include cricopharyngeal myotomy and bouginage (34–36). Injection of BTX-A into the posterior and both lateral sides of the cricopharyngeal muscle has been done using a rigid laryngoscope and a small butterfly cannula. One hundred units of BTX-A were diluted in 2.5 cc of sterile 0.9% saline without preservative. A total of 0.75 cc or 30 U of BTX-A (BOTOX) was injected (33). Hypopharyngeal retention or laryngeal penetration of barium was significantly reduced in four of seven patients. On follow-up at 4 to 6 weeks, clinical symptom scores improved in all patients. One patient was free of symptoms, mild dysphagia persisted in six patients, and moderate dysphagia persisted in three patients. The authors suggested that one reason for the still incomplete opening of the UES in the majority of patients may be the low dose of toxin used. However, the total dose injected into the UES is limited because of the proximity of the UES to the larynx and adjacent parts of the hypopharynx. The results of this study support the use of BTX-A for treatment of UES in selected patients with pure UES dysfunction and as a valuable diagnostic tool to identify patients who are unlikely to benefit from a cricopharyngeal myotomy (33).

Internal Anal Sphincter Disorders

Anismus. BTX-A has also been used in the treatment of disorders of the anal sphincters (1). Anismus is a disorder characterized by inappropriate contraction of the anal sphincters on straining. This can result in intractable constipation. Colonic resection for this disorder has had variable results. BTX-A has been injected into the puborectalis muscle in a group of patients with anismus to decrease paradoxical contraction of the puborectalis muscle (37). Significant improvement was seen in most patients with symptom scores and decrease of voluntary anal canal pressures.

Anal fissures. BTX-A has also been injected into the external or internal anal sphincters to transiently relieve pain and sphincter spasm facilitating complete healing of anal fissures (38–41). In a double-blind, placebo-controlled study of BTX-A for the treatment of chronic anal fissure in 30 consecutive symptomatic patients, 87% of patients had symptomatic relief after BTX-A injections and 73% were healed as compared with 27% and 13% in the saline injected groups, respectively (39). Transient fecal incontinence may occur with the injection of the toxin in the anal sphincters to treat anismus or fissures (38). Perianal thrombosis subsequent to BTX-A injection into the external anal sphincter has also been reported (42).

Hirschsprung's Disease

BTX-A has been used for persistent constipation in children after pull-through surgery for Hirschsprung's disease (43). Most children with Hirschsprung's disease have an excellent result after pull-through surgery. However, some experience persistent constipation caused by a hypertensive internal anal sphincter (IAS). Anal myectomy has been advocated for this problem, but it may result in permanent injury to the IAS and is not universally effective. The authors hypothesized that injection of BTX-A into the IAS should lower the pressure and produce the same functional result as anal myectomy but without the risk of permanent sphincter injury. Four-quadrant intrasphincteric BTX-A injections (total dose of 15 U) were performed in four children with Hirschsprung's disease. Resting IAS pressure decreased in all children 4 to 8 weeks after injection. These preliminary results suggest that BTX-A may be useful in the treatment of children with Hirschsprung's disease.

Sphincter of Oddi Dysfunction

Sphincter of Oddi dysfunction (SOD) is a disorder characterized by right upper-quadrant and epigastric pain occurring most commonly in postcholecystectomy patients (1). SOD results from either true sphincter stenosis or from a spasm of this sphincter. The treatment for this entity is problematic. Endoscopic sphincterotomy is performed in some of these patients to relieve the biliary obstruction caused by the stenosed or spastic sphincter of Oddi. Response to this treatment is not uniform and many patients have continued pain. Sphincterotomy is associated with major risks such as bleeding, pancreatitis, and perforation (44). An alternative approach to patients in whom the risk:benefit ratio of the treatment is uncertain is to use a diagnostic/therapeutic trial. The principle behind such a trial is to achieve the desired pathophysiologic effect (in this case reduction of SO pressure) in a simple noninvasive manner and then to observe the effects on the target symptoms (in this case pain). A positive association helps establish cause and effect and justifies the use of permanent, even if more invasive, treatment (in this case an endoscopic sphincterotomy). A negative association disproves a cause-and-effect relationship and avoids an unnecessary and risky procedure. Until recently, such a trial was difficult to conduct in patients with suspected SOD because of the lack of a reliable noninvasive method of achieving SO pressure reduction. Intrasphincteric BTX appears to offer a simple and relatively safe method of reducing SO pressure and its use as a therapeutic trial appears to have considerable potential. A pilot study of BTX-A injection into the sphincter of Oddi in patients with SOD documented a significant reduction in sphincter pressure and an improvement in bile flow (45). However, these patients showed no improvement in abdominal pain. In a more recent study, Wehrmann and colleagues (46) enrolled 22 patients with postcholecystectomy manometrically confirmed type III SOD patients. Patients received intrasphincteric BOTOX (100 U). Initial symptomatic responses were analyzed 6 weeks later. Overall, 11 of the 12 patients who responded to BTX injection, versus 2 of the 10 patients who did not gain pain relief after BTX injection, later benefitted from endoscopic sphincterotomy ($p < 0.01$). With the exception of one patient with mild pancreatitis (4.5%), no side effects were observed after endoscopic BTX injection The authors concluded that the clinical response to BTX injection can predict whether SOD patients will gain long-term benefit from endoscopic sphincterotomy.

Other authors have also reported encouraging data on the use of BTX-A in patients with idiopathic recurrent pancreatitis and suspected pancreatic sphincter dysfunction (47,48). Additional studies on the use of BTX-A for sphincter of Oddi dysfunction are eagerly awaited.

Trials of BTX are also underway in patients with diabetic and other forms of gastroparesis or delayed gastric emptying. The toxin is injected into the pylorus with the rationale that inappropriate spasm may contribute, at least in part, to the impairment in gastric emptying (49). Other suggested gastrointestinal indications for BTX-A include treatment of infantile hypertrophic pyloric stenosis and to transiently decrease gastric emptying as a treatment of obesity (50).

CONCLUSIONS

The demonstration that BTX could affect visceral smooth-muscle tone has opened an entirely new therapeutic area for this agent. As discussed in this review, the use of BTX for achalasia appears to be established. As gastroenterologists become more experienced and comfortable with BTX, new indications will continue to emerge in the near future. However, it must be pointed out that much needs to be learned about the biologic effects of this agent on the gastrointestinal tract, which cannot be simply extrapolated from the skeletal muscle literature.

REFERENCES

1. Bhutani MS. Gastrointestinal uses of botulinum toxin. *Am J Gastroenterol* 1997;92:929–933.
2. MacKenzie I, Burnstock G, Dolly JO. The effects of purified botulinum neurotoxin type A on cholinergic, adrenergic and non-adrenergic, atropine-resistant autonomic neuromuscular transmission. *Neuroscience* 1982; 7:997–1006.
3. Pasricha PJ, Ravich WJ, Kalloo AN. Effects of intrasphincteric botulinum toxin on the lower esophageal sphincter in piglets. *Gastroenterology* 1993;105: 1045–1049.
4. Csendes A, Smok G, Braghetto I, et al. Gastroesophageal sphincter pressure and histological changes in distal esophagus in patients with achalasia of the esophagus. *Dig Dis Sci* 1985;30:941–945.
5. Aggestrup S, Uddman R, Sundler F, et al. Lack of vasoactive intestinal peptide nerves in esophageal achalasia. *Gastroenterology* 1983;84:924.
6. Mearin F, Mourelle M, Guarner F, et al. Patients with achalasia lack nitric oxide synthase in the gastroesophageal junction. *Eur J Clin Invest* 1993;23:724.
7. Pasricha PJ, Ravich WJ, Hendrix TR, et al. Intrasphincteric botulinum toxin for the treatment of achalasia. *N Engl J Med* 1995;332:774–778.
8. Schiano T, Parkman H, Millier LS, et al. Use of botulinum toxin in the treatment of achalasia. *Dig Dis* 1998; 16:14–22.
9. Annese V, Bassotti G, Coccia G, et al. Comparison of two different formulations of botulinum toxin A for the treatment of oesophageal achalasia. *Aliment Pharmacol Ther* 1999;13:1347–1350.
10. Eaker, EY, Gordon, JM, Vogel, SB. Untoward effects of esophageal botulinum toxin injection in the treatment of achalasia. *Dig Dis Sci* 1997;42:724.
11. Bonavina L, Incarbone R, Antoniazzi L, et al. Previous endoscopic treatment does not affect complication rate and outcome of laparoscopic Heller myotomy and anterior fundoplication for oesophageal achalasia. *Ital J Gastroenterol Hepatol* 1999; 31(9):827–830.
12. Malnick SDH, Metchnik L, Somin M, et al. Fatal heart block following treatment with botulinum toxin for achalasia. *Am J Gastroenterol* 2000;95(11):3333–3334.
13. Annese V, Basciani M, Borrelli O, et al. Intrasphincteric injection of botulinum toxin is effective in long-term treatment of esophageal achalasia. *Muscle Nerve* 1998; 21:1540–1542.
14. Kolbasnik J, Waterfall WE, Fachnie B, et al. Long-term

efficacy of botulinum toxin in classical achalasia: a prospective study. *Am J Gastroenterol* 1999;94: 3434–3439.

15. Annese V, Bassotti G, Coccia G, et al. A multicentre randomized study of intrasphincteric botulinum toxin in patients with oesophageal achalasia. *Gut* 2000;46: 597–600.

16. Vaezi MF, Richter JE. Current therapies for achalasia. *J Clin Gastroenterol* 1998;27:21–35.

17. Vaezi MF. Achalasia: Diagnosis and management. *Semin Gastroint Dis* 1999;10:103–112.

18. Vaezi MF, Richter JE, Wilcox M, et al. Botulinum toxin versus pneumatic dilation in the treatment of achalasia: a randomized trial. *Gut* 1999;44:231–240.

19. Hoogerwerf WA, Pasricha PJ. Achalasia: treatment options revisited. *Can J Gastroenterol* 2000;14:406–409.

20. Annese V, Basciani M, Perri F, et al. Controlled trial of botulinum toxin injection versus placebo and pneumatic dilation in achalasia. *Gastroenterology* 1996;111: 1418–1424.

21. Vaezi M, Richter JE, Wilcox M, et al. One-year follow-up: pneumatic dilatation more effective than botulinum toxin. *Gastroenterology* 1997;112:A318.

22. Muehldorfer SM, Schneider TH, Hochberger J, et al. Esophageal achalasia: intrasphincteric injection of botulinum toxin A versus balloon dilation. *Endoscopy* 1999; 31:517–521.

23. Bansal R, Koshy S, Sheiman JM, et al. A randomized trial of Witzel pneumatic dilation versus intrasphincteric injection of botulinum toxin for achalasia. *Gastroenterology* 1995;110:A56.

24. Imperiale TF, O'Connor JB, Vaezi MF, et al. A cost-minimization analysis of alternative treatment strategies for achalasia. *Am J Gastroenterol* 2000;95:2737–2745.

25. Panaccione R, Gregor JC, Reynolds RP, et al. Intrasphincteric botulinum toxin versus pneumatic dilatation for achalasia: a cost minimization analysis. *Gastrointest Endosc* 1999;50:492.

26. Spiess AE, Kahrilas PJ. Treating achalasia. From whalebone to laparoscope. *JAMA* 1998;280:638–642.

27. Wehrmann T, Kokabpick H, Jacobi V, et al. Long-term results of endoscopic injection of botulinum toxin in elderly achalasic patients with tortuous megaesophagus or epiphrenic diverticulum. *Endoscopy* 1999;31: 352–358.

28. Gordon, JM, Eaker, EY. Prospective study of esophageal botulinum toxin injection in high-risk achalasia patients. *Am J Gastroenterol* 1997;92:1812.

29. Katzka, DA, Castell, DO. Use of botulinum toxin as a diagnostic/therapeutic trial to help clarify an indication for definitive therapy in patients with achalasia. *Am J Gastroenterol* 1999;94:637.

30. Annese V, Basciani M, Lombardi G, et al. Perendoscopic injection of botulinum toxin is effective in achalasia after failure of myotomy or pneumatic dilatation. *Gastrointest Endosc* 1996;44:461.

31. Hurwitz M, Bahar RJ, Ament ME, et al. Evaluation of the use of botulinum toxin in children with achalasia. *J Pediatr Gastroenterol Nutr* 2000;30:509–514.

32. Cassidy MJ, Schiano TD, Adrain AL, et al. Botulinum

toxin injection for the treatment of symptomatic diffuse esophageal spasm. *Am J Gastroenterol* 1996;91:1884.

33. Alberty J, Oelerich M, Ludwig D, et al. Efficacy of botulinum toxin A for treatment of upper esophageal sphincter dysfunction. *Laryngoscope* 2000;110: 1151–1156.

34. Lindgren S, Ekberg O. Cricopharyngeal myotomy in the treatment of dysphagia. *Clin Otolaryngol* 1990;15: 221–227.

35. Lernau OZ, Sherzer E, Mogle P, et al. Congenital cricopharyngeal achalasia treatment by dilatations. *J Pediatr Surg* 1984;19:202–203.

36. Blitzer A, Brin MF. Use of botulinum toxin for diagnosis and management of cricopharyngeal achalasia. *Otolaryngol Head Neck Surg* 1997;116:328–330.

37. Hallan RI, Williams NS, Melling J, et al. Treatment of anismus in intractable constipation with botulinum A toxin. *Lancet* 1988;2:714–717.

38. Gui D, Cassetta D, Anastasio G, et al. Botulinum toxin for chronic anal fissure. *Lancet* 1994;344:1127–1128.

39. Maria G, Cassetta E, Gui D, et al. A comparison of botulinum toxin and saline injection for the treatment of chronic anal fissure. *N Engl J Med* 1998;338:217–220.

40. Jost WH. One hundred cases of anal fissure treated with botulin toxin: early and long-term results. *Dis Colon Rectum* 1997;40:1029–1032.

41. Madalinski M, Jagiello K, Labon M, et al. Botulinum toxin injection into only one point in the external anal sphincter: a modification of the treatment for chronic anal fissure. *Endoscopy* 1999;31:S63.

42. Jost WH, Schanne S, Mlitz H, et al. Perianal thrombosis following injection therapy into the external anal sphincter using botulinum toxin. *Dis Colon Rectum* 1995;38: 781.

43. Langer JC, Birnbaum E. Preliminary experience with intrasphincteric botulinum toxin for persistent constipation after pull-through for Hirschsprung's disease. *J Pediatr Surg* 1997;32:1061–1062.

44. Sherman S, Ruffolo TA, Hawes RH, et al. Complications of endoscopic sphincterotomy. *Gastroenterology* 1991;101:1068–1075.

45. Pasricha PJ, Miskovsky EP, Kalloo AN. Intrasphincteric injection of botulinum toxin for suspected sphincter of Oddi dysfunction. *Gut* 1994;35:1319–1321.

46. Wehrmann T, Seifert H, Seipp M, et al. Endoscopic injection of botulinum toxin for biliary sphincter of Oddi dysfunction. *Endoscopy* 1998;30:702–747.

47. Muehldorfer SM, Hahn EG, Ell C. Botulinum toxin injection as a diagnostic tool for verification of sphincter of Oddi dysfunction causing recurrent pancreatitis. *Endoscopy* 1997;29:120–124.

48. Wehrmann T, Schmitt TH, Arndt A, et al. Endoscopic injection of botulinum toxin in patients with recurrent acute pancreatitis due to pancreatic sphincter of Oddi dysfunction. *Aliment Pharmacol Ther* 2000 14(11): 1469–1477.

49. Wiesel PH, Schneider R, Dorta G, et al. Botulinum toxin for refractory postoperative pyloric spasm. *Endoscopy* 1997;29(2):132.

50. Gui D, De Gaetano A, Spada PL, et al. Botulinum toxin injected in the gastric wall reduces body weight and food intake in rats. *Aliment Pharmacol Ther* 2000;14(6): 829–834.

Scientific and Therapeutic Aspects of Botulinum Toxin
edited by M.F. Brin, J. Jankovic, and M. Hallett
Lippincott Williams & Wilkins, Philadelphia, © 2002.

29

Treatment of Focal Hyperhidrosis with Botulinum Toxin A

Markus Naumann

Focal hyperhidrosis is a relatively common condition; it can be defined as excessive sweating of the palms and soles of the feet, axillae, and face. It may be both a distressing and a genuinely disabling condition. Usually it manifests itself during the second or third decade of life. A positive family history for the condition in 30% to 50% of cases suggests a genetic component (1). The pathophysiology of essential focal hyperhidrosis is unknown at present. The sweat glands and their innervation do not show any histologic abnormalities. A dysfunction of the central sympathetic nervous system is suspected (2,3).

Hyperhidrosis can be classified as generalized or focal. Only patients with focal hyperhidrosis are amenable to botulinum neurotoxin (BoNT) treatment. The most common form of focal hyperhidrosis is essential or *idiopathic focal hyperhidrosis* resulting from overactivity of the sweat glands of the palms, axillae, soles of the feet, and face. In about 60% of cases, the palms and soles of the feet (palmoplantar hyperhidrosis) are affected, and in 30% to 40% of cases, the axillae are affected (4). Facial sweating is less frequent and affects up to 10% of patients with idiopathic hyperhidrosis. A special form of focal hyperhidrosis is *gustatory sweating* occurring on the cheek in response to salivation. It is the result of misdirection of autonomic nerve fibers after surgery or diseases of the parotid gland and may be observed in some other rare conditions. Focal hyperhidrosis may also be associated with spinal cord injury and with some polyneuropathies. *Ross syndrome* is a rare form of focal hyperhidrosis of unknown etiology, which is characterized by progressive anhidrosis caused by degeneration of sudomotor fibers, and which may be associated with disabling compensatory hyperhidrosis, mostly at the trunk. *Generalized hyperhidrosis* with sweating occurring over the whole body can be secondary to a variety of metabolic diseases, chronic infections, alcoholism, and malignancy.

The consequences of hyperhidrosis include dehydration and maceration of the skin, which may result in secondary infections of the skin.

If there is no causal disease, or if the underlying disease cannot be controlled sufficiently, there are some therapeutic approaches: Current first-line treatment for focal hyperhidrosis is usually topical application of acids, aldehydes, and metal salts. Anticholinergic drugs are quite effective but have unpleasant side effects such as dry mouth and blurred vision. Tap-water iontophoresis is an option for patients suffering from palmar hyperhidrosis but is a time-consuming procedure. Many hyperhidrosis sufferers eventually resort to surgery. Excision and suction curettage of sweat glands are sometimes used in the axillae to remove the sweat coils in the skin. Since the introduction of transthoracic endoscopic sympathectomy, this operation has become an important treatment for severe cases of palmar hyperhidrosis because it provides a lasting relief in many cases. However, there may be some serious side effects (5,6).

BOTULINUM TOXIN TREATMENT OF HYPERHIDROSIS

Anhidrosis is a well known effect of botulism, as described in 1822 by Justinus Kerner (7,8), and was also noted as a side effect of BoNT serotype A (BoNT-A) used in treating hemifacial spasm. Subsequently, BoNT-A was shown to abolish physiologic sweating in healthy volunteers (9,10).

After the first report of BoNT-A use in a patient with palmar hyperhidrosis in 1997 (11), several smaller open and controlled studies were published (4,12–19). All these studies were mainly performed in axillary and palmar sweating, whereas reports on other indications such as plantar, truncal, or forehead sweating are sparse. Only recently, the results of two large placebo-controlled, double-blind studies on botulinum toxin type treatment of axillary hyperhidrosis were reported (20,21). Table 29.1 provides detailed information on the sites of injection, the doses used, and the duration of action after injections of BoNT-A for hyperhidrosis from the literature.

AXILLARY AND PALMAR SWEATING

The beneficial effect of BoNT-A on reducing *axillary hyperhidrosis* has been shown in several mainly open-label studies (4,13,14,17,22–25) and two recent large placebo-controlled, double-blind trials (20,21). In open studies, the doses required for the treatment of one axilla were quite constantly around 50 mouse units (mu) BOTOX or 250 mu DYSPORT. This was sufficient in most patients to completely abolish axillary sweating (Fig. 29.1). The duration of the BoNT-A action was at least 4 months and reached 7 to 12 months in many cases. Injection

of higher doses (24) had no convincingly prolonged effect on hyperhidrosis compared with lower doses (25) and is generally not recommended because it might lead to a higher rate of side effects and an increased risk of antibody formation. Side effects included painful injections and small local hematomas.

A large multicenter, randomized, placebo-controlled trial (20) enrolled 320 patients with persistent bilateral primary axillary hyperhidrosis. Patients were randomly assigned to receive either BoNT-A (BOTOX 50 U per axilla; $n = 242$) or placebo ($n = 78$) by 10 to 15 intradermal injections evenly distributed within the hyperhidrotic area of each axilla. The primary outcome was the percent of treatment responders (patients with an equal to or greater than 50% reduction from baseline of spontaneous sweat production, measured gravimetrically) in each treatment group. Satisfaction with the treatment was rated using a patient's global assessment of treatment satisfaction scale. BoNT-A was significantly superior to placebo at all posttreatment time points with respect to the incidence of responders, reduction in sweat production, reduction in area of sweating, and patient satisfaction ($p < 0.001$). At week 4, 93.8% of patients treated with BoNT-A were responders as compared with 35.9% of the placebo group, and by week 16 these values were 82% and 20.5%, respectively. The mean percentage reduction in sweat production at week 4 was 83.5% and 20.8% for the BoNT-A and the placebo-treated groups, respectively. Only few adverse events were reported. It was con-

TABLE 29.1. *Selection of larger studies (more than 10 patients) on BoNT-A treatment of focal axillary or palmar hyperhidrosis. One side placebo, other side BoNT-A*

Author	Year	Design	Region	No.	Dose per site	Duration
Naumann[13]	1998	open	palmar, axillary	11	30 to 50 U BOTOX	>5 mo
Glogau[22]	1998	open	axillary	12	50 U BOTOX	4 to 7 mo
Schnider[17]	1999	controlled	axillary	13	250 U DYSPORT	>3 mo
Naver[23]	1999	open	axillary	55	32 to 100 U BOTOX	3 to >14 mo
Karamfilov[25]	2000	open	axillary	24	200 U BOTOX	7 to 10 mo
Heckmann[21]	2001	controlled	axillary	140	100/200 U DYSPORT	>6 mo
Naumann[20]	2001	controlled	axillary	320	50 U BOTOX	mean 7 mo
Schnider[12]	1997	controlled	palmar	11	120 U DYSPORT	>3 mo
Naver[23]	1999	open	palmar	94	120 to 220 U BOTOX	3 to >14 mo
Solomon[26]	2000	open	palmar	20	165 U BOTOX	4 to 9 mo

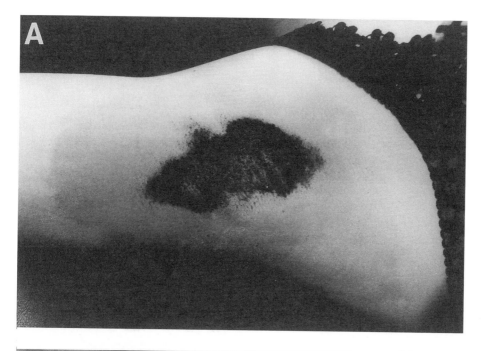

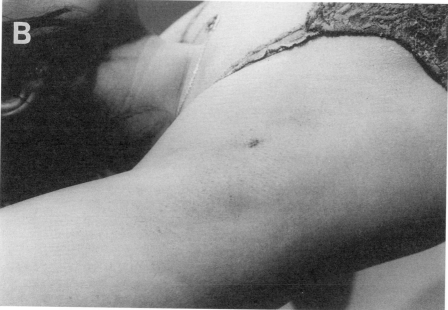

FIG. 29.1. Axillary hyperhidrosis (**A**) before treatment (Minor's iodine starch test) and (**B**) 2 weeks after intradermal injections of BoNT-A.

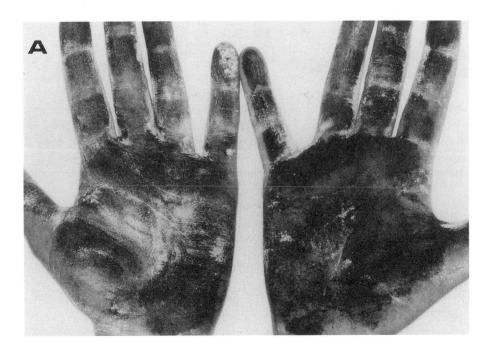

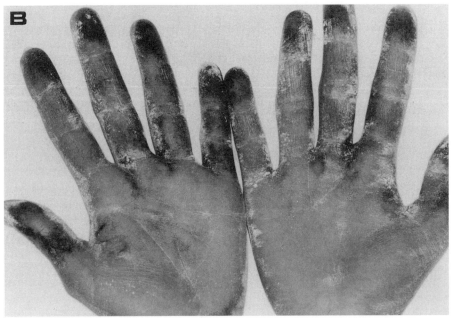

FIG. 29.2. Palmar hyperhidrosis (**A**) before treatment (Minor's iodine starch test) and (**B**) 2 weeks after intradermal injections of BoNT-A.

cluded that BoNT-A (BOTOX) is a safe and effective treatment for primary axillary hyperhidrosis with high patient satisfaction. Similar results were obtained by another controlled trial on 145 patients using 100 and 200 mu DYSPORT per axilla (one side was treated with placebo, the other side received BoNT-A) (21).

The positive effect of BoNT-A on *palmar hyperhidrosis* (Fig. 29.2) has been demonstrated by some open studies (4,13,14,18,23,27) and by one small double-blind placebo-controlled trial (12). The required total doses were higher than in the treatment of axillary hyperhidrosis because of the larger area to be injected (palms and fingers). In a few studies quantifying the sweat reduction after BoNT-A (4,12–14), a significant decrease of sweating could be demonstrated after injection, well in accordance with the subjective estimation by the patients (12). The duration of action varied between 4 and 12 months, but was mainly within a range of 4 to 6 months. Side effects included small hematomas, slight transient weakness of small hand muscles caused by diffusion of the toxin, and painful injections. Injection pain can be reduced by administering a local nerve block of the median and ulnar nerves.

GUSTATORY SWEATING AND OTHER INDICATIONS

One open-label study showed a significant decrease of sweat production on the forehead after intradermal injections of botulinum toxin A (28). BoNT-A (BOTOX) was injected at multiple sites evenly distributed over the forehead (mean, 86 mu). The effect lasted at least 5 months in nine of the ten patients. Patients with excessive compensatory sweating associated with Ross syndrome can effectively be treated with BoNT-A (28).

Gustatory sweating (Frey's syndrome). BoNT-A has also been used as a highly effective treatment for gustatory sweating. In a large open study of 45 patients, there was a significant reduction of local facial sweating after injection of 21 mu BOTOX on average (range, 5 to 72 mu) and no recurrence of sweating was observed during the follow-up period of 6 months (30). A marked long-lasting improvement ranging from 11 to 36 months after a single injection was also observed in three other open studies (31–33) (Table 29.2). Thus, BoNT-A obviously has a particularly long-lasting effect on gustatory sweating, which may be related to the specific etiology of the condition.

REINJECTION

Patients have been repeatedly injected over a period of 3 years with a relatively constant and reproducible effect (Naumann, personal observation). In treating dystonia, a primary concern about repeated BoNT-A injections is triggering an immune response to BoNT-A, thereby generating neutralizing antibodies. Therefore, reinjections should be strictly avoided within 3 months after injection.

CONCLUSIONS

All studies performed so far indicate that BoNT-A is a safe and effective treatment for focal hyperhidrosis of the axillae and palms, of gustatory sweating, and some other rare conditions associated with focal hyperhidrosis. There is class I evidence for the efficacy of BoNT-A in axillary hyperhidrosis, and class II evidence for gustatory and palmar sweating (classification according to reference 33). At present, it appears that the duration of treatment is 4 to 6 months or longer, thereby exceeding the duration of BoNT-

TABLE 29.2. *Selected studies (more than 10 patients) on BoNT-A treatment of gustatory sweating (Frey's syndrome)*

Author	Year	Design	No.	Dose (mean)	Duration
Naumann[30]	1997	open	45	21 mu BOTOX	>6 mo
Bjerkhoel[31]	1997	open	15	37 mu BOTOX	>13 mo
Laskawi[32]	1998	open	19	31 mu BOTOX	11 to 27 mo
Laccourreye[33]	1999	open	33	86 mu DYSPORT	12 to 36 mo

A treatment of muscle contraction. The optimal and lowest dose for the treatment of axillary and palmar hyperhidrosis still needs to be defined to minimize dose related side effects, to lower the costs of treatment, and to reduce the risk of antibody formation. BoNT-A has the potential to replace current invasive and surgical techniques and should at least be considered as a viable alternative.

REFERENCES

1. Mosek A, Korczyn A. Hyperhidrosis in palms and soles. In: Korczyn A, ed. *Handbook of autonomic nervous system dysfunction.* New York: Marcel Dekker, 1995: 167–177.
2. Sato K, Hang H, Saga K, et al. Biology of sweat glands and their disorders. I. Normal sweat gland function. *J Am Acad Dermatol* 1989:20:537–563.
3. Sato K, Hang H, Saga K, et al. Biology of sweat glands and their disorders. II. Disorders of sweat gland function. *J Am Acad Dermatol* 1989;20:713–726.
4. Naver H, Aquilonius S-M. The treatment of focal hyperhidrosis with botulinum toxin. *Eur J Neurol* 1997; 4(Suppl 2):S75–S79.
5. Claes G, Drott C. Hyperhidrosis. *Lancet* 1994;1: 247–248.
6. Drott C, Gothberg G, Claes G. Endoscopic transthoracic sympathectomy: an efficient and safe method for the treatment of hyperhidrosis. *J Am Acad Dermatol* 1995; 33:78–81.
7. Kerner J. *Das Fettgift oder die Fettsäure und ihre Wirkungen auf den thierischen Organismus, ein Beytrag zur Untersuchung des in verdorbenen Würsten giftig wirkenden Stoffes.* Stuttgart: Tübingen, Cotta 1822.
8. Erbguth F, Naumann M. Justinus Kerner (1786–1862) and the "sausage poison." The first systematic description of the effects of botulinum toxin on the neuromuscular and autonomic nervous system in medical history. *Neurology* 1999;53:1850–1853.
9. Bushara KO, Park DM. Botulinum toxin and sweating. *J Neurol Neurosurg Psychiatry* 1994;57:1437–1438.
10. Chesire WP. Subcutaneous botulinum toxin type A inhibits regional sweating: an individual observation. *Clin Auton Res* 1996;6:123–124.
11. Naumann M, Flachenecker P, Bröcker E-B, et al. Botulinum toxin for palmar hyperhidrosis. *Lancet* 1997;349: 252.
12. Schnider P, Binder M, Auff E, et al. Double-blind trial of botulinum toxin for the treatment of focal hyperhidrosis of the palms. *Br J Neurol* 1997;136:548–552.
13. Naumann M, Hofmann U, Bergmann I, et al. Focal hyperhidrosis: effective treatment with intracutaneous botulinum toxin. *Arch Dermatol* 1998;134:301–304.
14. Naumann M, Bergmann I, Hofmann U, et al. Botulinum toxin for focal hyperhidrosis: technical considerations and improvements of application. *Br J Dermatol* 1998; 139:1123–1124.
15. Odderson IR. Axillary hyperhidrosis: treatment with botulinum toxin A. *Arch Phys Med Rehabil* 1998;79: 350–352.
16. Naumann M, Hamm H, Kinkelin I, et al. Botulinum toxin type A in the treatment of focal, axillary and palmar hyperhidrosis and other hyperhidrotic conditions. *Eur J Neurol* 1999;6:S111–S115.
17. Schnider P, Binder M, Kittler H, et al. A randomized, double-blind, placebo-controlled trial of botulinum toxin for severe axillary hyperhidrosis. *Br J Dermatol* 1999;140:677–680.
18. Shelley WB, Talanin NY, Shelley ED. Botulinum toxin therapy for palmar hyperhidrosis. *J Am Acad Dermatol* 1998;38:227–229.
19. Naumann M, Jost W, Toyka KV. Botulinum toxin in the treatment of neurological disorders of the autonomic nervous system. *Arch Neurol* 1999;56:914–916.
20. Naumann M, Lowe N, for the hyperhidrosis study group. A randomized, placebo-controlled, double-blind study of botulinum toxin type A in bilateral axillary hyperhidrosis. *BMJ* 2001;323:596–579.
21. Heckmann M, Ceballos-Baumann A, Plewig G. Botulinum toxin A for axillary hyperhidrosis (excessive sweating). *N Engl J Med* 2001;344:488–493.
22. Glogau RG. Botulinum A neurotoxin for axillary hyperhidrosis. *Dermatol Surg* 1998;24:817–819.
23. Naver H, Swartling C, Aquilonius S. Treatment of focal hyperhidrosis with botulinum toxin type A. Brief overview of methodology and 2 years' experience. *Eur J Neurol* 1999;6:S117–S120.
24. Heckmann M, Breit S, Ceballos-Baumann A, et al. Side-controlled intradermal injection of botulinum toxin A in recalcitrant axillary hyperhidrosis. *J Am Acad Dermatol* 1999;41:987–990.
25. Karamfilov T, Konra H, Karte K, et al. Relapse rate of botulinum toxin A therapy for axillary hyperhidrosis by dose increase. *Arch Dermatol* 2000;136:487–490.
26. Naver H, Swartling C, Aquilonius S-M. Palmar and axillary hyperhidrosis treated with botulinum toxin: one-year clinical follow-up. *Eur J Neurol* 2000;7:55–62.
27. Solomon B, Hayman R. Botulinum toxin type A therapy for palmar and digital hyperhidrosis. *J Am Acad Dermatol* 2000;42:1026–1029.
28. Kinkelin I, Hund M, Naumann M, et al. Effective treatment of frontal hyperhidrosis with botulinum toxin A. *Br J Dermatol* 2000;143:824–827.
29. Bergmann I, Dauphin M, Naumann M, et al. Selective degeneration of sudomotor fibers in Ross syndrome and successful treatment of compensatory hyperhidrosis with botulinum toxin. *Muscle Nerve* 1998;21: 1790–1793.
30. Naumann M, Zellner M, Toyka KV, et al. Treatment of gustatory sweating with botulinum toxin. *Ann Neurol* 1997;42:973–975.
31. Bjerkhoel A, Trobbe O. Frey's syndrome: treatment with botulinum toxin. *J Laryngol Otol* 1997;111: 839–844.
32. Laskawi R, Drobik C, Schönebeck C. Up-to-date report of botulinum toxin type A treatment in patients with gustatory sweating (Frey's syndrome). *Laryngoscope* 1998;108:381–384.
33. Laccourreye O, Akl E, Gutierrez-Fonseca R, et al. Recurrent gustatory sweating (Frey's syndrome) after intracutaneous injection of botulinum toxin type A. *Arch Otolaryngol Head Neck Surg* 1999;125:282–286.
34. Deleted in proof.

Scientific and Therapeutic Aspects of Botulinum Toxin
edited by M.F. Brin, J. Jankovic, and M. Hallett
Lippincott Williams & Wilkins, Philadelphia, © 2002.

30

The Use of Botulinum Toxins in the Management of Myofascial Pain and Other Conditions Associated with Painful Muscle Spasm

Mike A. Royal

Botulinum toxins (BTX) are potent neurotoxins produced by *Clostridium botulinum* that block acetylcholine (ACh) release at the neuromuscular junction to produce flaccid paralysis. In controlled amounts, they produce temporary and fully reversible chemodenervation (typically lasting several months) with minimal risk of systemic adverse effects. These advantages have prompted clinicians to use BTX in a wide variety of conditions associated with muscle spasm or hypertonicity (1), including focal dystonia (2), cervical dystonia (3), spasmodic dysphonia (4), oromandibular dystonia (5), and temporomandibular disorder (6). Additionally, BTX are helpful in other pain conditions such as tension-type (7) and migraine (8) headache and refractory myofascial pain syndrome (9). Although cosmetic injection to reduce facial wrinkling (10) is likely the most familiar application for BTX, there has been tremendous interest in and clinical study of their potential for therapeutic efficacy in chronic pain and headache (12–16), especially because clinical observations and animal data point to a potential direct antinociceptive effect for BTX in addition to any muscle-tone reduction. This chapter summarizes the clinical studies evaluating botulinum toxins as potential therapeutic agents in refractory cases of myofascial pain or other conditions associated with painful muscle spasm.

Historically, BOTOX [Botulinum toxin type A (BTX-A), Allergan] has been the only commercially available BTX in the United States, but the recent addition of MYOBLOC [Botulinum toxin type B (BTX-B), Elan Pharmaceuticals] and the potential introduction of DYSPORT (BTX-A, Ipsen) give clinicians a choice in BTX use. Although the net effect of each BTX is to block acetylcholine release, one must be careful, until more data specific to BTX-B is developed, in taking data derived from clinical studies of BTX-A and applying it to BTX-B. There may be more than just potency differences to take into account. Although each of the commercially available BTX ultimately block acetylcholine release, structures, target sites for activity, commercial formulations, storage and handling guidelines, approved indications, and dosing are quite different. Additionally, although the data is somewhat limited, antibody responses may be different as well. BTX-A has been around much longer and all of the published pain and headache clinical research used BTX-A (either BOTOX or DYSPORT).

MYOFASCIAL PAIN SYNDROME

Myofascial pain syndrome (MPS) (17) is a regional pain syndrome defined by the presence of a localized, hyperirritable trigger point, a palpable knot or mass (usually 3 to 6 mm in diameter), in a taut band of muscle associated with

---

Mike A. Royal became an employee of Elan Corporation in 2002, subsequent to the international meeting in 1999.

tenderness and referred pain into well-defined areas remote from the trigger point area (18,19). Myofascial pain syndrome is characterized by chronic, focal muscle pain, associated with stiffness, tenderness, and fatigue (20). An active myofascial trigger point has been defined as a well-localized, highly irritable taut band of skeletal muscle fibers that responds with a twitch response and referred pain distribution pattern to palpation (21). Latent trigger points are clinically silent, but may cause pain on palpation. Laboratory testing, radiographic studies or other standard tests, including diagnostic ultrasound (22), are not helpful in making a diagnosis of MPS (23). Such testing is useful only to exclude other diagnoses.

Most clinicians now treat fibromyalgia (FM) and MPS as distinct conditions. By the American College of Rheumatology 1990 Criteria (24), FM is a more widespread pain condition (three or more body regions above and below the waist) that lasts for 3 or more months and is associated with pain in at least 11 of 18 tenderpoint sites on digital palpation with a force of approximately 4 kg (8.8 lb). Myofascial trigger points should be distinguished from fibromyalgia tender points. Tender points are not associated with a "twitch" on palpation and are usually clinically silent unless stimulated by palpation. Tender points typically do not cause a referred pain pattern on palpation (20). Patients with FM tend to have more constitutional symptoms than do patients with MPS. Table 30.1 lists characteristics of FM and MPS.

Without a well-understood pathophysiologic etiology and with a lack of specific diagnostic tests and a paucity of objective physical signs, the diagnosis of MPS has become suspect for some and overly diagnosed for others (27). The pathogenesis of trigger points is unknown but several hypotheses exist (28). The *energy crisis* model of MPS proposes that direct injury or repetitive overloading of muscle results in sustained release of intracellular calcium and focal muscle hypercontraction, possibly caused by disruption of the sarcoplasmic reticulum (29). The localized spasm induces release of nociceptive and inflammatory mediators that produces a positive feedback process leading to focal ischemia (depletion of ATP), lactic acidosis, and eventual fibrosis. However, pathologic and histologic analyses do not support this theory (30).

The *dysfunctional muscle spindle* and the *irritable motor endplate* models grew out of different interpretations of electromyographic (EMG) evaluations of trigger points. Durette et al. studied 21 patients with MPS and found no evidence of spontaneous fibrillation or positive

TABLE 30.1. *Distinguishing fibromyalgia from myofascial pain syndrome (26)*

Characteristic	Fibromyalgia syndrome	Myofascial pain syndrome
Prevalence	4% to 6% of general medical patients	30% to 60% of pain clinic patients
Sex	10:1 female	1:1
Onset	50% idiopathic; 20% physical trauma; 20% viral; 10% emotional	Trauma or strain
Sleep disorder, fatigue	Always	Often
Pain	Diffuse	Localized
Pain referral (trigger point)	?	Localized
Tenderness (tender point)	Multiple spots at tendon insertion, in muscle belly or over bone	Few spots in muscle belly only
Palpable taut band with twitch response	?	Present
Interrater reliability	Good for palpation or algometry	Good for tenderness to palpation, poor for other features
Fatigue	Common	Uncommon
Irritable bowel symptoms	Common	Uncommon
Treatment	Medications, exercise	Local myofascial release
Local injections	Uncertain	Good results in case series
Outcome	Usually chronic	Usually self-limited

sharp-wave potentials (31). In contrast, Hubbard and Berkoff examined EMGs in the upper portion of the trapezius muscle in individuals with fibromyalgia or tension-type headaches (32). Trigger points were identified with digital palpation of the taut muscular band and characteristic pain referral pattern. A monopolar EMG needle was inserted directly over the trigger point and advanced incrementally until the patient described his typical pain and referral pattern. One millimeter adjustments in the needle were enough to make the pain/referral disappear. A second control needle was placed 1 cm away. Sustained spontaneous EMG activity was found at the trigger point, but not at the control point. This low-level electrical activity was not blocked by tubocurarine (which blocks cholinergic motor activity) but was by sympatholytics such as phentolamine (which blocks muscle-spindle afferents). Latent trigger points showed similar findings, but to a lesser degree. No fibrillation potentials or positive sharp-wave potentials were noted in trigger points or control points. The authors hypothesized that the EMG activity was generated from sympathetically stimulated intrafusal muscle fibers. Simons et al. used a similar technique and found active loci of spontaneous EMG activity much like that seen in the endplate region (33). They postulated that the electrical activity was due to the result of abnormally increased motor endplate activity with excessive release of acetylcholine at the neuromuscular junction resulting in extrafusal muscle contraction in the immediate vicinity of the extrafusal motor endplates.

The *peripheral sensitization model* proposes that peripheral silent afferents become activated after injury by the release of peripheral nociceptive mediators (34), whereas the *central sensitization model* proposes that the repetitive incoming nociceptive traffic induces neuroplastic changes in the dorsal horn (*N*-methyl-D-aspartate receptor or NMDA-mediated process) (35). It is likely that many of these proposed processes are occurring simultaneously.

MPS treatment goals are directed toward interrupting the pain/spasm cycle, treating underlying conditions when MPS is superimposed on another process, and decreasing and eliminating maladaptive behaviors by using cognitive-behavioral approaches (36). Travell and Simons popularized the spray and stretch technique as the mainstay of treatment for MPS (37). The purpose is to desensitize the trigger point, and to then stretch and relax the taut band of muscle. Ice may be used instead of vapocoolant sprays. Whether trigger-point injections are better than spray and stretch is unclear, but it certainly makes sense to use this noninvasive technique as an adjunct to other therapies, especially where the patient and family can be trained in the technique and the patient is cooperative and willing to do the posttreatment exercises.

Along with spray and stretch techniques, physical therapy (PT) and PT modalities are probably the most commonly used approaches in early MPS. Therapeutic heat and cold therapy, transcutaneous nerve stimulation, electrical muscle stimulation, ultrasound, iontophoresis, myofascial release, massage, hydrotherapy, stretching and strengthening exercises (passive and active), and acupuncture can be very helpful.

Borg-Stein and Stein reviewed the medical literature of trigger-point injections and concluded that although such injections have widespread clinical acceptance, evaluating their efficacy is hindered by difficulties in definitions as well as variations in technique (38). Gerwin et al. noted that although interrater reliability in identifying trigger points is somewhat suspect, it improves significantly with a few hours of training (39). Obviously, training in injection technique is important, as is ensuring that whatever is injected is delivered to the trigger-point region.

Short-term efficacy has been demonstrated with dry needling (40), sterile water (41), lidocaine (plain 1% and 2%) (42,43), bupivacaine (44), diclofenac (45), and prednisone or methylprednisolone. It appears that the nature of the injected substance is not a critical factor and it is unclear whether any therapeutic substance injected provides more benefit than dry needling alone. Of course, dry needling is not reimbursable under current payment guidelines unless it is being performed as part of an acupuncture treatment. The needle is presumed to cause a mechanical disruption of the trigger-point zone and stretch of adjacent muscle fibers. Local anesthetics, when injected, do reduce postinjection soreness, and for that reason are most commonly used. All local anesthetics have the potential for myotoxicity, with lidocaine 0.5% to 1.0% having less potential for this than bupivacaine 0.25% to 0.5%, but significant myotoxicity rarely occurs absent excessive use of this modality. Epinephrine may prolong the block from the local anesthetic, but is not necessary for trigger-point release. Most clinicians feel that steroids are not indicated unless there is an associated inflammatory process such as bursitis, tendonitis, or scar neuroma. Trigger point injections should be part of a comprehensive treatment program and not a sole treatment initiative.

Pharmacotherapy for MPS has included skeletal muscle relaxants (although many of these produce unwanted sedation and side effects), antispastic agents (such as baclofen and tizanidine), antidepressants (especially tricyclic antidepressants), anticonvulsants (especially those producing reduction in muscle spasm such as the benzodiazepines clonazepam, diazepam, and gabapentin), and traditional analgesics (46). None of these agents is particularly effective, but may be useful as adjuncts to other treatments. Unfortunately, much of the published literature discussing pharmacotherapy options lumped MPS and FM together, without speaking specifically to the response of MPS, making it difficult to make anything more than general recommendations.

BOTULINUM TOXINS IN MYOFASCIAL PAIN AND CONDITIONS WITH MUSCLE SPASM: CLINICAL DEVELOPMENTS

When conservative therapies fail to improve refractory myofascial pain, BTX may be quite helpful in reducing the spasm to a point where conservative measures can be reinstituted with greater effect to resolve the process. There seems little doubt that BTX injections can produce a much longer duration response than local anesthetic or steroid plus local anesthetic trigger-point injections. However, it was only relatively recently that this fact was firmly established.

Lalli et al. looked at lidocaine versus BTX-A in the treatment of myofascial pain in a double-blind randomized trial of 20 patients (15 female) who received 50 U of BTX-A (BOTOX) or 1% lidocaine (47). BTX-treated patients showed statistically significant improvement at 2 and 4 weeks as measured by visual analog scales and palpable muscle spasm. No major side effects were seen.

Porta et al. examined the effects of lidocaine/methylprednisolone versus BTX-A (BOTOX) in 40 patients with MPS in the psoas, piriformis, and scalenus anterior muscles in a single-blind, randomized trial (48). Patients received BTX (80 to 150 U) or similar volume of steroid/local anesthetic as a compartment injection into the affected muscle. The reduction in pain scores was better in the BTX-treated group at 30 days ($p = 0.0598$) but did not reach significance until 60 days ($p = 0.0001$). No major side effects were observed.

Patel et al. presented their preliminary results from a randomized double-blind, placebo-controlled study comparing trigger point injections with saline, bupivacaine, or BTX-A (BOTOX) (49). Twelve patients had completed the study at the time of the poster presentation. The preliminary data with this small number of patients showed a trend toward significance for the BTX-A group.

It was in 1994 that initial clinical reports hinted at the potential of BTX in improving myofascial pain. As seems to be the case in other new areas for use of a product, initial reports were either anecdotal case reports or flawed by small numbers of patient participants, but were valuable nonetheless in prompting others to conduct larger trials. Acquadro and Borodic reported on the use of BTX-A (BOTOX) in two female patients with refractory trapezius and splenius capitis myofascial pain (50). The first injection of 50 U provided the patients with slight improvement, and the second of 150 U 4 weeks later provided what was reported as dramatic improvement.

Cheshire et al. described responses to BTX-A (BOTOX) trigger-point injections in six patients with chronic myofascial pain in a randomized double-blind, placebo-controlled study (51). Cervical paraspinal or shoulder girdle trigger points were injected with either saline or 50 U of BTX-A reconstituted in 4 mL of preservative-free saline injected equally into two or three sites. Responses were measured over 8 weeks by verbal pain descriptors, visual analog scales (VAS), pressure algometry, and palpable muscle spasm or firmness. Four of six subjects experienced reduction in pain and spasm following BTX, but not saline, injections. Onset of responses occurred within the first week following BTX injections with a mean duration of 5 to 6 weeks.

In 1997, Alo and colleagues reported on their prospective but uncontrolled study of 52 patients (29 to 83 years old) with refractory MPS (cervicothoracic $n = 33$, low back/gluteal $n = 19$). The patients received fluoroscopically-directed injections of BTX-A (BOTOX) 10 U/cc in preservative-free saline (10 to 300 U BTX-A were used in the cervicothoracic MPS patients and 90 to 300 U BTX-A were used in the low back/gluteal MPS patients) (52). Up to three treatments were given 4 weeks apart if persistent spasm and pain were noted; present guidelines, however, suggest that injections more frequent than every 3 months should be avoided to reduce the risk of antibody formation. Greater than 50% reduction in spasm and symptoms were achieved in 63% of the cervicothoracic and 43% of the lumbar/gluteal patients. A very mild, short-lived flu-like syndrome was seen in 62% of patients with the first injection and not observed subsequently to this extent, and only one patient suffered transient dysphagia. The rather high incidence of flu-like syndrome has not been reported by other authors and may have been a result of the use of contrast for targeting the injections under fluoroscopy.

Grana reported on 5 patients with cervical MPS who received BTX-A (BOTOX) 50 U in 4 cc of preservative-free normal saline in divided doses into the upper and middle trapezius, scalene, levator scapulae, and sternocleidomastoid muscles after achieving less than 1 week of relief with standard trigger-point injections with local anesthetics (53). All five patients reported improved VAS pain scores 2 weeks post–BTX-A and four of five patients still had VAS reductions at 3 months.

In the first large prospective, controlled study of BTX-A in chronic muscular low back pain (without prior surgery or other identifiable spine pathology), Knusel et al. presented data on the use of BTX-A (BOTOX) in 70 patients randomized into four groups (placebo, 120, 180, or 240 U of BTX-A) (54). Patients in all groups improved in all outcome measures. The BTX-A 240 U group showed statistical significance over placebo at weeks 6, 9, and 12 for muscle spasm and at weeks 6 and 12 for physician global assessment. No adverse events of significance were noted.

These data and subsequent unpublished data derived from other studies conducted by Allergan on low-back pain point to the difficulty of assessing a new modality of treatment in a rather amorphous condition. Low-back pain is a rather broad diagnostic category that makes it difficult to be sure that any patient group is relatively homogenous. Recruiting patients who have not had surgery, who have no spine pathology, who have no pending litigation, disability, or workers' compensation claims, and who have had no significant interventions whatsoever collects a group of patients who are not clinically relevant and who are likely to respond to simple modalities, such as trigger-point injections, creating the potential for high placebo response rates. The other variable not resolved in most of these multicentered trials is ensuring a uniform application of diagnostic criteria and injection techniques. Additionally, because the lower back muscles are much larger than those in the cervical region, dosing guidelines used in these early studies probably were insufficient and part of the reason for uninspiring results. Perhaps if different inclusion/exclusion criteria and a higher total dose were used and standardization of examination findings and injection techniques was ensured, better results might have been seen.

Porta et al. performed a preliminary trial of BTX-A (BOTOX) and physical therapy on 38 patients (24 women, 14 men; age range, 18 to 73 years; 3 with fibromyalgia) with piriformis ($n = 27$), iliopsoas ($n = 9$), and scalenus ($n = 2$) myofascial pain (55). Injections into the piriformis and iliopsoas were performed with CT guidance, while other injections were done by palpation alone. Efficacy and safety were evaluated at 1 month. Seventeen patients (45%) reported pain relief and six (16%) reported improvement. Eight of the 15 who had no improvement admitted to failing to comply with the therapy requirements, suggesting that BTX treatments do not work in a vacuum but must be part of a treatment continuum.

Wheeler et al. reported the lack of efficacy of BTX-A (BOTOX) over placebo when injected into trigger points in 33 patients with cervicothoracic myofascial pain in a randomized, double-blind study (56). Participants were divided into three groups receiving 50 or 100 U of BTX-A diluted in 2 mL of preservative-free normal saline or normal saline and were evaluated over a 4-month period in a standard fashion. The most tender trigger point (if there were several) was chosen as the injection site. Participants were followed regularly and algometer measurements of the trigger point injected as well as subjective assessment of improvement, visual analog scale measurements, and physical examinations were performed. A second injection of 100 U of BTX in 2 mL of normal saline was given to 11 patients in the same site and to 2 patients in an adjacent symptomatic site.

Although by their strict criteria for improvement (absence of pain simultaneously on three different measures: Neck Pain and Disability Scale, pressure algometer, and patient's global assessment), similar clinical improvement rates across the three groups were seen, there were notable differences among the groups in response to the second injection. The number of patients determined to be asymptomatic was higher in the BTX groups. The authors noted that further investigation with higher doses and sequential injections might have reached clinical significance. Certainly the use of 50 U of BoNT-A, while reasonable for a single injection site, is insufficient if several muscles are involved. Additionally, the study design of injecting only the most tender trigger point even if several active trigger points were identified seems to run counter to typical approaches used by most pain clinicians who would opt to "deactivate" all of the active trigger points in order to give the patient better relief and to avoid secondary active pain sources from perpetuating the patient's symptoms.

Royal et al. presented their retrospective data on 104 patients (age range, 18 to 85 years old) who received 187 BTX-A injections over a 4-year period. These patients had previously failed traditional conservative measures and had experienced only short-term improvement with standard trigger-point injections (57). Areas of MPS involvement were cervical (64.1%), thoracic (10.9%), lumbar (10.4%), gluteal (3.6%), piriformis (7.7%), and extremity (3.2%). Six patients were excluded from analysis because of insufficient follow-up information. Of the 187 injections, 135 (72.2%) produced at least a 50% reduction in patient global responses. BOTOX dosing ranges for specific muscle groups were as follows: trapezius: 20 to 100 U; levator scapulae: 15 to 40 U; splenius capitis: 20 to 50 U; sternocleidomastoid: 25 to 100 U; quadratus lumborum: 20 to 60 U; piriformis: 30 to 100 U; rhomboid: 20 to 120 U; thoracic and lumbar paraspinals: 20 to 40 per segment.

The BTX-A injections were performed as standard trigger-point injections with the BOTOX reconstituted in local anesthetic, typically bupivacaine 0.5%, in a final concentration of 10 U/cc. Each trigger point received 2 to 4 cc of total volume infiltrated in a standard fashion under direct digital palpation using a 25-gauge 1.5-inch needle with 1 to 2 cc directly into the trigger point and additional amounts in the surrounding taut band of muscle. Patients received 100 to 300 U of BTX-A (the majority received 100 U for unilateral pain and 200 U for bilateral pain) at any injection session with the dosing amount determined by the number of involved muscles and severity of spasm. Only patients with a good to excellent response were offered repeat BTX-A injections when the first wore off. The complication rate was exceedingly low. One patient had transient neck muscle weakness within the first week that resolved completely after a few days. One patient developed transient tension-type headache symptoms in the first few days of the injection that was felt to be caused by the injection itself.

A positive response was defined as at least a 30% reduction in symptoms from baseline. An excellent response was defined as at least 70% reduction from baseline. A good response was defined as a 50% to 69% reduction and a fair response as a 30% to 49% reduction. No relief or minimal relief was defined as a response less than 30% from baseline. The Table 30.2 provides a breakdown of the responses and durations of response. Ten percent of the patients injected were "cures" with complete resolution of symptoms at 1-year follow up. Certain population subtypes appeared to have greater likelihood of positive response. Of those patients with posttraumatic myofascial pain, 67% had at least a 50% improvement in symptoms. Of those with failed back surgery syndrome (persistent pain after significant lumbar surgery) and piriformis syndrome, 71% and 56%, respectively, had at least a 50% reduction in symptoms. Insurance coverage appeared not to have an affect on patient response.

Freund and Schwartz reported on the treatment of whiplash-associated neck pain with botulinum toxin in a randomized, double-blind, placebo-controlled trial of 26 patients (58). Fourteen of the patients received 100 U of BTX-A (BOTOX) in 1 mL of saline, while 12 patients received placebo (1 mL of saline). Five trigger points received 0.2 mL each via a 30-gauge needle. The treatment group showed a trend toward improvement in range of motion and reduction in pain at 2 weeks postinjection. At 4 weeks postinjection, the treatment group was significantly improved ($p < 0.01$).

Bahman Jabbari and colleagues at the Department of Neurology, Walter Reed Army Medical Center/Uniformed Services University, Bethesda, Maryland, have studied the use of 200 U of BTX-A (BOTOX), 40 U/site, versus saline placebo at five lumbar paravertebral levels on 31 patients with chronic unilateral low-back pain using a randomized, double-blind design (59). Visual analog scores and the Oswestry's Low Back Pain Questionnaire (OLBPQ) were used to follow the patients. At 3 weeks, 11 of 15 patients who received BTX-A (73%) showed significant (greater than 50%) pain relief versus 4 of 16 (25%) in the NS group ($p = 0.012$). At 8 weeks, 9 of 15 in the BTX-A group (60%) and 2 of 16 (13%) of NS group reported relief ($p = 0.009$). Repeat OLBPQ at 8 weeks showed improvement in 10 of 15 (67%) in the BTX-A group versus 3 of 16 (19%) in the NS group ($p = 0.011$). No patient experienced side effects.

Jabbari's study should be contrasted with the relatively mediocre results seen in other studies, particularly the multicentered trial by Knusel et al. evaluating low-back MPS (54). Perhaps the asymmetric nature of the patients' symptoms or the larger total dose of BTX used was the reason for the greater response.

Lang published her data on 72 patients who received 95 BTX-A (BOTOX) injections for MPS via a novel grid pattern into the mid-belly of the muscles (60). The median BTX-A dose was 200 U. Outcomes were good to excellent in 65%, fair in 24%, and poor in 12% of the patients. There were two cases of transient weakness and one case of transient flu-like syndrome. Insurance type seemed not to be predictive of outcome. Comparing her results with those of others using standard trigger-point injection techniques suggests that a grid pattern may not be necessary.

Although the data on BTX use in myofascial pain and conditions associated with painful muscular spasm can be challenged on the basis that most of the studies were retrospective or uncontrolled, the sheer number of studies showing positive results along with similar findings in the few controlled prospective studies suggest that there is something of value to consider.

TABLE 30.2. *Response and duration of response to BTX-A injection in 104 patients*

187 injections in 104 patients	# of injections	%	% of total patients	M:F (# patients)	Response duration in months (range)
Excellent (greater than 70% improvement)	104	55.6	48.1	13:40	3.6 (1–18)
Good (50–69% better)	31	16.6	16.3	7:10	2.5 (1–8)
Fair (30–49% better)	33	17.6	24.0	11:14	2.4 (0.5–3)
No/minimal (less than 30% better)	19	10.2	11.6	3:6	–

ANTINOCICEPTIVE MECHANISMS

The mechanism of action for BTX in migraine may be less likely a result of blocking muscle contraction and thus removing a migraine trigger and more likely a result of blocking release of pain-mediating neurotransmitters or peptides or some other central effect. There is considerable supporting data from the cervical dystonia and spasticity literature for the position that BTX reduces pain from some mechanism other than effects on alpha motor neurons even before the chemodenervation effects occur. Jankovic and Schwartz noted that pain consistently improved, often within hours after the BTX-A injection, well before any reduction in muscle spasm could be detected in their large series of cervical dystonia patients (61). Most clinicians treating cervical dystonia with BTX-A have observed that pain relief typically outweighs the degree of spasm reduction seen (62). Fillippi et al. demonstrated that gamma motor endings of isolated rat masseter muscles could be blocked within 80 minutes by BTX thereby reducing the Ia afferent signal from the muscle spindles and muscle tone via a reflex mechanism (63). Subsequent intrafusal and extrafusal atrophy from chemodenervation prolongs the effect (64). Giladi also postulates that a central reorganization takes place because of the prolonged reduced spindle feedback (65).

In the 1970s, Wiegand et al. demonstrated retrograde axonal spread of radiolabeled BTX injected near the sciatic nerve within 48 hours (66). The authors noted that they could not confirm whether the retrograde radioactivity was unchanged toxin or breakdown products. Aoki confirmed the findings of Wiegand et al. in a study in which rats were injected unilaterally in the gastrocnemius muscle with radiolabeled BTX-A (67). Radioactivity remained at the injection site for at least 2 hours and disappeared by 48 hours, having appeared in the sciatic nerve and spinal cord. However, Aoki was able to show that the retrograde radioactive spread was caused by breakdown products and not intact toxin transport.

Because colocalization of vasoactive intestinal peptide and neuropeptide Y with acetylcholine has been demonstrated in parasympathetic neurons, inhibition of synaptosomal-associated protein of 25 kDa (SNAP-25) or vesicle-associated membrane protein (VAMP, also known as synaptobrevin) by BTX could block neurotransmitter exocytosis and reduce pain (68). In a study of rat dorsal root ganglia neurons and isolated rabbit iris sphincter and dilatory muscles, BTX-A was shown to inhibit neuropeptide release (69). Additionally, BTX-A can block the *in vitro* release of substance P and acetylcholine, but not norepinephrine, from rabbit ocular tissue (70). Aoki and Cui demonstrated that BTX-A (3.5 or 7.0 U/kg/paw) blocked the neuropathic pain component (rat hind paw formalin model) in a dose-dependent fashion (71). Rats were challenged with subcutaneous 5% formalin in one hind paw at 5 days, and in the opposite hind paw at 12 days post–BTX-A. BTX-A efficacy was slightly less at day 12 than at day 5. The animals showed no obvious motor weakness or weight loss. These data provide interesting topics for discussion, but answers must await further study.

TECHNICAL CONSIDERATIONS

After the decision is made to consider BTX for the treatment of MPS or other muscle spasm conditions, the key questions become which patient will best benefit from this therapy, what dose to administer (in what concentration and in what diluent), and how to administer it. Unfortunately, the answers to many of these questions are still somewhat uncertain. Until more studies are performed, only general guidelines are available from the currently available literature.

Patient Selection

As with any new therapy, especially one that is expensive, it makes sense to use BTX only in more refractory cases until the treatment becomes established and pharmacoeconomic data is supportive. For patients with MPS in the cervical and thoracic region, results from numerous retrospective case series and prospective trials demonstrate the potential for significant reduction in medication use and complete resolution of symptoms in a substantial portion of refractory cases. Quality of life and functional improvement can be measurably improved in many patients. This creates a strong argument in support of BTX use in such patients. In the lower back, retrospective data and large multicentered trials seem to indicate that such patients respond less well than those with cervicothoracic involvement. However, Jabbari's prospective study seems to indicate that there is a patient population with chronic low back MPS that responds well. Some of the factors that may contribute to the disparate results have been discussed and we will have to await additional trials for the final answer.

From a review of the currently available studies some trends appear that may provide clinicians with some help with patient selection. Single muscle involvement (55) or more focal symptoms/examination findings (e.g., Jabbari's study with more unilateral involvement) seem to respond better. Finding more muscle spasm on examination may also be a good predictor of response (72). Patients who have had extensive lumbar surgery and who develop very tender paraspinal muscles with palpable spasm may respond well (73). Posttraumatic cases also seem to do better (58).

Injection Technique

With MPS, most investigators have injected active trigger points directly or used a grid pattern (Lang's method) around them to get more diffuse spread through the involved muscle. Results from trials indicate that a grid technique is unnecessary. Most practitioners now inject trigger points or areas of tenderness/spasm in muscle. Yue also has demonstrated that scalene or psoas compartment injections under fluoroscopic guidance can be used with success to target adjacent muscles (74). However, this technique appears to run the risk of spread to uninvolved muscles and probably offers little advantage to directed injections into the involved muscles.

Success in reducing patients' symptoms using local anesthetic trigger-point injections performed by palpation appears to be predictive of greater response with BTX injections and gives the clinician feedback that EMG or fluoroscopy use for targeting probably is not necessary. Posterior neck strap muscles typically are easily palpable and present little challenge for clinicians comfortable with performing trigger-point injections. However, in the lower back, trigger points in deeper paraspinals may not be as easily felt, especially in those with greater subcutaneous tissue, and may require some type of targeting technique.

The use of fluoroscopic or EMG guidance to identify the muscle or to localize the motor endplate prior to injections appears to be a benefit in some situations. Targeting motor endplates with EMG to allow for lower toxin doses and to increase success has not been shown to be necessary in MPS. When injecting in the anterior neck for cervical dystonia or MPS, it is important to keep volumes low and to use precise targeting as the muscles are smaller and spread to adjacent structures creates the potential for dry mouth, dysphonia, and dysphagia. With deeper paraspinal muscles (multifidus and psoas) and gluteal muscles (piriformis), it is probably better to use a targeting method to maximize success. Fluoroscopic or CT guidance with or without EMG can be very helpful for injections of these deeper muscles. EMG guidance should be used when targeting extremity muscles or neck muscles that cannot reliably be identified with palpation.

Dosing Guidelines

Dystonia and spasticity data has been used as a starting point for BTX-A dose calculations for other conditions (Table 30.3). Adjustments are made depending upon the size of the muscle and degree of spasm; in other words, muscle-specific, not disease-specific, dosing seems appropriate for BTX injections. Clinical experience with BTX-A seems to support this extrapolation to MPS/headache, but we need published data to confirm that this is the case for BTX-B as well. Thus, with BTX-B, it will be important to be cautious at first starting at a maximum of 2,500 to 5,000 U and moving upward, depending upon clinical response, until data from current

TABLE 30.3. *Recommended unit dose ranges for BXT-A (BOTOX)*

Frontalis:	6 to 10 per side	Trapezius:	25 to 100	Iliopsoas:	50 to 100
Corrugator:	3 to 5	Levator scapulae:	25 to 50	Lumbar paraspinals:	50 per segment (300 to 400)
Procerus:	3 to 5	Latissimus dorsi:	50 to 100	Quadratus lumborum:	50 to 100
Obicularis oculi:	3 to 5	Teres major:	25 to 75	Piriformis	50 to 100
Temporalis:	6 to 10	Brachioradialis:	25 to 75	Medial hamstrings:	50 to 150
Sternocleidomastoid:	50 to 100	Biceps:	75 to 125	Gastrocnemius:	50 to 100
Scalene:	25 to 50	Brachialis:	25 to 50	Lateral hamstrings:	75 to 150
Splenius capitis:	10 to 30	Flexor carpi radialis:	10 to 50	Soleus:	25 to 75
Semispinalis capitis:	10 to 30	Flexor carpi ulnaris:	10 to 50	Tibialis posterior:	75 to 125
Splenius cervices:	10 to 30	Iliocostalis thoracis:	100 to 200	Tibialis anterior:	50 to 100

studies provides confirmation of dose-response in MPS.

The total maximum dose per visit for BTX-A (BOTOX) typically should not exceed the 300 to 400 U range (although many have gone as high as 600 to 700 U safely for numerous involved muscles as in diffuse spasticity/dystonia) and intervals between doses should be no more frequent than every 3 months. Following these general guidelines will reduce adverse events (primarily weakness) and antibody formation. Little data is available to help one decide on BTX-B dosing outside of cervical dystonia (Table 30.4). It appears to be about 40 to 50 times less potent than BTX-A with very few patients having received doses at or above 20,000 U, although these doses appear to be well tolerated. In the cervical dystonia data, BTX-B produced a clinical response duration of between 12 and 16 weeks, which is similar to that seen with BTX-A.

What to Use as Diluent?

Current recommendations are that only preservative-free saline (PFNS) be used as the diluent for BTX-A (BOTOX). After BOTOX is reconstituted, recommendations are for it to be used within 4 hours because of dual concerns of protein denaturation and infection risk. MYO-BLOC, although stable for months at room temperature, should be used within 4 hours once the vial has been opened because of infection concern. Because the pH of 5.6 in the MYO-BLOC preparation might cause local injection discomfort, perhaps more than that seen with the more neutral pH of BTX-A, the author recommends that preservative-free lidocaine or bupivacaine be used to dilute the BTX to provide a local anesthetic effect. Another innovation is to freeze one's injection needles to obtain a "cryo-analgesic" effect. Topical local anesthetics such as EMLA or Lidoderm patches also may be helpful for providing local numbness preinjection in squeamish patients.

The use of preservative-free local anesthetic (with or without contrast such as Isoview or Omnipaque) as a diluent, although outside of labeling from the manufacturers, does not appear to denature the protein (as long as not too much bicarbonate is added to alkalinize the acidic pH needed to avoid toxin denaturation) and cer-

TABLE 30.4. *Recommended unit dose ranges for BTX-B (MYOBLOC) (75)*

Doses per muscle with 2,500 U total		Doses per muscle with 5,000 U total		Doses per muscle with 10,000 U total	
Semispinalis capitis:	608 to 1,500	Semispinalis capitis:	1,000 to 3,750	Semispinalis capitis:	2,000 to 7,500
Trapezius:	300 to 1,250	Trapezius:	500 to 2,500	Trapezius:	1,000 to 6,500
Sternocleidomastoid:	270 to 1,250	Sternocleidomastoid:	500 to 1,500	Sternocleidomastoid:	1,000 to 9,000
Levator scapulae:	250 to 825	Levator scapulae:	625 to 1,500	Levator scapulae:	1,000 to 4,000
Splenius capitis:	625 to 1875	Splenius capitis:	1,000 to 4,250	Splenius capitis:	1,250 to 7,000
Scalene complex:	500 to 838	Scalene complex:	500 to 2,250	Scalene complex:	1,800 to 3,750

tainly seems to help with local injection pain with the BTX-B formulation (74). In MPS, numerous studies have documented that local anesthetics seem not to interfere with toxin efficacy, although studies comparing local anesthetics versus PFNS have not been done. Additionally, whether volume of diluent makes a difference in efficacy is not known, although studies are in progress to answer this question as well.

CONCLUSIONS

BTX appear to be a useful treatment in refractory MPS and other conditions associated with painful muscle spasms. Presumably BTX work by breaking the spasm/pain cycle, giving the patient a "window of opportunity" for traditional conservative measures to have a greater beneficial impact, but several studies suggest that a direct antinociceptive effect distinct from any reduction in muscle spasm may be at play. The major benefit of BTX compared with standard therapies is duration of response. The author does not advocate that BTX be used as a first line treatment for MPS. However, in refractory cases where nothing else has worked, it may offer a chance for improvement or cure not otherwise available. Soon some very good data should be available from studies presently being conducted to help decide where to place BTX in our pain treatment continuum. For now, it remains an off-label, but increasingly accepted, approach in patients with refractory myofascial or muscular pain who, despite multidisciplinary approaches, continue to suffer.

REFERENCES

1. Raj PP. Botulinum toxin in the treatment of pain associated with musculoskeletal hyperactivity. *Curr Rev Pain* 1997;1:403–416.
2. Jankovic J, Brin MF. Therapeutic uses of botulinum toxin. *N Engl J Med* 1991;324:1186–1194.
3. Jankovic J, Schwartz K. Botulinum toxin injections for cervical dystonia. *Neurology* 1990;40:277–280.
4. Ludlow CL, Naunton RF, Sedory SE, et al. Effects of botulinum toxin injections on speech in adductor spasmodic dysphonia. *Neurology* 1988;38:1220–1225.
5. Soulayrol S, Capean A, Penot-Ragon C, et al. Local botulinum toxin injection therapy in neurology. *Presse Med* 1993;22:957–963.
6. Freund B, Schwartz M, Symington JM. The use of botu-
linum toxin for the treatment of temporomandibular disorders: preliminary findings. *J Oral Maxillofac Surg* 1999;57:916–920.
7. Relja M. Botulinum toxin type A in the treatment of tension-type headache. Presented at the 9th World Congress on Pain, Aug 22–27, 1999, Vienna, Austria, and at the International Conference 1999: Basic and Therapeutic Aspects of Botulinum and Tetanus Toxins, Nov 16–18, 1999, Orlando, Florida.
8. Brin MF, Binder WJ, Blitzer A, et al. Botulinum toxin or headache: data and review. Presented at the International Conference 1999: Basic and Therapeutic Aspects of Botulinum and Tetanus Toxins, Nov 16–18, 1999, Orlando, Florida.
9. Childers MK, Wison DJ, Galate JF, et al. Treatment of painful muscle syndromes with botulinum toxin: a review. *J Back Musculoskel Rehabil* 1998;10:89–96.
10. Benedetto AV. The cosmetic uses of Botulinum toxin type A. *Int J Dermatol* 1999;38:641–655.
11. Deleted in proof.
12. Jankovic J, Hallett M, eds. *Therapy with botulinum toxin.* New York: Marcel Dekker, 1994.
13. Racz GB. Botulinum toxin as a new approach for refractory pain syndromes. *Pain Dig* 1998;8:353–356.
14. Porta M, Perretti A, Gamba M, et al. The rationale and results of treating muscle spasm and myofascial syndromes with botulinum toxin type A. *Pain Dig* 1998;8:346–352.
15. Abrams BM. Tutorial 36: myofascial pain syndrome and fibromyalgia. *Pain Dig* 1998; 8:264–272.
16. Lang AM. Botulinum toxin for myofascial pain. In: *Advancements in the treatment of neuromuscular pain.* Baltimore, MD: Johns Hopkins University Office of Continuing Medical Education Syllabus, October 1999: 23–28.
17. Travell JG. Referred pain from skeletal muscle. *N Y State J Med* 1952;55:331–339.
18. Travell JG, Simons DG. *Myofascial pain and dysfunction: the trigger point manual.* Baltimore, MD: Williams & Wilkins, 1983.
19. Simons DG. Referred phenomena of myofascial trigger points. In: Vechiet L, Albe-Fessard D, Lindblom U, eds. *New trends in referred pain and hyperalgesia.* Amsterdam: Elsevier, 1993:341.
20. Wolfe F, Simons DG, Friction J, et al. The fibromyalgia and myofascial pain syndromes: a preliminary study of tender points and trigger points in persons with fibromyalgia, myofascial pain syndrome and no disease. *J Rheumatol* 1992;19:944–951.
21. Travell JG, Simons DG. *Myofascial pain and dysfunction: the trigger point manual, Vol 1.* Baltimore, MD: Williams & Wilkins, 1983.
22. Lewis J, Tehan P. A blinded pilot study investigating the use of diagnostic ultrasound for detecting active myofascial trigger points. *Pain* 1999;79:39–44.
23. Kadi F, Waling K, Sundelin G, et al. Pathological mechanisms implicated in localized female trapezius myalgia. *Pain* 1998;78:191–196.
24. Wolfe F, Smythe HA, Yunus MB, et al. The American College of Rheumatology 1990 criteria for the classification of fibromyalgia: report of the Multicentre Criteria Committee. *Arthritis Rheum* 1990;33:160–172.
25. Deleted in proof.
26. Goldenberg DL. Controversies in fibromyalgia and myofascial pain syndromes. In: Aronoff GM, ed. *Evalua-*

tion and treatment of chronic pain. Baltimore, MD: Williams & Wilkins, 1999.

27. Bohr T. Problems with myofascial pain syndrome and fibromyalgia syndrome. *Neurology* 1996;46:593–597.

28. Simons DG. Clinical and etiological update of myofascial pain from trigger points In: Russell JJ, ed. *Clinical overview and pathogenesis of fibromyalgia syndrome, myofascial pain syndrome, and other pain syndromes.* Binghamton, NY: Hayworth Medical Press, 1996: 93–121.

29. Travell JG, Rinzler SH. The myofascial genesis of pain. *Postgrad Med* 1952;11:425–434.

30. Kravis M, Munk P, McCain G, et al. MR imaging of muscle and tender points of fibromyalgia. *J Mag Reson Imag* 1993;3:669–670.

31. Durette MR, Rodriques AA, Agre JC, et al. Needle electromyographic evaluation of patients with myofascial or fibromyalgic pain. *Arch Phys Med Rehabil* 1991;70: 154–156.

32. Hubbard DR, Berkoff GM. Myofascial trigger points show spontaneous needle EMG activity. *Spine* 1993;18: 1803–1807.

33. Simons, DG. Fibrositis/fibromyalgia: a form of myofascial trigger points? *Am J Med* 1986;81(Suppl 3A): 93–98.

34. Michaelis M, Habler H-J, Janig W. Silent afferents: a separate class of primary afferents? *Clin Exp Pharmacol Physiol* 1996;23:99–105.

35. Mense S. Biochemical pathogenesis of myofascial pain. *J Musculoskel Pain* 1996;4:93–121.

36. Johnson MH, Petrie SM. The effects of distraction on exercise and cold pressor tolerance for chronic low back pain sufferers. *Pain* 1997;69:43–48.

37. Travell JG, Simons DG. *Myofascial pain and dysfunction: the trigger point manual.* Baltimore, MD: Williams & Wilkins, 1983.

38. Borg-Stein J, Stein J. Trigger points and tender points. *Rheum Dis Clin North Am* 1996;22:305–322.

39. Gerwin RD, Shannon S, Hong C-Z. Identification of myofascial trigger points: interrater agreement and effect of training. *J Musculoskel Pain* 1995;3(Suppl 1): 55.

40. Hong C-Z. Lidocaine injection versus dry needling to myofascial trigger point: the importance of the local twitch response. *Am J Phys Med Rehabil* 1994;73: 256–263.

41. Byrn C, Olsson I, Falkheded L, et al. Subcutaneous sterile water injections for chronic neck and shoulder pain following whiplash injuries. *Lancet* 1993;341:449–452.

42. Bourne IHJ. Treatment of chronic back pain comparing corticosteroid-lignocaine injections with lignocaine alone. *Practitioner* 1984;228:333–338.

43. Delin C. Treatment of sciatica with injections of novocaine into tender points along the sciatic nerve, 132 cases. *J Tradit Chin Med* 1994;14:32–34.

44. Garvery TA, Marks MR, Wiesel SW. A prospective, randomized, double-blind evaluation of trigger point injection therapy for low-back pain. *Spine* 1989;14: 962–964.

45. Drewes AM, Andreasen A, Poulsen LH. Injection therapy for treatment of chronic myofascial pain: a double-blind study comparing corticosteroid versus diclofenac injections. *J Musculoskel Pain* 1993;1:289–294.

46. Esenyel M, Caglar N, Aldemir T. Treatment of myofascial pain. *Am J Phys Med Rehabil* 2000;9:48–52.

47. Lalli F, Gallai V, Tambasco N, et al. Botulinum A toxin versus lidocaine in the treatment of myofascial pain: a double-blind randomized study. Presented at the International Conference 1999: Basic and Therapeutic Aspects of Botulinum and Tetanus Toxins, Nov. 16–18, 1999, Orlando, Florida.

48. Porta M, Loiero M, Gamba M, et al. Botulinum toxin type A versus steroid for the treatment of myofascial pain syndromes. Presented at the International Conference 1999: Basic and Therapeutic Aspects of Botulinum and Tetanus Toxins, Nov. 16–18, 1999, Orlando, Florida. See also: Porta M. A comparative trial of botulinum toxin type A and methylprednisolone for the treatment of myofascial pain syndrome and pain from chronic muscle spasm. *Pain* 2000;85:101–105.

49. Patel RK, Cianca JC, Nguyen D. Therapeutic efficacy of botulinum toxin A trigger point injections for patients with myofascial pain. *Arch Phys Med Rehab* 1998;79: 1173–1174.

50. Acquadro MA, Borodic GE. Treatment of myofascial pain with botulinum A toxin [Letter]. *Anesthesiology* 1994;80:705–706.

51. Cheshire WP, Abashian SW, Mann JD. Botulinum toxin in the treatment of myofascial pain syndrome. *Pain* 1994;59:65–69.

52. Alo KM, Yland MJ, Kramer DL, et al. Botulinum toxin in the treatment of myofascial pain. *Pain Clin* 1997;10: 107–116.

53. Grana EA. Treatment of chronic cervical myofascial pain with botulinum toxin. *Arch Phys Med Rehabil* 1998;79:1172.

54. Knusel B, DeGryse R, Grant M, et al. Intramuscular injection of botulinum toxin type A (BOTOX) in chronic low back pain associated with muscle spasm. Data presented at 17th Annual Scientific Meeting, American Pain Society, Nov 5–8, 1998, San Diego, California.

55. Porta M, Perretti A, Gamba M, et al. The rationale and results of treating muscle spasm and myofascial syndromes with botulinum toxin type A. *Pain Dig* 1998;8: 346–352.

56. Wheeler AH, Goolkasian P, Gretz SS. A randomized, double-blind, prospective pilot study of botulinum toxin injection for refractory, unilateral, cervicothoracic, paraspinal, myofascial pain syndrome. *Spine* 1998;23: 1662–1667.

57. Royal MA, Gunyea I, Bhakta B, et al. Botulinum toxin type A (BOTOX) in the treatment of refractory myofascial pain. Abstract presented at the 2nd World Congress of the World Institute of Pain: Pain Management in the 21st Century, June 27–30, 2001, Istanbul, Turkey.

58. Freund BJ, Schwartz M. Treatment of whiplash-associated neck pain with botulinum toxin A: A pilot study. Presented at the International Conference 1999: Basic and Therapeutic Aspects of Botulinum and Tetanus Toxins, Nov. 16–18, 1999, Orlando, Florida. See also: Freund BJ, Schwartz M. Treatment of whiplash-associated neck pain with botulinum toxin A: a pilot study. *Headache* 2000;40:231–236 and *J Rheum* 2000;27: 481–484.

59. Foster L, Clapp L, Erickson M, et al. Botulinum toxin A and chronic low back pain: a randomized double blind study. *Neurology* 2000;54(7 Suppl 3):A178.

60. Lang AM. A pilot study of botulinum toxin type A (BOTOX), administered using a novel injection tech-

nique, for the treatment of myofascial pain. *Am J Pain Mgt* 2000;10:108–112.

61. Jankovic J, Schwartz K. Botulinum toxin injections for cervical dystonia. *Neurology* 1990;40:277–280.

62. Brin MF, Fahn S, Moskowitz C, et al. Localized injections of botulinum toxin for the treatment of focal dystonia and hemifacial spasm. *Mov Disord* 1997;12: 722–726.

63. Fillippi GM, Errico P, Santarelli R, et al. Botulinum toxin effects on rat jaw muscle spindles. *Acta Otolaryngol* 1993;113:400–404.

64. Rosales RL, Arimura K, Takenaga S, et al. Extrafusal and intrafusal muscle effects in experimental botulinum toxin type A injection. *Muscle Nerve* 1996;19:488–496.

65. Giladi N. The mechanism of action of botulinum toxin type A in focal dystonia is most probably through its dual effect on efferent (motor) and afferent pathways at the injected site. *J Neurol Sci* 1997;152:132–135. See also: Moreno-Lopez B, Pastor AM, de la Cruz RR, et al. Dose-dependent, central effects of botulinum neurotoxin type A: a pilot study in the alert behaving cat. *Neurology* 1997;48:456–464.

66. Wiegand H, Wellhoner HH. The action of botulinum A neurotoxin on the inhibition by antidromic stimulation of the lumbar monosynaptic reflex. *Naunym Schmiedebergs Arch Pharmacol* 1977;298:235–238.

67. Aoki R. The development of BOTOX—its history and pharmacology. *Pain Dig* 1998; 8:337–341.

68. Hohne-Zell B, Galler A, Schepp W, et al. Functional importance of synaptobrevin and SNAP-25 during exocytosis of histamine by rat gastric enterochromaffin-like cells. *Endocrinology* 1997;138:5518–5526.

69. Welch MJ, Purkiss JR, Foster KA. Sensitivity of embryonic rat dorsal root ganglia neurons to clostridium botulinum neurotoxins. *Toxicon* 2000;38:245–258.

70. Ishikawa H, Mitsui Y, Yoshitomi T, et al. Presynaptic effects of botulinum toxin type A on the neuronally evoked response of albino and pigmented rabbit iris sphincter and dilator muscles. *Jpn J Ophthalmol* 2000; 44:106–109.

71. Aoki KR, Cui M. Botulinum toxin type A: potential mechanism of actions in pain relief. Presented at 37th Annual Meeting of the Interagency Botulism Research Coordinating Committee, Oct. 17–20, 2000, Asilomar, California.

72. Davis D, Jabbari B. Significant improvement of stiff-person syndrome after paraspinal injection of botulinum toxin A. *Mov Disord* 1993;8:371–373.

73. Ghika J, Nater B, Henderson J, et al. Delayed segmental axial dystonia of the trunk on standing after lumbar disk operation. *J Neurol Sci* 1997;152:193–197.

74. Yue SK. Compartment approach to the treatment of myofascial pain syndrome of the shoulder and pelvic girdles (including low back pain). Presented at the 8th World Congress on Pain, August 17–22, 1996, Vancouver, BC, Canada.

75. MYOBLOC Product Monograph, Elan Pharmaceuticals, February 2001:38.

Scientific and Therapeutic Aspects of Botulinum Toxin
edited by M.F. Brin, J. Jankovic, and M. Hallett
Lippincott Williams & Wilkins, Philadelphia, © 2002.

31

Botulinum Toxin Treatment in Tremors

Jyh-Gong Hou and Joseph Jankovic

Tremor, the most common movement disorder, is defined as a rhythmic, oscillatory movement of a body part produced by alternating or synchronous contractions of agonist and antagonist muscles. It ranges from a normal, barely noticeable, physiologic phenomenon to a severe, disabling movement disorder. Tremors can be classified according to their phenomenology, distribution, frequency, amplitude, or etiology (1,2). Phenomenologically, tremors are subdivided into two major categories: rest tremors and action tremors. Rest tremors occur when the body part is fully supported against gravity and not actively contracting. It is present predominantly in Parkinson's disease (PD), but may also occur in other conditions such as various forms of parkinsonisms, severe essential tremor (ET) and midbrain lesions. Action tremors manifest during voluntary muscle contraction while holding an antigravity posture (postural tremor) or during a goal-directed movement (kinetic tremor). Postural tremors are typically caused by physiologic tremor, enhanced physiologic tremor, and ET (3). Task- or position-specific tremors are action tremors that occur only during specific motor activities, such as writing ("primary writing tremor") or while maintaining a certain specific posture. Kinetic tremors exist in cerebellar or midbrain disorders. Isometric tremor is seen during a voluntary isometric contraction, such as making a tight fist or contracting abdominal muscles. Tremors associated with parkinsonism, dystonia, myoclonus, tardive dyskinesia, and other movement disorders may exhibit mixed phenomenology. The term "dystonic tremor" is used to describe a tremor that occurs in the same anatomic location involved with dystonia. It is often irregular in frequency and is most prominent when the patient attempts to resist the abnormal posture or tries to maintain a primary position.

Oral medications are usually the first-line treatment for most tremors, although surgical interventions, particularly deep brain stimulation, offer a remarkable benefit in patients whose tremor is troublesome or disabling despite optimal medical therapy (4). This review focuses on treatment of tremor with botulinum toxin (BTX) type A (BTX-A) injections.

Almost all types of tremor have been reported to benefit from BTX injections (Table 31.1). Since its introduction in 1980s, BTX, with its ability to relieve inappropriate muscle contractions, has revolutionized the treatment of various disorders associated with inappropriate muscle contractions, including dystonia and tremors. Initially used in the treatment of dystonia, BTX was observed to improve not only the abnormal movement and posturing, but also the accompanying dystonic tremor (5). This observation stimulated interest in BTX as a treatment modality for different types of tremors (6). In an initial pilot study, 35 (67%) of patients with disabling head-neck (42 patients) and hand (10 patients) tremor noted moderate to marked functional improvement and a reduction in the amplitude of the tremor. This chapter organizes the review of BTX in tremor according to anatomic distribution.

BTX TREATMENT OF HEAD TREMOR

Head tremor is usually caused by ET and generally does not respond well to medications, such as propranolol and primidone, which are most

TABLE 31.1. *Medical treatment of tremor variants*

Variant	Treatment		
Rest tremor	T, L, PH	BTX	DBS
Postural hand/arm tremor	P, PRI, A, PH	BTX	DBS
Head tremor	C, PRI, P	BTX	—
Voice tremor	P	BTX	—
Facial/tongue tremor	P, PRI, L	BTX	—
Task-specific tremor	T, P, PRI	BTX	—
Orthostatic tremor	G, C, PRI, PH, L	—	—
Kinetic hand/arm tremor	C, P, PRI, BU, PH	BTX	DBS

A, alprazolam; BTX, botulinum toxin; BU, buspirone; C, clonazepam; DBS, deep-brain stimulation; G, gabapentin; L, levodopa; P, propranolol; PH, phenobarbital, PRI, primidone; T, trihexyphenidyl

frequently used in the treatment of ET involving the hands. Intractable head tremor, therefore, is particularly suited for treatment with BTX injections (Table 31.2). Besides ET, head-neck tremor is also present in up to 68.4% of patients with cervical dystonia (CD) (5,7). In early reports, BTX treatment of CD was found to improve head tremor in 50% to 65% of CD patients (8,9).

In the first systematic study of BTX in the treatment of head tremor, Jankovic and Schwartz injected both splenius capitis muscles if patients had lateral oscillation of the head, and one or both sternocleidomastoid muscles if they had anterior-posterior oscillation (6). In the 42 patients with head tremor treated by this approach, the average BTX-A dosage was 107 ± 38 U. Onset of effect had an average latency of 6.8 days; the average duration of total response was 12.5 weeks and the duration of maximum response was 10.5 weeks. The improvement in tremor severity was 3.0 ± 1.1 on a 0 to 4 scale, where 4 means total abolishment of tremor. This improvement was better than that in hand tremor treated similarly (2.0 ± 1.7), but the difference was not statistically significant. The clinical improvement was accompanied by a marked reduction in the recorded electromyographic (EMG) burst amplitude in splenius capitis muscles. The frequency, burst duration, interburst intervals, and synchronicity of EMG activity were not changed (Fig. 31.1B). The side effects included weakness of neck muscles in 9.5% and dysphagia in 28.6% of patients. These side effects, however, were mild and transient,

with neck weakness persisting for 21.8 days and dysphagia lasting only 8.4 days.

Pahwa et al. conducted a double-blind, placebo-controlled study of BTX-A treatment in ten ET patients with intractable head tremor (10). All manifested lateral oscillation of the head. Each subject received normal saline as placebo or BTX injection 3 months apart. Under EMG guidance, BTX 40 U (BOTOX) was injected into each sternocleidomastoid muscle and BTX 60 U was injected into the splenius capitis. Rating by "blinded" examiners showed that 50% had moderate to marked improvement with BTX as compared to only 10% improvement in patients who received placebo. Subjective moderate to marked improvement also occurred in 50% of patients treated with BTX as compared to 30% in those who received placebo. However, there was no statistically significant difference between the two groups when the tremor was measured by accelerometry. Side effects were again transient and mild, mainly neck weakness, swallowing difficulty, and headache.

A case report by Finsterer et al. described a 67-year-old man who developed a "yes–yes" head tremor without appendicular tremor, dystonia, or titubation 6 weeks after right occipital and bilateral cerebellar infarction (11). EMG revealed rhythmic, synchronous agonist/antagonist activity in both splenius capitis and sternocleidomastoid muscles. The tremor was markedly improved after 120 U of BTX was injected into the former and 80 U into the latter muscles, but 5 weeks after the injection the tremor worsened again. After a booster injec-

TABLE 31.2. *BTX injections for head tremors*

Year	Authors	Number of patients	Muscles injected	Dose (units)	Results	Side effects
1991	Jankovic and Schwartz (6)	42	Splenius capitis for lateral oscillation; sternocleidomastoid for anterior-posterior tremor	107±38 (B)	Improvement of 3.0±1.1 on a 4-point scale; significantly reduced EMG burst amplitude on splenius capitis	29% with dysphagia; 10% with transient weakness; 5% with local pain
1995	Pahwa et al. (10)	10 (Head ET)	Sternocleidomastoid	40 (B)	50% had moderate to marked improvement (vs 10% in controls) on clinical ratings and on subjective ratings	60% had transient neck weakness; 20% had headache; 30% had swallowing difficulty
1996	Finsterer, Muellbacher, and Mamoli (11)	1 (case report)	Splenius capitis Sternocleidomastoid	60 (B) 80 (B)	Tremor markedly improved and vanished completely after a booster	Not mentioned
1997	Wissel et al.(12)	43 (29 with CD; TCD)	Splenius capitis Splenius capitis, sternocleidomastoid and trapezoid	120 (B) 500 (320 to 720) (D)	Tsui and pain scales, amplitude all decreased, subjective improvement in 26 of 29 patients	Local pain, neck weakness, dysphagia in 39%
		(14 without CD; HT)		400 (160 to 560) (D)	All significantly decreased	Similar side effects in 40%

B, BOTOX; CD, cervical dystonia; D, DYSPORT; ET, essential tremor; HT, head tremor; TCD, tremulous cervical dystonia

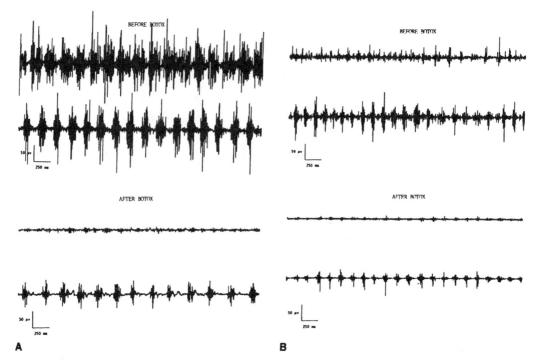

FIG. 31.1. Reduction in tremor amplitude after BTX injections into (**A**) forearm muscles in a patient with postural hand tremor and (**B**) into splenius capitis muscles in a patient with lateral head oscillation. (Adapted from Jankovic J, Schwartz K. Botulinum toxin treatment of tremors. *Neurology* 1991;41: 1185–1188.)

tion, the tremor completely disappeared 3 weeks later.

Wissel et al. assessed 43 patients with head tremor: 29 suffered from tremulous cervical dystonia (TCD) and 14 had essential head tremor (HT) without dystonia (12). Mean BTX-A (DYSPORT) dosages were 500 U (range 320 to 720 U) in TCD and 400 U (range 160 to 560 U) in HT. All HT patients received only bilateral splenius capitis injections, whereas most TCD patients received injections into splenius capitis, sternocleidomastoid, trapezius, levator scapulae, or semispinalis cervicis muscles. After 2 to 3 weeks, subjective improvements occurred in 100% of HT and 89.7% of TCD (26 of 29 patients). Tsui scores (5-point) decreased from 3.1 to 1.1 in HT patients and from 10.2 to 5.2 in TCD; pain scores (4-point) decreased from 1.0 to 0.4 in HT and 1.5 to 0.8 in TCD; all were statistically significant. The authors found no

significant changes in head oscillation frequency after BTX injections in either TCD or HT patients. The tremor amplitudes of the mean peak power measured by accelerometer before and after treatment showed significant reductions (0.079 to 0.026 in HT, $p < 0.05$; 0.088 to 0.025 in TCD, $p < 0.001$). Side effects were mild and transient, and included local pain, neck weakness, and dysphagia in 40% of HT and 39% of TCD patients.

In summary, essentially all patients with head tremor of various etiologies (ET, CD, or cerebellorubral lesions) seem to benefit from BTX injections. Sternocleidomastoid and splenius capitis muscles are often the target muscles. According to different studies, at least half of the patients improve on objective examinations or measurements, while subjective improvement percentages can be even more robust. Response typically occurs a week after the injection and may last for 8 to 12 weeks. Common side effects are mostly mild and transient, including neck weakness, dysphagia, and local pain.

BTX TREATMENT OF LIMB TREMOR

The first-line treatments in patients with hand tremor are usually oral tremorlytic medications. In ET, β-blockers, primidone, and benzodiazepines are the most frequently used drugs (Table 31.3). For refractory tremor, BTX treatment is usually effective in reducing the tremor amplitude before considering surgical intervention. In the pilot study by Jankovic and Schwartz, ten patients with hand tremor (four essential, one dystonic, three combination, one parkinsonian, one peripherally induced) were injected with an average of 95 ± 38 U of BTX-A in the wrist extensors (extensor carpi radialis and ulnaris) and flexors (flexor carpi radialis and ulnaris) (6). The reduction of tremor severity was 2.0 ± 1.7 on a 0 to 4 rating scale (4 = total abolishment of tremor). This reduction was less than that in head tremor, but there was no statistically significant difference between the two groups. Many patients reported marked functional improvement in handwriting and other daily activities (Figs. 31.1A and 31.2A, B). EMG findings, as with head tremor, showed reductions in burst amplitude in forearm muscles but no change in frequency, burst duration, interburst intervals, or synchronicity of EMG activity (Fig. 31.1A, B). Complication of local hand weakness occurred in 60% of patients and lasted for an average 23.9-day transient period. Since the initial, exploratory study, we have modified our approach and no longer inject the wrist extensor or inject with very low doses. As a result, extensor finger or wrist weakness is almost never observed in our tremor patients.

In an open-label study, Trosch and Pullman treated 12 patients with PD and 14 with ET for their hand tremors (13). The target muscles were selected by clinical examination and EMG, and included extensor carpi radialis, extensor carpi ulnaris, flexor carpi radialis, and flexor carpi ulnaris. In addition, extensor digitorum communis, pronator teres, biceps, and triceps were also injected if more proximal muscles were involved. Average doses of BOTOX in the distal muscles were between 10 and 25 U and in the proximal muscles were approximately 60 to 75 U. Average dose per patient was 107.5 U for PD and 108.6 U for ET. Six weeks after the injection, five patients, each with PD and ET, reported improvement of 3 or greater on a 4-point scale. Significant improvement on Webster Tremor and Global Assessment scales were found in ET, but not in PD patients. Quantitative tremor measurements showed that 2 PD and 3 ET patients had a greater than 50% reduction in amplitude. On average, PD rest tremor amplitude decreased by 15% and postural tremor by 11%. However, none of the results was significantly different, and there was no significant change in tremor frequency. The only adverse reaction was weakness of digit extension, noted on examination in all patients, but this did not result in functional impairment.

A single-blinded, placebo-controlled study by Henderson et al. evaluated BTX injections in patients with nondystonic tremors (14). They subdivided 17 patients into eight ET-like tremors and nine PD-like tremors, which included cases of PD, multiple-system atrophy (MSA), PD/ET combination, and midbrain tremor. All patients were initially injected with placebo followed by BTX injections 4 to 6 weeks later. Average dose of BOTOX was 25 U to each extensor or flexor muscle. By using accelerometry, both groups of ET- and PD-like tremors demonstrated large placebo effects ($\geq$30%) on resting and postural tremors. After BTX injections, there was no further improvement on resting tremor, but postural tremor improved 40% from baseline in PD-like and 57% in the ET-like groups, about a twofold improvement relative to placebo. At the second follow-up 3.7 months after BTX injection, there was still an improvement in the ET-like group by accelerometry and $\geq$20% improvement in both groups by clinical scores. There was a small (1 Hz) frequency variation in both groups when compared with placebo. The only side effect was transient forearm extensor weakness. The authors suggested that distributing the total BTX

TABLE 31.3. *BTX injections on limb tremors*

Year	Authors	Number of patients	Muscles injected	Dose (units) BOTOX	Results	Side effects
1991	Jankovic, Schwartz (6)	10	Wrist flexors and wrist extensors	95±38	Improvement of 2.0±1.7 on a 4-point scale; significantly reduced EMG burst amplitude on forearm muscles	60% had transient hand weakness
1994	Trosch, Pullman (13)	26				
		12 PD	Flexors and extensors	PD: 107.5	17% PD and 21% ET had greater than 50% amplitude reduction; average amplitude reduction was less than 25% ($p > 0.05$); 38% (5 PD, 5ET) had moderate to marked subjective functional benefit	One patient with excessive weakness of third-digit extension
		14 ET	Biceps and triceps	ET: 108.6		
1996	Henderson et al. (14)	17 (BTX vs control)	Flexors and extensors	25 to each muscle	Strong placebo effects in both groups; no further improvement on rest tremor from placebo; twofold improvement on postural tremor from placebo	9 of 17 patients had significant extensor muscle weakness
1996	Jankovic et al. (16)	25 (BTX vs control)	Wrist flexors and extensors	50; 4 weeks later, 100 booster	75% had mild to moderate ($\geq$2 rating scales); 9 of 12 patients had a $\geq$30% reduction of amplitude; no significant functional rating scale improvement	All had some degree of finger weakness; no severe, irreversible, or unexpected adverse effects
1996	Pullman, Greene, Fahn, Pedersen (15)	37 (Open label)	Wrist flexors and extensors	PD: 107.5 ET: 108.6 CBL: 278.4	PD: 13% amplitude reduction ET: 25% amplitude reduction CBL: 19% amplitude reduction	Finger flexors weakness
2001	Brin et al. (17)	133 (BTX low, high doses vs control)	Wrist flexors and extensors	50 (low)	0.6 to 0.7 scale improved on postural tremor from weeks 6 to 16; 0.4 improved on kinetic tremor only on week 6	30% had handgrip weakness
				100 (high)	0.7 to 1.0 scale improved on postural tremor from weeks 6 to 16; 0.6 improved on kinetic tremor only on week 6	70% had handgrip weakness

CBL, cerebellar tremor

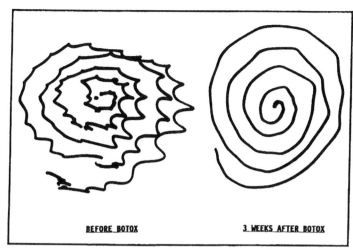

FIG. 31.2. A: Improvement in handwriting after BTX injection into wrist flexors in extensors of a patient with essential tremor. (Adapted from Jankovic J, Schwartz K. Botulinum toxin treatment of tremors. *Neurology* 1991;41:1185–1188.) **B:** Improvement in drawing of a spiral after BTX injection into wrist flexors in a patient with essential tremor during a 150-day follow-up showing marked improvement during days 10 to 60.

A

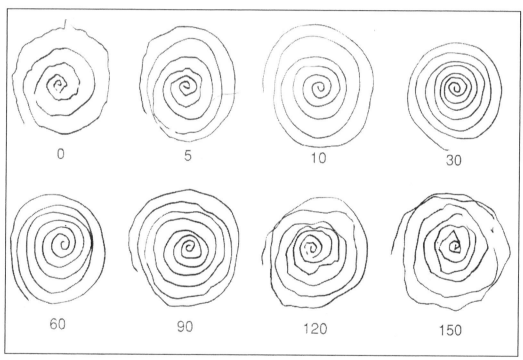

B

dose in a 2:1 flexor/extensor ratio might reduce the risk of extensor weakness.

Pullman et al. conducted a large series of BTX injections in 187 patients with various disorders involving the upper and lower limbs; 15 patients had PD, 17 had ET, and 5 had cerebellar tremor (15). Two of the 15 PD patients (13.3%) and 3 of the 17 ET patients (17.6%) had marked subjective improvements and significant decrement (greater than 50% reduction) in tremor amplitudes. The largest decrease in tremor amplitude was seen in ET patients (25% reduction), as compared with a 13% reduction in PD and a 19% reduction in cerebellar tremor patients. The overall improvement of disability was greatest in cerebellar tremor (50.6%) and lowest in PD tremors (35.7%). Generally, the BTX improvement on clinical disability ratings and the combined efficacy scores in tremors were not as great as in dystonia or spasticity, but showed slightly better average global functional improvement as compared with dystonia.

Jankovic et al. conducted the first double-blinded, placebo-controlled study in patients with ET hand tremor (16). Twenty-five patients with 2 + to 4 + tremor severity score were randomized to receive placebo (12 patients) or 50 U of BOTOX (13 patients) injections into the wrist flexors and extensors. Patients received a booster of 100 U 4 weeks later if they failed to respond the initial injections. Eleven of the placebo-treated subjects and only one in the BTX-treated group needed the booster. During the period of 4 to 16 weeks after the injections, the BTX group enjoyed an average improvement of 2.00 ± 0.95 versus 0.55 ± 1.04 in placebo group on a 4-point tremor scale, a statistically significant difference ($p < 0.05$). Furthermore, 75% of BTX-treated patients versus 27% of placebo-treated patients ($p < 0.05$) reported improvement with peak effect rating ≥ 2. Postural accelerometry showed a $\geq 30\%$ reduction in amplitude in nine BTX-treated patients and in only one placebo-treated patient ($p < 0.05$). All postural, kinetic, and composite tremors had significant decrease on tremor ratings. Functional rating scales, however, did not significantly improve. Improvement trends were found in some items such as feeding, handwriting, straight/sine wave drawings, and composite score for drawing. Adverse reaction was mild to moderate finger weakness in about half of the BTX-treated patients at week 4, and persisted in some patients to week 16, but no patient reported interference with their daily functions or activities.

Brin et al. conducted a similar placebo-controlled trial, involving 133 patients with hand ET recruited from ten centers in North America (17). The patients were randomized to one of three treatment groups—low-dose BTX, high-dose BTX, and placebo—and then followed up for 16 weeks. The postural tremor was rated ≥ 2

on 0 to 4 scales. For the low-dose group, 15 U were injected into flexor carpi radialis and ulnaris and 10 U into extensor carpi radialis and ulnaris. For the high-dose group, 30 U were injected into the flexors and 20 U into the extensors. The control group was injected with the comparable volume containing albumin and sodium chloride solution. Based on tremor rating, both low- and high-dose BTX groups improved significantly by physician and subjective ratings (0.6 to 0.7 scale improvement in low-dose; 0.7 to 1.0 scale improvement in high dose), with peak effect at 6 to 16 weeks. Kinetic tremors only slightly improved at week 6. The improvement in functional ratings was mild and not very consistent; it improved mainly in drawing a spiral and straight line (at high dose group), although on other tasks including feeding, dressing, and drinking, both groups showed about equal improvement. Quality of life by Sickness Impact Profile (SIP) scale did not show any improvement. Hand weakness was the most common side effect; 30% of the low-dose group and 70% of the high-dose group complained of decreased grip strength. Other adverse reactions included rash, pain, stiffness, cramping, hematoma, and paresthesias.

In summary, essential hand tremor has a favorable response to BTX treatment with minimal side effects, consisting chiefly of forearm muscle weakness. This complication can be markedly reduced or prevented by substantially reducing BTX dosage in wrist extensors. Fewer studies have been conducted on rest or kinetic tremors, and their results showed mixed responses. There are virtually no studies on lower limb tremors. Proximal arm muscles require larger doses than do the hands or forearms.

BTX TREATMENT IN VOICE TREMOR

Spasmodic dysphonia (SD) had long been successfully treated with EMG-guided injections of BTX (18,19). The response of BTX injection on essential voice tremor (VT), however, has not been thoroughly studied until recently (Table 31.4). The clinical manifestations of SD and VT can be confusing. In fact, 25% to 65% of patients

TABLE 31.4. *BTX injections on voice tremor*

Year	Authors	Number of patients	Muscles injected	Dose (units)	Results	Side effects
2000	Hertegard, Granqvist, Lindestad (30)	15	Thyroarytenoid muscles	0.6 to 5	67% had subjective improvement; significant decrease in voice tremor in perceptual evaluations; significant decrease in fundamental frequency on sustained vowel phonation	12 of 15 patients had breathy and weak voice for 1 to 2 weeks; 3 of 15 had hoarseness for 4 weeks
			Cricothyroid or thyrohyoid	1.25		
2000	Warrick et al. (31)	10	Thyroarytenoid	2.5 bilateral	3 of 10 patients had reduced voice tremor (8 of 10 subjectively improved)	3 patients had severe lengthy breathiness
				15 unilateral	2 of 9 patients had reduced voice tremor (8 of 10 subjectively improved)	2 patients had moderate lengthy breathiness
2000	Warrick et al. (29)	1	Thyroarytenoid (bilateral)	2.5 each side	Reduction in frequency and tremor amplitude from 1 to 10 weeks; reduction in airflow resistance	Mild hoarseness

with SD also have VT (20). VT is caused by oscillation of the vocalis muscle complex or posterior pharyngeal muscles with frequency about 5 to 7 Hz, most noticeable during sustained vowels. EMG recordings have shown that the intrinsic laryngeal muscles, specifically thyroarytenoid, are the most frequently involved (21). While the voice of SD is characterized by a strained, choked, strangled, and abrupt character (adductor type) or by a breathy, whispering voice (abductor type), VT is characterized by pitch breaks and vocal arrests, with excessive or interrupted glottal airflow (22). Although VT may concomitantly occur with SD, ET is the most common cause of pure VT. Approximately 25% of patients with ET have VT (23). In the study of Brown and Simonson of 31 patients with VT, 6 had isolated VT and 25 had involvement of other tremors. Sixteen (52%) had family history of tremors (24).

The mechanism by which VT is reduced with BTX injections is not completely clear. Several groups have conducted various aerodynamic studies on vocal cords of SD. BTX injection was shown to improve the airflow (25–27). The experiment by Finnegan et al. revealed that the improvement of VT was a result of increased stability of airflow after BTX injection rather than simply an increase in airflow (28). They studied five patients (one with SD; others with adductor SD and VT) and found that the mean airflow was similar to controls, but the airflow stability was decreased. After BTX injections, both mean airflow and airflow stability increased substantially. The authors proposed that increasing the stability of the laryngeal and respiratory systems leads to improved airflow stability and a reduction in VT.

Warrick et al. reported a 65-year-old patient suffering from periodic tremor and severe voice breaks (29). He was injected bilaterally into thyroarytenoid muscles with 2.5 U of BTX on each side. Acoustic analysis revealed a reduction in tremor frequency and amplitude during weeks 1 to 10. Perceptual ratings by three speech-language pathologists of tremor, voice break, and perceived vocal effort were all decreased during (approximately) weeks 2 to 10. Nasopharyngoscopy found that abductor-adductor, superior-in-ferior tremor, supraglottic hyperfunction, and vocal fold adduction were markedly reduced until weeks 10 to 16 after BTX injection. Hoarseness was briefly present and disappeared by the sixth week. Authors also demonstrated that laryngeal airflow dramatically increased and the estimated laryngeal resistance dropped markedly after BTX injection.

Hertegard et al. studied BTX injections in 15 patients with essential VT (30). Acoustic analysis of sustained vowel /a/ for these patients revealed tremor and falsetto phonation. Ordinary voice quality was tremulous to various degrees. All patients were injected into thyroarytenoid muscles with additional cricothyroid or thyrohyoid muscles in some patients. Ten patients (67%) reported subjective improvement 1 month after the injection. Patients were also tested by perceptual evaluations by recording their connected speech (in Swedish) and sustained vowels on the digital audiotapes and rated by two phoniatricians. This evaluation showed a significant decrease in voice tremor during connected speech. Acoustic analyses by computers showed a nearly significant decrease in the fundamental frequency variations ($p = 0.06$) and a significant decrease in fundamental frequency during sustained vowel phonation. The results of perceptual evaluation coincided most closely with the subjective judgment. Twelve of 15 patients had a temporarily breathy and weak voice for 1 to 2 weeks. Three patients had hoarseness lasting up to 4 weeks. The authors concluded that the treatment was successful in 50% to 65% of patients depending on the method of evaluation.

Warrick et al. further evaluated the relative efficacy of unilateral versus bilateral injections of BTX in the treatment of VT (31). They injected 10 patients with essential VT in an open-label trial. Five patients received 15 U of BOTOX injected into the unilateral vocalis muscle first, followed by bilateral 2.5-U injections at 16 to 18 weeks. The other five patients received bilateral injections followed by unilateral injections. Using objective acoustic measures, only a small portion of patients achieved reduction in tremor severity and there were no significant differences between unilateral and bilateral injections (two of nine in unilateral and three of ten in bilateral injections). Eight of ten patients reported subjective reduction in vocal effort and wanted to be reinjected. The aerodynamic estimation of laryngeal airway resistance decrease was correlated with the patients' perception of vocal effort. The only obvious side effect was lengthy breathiness in three patients rated 8.0 on the ten-point scale; five rated 5.0. One patient refused to continue injection because of this side effect. No difference in the frequency of side effects was found between unilateral and bilateral injections.

In summary, about 30% to 50% of VT patients improve based on objective acoustic analysis, and 65% to 80% of patients improve by subjective assessments. The objective response rates in patients with VT are not as robust as those in SD, especially the adductor type (32,33). This is mainly because different factors in laryngeal, respiratory, and orofacial systems contribute to the generation of VT. The beneficial effect of BTX injection is limited to the effect on the thyroarytenoid muscle, the most frequently injected muscle. BTX injection reduces the airflow resistance and increases the stability of airflow. The side effects are mostly mild and temporarily, include hoarseness, breathiness, and weak voice. There does not appear to be a significant difference in result between unilateral versus bilateral injections. These studies suggest that BTX injection is an ideal therapeutic option for patients with VT who usually fail to obtain satisfactory response to oral medical treatment.

BTX INJECTIONS FOR MISCELLANEOUS TYPES OF TREMORS

Two case reports discussed the effects of BTX injections on hereditary trembling chin. This is a relatively rare autosomal-dominant disorder presenting with intermittent trembling of mentalis muscles (34,35). The tremor frequency ranges between 2 and 11 Hz with variable amplitudes. It occurs at rest and may be precipitated by emotional changes. The tremor is often socially embarrassing to the patient because it is often misinterpreted as revealing an emotional upset. Traditional treatments, including faradic current, ultraviolet light, sedatives, and anticonvulsants are usually unsatisfactory (36). Gordon et al. injected 5 U of BOTOX bilaterally into mentalis muscles in one patient with this disorder and in his two affected sons (37). This effectively obliterated the symptoms with benefits lasting for 2 to 3 months. No side effects were reported. The patients continued to receive BTX injections every 3 months for more than 5 years with satisfactory results. Bakar et al. treated a 28-year-old man with hereditary chin tremor since birth (36). He had a positive family history involving his mother and grandmother. Mentalis, mylohyoid, and orbicularis oris muscles were all affected. BOTOX at 25 U was injected into each mentalis muscle. The paralysis of both mentalis muscles occurred within 2 days and lasted for 5 months. Local spread of BTX to surrounding muscles caused a side effect of distortion of the mouth lasting for about 30 to 45 days. This was later corrected by reducing the volume but leaving the BTX dose the same to minimize the spreading to adjacent muscles. The mother later received the injection and also enjoyed a similar result.

Palatal tremor (more frequently referred to as palatal myoclonus) is another disorder that benefits from BTX injections. Deuschl et al. reported a patient who had a rhythmic, continuous ear click caused by palatal tremor (38). They found that the ear click occurred during contraction of the tensor veli palatini, which opens the eustachian tube, and the disorder was attributed to involvement of the trigeminal nucleus. When BTX was injected into that muscle it successfully alleviated the ear click. Jamieson et al. reported a similar case of an ear click caused by palatal tremor (39). However, surgical division of the tensor veli palatini tendon failed to provide symptomatic relief. Using EMG guidance, the authors injected 20 U of BOTOX into the deep soft palate in close proximity to the insertion of levator veli palatini muscle. This eliminated the ear click within 3 days and the benefit was sustained for about 5 weeks. The authors suggested that in this patient the nucleus ambiguous or facial nucleus were responsible for the palatal tremor. Despite some controversy about the origins of palatal tremor, BTX injection has proven to be an effective treatment for this disorder. Needle EMG to detect the affected muscle is important, but local diffusion of BTX in the palate may still provide partial relief, even if the involved muscles are not precisely targeted.

MECHANISMS OF ACTION OF BTX ON REDUCING TREMOR

BTX acts at the neuromuscular junction by binding to presynaptic cholinergic nerve terminals and inhibiting the exocytosis of acetylcholine by interfering with acetylcholine release, thus relieving the abnormal muscle contractions or spasms (40). The mechanisms by which BTX reduces tremor, however, are not well understood. Different tremors respond to BTX treatment differently, suggesting various pathophysiologic mechanisms among tremors. ET has been proposed to originate from the disruption of neuron firing between the inferior olivary nucleus and cerebellar Purkinje cells (2,41). Peripherally, disruption of reciprocal inhibition between antagonist muscles may also play a role in ET (42). Modugno et al. studied BTX injection effects on the reciprocal inhibition circuitry in ET patients (43). Ten patients with ET were shown to have a reduced presynaptic phase of reciprocal inhibition by measuring H reflex, M response and H/M ratio at a regular interval-stimulation (every 10 ms). The patients received BTX injections into forearm flexor and extensor muscles at an average dose of 80 to 100 U. although BTX injections produced a 20% functional improvement in tremor on a 44-point scale, it also markedly restored the previously reduced presynaptic phase of reciprocal inhibition. Both the sizes of H reflex and M wave were reduced, but H:M ratio remained unchanged. The authors proposed that BTX reduced the amplitude of ET by inhibiting the extrafusal and intrafusal fibers simultaneously, thus decreasing the spindle afferent input to the spinal cord. A similar mechanism was proposed for the effects of BTX on dystonic tremor (44).

REFERENCES

1. Deuschl G, Krack P. Tremors: differential diagnosis, neurophysiology, and pharmacology. In: Jankovic J, Tolosa E, eds. *Parkinson's disease and movement disorders*. Baltimore, MD: Williams and Wilkins, 1998: 419–452.
2. Deuschl G, Raethjen J, Lindemann M, et al. The pathophysiology of tremor. *Muscle Nerve* 2001;24:716–735.
3. Lou JS, Jankovic J. Essential tremor: clinical correlates in 350 patients. *Neurology* 1991;41:234–238.
4. Jankovic J. Surgery for Parkinson's disease and other movement disorders: benefits and limitations of ablation, stimulation, restoration, and radiation. *Arch Neurol* 2001;58:1970–1972.
5. Jankovic J, Leder S, Warner D, et al. Cervical dystonia: clinical findings and associated movement disorders. *Neurology* 1991;41:1088–1091.
6. Jankovic J, Schwartz K. Botulinum toxin treatment of tremors. *Neurology* 1991;41:1185–1188.
7. Pal PK, Samii A, Schulzer M, et al. Head tremor in cervical dystonia. *Can J Neurol Sci* 2000;27:137–142.
8. Borodic GE, Mills L, Joseph M. Botulinum A toxin for the treatment of adult-onset spasmodic torticollis. *Plast Reconstr Surg* 1991;87:285–289.
9. Boghen D, Flanders M. Effectiveness of botulinum toxin in the treatment of spasmodic torticollis. *Eur Neurol* 1993;33:199–203.
10. Pahwa R, Busenbark K, Swanson-Hyland EF, et al. Botulinum toxin treatment of essential head tremor. *Neurology* 1995;45:822–824.
11. Finsterer J, Muellbacher W, Mamoli B. Yes/yes head tremor without appendicular tremor after bilateral cerebellar infarction. *J Neurol Sci* 1996;139:242–245.
12. Wissel J, Masuhr F, Schelosky L, et al. Quantitative assessment of botulinum toxin treatment in 43 patients with head tremor. *Mov Disord* 1997;12:722–726.
13. Trosch RM, Pullman SL. Botulinum toxin A injections for the treatment of hand tremors. *Mov Disord* 1994;9: 601–609.
14. Henderson JM, Ghika JA, Van Melle G, et al. Botulinum toxin A in non-dystonic tremors. *Eur Neurol* 1996;36: 29–35.
15. Pullman SL, Greene P, Fahn S, et al. Approach to the treatment of limb disorders with botulinum toxin A: experience with 187 patients. *Arch Neurol* 1996;53: 617–624.
16. Jankovic J, Schwartz K, Clemence W, et al. A randomized, double-blind, placebo-controlled study to evaluate botulinum toxin type A in essential hand tremor. *Mov Disord* 1996;11:250–256.
17. Brin MF, Lyons KE, Doucette J, et al. A randomized, double-masked, controlled trial of botulinum toxin type A in essential hand tremor. *Neurology* 2001;56: 1523–1528.
18. Brin MF, Blitzer A, Fahn S, et al. Adductor laryngeal dystonia (spastic dysphonia): treatment with local injections of botulinum toxin (BOTOX). *Mov Disord* 1989; 4:287–296.
19. Blitzer A, Brin MF, Stewart C, et al. Abductor laryngeal dystonia: a series treated with botulinum toxin. *Laryngoscope* 1992;102:163–167.
20. Blitzer A, Brin MF, Fahn S. Clinical and laboratory characteristics of focal laryngeal dystonia. Study of 110 cases. *Laryngoscope* 1988;98:636–640.

21. Koda J, Ludlow CL. An evaluation of laryngeal muscle activation in patients with voice tremor. *Otolaryngol Head Neck Surg* 1992;107:684–696.
22. Aronson AE, Hartman DE. Adductor spasmodic dysphonia as a sign of essential voice tremor. *J Speech Hear Disord* 1981;46:52–58.
23. Koller WC, Busenbark K, Miner K. The relationship of essential tremor to other movement disorders: report on 678 patients. Essential tremor study group. *Ann Neurol* 1994;35:717–723.
24. Brown JR, Simonson J. Organic voice tremor: a tremor of phonation. *Neurology* 1963;13:520–525.
25. Briant TDR, Blair RL, Cole P, et al. Laboratory investigation of abnormal voice. *J Otolaryngol* 1983;12:285–290.
26. Woo P, Colton R, Casper J, et al. Analysis of spasmodic dysphonia by aerodynamic and laryngostroboscopic measurements. *J Voice* 1992;6:344–351.
27. Zwirner P, Murry T, Swenson M, et al. Effects of botulinum toxin therapy in patients with adductor spasmodic dysphonia: acoustic, aerodynamic, and videoendoscopic findings. *Laryngoscope* 1992;102:400–406.
28. Finnegan E, Luschei ES, Gordon J, et al. Increased stability of airflow following botulinum toxin injection. *Laryngoscope* 1999;109:1300–1306.
29. Warrick P, Dromey C, Irish J, et al. The treatment of essential voice tremor with botulinum toxin A: a longitudinal case report. *J Voice* 2000;14:410–421.
30. Hertegard S, Granqvist S, Lindestad PA. Botulinum toxin injections for essential voice tremor. *Ann Otol Rhinol Laryngol* 2000;109:204–209.
31. Warrick P, Dromey C, Irish J, et al. Botulinum toxin for essential tremor of the voice with multiple anatomical sites of tremor: a crossover design study of unilateral versus bilateral injection. *Laryngoscope* 2000;110:1366–1374.
32. Truong DD, Rontal M, Rolnick M, et al. Double-blind controlled study of botulinum toxin in adductor spasmodic dysphonia. *Laryngoscope* 1991;101:630–634.
33. Blitzer A, Brin MF. The evaluation and management of abductor laryngeal dystonia. In: Jankovic J, Hallett M, eds. *Therapy with botulinum toxin.* New York: Marcel Dekker, 1994:451–459.
34. Laurence BM, Mattlows WB, Diggle JH. Hereditary quivering of the chin. *Arch Dis Child* 1968;43:249–251.
35. Alsager DE, Bowen P, Bamforth JS. Trembling chin—a report of the inheritable dominant character in a four generation Canadian family. *Clin Genet* 1991;40:186–189.
36. Bakar M, Zarifoglu M, Bora I, et al. Treatment of hereditary trembling chin with botulinum toxin. *Mov Disord* 1998;13:845–850.
37. Gordon K, Cadera W, Hinton G. Successful treatment of hereditary trembling chin with botulinum toxin. *J Child Neurol* 1993;8:154–156.
38. Deuschl G, Lohle E, Heinen F, et al. Ear click in palatal tremor: its origin and treatment with botulinum toxin. *Neurology* 1991;41:1677–1679.
39. Jamieson DRS, Mann C, O'Reilly B, et al. Ear clicks in palatal tremor caused by activity of the levator veli palatini. *Neurology* 1996;6:1168–1169.
40. Simpson LL. The origin, structure, and pharmacologic activity of botulinum toxin. *Pharmacol Rev* 1981;33:155–188.
41. Jankovic J. Essential tremor: clinical characteristics. *Neurology* 2000;54(Suppl 4):S21–S25.
42. Mercuri B, Berardelli A, Modugno N, et al. Reciprocal inhibition in forearm muscles in patients with essential tremor. *Muscle Nerve* 1997;41:553–556.
43. Modugno N, Priori A, Berardelli A, et al. Botulinum toxin restores presynaptic inhibition of group Ia afferents in patients with essential tremor. *Muscle Nerve* 1998;21:1701–1705.
44. Priori A, Berardelli A, Mercuri B, et al. Physiological effects produced by botulinum toxin treatment of upper limb dystonia. Changes in reciprocal inhibition between forearm muscles. *Brain* 1995;118:801–807.

Scientific and Therapeutic Aspects of Botulinum Toxin
edited by M.F. Brin, J. Jankovic, and M. Hallett
Lippincott Williams & Wilkins, Philadelphia, © 2002.

32

Botulinum Toxin in the Treatment of Tics

Carolyn H. Kwak and Joseph Jankovic

CLINICAL PHENOMENOLOGY OF TICS

Tics are among the most common movement disorders, estimated to affect as many as 3.5% of children (1,2). Motor tics are characterized by abrupt, rapid, frequently repetitive movements that wax and wane in intensity and frequency (3) and are commonly preceded by a premonitory urge or sensation (4). The term "unvoluntary" or "semivoluntary" has been used to describe the motor component of a tic that is a response to an involuntary premonitory sensation (5). Common motor tics include eye blinking, oculogyric deviation, facial grimacing, neck popping or stretching, shoulder shrugging and a variety of other complex maneuvers. Phonic tics involve the nasal and oropharyngeal passages and manifest as throat clearing, sniffing, coughing, grunting, inhaling, lip smacking, blowing, sucking, barking, screaming, squealing, and other sounds. Tic exacerbation commonly occurs with anxiety, fatigue, hunger, stress, suggestion, and central nervous system stimulants (6–9), whereas concentration, distraction, and physical activity tend to improve tics.

Tics are most frequently observed in patients with Tourette syndrome (TS), a neurologic movement disorder associated with neurobehavioral comorbidities, such as attention deficit hyperactivity disorder (ADHD), obsessive-compulsive disorder (OCD), and impulse control problems. Motor and phonic tics are classified as simple or complex in TS patients (3). Simple tics involve an isolated muscle group, whereas complex motor tics involve integration of a variety of learned, sequenced movements such as

touching, tapping, jumping, socially inappropriate gestures (copropraxia), or self-injurious behaviors. Shouting of obscenities (coprolalia) and repetition of one's own words (palilalia) or others' words (echolalia) are complex phonic tics included in the spectrum of vocalizations seen in about half of TS patients (10).

Frequently tics are preceded by premonitory sensations commonly described as an urge to move, stretch, or apply pressure to the muscle, internal tension, or an urge to move until it feels "just right" (11). The presentation of OCD in TS is complex yet unique in that obsessive compulsive symptomatology may be integrated in the phenotypic expression of the tics. Although premonitory sensation may be present in other movement disorders such as dystonia, the occurrence is less consistent and much less common than the 90% frequency of this phenomenon in patients with tics (12).

PATHOPHYSIOLOGY OF TICS AND TOURETTE SYNDROME

Because dopamine receptor-blocking drugs (neuroleptics) such as fluphenazine, haloperidol, pimozide, and risperidone reduce motor and phonic tics, dopaminergic overactivity has been postulated as an important biochemical-pharmacologic mechanism of tics. Dysfunction of any of five distinct fronto-subcortical pathways has been implicated in TS pathology: the motor circuit originating from the supplementary motor area (SMA) projecting to the putamen (motor tics); the oculomotor circuit projecting from the frontal eye fields to the central caudate (ocular deviations); the dorsolateral prefrontal circuit linking Brodmann's areas 9 and 10 to the dorsolateral head of the caudate (ADHD in TS); the lateral orbitofrontal circuit projecting from the inferolateral prefrontal cortex to ventromedial caudate; and the anterior cingulate/limbic circuit originating in the cingulate gyrus projecting to the ventral striatum (OCD associated with TS). In addition to dysregulation of dopamine, abnormalities of acetylcholine, gamma-aminobutyric acid (GABA), norepinephrine, and serotonin of the frontal subcortical circuits have also been suggested (13–17).

Although clinical evidence predominantly supports a dopaminergic dysfunction, supported by the observation that dopamine-receptor antagonists or dopamine-depleting agents alleviate tics, an interrelated chemical imbalance involving several neurotransmitters depicts a more probable neurochemical pathology. The current dopaminergic hypothesis proposes involvement of supersensitive postsynaptic dopamine receptors, hyperinnervation of dopaminergic neurons in the striatum, and presynaptic excessive dopamine synthesis (18–20).

TREATMENT OF TICS WITH BOTULINUM TOXIN

Dopamine antagonists are the most commonly prescribed medications to reduce tic frequency and severity. Fluphenazine, haloperidol, pimozide, and risperidone are the most frequently used neuroleptics. Although tic reduction of up to 80% has been noted with these drugs (21–23), 70% to 80% of patients have reported some side effect (24,25). Sedation, weight gain, lethargy, and mood alterations are the most common troublesome side effects. The more serious side effects, such as acute dystonic reaction, parkinsonism, tardive dyskinesia, and hepatotoxicity, are rare but more disabling. Tetrabenazine, a monoamine depleter and dopamine-receptor blocker, also improves tics but without the side effect of tardive dyskinesia (26).

Botulinum toxin (BTX), the most potent biologic toxin, effectively treats several neurologic conditions characterized by involuntary movements such as dystonia, tremors, spasticity, and tics. The use of BTX as an effective and safe treatment for tics was first demonstrated in a pilot study of ten TS patients (27). The sites of injection included the orbicularis oculi, eyebrow, masseter, rhomboid, splenius, and trapezius muscles with reported side effects of transient ptosis (one patient), neck pain (two patients), neck stiffness (one patient), and neck weakness (two patients). All patients improved to some degree with the mean "peak-effect" score of 3.76 (0, no effect; 1, mild effect but no functional improvement; 2, moderate change but no functional improvement; 3, moderate change in both severity and function; 4, marked improvement in both severity and function). The mean global score, defined as the peak-effect score subtracted by the degree of the side effect (−1 for nondisabling and −2 for disabling) was also assessed for each patient. The latency to initial response was 3 to 7 days, the duration of clinical benefit was 2 to 20 weeks. The mean dose per session for the upper face was 56.7 mouse units (U) BOTOX, 141.7 U for cervical tics, and 62.5 U for the masseter muscles. An interesting finding from this pilot study was the reduction of the premonitory sensation preceding the tic in all patients.

In a follow up study of 35 patients with tics and TS (28), 29 of 35 patients (83%) reported improvement of tics, with 23 reporting a peak effect of 3 or higher (markedly improved function); mean peak-effect score of 2.8, latency of 3.8 days; and duration of effect of 14.4 weeks. Five patients experienced complete resolution of tics, defined as tic remission for a period of more than 1 year. The mean dose per injection site per session was 149.6 U in cervical muscles, 57.4 U in upper face, 79.3 U in lower face, 17.8 U in vocal cords, and 121.7 U in other muscles such as the shoulder, forearm, or scalp. The side effects included mild and transient neck weakness (four patients), ptosis (two patients), mild and transient dysphagia (two patients), nausea (one patient), generalized weakness (one patient), fatigue (one patient) and hypophonia (one patient). Interestingly, 84% of patients also reported a reduction of premonitory sensations after the BTX injections.

In addition to these results in patients with motor and phonic tics, Scott (29) and Trimble (30) reported considerable improvement in two

TABLE 32.1. *Studies of botulinum toxin in treatment of tics*

Study (first author, year)	n	Site of injection (n)	Results	Side effects (n) *	Comment
Marras et al, 2001 (35)	18	Cervical (8), upper face (10), lower face (2), shoulder (1)	15/17 improved based on rating of a video; 9/13 had an improvement in premonitory "urge score." Despite reduction in rating scores, patients did not report overall improvement	Unspecified weakness (12), neck discomfort (3), blurred vision (1), swallowing difficulty (2), motor restlessness (2), increased urge to tic (1), onset of new tics to replace treated tic (2)	Patients had mild tics (median global TS score of 9.3 of 100)
Kwak et al, 2000 (28)	35	Cervical (17), upper face (14), lower face (7), vocal cords (4), other (3)	29/35 (83%) improved; 21/25 (84%) with premonitory sensations improved	Neck weakness (4), transient ptosis (2), mild dysphagia (2), nausea (1), fatigue (1), hyphonia (1)	Open label
Awaad et al, 1999 (31)	186	Face, cervical, vocal cords (n not specified)	Degree of improvement in tics or premonitory sensation not well specified	Soreness (5), transient neck weakness (4), ptosis (3)	Open label, methods of patient selection and assessments not well defined (38)
Trimble et al, 1998 (30)	1	Vocal cords	Improved coprolalia	Hypophonia	Case report coprolalia
Adler et al, 1996 (32)	1	Cervical	Improved	None reported	Case report cervical myelopathy secondary severe tics
Salloway et al, 1996 (33)	1	Vocal cords	Improved phonic tic	Hypophonia	case report refractory phonic tics
Scott et al, 1996 (29)	1	Vocal cord	Improved coprolalia	Hypophonia	case report; coprolalia
Krauss et al, 1996 (34)	1	Cervical	Improved tics and premonitory sensation	None reported	case report; cervical myelopathy secondary severe tics
Jankovic, 1994 (27)	10	Upper face (5), cervical (5)	All patients improved (peak effect 3.8; 4 = total abolishment).	Premonitory sensation improved in all	Transient ptosis (2), neck weakness (3)

* All side effects were reported as transient and non-functionally disabling.

TS patients treated with BTX for severe, disabling coprolalia. In these two cases, BTX was injected into the vocal cord (bilateral thyroarytenoid) and intralaryngeal muscles respectively. A dose of 3.75 U into each thyroarytenoid in the first case was highly beneficial for the patient who was able to integrate his vocalizations into sentences without social embarrassment after the injections. The premonitory urge to scream obscenities was also reported to diminish. However, repeated injections with 5 U on each side at 3 and 6 months were required for continued therapeutic effect. A transient breathy voice and very mild aspiration with drinking liquids were the only reported side effects. In the latter case, the reduction in volume of coprolalia resulted in reduction of stress in his social environment and subsequent mitigation of other tics as well for a duration of 18 months.

Only one randomized, double-blind study involving 18 patients (35) has evaluated the efficacy of BTX injections in the treatment of tics. Although a significant reduction in the frequency and severity of tics was reported based on tic count through videotaped analysis rated by board-certified neurologists (a 39% reduction as compared to a 5.8% increase in tics with placebo injections), the study also concluded that patients failed to show subjective "overall benefit" after the injection. However, there were several limitations to this study, including a small sample size ($n = 18$), very mild severity of tics at baseline (median TS global score of 9.3 out of 100, median premonitory sensation score of 0.5 out of 4, and 10 of 20 patients did not currently require medications), and the method of measuring outcome variables. Because of the fluctuating course of a tic disorder, controlling for confounding variables in any double-blind controlled study is difficult. Tics wax and wane in severity and frequency depending on the level of stress, anxiety, suggestibility, or other exacerbating stimuli. In this double-blind study, the primary outcome measure of change in tic frequency (count) was assessed between baseline and week 2. However, the latency and peak-effect response to BTX are highly variable for individual patients, with some experiencing delay in observed peak effect for up to 4 weeks and,

therefore, some patients may not have been observed at the time of their optimal benefit. Despite this limitation, 15 of 17 patients were reported improved based on a rating of a 12-minute video taken 2 weeks after the injection. Furthermore, because of the crossover design, it is possible that there was a carryover effect into the second phase of the study, thus obscuring the difference in response between the two phases. All side effects, such as muscle weakness, swallowing difficulty, and visual changes were reported as transient and nondisabling. However, the presence of weakness, noted by examination in 12 patients, could have potentially unblinded the study. An interesting finding in this study was the report of a new onset of tics following the resolution of the injected tic in some patients. It should, however, be noted that as part of the natural history of tics, new tics emerge as old tics disappear and, therefore, this finding may not necessarily indicate that the new tic was caused by BTX-induced resolution of a tic. Furthermore, in more than 100 patients with tics treated in our clinic over the past 8 years, we have not consistently observed an emergence of new tics after BTX treatment.

Consistent with previous studies, a significant attenuation of premonitory sensations was noted with BTX as compared to placebo ($p < 0.02$); 9 of 13 patients reported improvements in "urge score" 2 weeks after injection. The mechanism by which BTX improves premonitory sensation is unknown. Although a previous study found no premotor cortical potential in patients during spontaneous tics, suggesting that tics are truly involuntary (36), Karp et al. showed that some (two of five) patients had premotor negativity with spontaneous tics, similar to the observation when patients were simulating their tics voluntarily (37). It is possible that the premonitory sensations represent or correlate with subclinical isometric muscle contraction; hence, it would be expected to respond to BTX.

REFERENCES

1. Mason A, Banergee S, Zeitlin H, et al. The prevalence of Tourette syndrome in a mainstream school population. *Dev Med Child Neurol* 1998;40:292–296.

2. Costello E, Angold A, Burns B, et al. The Great Smokey Mountains study of youth: goals, design, method, and the prevalence of DSM-III-R disorders. *Arch Gen Psychiatry* 1996;53:1129–1136.

3. Jankovic J. Phenomenology and classification of tics. *Neurol Clin* 1997;15:267–275.

4. Leckman J, Walker D, Cohen D. Premonitory urges in Tourette's syndrome. *Am J Psychiatry* 1993;150: 98–102.

5. Jankovic J. Differential diagnosis and etiology of tics. In: Cohen D, Jankovic J, Goetz C, eds. Tourette syndrome. *Adv Neurol* 2001:85;15–30.

6. Gadow KD, Nolan EE, Sverd J. Methylphenidate in hyperactive boys with comorbid tic disorder: II. Short-term behavioral effects in school settings. *J Am Acad Child Adolesc Psychiatry* 1992;31:462–471.

7. Gadow KD, Nolan E, Sprafkin J, et al. School observations of children attention-deficit hyperactivity disorder and comorbid tic disorder: effects of methylphenidate treatment. *J Dev Behav Pediatr* 1995;16:167–176.

8. Borcherding BG, Keysor CS, Rapoport JL, et al. Motor/vocal tics and compulsive behaviors on stimulant drugs: is there a common vulnerability? *Psychiatry Res* 1990; 33:83–94.

9. Castellanos FX, Giedd JN, Elia J, et al. Controlled stimulant treatment of ADHD and comorbid Tourette's syndrome: effects of stimulant and dose. *J Am Acad Child Adolesc Psychiatry* 1997;36:589–596.

10. Robertson M. Tourette syndrome, associated conditions and the complexities of treatment. *Brain* 2000;123: 425–462.

11. Leckman JF, Walker DE, Goodman WK, et al. "Just right" perceptions associated with compulsive behavior in Tourette's syndrome. *Am J Psychiatry* 1994;151: 675–680.

12. Leckman J, Walker D, Cohen D. Premonitory urges in Tourette's syndrome. *Am J Psychiatry* 1993;150: 98–102.

13. Castellanos F. Neural substrates of attention-deficit hyperactivity disorder. In: Cohen D, Jankovic J, Goetz C, eds. Tourette syndrome. *Adv Neurol* 2001;85:197–206.

14. Peterson, B. Neuroimaging studies of Tourette syndrome: a decade of progress. In: Cohen D, Jankovic J, Goetz C, eds. Tourette syndrome. *Adv Neurol* 2001;85: 179–196.

15. Alexander G, DeLong M, Strick P. Parallel organization of functionally segregated circuits linking basal ganglia and cortex. *Annu Rev Neurosci* 1986;9:57–81.

16. Cummings J. Frontal-subcortical circuits and human behavior. *Arch Neurol* 1993;50:873–880.

17. Singer HS. Neurobiology of Tourette syndrome. *Neurol Clin* 1997;15:357–379.

18. Singer HS, Butler IJ, Tune LE. Dopaminergic dysfunction in Tourette syndrome. *Ann Neurol* 1982;12: 361–366.

19. Singer HS, Hahn I-H, Moran TH. Abnormal dopamine uptake sites in postmortem striatum from patients with Tourette syndrome. *Ann Neurol* 1991;30:558–562.

20. Cohen DJ, Shaywitz BA, Caparulo BK. Chronic, multiple tics of Gilles de la Tourette disease: CSF acid monoamine metabolites after probenecid administration. *Arch Gen Psychiatry* 1978;35:245–250.

21. Sallee F, Nesbit L, Jackson C. Relative efficacy of haloperidol and pimozide in children and adolescents. *Am J Psychiatry* 1997;154:1057–1062.

22. Bruun R, Budman C. Risperidone as a treatment for Tourette's syndrome. *J Clin Psychiatry* 1996;57:29–31.

23. Jankovic J, Pohaidy H. Motor, behavioral and pharmacological findings in Tourette's syndrome. *Can J Neurol Sci* 1987;14:541–546.

24. Kurlan R. Tourette syndrome. Treatment of tics. *Neurol Clin* 1997a;15:403–409.

25. Lang A. Update on the treatment of tics. In: Cohen D, Jankovic J, Goetz C, eds. Tourette syndrome. *Adv Neurol* 2001;85:355–362.

26. Jankovic J, Beach J. Long-term effects of tetrabenazine in hyperkinetic movement disorders. *Neurology* 1997; 48:358–362.

27. Jankovic J. Botulinum toxin in the treatment of dystonic tics. *Mov Disord* 1994;9:347–349.

28. Kwak CH, Hanna PA, Jankovic J. Botulinum toxin in the treatment of tics. *Arch Neurol* 2000;57:1190–1193.

29. Scott BL, Jankovic J, Donovan DT. Botulinum toxin injection into vocal cord in the treatment of malignant coprolalia associated with Tourette's syndrome. *Mov Disord* 1996;11:431–433.

30. Trimble MR, Whurr R, Brookes G, et al. Vocal tics in Gilles de la Tourette syndrome treated with botulinum toxin injections. *Mov Disord* 1998;13:617–619.

31. Awaad Y. Tics in Tourette syndrome: new treatment options. *J Child Neurol* 1999;14:316–319.

32. Adler CH, Zimmerman RS, Lyons MK, et al. Perioperative use of botulinum toxin for movement disorder-induced cervical spine disease. *Mov Disord* 1996;11: 79–81.

33. Salloway S, Stewart CF, Israeli L, et al. Botulinum toxin for refractory vocal tics. *Mov Disord* 1996;11:746–748.

34. Krauss JK, Jankovic J. Severe motor tics causing cervical myelopathy in Tourette's syndrome. *Mov Disord* 1996;11:563–566.

35. Marras C, Andrews D, Sime E, et al. Botulinum toxin for simple motor tics: a randomized, double-blind, controlled clinical trial. *Neurology* 2001;56:605–610.

36. Obeso J, Rothwell J, Marsden C. Simple tics in Gilles de la Tourette's syndrome are not prefaced by a normal premovement EEG potential. *J Neurol Neurosurg Psychiatry* 1981;44:735–738.

37. Karp B, Porter S, Toro C, et al. Simple motor tics may be preceded by a premotor potential. *J Neurol Neurosurg Psychiatry* 1996;61:103–106.

Scientific and Therapeutic Aspects of Botulinum Toxin
edited by M.F. Brin, J. Jankovic, and M. Hallett
Lippincott Williams & Wilkins, Philadelphia, © 2002.

33

Botulinum Toxin Type A in the Management of Oromandibular Dystonia and Bruxism

Ron Tintner and Joseph Jankovic

Oromandibular dystonia (OMD) refers to involuntary spasms of masticatory, lingual, and pharyngeal muscles. Phenomenologically, there are seven types of OMD: jaw-closing dystonia (JCD); jaw-opening dystonia (JOD); jaw-deviation dystonia (JDD); lip and perioral dystonia; lingual dystonia; pharyngeal dystonia; and combination OMD (1). OMD may be seen in isolation (focal dystonia), as part of a more widespread segmental cranial dystonia, or as part of a multisegmental or generalized dystonia. In 1910, the French neurologist Henry Meige described a syndrome, sometimes still referred to as Meige's syndrome, that occurred predominantly in middle-aged women and consisted of spasms of the eyelids as well as contractions of the pharyngeal, jaw, and tongue muscles (2). Because Meige was not the first to describe the disorder (Horatio Wood, a Philadelphia neurologist, described facial and oromandibular dystonia in 1887) (3), the syndrome is now more accurately referred to as cranial dystonia.

The etiologies of OMD are diverse (Table 33.1). The leading cause is primary (idiopathic) dystonia, which is often associated with other dystonias, particularly cervical and cranial. Some cases of OMD may be manifestations of inherited disorders; however, DYT1 dystonia, caused by a mutation of the torsinA gene on chromosome 9q34, the most common form of inherited dystonia, rarely involves the cranial structures (4). A patient with adult-onset OMD and no obvious family history of dystonia has been reported with a mutation of the gene for GTP cyclohydrolase 1, which causes the syndrome of dopa-responsive dystonia (5). The patient responded well to treatment with L-dopa. In addition to the primary dystonias, other common causes of OMD are drugs (tardive OMD) and peripheral injury, such as dental procedures and jaw trauma (6,7).

Until the advent of botulinum toxin (BTX) therapy, systemic pharmacologic agents were the traditional mainstay of treatment for OMD. Anticholinergics (e.g., trihexyphenidyl, benztropine), benzodiazepines (e.g., clonazepam, lorazepam, diazepam), baclofen, and tetrabenazine (which deplete dopamine and block dopamine receptors), were useful in some patients (8). Chronic systemic pharmacotherapy, however, is largely unsatisfactory because of modest improvements and frequent side effects, resulting in a low therapeutic ratio. Dental appliances have occasionally been helpful (9). There are no effective regional denervating surgical procedures, such as those used for cervical dystonia or blepharospasm. Central stereotactic surgery, such as pallidotomy (10) and deep brain stimulation (11) have been used successfully for treatment of generalized and hemidystonias, but there is no information regarding their use for more limited craniofacial dystonias. The remainder of this review focuses on regional procedures, particularly chemodenervation with BTX.

The pharmacology of BTX and the mechanisms by which this potent biologic toxin produces local chemodenervation, benefiting patients with involuntary muscular spasms such as

---

Throughout this chapter n ± m refers to mean ± SD, unless indicated otherwise.

TABLE 33.1. *Etiology of abnormal jaw and mouth movements*

Dystonias
Primary (idiopathic) dystonia
Inherited dystonia syndromes
   X-linked dystonia parkinsonism (Lubag); locus: DYT3
   Dopa-responsive dystonia; locus: DYT5
   Adult-onset idiopathic torsion dystonia of mixed type; locus: DYT6
   Focal, adult-onset idiopathic torsion dystonia; locus: DYT7
   Adult- and juvenile-onset idiopathic torsion dystonia of mixed type and mild severity; locus: DYT13
Secondary dystonias
   Drug-induced (dopamine receptor-blocking drugs, levodopa, and some serotonin reuptake inhibitors)
   Anoxic brain damage
   Peripheral dystonia (posttraumatic after oromandibular or dental injury or surgery)
Neurodegenerative disorders with dystonia
   Parkinson's disease (jaw tremor and levodopa-induced dyskinesias)
   Multiple system atrophy (especially that caused by levodopa-induced dyskinesias)
   Progressive supranuclear palsy
   Huntington's disease
Bruxism (idiopathic, diurnal, mental retardation, neurodegenerative disorders)
Hemimasticatory spasm
Hemifacial spasm
Satoyoshi's syndrome

can transiently alter intracortical inhibition (18) and normalize distorted primary motor cortex projections to hand and forearm muscles. Secondary alteration of central sensorimotor physiology and an additional primary effect on muscle spindle function are probably critical in the long-term efficacy of BTX in dystonia (19,20). To test this hypothesis directly, blockade of muscular afferents has been performed. Yoshida et al. (21) treated 13 patients with OMD resistant to pharmacotherapy or dental treatment by injecting diluted lidocaine and alcohol intramuscularly to reduce muscle spindle afferent activity. All patients reportedly showed clinical improvement after this therapy with reduced electromyographic (EMG) activities in the affected muscles. The overall subjective improvement was $57.7\% \pm 25.1\%$ (mean $\pm$ SD) on a self-rating scale. There was a 70% mean improvement in JCD, which was significantly higher than the 38% improvement in JOD. This mode of therapy may turn out to be useful when more experience is obtained and should ultimately be compared directly with BTX.

MUSCLE SELECTION

Ideally, one should be able to determine which muscles are primarily involved in the abnormal movements, and inject these muscles with the appropriate dose of BTX, thus affecting only those actions involved in the production of the abnormal movement or posture. Table 33.2 lists

those seen in OMD, are discussed elsewhere in this volume and in other reviews (12–14). Although denervation of motor endplates has been proposed as the leading mechanism of action of BTX in dystonia, including OMD (15), there are certain paradoxes about its action that are not fully explained (16). First, the clinical effect of BTX appears to continue beyond the point of inducing weakness. Second, although BTX has been thought to affect muscle spindles, it is effective in the treatment of facial spasms, even though facial muscles are void of muscle spindles (17). Third, BTX treatment decreases sensory symptoms, including premonitory sensations experienced by patients with tics and dystonia (see Chapter 32 regarding the treatment of tics with BTX). Finally, there is controversy as to the role of central effects of BTX in patients with dystonia. Transcranial magnetic stimulation of the motor cortex in patients with limb dystonia has been used to demonstrate that BTX

TABLE 33.2. *Muscles affecting jaw and tongue movement*

Muscle	Actions
Masseter	Jaw closing
Temporalis	Jaw closing; anterior fibers assist in jaw opening and deviation
Internal pterygoid	Jaw closing
Digastric	Jaw opening
External pterygoid	Jaw opening; jaw deviation to opposite side and protrusion
Genioglossus	Tongue protrusion
Hyoglossus	Tongue protrusion
Geniohyoid	Jaw opening
Mylohyoid	Elevation of hyoid; jaw opening

the muscles involved in oromandibular function and their actions.

As can be seen, any given movement can be produced by several muscles. The masseters, temporalis or internal (medial) pterygoids represent potential injection targets for JCD, and the submental muscles or external (lateral) pterygoids for JOD. Palpation may be helpful in this approach, but not all muscles are palpable. Another approach might be to monitor muscle activity by EMG and inject those muscles that show increased activity during the particular abnormal movement or posture. This is, however, not always possible because EMG recordings of all involved muscles during action dystonia, such as OMD, are technically difficult. In some forms of focal dystonia, the pattern of muscle involvement may change over time (22). Furthermore, dystonia is a disorder of the CNS and specified at the level of movements, not muscles, adding to the complexity of treatment. These issues remain unresolved and studies directly comparing various modes and dosage of BTX administration remain to be done. Thus, different methods of muscle selection, techniques of injection, and assessment of response account for the observed differences across different studies.

RESULTS OF TRIALS OF BTX IN OMD

Many anecdotal and small case series detailing response of OMD to BTX have been reported (23–27), including one using a primary quality-of-life measure (28). We restrict our discussion, however, to the two large case series published. These reports also have the advantage of being relatively recent; i.e., after preliminary experience has allowed refinement of techniques and assessments of results. In the experience reported by the group at Columbia University College of Physicians and Surgeons (CPS), muscle selection was made using EMG and a relatively large number of muscles were considered (29). In the other study, conducted at Baylor College of Medicine (BCM), muscle selection was based on clinical observation and examination coupled with extensive, long-term experience (30). Both groups used BOTOX (Allergan Pharmaceuticals) preparation of BTX type A (BTX-A).

Brin et al. (29) described their experience with 96 patients with OMD. Onset was generally when the patients' ages were in the mid-40s, but the ages at injection and duration of symptoms are not given. More than 70% of patients in all movement groups had idiopathic OMD. Response was rated primarily by a subjective "linear" scale, in which subjects were asked to assess their percent normal function from 0% to 100%. All muscles involved in jaw motion were considered for injection. EMG was always used to inject the pterygoids and usually to inject the other muscles. In all movement categories, patients' function improved from about 30% of normal function to about 74% after BTX-A treatment. JDD patients started from a higher baseline (39%) with the same final functional status, and thus showed less percent change; however, only five patients were treated. Adverse effects were seen in 13 of 96 (14%) patients and at 29 of 481 (6%) visits. Of 14 instances of dysphagia, only one was severe enough to require a change in diet. Most of the cases of dysphagia were seen in patients with JOD and were associated with injection of the digastrics. The details of the demographics and response of individual subgroups and muscles are given in Tables 33.3, 33.4, and 33.5. The au-

TABLE 33.3. *Distribution of types of oromandibular dystonia in case series from Columbia University College of Physicians and Surgeons (CPS) and Baylor College of Medicine (BCM)*

Distribution	BCM Percent (number)	CPS Percent (number)
Jaw-closing dystonia	52.5% (85)	53.1% (51)
Jaw-opening dystonia	21.6 (35)	41.7 (40)
Jaw-deviation dystonia	1.9 (3)	5.2 (5)
Mixed jaw-movement dystonia	24.0 (39)	

TABLE 33.4. *BTX-A doses in JCD and JOD in case series from Columbia University College of Physicians and Surgeons (CPS) and Baylor College of Medicine (BCM)*

Muscle	BCM (BOTOX Units)	CPS (BOTOX Units)
Masseter	54.2 (25 to 100)	24.5 (2 to 100)
Temporalis	—	18.5 (2 to 75)
Medial pterygoid	—	16.3 (5 to 40)
Lateral pterygoid	—	15.9 (2.5 to 60)
Anterior digastric	—	9.8 (3.75 to 30)
Submentalis	28.6 (10 to 200)	—

thors do not describe how they verified the placement of the EMG electrode in a particular muscle. For other aspects of the controversy associated with EMG-guided BTX injections, the reader is referred to a recently published review (31).

Tan and Jankovic (30) reported their long-term experience with BTX-A for OMD. Of 202 patients seen from 1988 through 1998, diagnosed clinically to have OMD in a movement disorders clinic over a period of 10 years, 162 patients satisfied the study inclusion criteria of being refractory to other treatments, having at least one follow-up visit and having symptoms of sufficient severity to interfere with swallowing, speech or chewing. The mean age was 57.9 ± 15.3 years and the mean follow-up period was 4.4 ± 3.8 years. The masseters and submental muscles were the only two muscle groups injected with BTX-A for JCD and JOD, respectively, in this group of patients. More than half (52.5%) of the patients had JCD. A total of 2,529 BTX-A treatments were administered into the masseter muscles, submental muscles, or both during a total of 1,213 treatment visits. The mean doses of BTX-A (per side) were 54.2 ± 15.2 U for the masseters and 28.6 ± 16.7 U for the submental muscles. The overall mean total duration of response was 16.4 ± 7.1 weeks. The primary efficacy variable was the global effect of BTX-A. To calculate the global effect score, the "peak effect" (range 0 to 4, where 4 = complete abolition of the dystonia and 0 = no effect) is decreased by 1 if mild adverse effect occurred and by 2 if more severe adverse effect was experienced. The mean global effect of BTX-A was 3.1 ± 1.0. Of the JCD patients, 80% (68 of 85) responded with a score ≥ 3 (i.e., moderate to marked improvement); 40% (14 of 35) of JOD, 33% (1 of 3) of JDD, and 52% (16 of 31) of the mixed patients. Fifty-one (31.5%) patients reported adverse effects with BTX-A in at least one visit. Complications such as dysphagia and dysarthria were reported in 135 (11.1%) of all treatment visits. There was a poorer re-

TABLE 33.5. *Therapeutic and adverse effects of BTX-A in JCD and JOD in case series from Columbia University College of Physicians and Surgeons (CPS) and Baylor College of Medicine (BCM)**

	BCM	CPS
Jaw-closing dystonia		
Effect (ultimate % normal function)	80.0	72.0
Duration (weeks; mean ± SD)	16.3±8.1	14.6±2.1
Adverse events: % of patients	18.8	11.8
Adverse events: % of visits	6.2	4.1
Jaw-opening dystonia		
Effect (ultimate % normal function)	72.5	73.8
Duration (weeks; mean ± SD)	16.6±6.9	11.8±2.1
Adverse events: % of patients	40	17.5
Adverse events: % of visits	15.7	9.9

*A comparison of the two studies is not entirely appropriate because of different methods of patient selection, assessment of results and adverse effects, injection techniques, and other differences.

sponse and higher complication rate with JOD than with the other types of OMD (Tables 33.3–33.5).

Because of different methods of patient and muscle selection, different methods of assessing severity, response, and adverse effects, and different injection techniques, it is impossible to compare the two studies; the overall results, however, appear to be similar. Both studies found that, as compared to JCD, JOD is associated with a higher frequency of adverse effects. While the BCM group reported a longer duration of benefit as compared to the CPS group, there was a higher frequency of adverse effects, probably related to higher dose of BTX-A, higher sensitivity of reporting adverse effects, or both. The higher dose may have been necessitated by greater severity of OMD in the BCM patient population. During the past several years we have modified our technique by directing the injection needle and administering the total dosage as a single bolus into the most anterior portion of the submental complex; this has resulted in a marked reduction in dysphagia and other complications. The CPS group preferentially injects the external pterygoids, and if necessary, adds the digastrics and submentals.

TONGUE PROTRUSION DYSTONIA

Tongue protrusion dystonia (TPD) usually interferes with speech and chewing and is most frequently seen in patients with tardive dystonia and with primary (idiopathic) cranial dystonia, but this form of lingual dystonia is also typically present in patients with neuroacanthocytosis. Treatment of this form of focal dystonia is particularly challenging because medications are universally ineffective (except possibly tetrabenazine in tardive lingual dystonia), and BTX-A injections into the tongue muscles can result in severe dysarthria and dysphagia, which are rarely associated with aspiration requiring intubation for airway protection (32).

Gelb et al. reported their experience with 13 patients with TPD (21). They injected an average of 18.3 U (range, 10 to 27) into the genioglossus and hypoglossus muscles, although the exact location of the EMG needle could not be confirmed. The patients' function improved from 32% to 76% of normal function and the effect lasted 11.2 ± 1.9 weeks. Adverse events were seen in 38.5% of patients and 13% of visits. Five patients developed dysarthria and dysphagia, requiring a change in diet; one developed aspiration pneumonia.

Charles et al. (33) performed a retrospective analysis of clinical findings and results of BTX-A treatment in 9 patients treated at Vanderbilt between 1989 and 1995. After unsuccessful treatment with conventional oral medications the patients were injected with BTX-A into their "genioglossus muscles" at four sites via a submandibular approach. A marked reduction in tongue protrusion was achieved in six patients (67%). Of 35 consecutive injections, 83% were successful at reducing tongue protrusion. Mild dysphagia complicated 14% of the injections. The average dose injected was 34 ± 3 U and the average duration of effect was 15 ± 2 weeks.

Because the various muscles involved in tongue protrusion cannot be reliably differentiated clinically or by EMG sampling, we prefer the term "submental muscles" rather than naming individual muscles layered in the submental area. These muscles are involved in various functions, including tongue protrusion and jaw opening.

BRUXISM AND OTHER OROMANDIBULAR SYNDROMES

Bruxism is a diurnal or nocturnal activity that consists of clenching, grinding, bracing, and gnashing of the teeth. Its exact prevalence is unknown, but it is probably much more common than thought because the vast majority of patients with bruxism probably never seek medical attention and the disorder is often misdiagnosed as TMJ (temporomandibular joint) syndrome, although TMJ may occur as a secondary complication of bruxism. Some view bruxism as a form of OMD; it was present in 78.5% of 79 patients with cranial-cervical dystonia (34). Besides dystonia, bruxism can also be seen in a variety of other disorders, particularly mental retardation and other forms of CNS damage, as well as neurodegenerative disorders such as Huntington's disease (35). In an open trial, Tan and Jankovic (36) studied 18 subjects with severe bruxism lasting an average of 14.8 ± 10.0 years (range, 3 to 40). A total of 241 injections of BTX-A were administered in the masseter muscles during 123 treatment visits. The mean dose of the BTX-A was 61.7 ± 11.1 U (range, 25 to 100 U) per masseter muscle on one side. The mean total duration of response was 19.1 ± 17.0 weeks (range, 6 to 78), and the mean peak effect on a scale of 0 to 4, in which 4 is equal to total abolishment of grinding, was 3.4 ± 0.9. Only one subject (5.6%) reported having experienced dysphagia.

OTHER OROMANDIBULAR CONDITIONS

Freund et al. (37) evaluated subjective and objective responses to treatment with BTX-A in an uncontrolled study of a group of 46 patients with various "TMJ" disorders. Both masseter muscles were injected with 50 U each and both temporalis muscles with 25 U each under EMG guidance. Subjects were assessed at 2-week intervals for 8 weeks. Outcome measures included subjective assessment of pain by visual analog scale (VAS), measurement of mean maximum voluntary contraction (MVC), interincisal oral opening, tenderness to palpation, and a functional index based on multiple VAS. There were significant differences in all median outcome measures between the pretreatment assessment and the four follow-up assessments except for MVC. Although MVC was significantly reduced midway through the study, it had returned to pretreatment values by the final two assessments. All other outcome measures remained significantly different from the pretreatment findings. Paired correlation of variables including age, sex, diagnosis, depression index, and time of onset showed no significant differences. BTX-A injections produced significant improvements in pain, function, mouth opening, and tenderness to palpation. MVC initially diminished and then returned to the initial values. Reduced severity of symptoms and improved

functional abilities seemed to have extended beyond the period of the muscle-relaxing effects of BTX-A.

A case of recurrent dislocations of the TMJ because of spasticity from multiple sclerosis has been reported (38). This resolved for periods of up to 4 months following chemodenervation of the masseter and pterygoid muscles with injections of BTX-A.

Hemimasticatory spasm is a rare disorder of the trigeminal nerve that produces involuntary jaw closure as a result of unilateral contractions of jaw-closing muscles (39). It is sometimes associated with facial hemiatrophy. The masseter inhibitory reflex is absent during periods of spasm. Needle EMG demonstrates irregular bursts of motor unit potentials that are identical to the pattern observed in hemifacial spasm. The electrophysiologic findings suggest ectopic excitation of the trigeminal motor root or its nucleus, an abnormality that is analogous to ectopic excitation of the facial nerve in hemifacial spasm. This ectopic excitation can be caused by peripheral irritation of the trigeminal nerve itself, entrapment of the motor branches in the infratemporal fossa or focal demyelination of motor branches of the trigeminal nerve. Hemimasticatory spasm has been reported to respond to BTX-A in several case reports (30–42). Masticatory muscle spasms caused by Satoyoshi's syndrome have also been successfully treated with BTX-A (43).

CONCLUSIONS AND REMAINING QUESTIONS

In summary, BTX-A is now considered the treatment of choice for OMD. Injection into the masseter (and possibly temporalis and internal pterygoids) usually results in marked improvement of JCD and associated bruxism. In JOD, injection of BTX-A into the submental muscles and/or the external pterygoids is usually associated with a robust improvement in jaw opening and dysarthria, although a small percentage of patients may develop transient dysphagia, which can be minimized by directing the injection into the most anterior portion of the submental complex. BTX-A treatment of TPD is also usually highly successful, although this procedure carries a risk of dysphagia.

There are many unanswered questions that should be addressed by future studies. How do we optimize the therapeutic ratio, especially in JOD and TPD? What is the best method of identifying and selectively injecting the most appropriate muscles? Can additional benefit be obtained by injecting more than one muscle (e.g., injecting temporalis muscles in addition to the masseter muscles in patients with JCD, or injecting pterygoids in addition to submental muscles in patients with JOD)? Because individual muscles in the submental complex are difficult to differentiate by palpation (and even with EMG), what is the role of EMG or ultrasound (44) in locating the muscles responsible for the abnormal jaw movements and postures? What is the role of ethanol and lidocaine (muscle-afferent blockers) (45) in conjunction with BTX-A in the treatment of OMD? Why is dryness of mouth a rarely reported side effect of BTX-A treatment for OMD, even though BTX-A injection into salivary glands, adjacent to the muscles injected in patients with OMD, is increasingly used for the treatment of sialorrhea (46,47)? These and other questions need to be addressed by properly designed trials. It is clear, however, that even without the benefit of all the answers, the use of BTX-A has been accepted as the treatment of choice not only for focal dystonias, such as OMD, but also for a rapidly expanding number of disorders associated with excessive or inappropriate muscle contractions (48).

REFERENCES

1. Cardoso F, Jankovic J. Oromandibular dystonia. In: Tsui J, Calne D, eds. *Handbook of dystonia*. New York: Marcel Dekker; 1995:181–190.
2. Meige H. Les convulsions de la face: Une forme clinique de convulsions faciales, bilaterale et mediane. *Rev Neurol (Paris)* 1910;21:437–443.
3. Wood HC. *Nervous diseases and their diagnosis*. Philadelphia, PA: JB Lippincott, 1887:137.
4. Bressman SB, de Leon DDR, Ozelius L, et al. Clinical-genetic spectrum of primary dystonia. *Adv Neurol* 1998;78:79–91.
5. Steinberger D, Topka H, Fischer D, et al. GCH1 mutation in a patient with adult-onset oromandibular dystonia. *Neurology* 1999;52:877–879.
6. Sankhla C, Lai EC, Jankovic J. Peripherally induced oromandibular dystonia. *J Neurol Neurosurg Psychiatry* 1998;65:722–728.
7. Tan EK, Jankovic J. Tardive and idiopathic oromandibular dystonia: a clinical comparison. *J Neurol Neurosurg Psychiatry* 2000;68:186–190.
8. Jankovic J. Medical therapy and botulinum toxin in dystonia. *Adv Neurol* 1998;78:169–183.
9. Sutcher H, Underwood R, Beatty R, et al. Orofacial dyskinesia: a dental dimension. *JAMA* 1971;216:1459–1463.
10. Ondo WG, Desaloms JM, Jankovic J, et al. Pallidotomy for generalized dystonia. *Mov Disord* 1998;13:693–698.
11. Coubes P, Roubertie A, Vayssiere N, et al. Treatment of DYT1-generalised dystonia by stimulation of the internal globus pallidus. *Lancet* 2000;355:2220–2221.
12. Humeau Y, Doussau F, Grant NJ, et al. How botulinum and tetanus neurotoxins block neurotransmitter release. *Biochimie* 2000;82:427–446.
13. Huang W, Foster JA, Rogachefsky AS. Pharmacology of botulinum toxin. *J Am Acad Dermatol* 2000;43:249–259.
14. Schiavo G, Matteoli M, Montecucco C. Neurotoxins affecting neuroexocytosis. *Physiol Rev* 2000;80:718–766.
15. American Academy of Neurology. Assessment: the clinical usefulness of botulinum toxin-A in treating neurologic disorders. Report of the Therapeutics and Technology Assessment Subcommittee of the American Academy of Neurology. *Neurology* 1990;40:1332–1336.
16. Giladi N. The mechanism of action of botulinum toxin type A in focal dystonia is most probably through its dual effect on efferent (motor) and afferent pathways at the injected site. *J Neurol Sci* 1997;152:132–135.
17. Filippi GM, Errico P, Santarelli R, et al. Botulinum A toxin effects on rat jaw muscle spindles. *Acta Otolaryngol* 1993;113:400–404.
18. Gilio F, Curra A, Lorenzano C, et al. Effects of botulinum toxin type A on intracortical inhibition in patients with dystonia. *Ann Neurol* 2000;48:20–26.
19. Kaji K. Facts and fancies on writer's cramp. *Muscle Nerve* 2000;23:1313–1315.
20. Hallett M. How does botulinum toxin work? *Ann Neurol* 2000;48:7–8.
21. Yoshida K, Kaji R, Kubori T, et al. Muscle afferent block for the treatment of oromandibular dystonia. *Mov Disord* 1998;13:699–705.
22. Gelb DJ, Yoshimura DM, Olney RK, et al. Change in pattern of muscle activity following botulinum toxin injections for torticollis. *Ann Neurol* 1991;29:370–376.
23. Van den Bergh P, Francart J, Mourin S, et al. Five-year experience in the treatment of focal movement disorders with low-dose DYSPORT botulinum toxin. *Muscle Nerve* 1995;18:720–729.
24. Heise GJ, Mullen MP. Oromandibular dystonia treated with botulinum toxin: report of case. *J Oral Maxillofac Surg* 1995;53:332–335.
25. Berardelli A, Formica A, Mercuri B, et al. Botulinum toxin treatment in patients with focal dystonia and hemifacial spasm. A multicenter study of the Italian Movement Disorder Group. *Ital J Neurol Sci* 1993;14:361–367.
26. Hermanowicz N, Truong DD. Treatment of oromandibular dystonia with botulinum toxin. *Laryngoscope* 1991;101:1216–1218.

27. Maurri S, Brogelli S, Alfieri G, et al. Use of botulinum toxin in Meige's disease. *Riv Neurol* 1988;58:245–248.

28. Bhattacharyya N, Tarsy D. Impact on quality of life of botulinum toxin treatments for spasmodic dysphonia and oromandibular dystonia. *Arch Otolaryngol Head Neck Surg* 2001;127:389–392.

29. Brin M, Blitzer A, Herman S, et al. Oromandibular dystonia: treatment of 96 cases with botulinum A. In: Jankovic J, Hallett M, eds. *Therapy with botulinum toxin.* New York: Marcel Dekker; 1994:429–435.

30. Tan EK, Jankovic J. Botulinum toxin A in patients with oromandibular dystonia: long-term follow-up. *Neurology* 1999;53:2102–2107.

31. Jankovic J. Needle EMG guidance is rarely required. *Muscle Nerve* 2001;24:1568–1570.

32. Blitzer A, Brin MF, Fahn S. Botulinum toxin injections for lingual dystonia [Letter]. *Laryngoscope* 1991;101: 799.

33. Charles PD, Davis TL, Shannon KM, Hook MA, Warner JS. Tongue protrusion dystonia: treatment with botulinum toxin. *South Med J* 1997;90:522–525.

34. Watts MW, Tan EK, Jankovic J. Bruxism and cranial-cervical dystonia: is there a relationship? *Cranio* 1999; 17:196–201.

35. Tan EK, Jankovic J, Ondo W. Bruxism in Huntington's disease. *Mov Disord* 2000;15:171–173.

36. Tan EK, Jankovic J. Treating severe bruxism with botulinum toxin. *J Am Dent Assoc* 2000;131:211–216.

37. Freund B, Schwartz M, Symington JM. Botulinum toxin: new treatment for temporomandibular disorders. *Br J Oral Maxillofac Surg* 2000;38:466–471.

38. Daelen B, Thorwirth V, Koch A. Treatment of recurrent dislocation of the temporomandibular joint with type A botulinum toxin. *Int J Oral Maxillofac Surg* 1997;26: 458–460.

39. Jankovic J. Etiology and differential diagnosis of bleph-arospasm and oromandibular dystonia. In: Jankovic J, Tolosa E, eds. *Facial dyskinesias.* New York: Raven Press, 1988:103–116.

40. Auger R, Litchy W, Cascino T, et al. Hemimasticatory spasm: clinical and electrophysiologic observations. *Neurology* 1992;42:2263–2266.

41. Kim HJ, Jeon BS, Lee KW. Hemimasticatory spasm associated with localized scleroderma and facial hemiatrophy. *Arch Neurol* 2000;57:576–580.

42. Ebersbach G, Kabus C, Schelosky L, et al. Hemimasticatory spasm in hemifacial atrophy: diagnostic and therapeutic aspects in two patients. *Mov Disord* 1995;10: 504–507.

43. Merello M, Garcia H, Nogues M, et al. Masticatory muscle spasm in a non-Japanese patient with Satoyoshi syndrome successfully treated with botulinum toxin. *Mov Disord* 1994;9:104–105.

44. Emshoff R, Bertram S, Strobl H. Ultrasonographic cross-sectional characteristics of muscles of the head and neck. *Oral Surg Oral Med Oral Pathol Oral Radiol Endod* 1999;87:93–106.

45. Mezaki T, Matsumoto S, Sakamoto T, et al. [Cervical echomyography in cervical dystonia and its application to the monitoring for muscle afferent block (MAB).] *Rinsho Shinkeigaku* 2000;40:689–693.

46. Pal PK, Calne DB, Calne S, et al. Botulinum toxin A as treatment for drooling saliva in PD. *Neurology* 2000; 54:244–247.

47. Porta M, Gamba M, Bertacchi G, et al. Treatment of sialorrhoea with ultrasound guided botulinum toxin type A injection in patients with neurological disorders. *J Neurol Neurosurg Psychiatry* 2001;70:538–540.

48. Thomas M, Jankovic J. Botulinum toxin treatment of tics, myoclonus, stiff-person syndrome, gait freezing and rigidity. In: Moore P, Naumann M, eds. *Handbook of botulinum toxin treatment, 2nd ed.* London: Blackwell Science, 2002 *(in press).*

Scientific and Therapeutic Aspects of Botulinum Toxin
edited by M.F. Brin, J. Jankovic, and M. Hallett
Lippincott Williams & Wilkins, Philadelphia, © 2002.

34

Use of Botulinum Toxin in Urologic Disorders

Dennis D. Dykstra

Botulinum toxin inhibits release of acetylcholine from the neuromuscular junction. It is used successfully to treat abnormal skeletal and smooth-muscle activity in patients. This chapter discusses its use in patients with detrusor-sphincter dyssynergia and detrusor hyperreflexia.

ANATOMY AND PHYSIOLOGY OF MICTURITION

The two functions of the urinary bladder are storage and active expulsion of urine (1). During bladder filling, intravesical pressure rises slowly despite an increase in volume, a phenomenon that is caused, initially at least, by the viscoelastic properties of the smooth muscle and connective tissue of the bladder wall. There is little neural efferent activity to the bladder until a critical intravesical pressure is reached, after which any further pressure increase stimulates a reflex arc. The afferent impulses of this reflex arc travel via the pelvic nerve and the efferent impulses travel via the hypogastric nerve (Fig. 34.1). This sympathetic spinal reflex results in active stimulation of the functional internal sphincter; in addition, it inhibits bladder activity by a direct effect on smooth muscle and an indirect effect on parasympathetic ganglia, which allow more complete bladder filling.

Although many factors are involved in the micturition reflex, it is intravesical pressure, producing the sensation of distention, that primarily initiates bladder contraction. The pelvic nerve, which is the parasympathetic neural outflow to the bladder, has its origin in the sacral spinal cord. However, it appears that the actual organizational center for the micturition reflex is in the brainstem and that the complete neural circuit

for normal micturition includes ascending and descending spinal cord pathways to and from this area. The final step in micturition involves a highly coordinated, parasympathetically induced contraction of the bladder body, the shaping or funneling of a relaxed bladder outlet, the depression of the sympathetic inhibitory outflow and the inhibition of the tonic somatic discharge to the striated pelvic floor musculature surrounding the bladder neck and urethra. Other reflexes that are elicited by bladder contraction and the passage of urine through the urethra may reinforce these primary reflexes and facilitate complete bladder emptying. Superimposed on the autonomic and somatic reflexes are complex modifying supraspinal inputs from other central neuronal networks. These facilitatory and inhibitory impulses, which originate at several levels of the nervous system—including the brainstem, the cerebellum, and the cerebral cortex—allow for full conscious control of micturition.

Detrusor hyperreflexia is characterized by involuntary detrusor contractions during bladder filling that cannot be consciously suppressed and that produce an increase in intravesical pressure greater than 15 cm H_2O (2). Other terms that have been used to describe this disorder include motor unstable bladder, automatic bladder, and uninhibited neurogenic bladder (3). Detrusor hyperreflexia may be associated with a variety of clinical entities (4). Neurogenically induced detrusor hyperreflexia is almost always associated with a lesion that affects the sacral cord outflow.

Several theories have been offered to explain the neurophysiologic basis of detrusor hyperreflexia following suprasacral neurologic lesions.

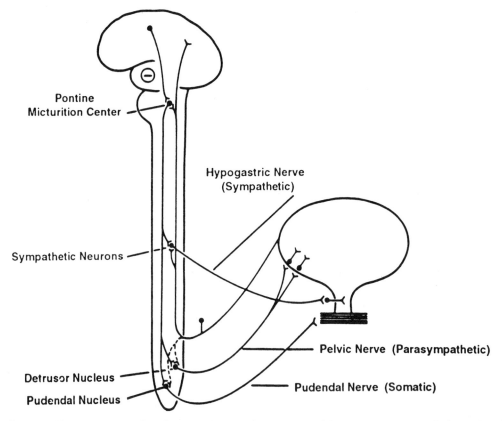

FIG. 34.1. Neuronal interactions between lower urinary tract and the nervous system. Before micturition, vesical afferents ascend to the pontine micturitional center, which is normally inhibited by higher centers. Efferents from the pons descend to the thoracolumbar sympathetic center and the detrusor and pudendal nuclei to coordinate vesical contraction with relaxation of the smooth muscle and striated muscle sphincter. (From Krane FJ, Siroky MD. Classification of neuro-urologic disorders. In: Krane FJ, Siroky MD, eds. *Clinical neuro-urology.* Boston: Little Brown, 1976:144–147, with permission.)

The normal micturitional reflex is not a simple segmental phenomenon; rather, it involves synapsing of long spinal tracts, presumably in the region of the pontine reticular formation (5–7). After suprasacral spinal cord transection, the micturitional reflex changes in nature from a long-tract reflex to a segmental reflex. Whether this segmental pathway is normally present in humans and is unmasked by a suprasacral lesion, or whether it represents a new reflex pathway formed by collateral sprouting, is not known (8,9). Whatever the cause, the end result is a new micturitional reflex center located in the sacral cord. The threshold for firing of this reflex center

is reduced, which accounts for involuntary detrusor contractions at low intravesical volumes.

Reflex interactions between the detrusor and the external striated urethral sphincter must also be taken into account. Bladder filling will lead to increased external urethral sphincter activity. Conversely, a bladder contraction will normally be associated with reflex inhibition of all activity in the external urethral sphincter (10–12). In an intact nervous system, reflex coordination between the bladder and the external sphincter is thought to occur at a suprasacral level. Experimentally, it is known that centers for coordination of such long-tract reflexes exist in the region of the pons (5–7). Thus, suprasacral lesions between the sacral cord and pons (i.e., spinal cord injury) may result not only in detrusor hyperreflexia as described above, but also in lack of appropriate coordination between the detrusor and external sphincter (vesicosphincter dyssynergia) (13). As may be the case for detrusor hyperreflexia, vesicosphincter dyssynergia may represent unmasking of a facilitative reflex between the detrusor and external sphincter or the formation of a new reflex by neural reorganization (collateral sprouting).

On rare occasions, detrusor hyperreflexia may be associated with a neurogenically mediated obstruction at the level of the smooth muscle sphincter (14,15). A detrusor contraction is normally accompanied by synchronous neurogenic relaxation of the smooth muscle sphincter. A lesion situated above the sympathetic spinal cord outflow (T6) may result in a loss of this appropriate inhibition of sympathetic discharge to the smooth muscle sphincter.

DETRUSOR-SPHINCTER DYSSYNERGIA

Detrusor-sphincter dyssynergia (DSD) is defined as inappropriate contractions of the urethral sphincter coincident with detrusor contractions (13). DSD is a significant problem for spinal cord injury patients. The resulting high intravesical pressures and poor bladder emptying may lead to autonomic dysreflexia, serious urinary tract infection, renal damage and prema-

ture death (16). DSD is typically managed with medication, condom or indwelling catheters, intermittent catheterization and electrical stimulation, or surgery to destroy sphincter function. All of these treatment methods have associated complications. Use of botulinum neurotoxin type A (BoNT-A) injections offer a safe, effective and reversible treatment that allows low-pressure bladder drainage.

Use of Botulinum Toxin

We evaluated the ability of BoNT-A to denervate and relax the spastic external striated urethral sphincter in 11 men with spinal cord injury and DSD (17). Toxin concentration, injection volume, percutaneous versus cystoscopic injection of the sphincter (Figs. 34.2 and 34.3) and number of injections were evaluated in three treatment protocols. The ten patients who were evaluated by electromyography after injection showed signs of sphincter denervation. Bulbosphincteric reflexes in these ten patients were more difficult to obtain and they showed a decreased amplitude and normal latency. In the seven patients in whom it was measured, the urethral pressure profile before and after treatment decreased an average of 27 cm H_2O after toxin injections. In eight patients, postvoiding residual urine volume decreased by an average of 146 mL after the toxin injections. In the eight patients for whom it could be determined, toxin effects lasted an average of 50 days. The toxin

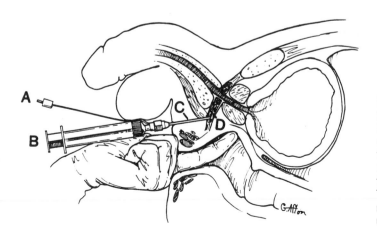

FIG. 34.2. Percutaneous technique used to inject toxin into the external urethral sphincter. **A:** Electrode to electromyography machine. **B:** Syringe containing toxin for injection. **C:** 23-gauge, 3.5-cm, Teflon-coated monopolar needle electrode. **D:** External urethral sphincter.

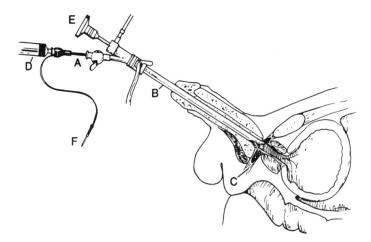

FIG. 34.3. Technique used to inject toxin into the external urethral sphincter with a cystoscope. **A:** 23-gauge, 35-cm, Teflon-coated monopolar needle electrode. **B:** Cystoscope. **C:** External urethral sphincter. **D:** Syringe containing toxin for injection. **E:** Eyepiece of cystoscope. **F:** Electrode to electromyography machine.

also decreased autonomic dysreflexia in five patients.

The ability of BoNT-A to denervate and relax a spastic external urethral sphincter was further evaluated in a double-blind study involving five men with high spinal cord injuries and DSD (18). The sphincter was injected with either 140, 240, or 240 U BOTOX or normal saline once a week for 3 weeks. Electromyography of the external urethral sphincter indicated denervation in the three patients who received toxin injections. The urethral pressure profile decreased an average of 25 cm H$_2$O, postvoiding residual volume of urine decreased an average of 125 mL, and bladder pressure during voiding decreased to an average of 30 cm H$_2$O. Bulbosphincteric reflexes were more difficult to obtain and they showed decreased amplitude with normal latency. In the two patients who received normal saline injections, parameters were unchanged from baseline values until subsequent injection with BoNT-A once a week for 3 weeks, when their responses were similar to those of the other three patients. Mild, generalized weakness lasting 2 to 3 weeks was reported by three patients after initial toxin injections. The duration of the toxin's effect on bladder function averaged 2 months.

Transurethral versus transperineal BoNT-A injections into the external urethral sphincter were performed in 24 male spinal cord injury patients with DSD and the respective efficacy was compared (19). In 21 of 24 patients, DSD

was significantly improved with a concomitant decrease in postvoid residual volumes in most cases. Transurethral injections appeared to be more effective on maximum urethral pressure during DSD than did transperineal injections. A protocol of three repeated injections of 100 U BOTOX at monthly intervals seemed to yield the best results. Immunity to BoNT-A did not occur, and there were no significant side effects. Botulinum A toxin effects lasted 3 to 9 months, making reinjections necessary. The authors concluded that BoNT-A injections for DSD appear to be a valid alternative for patients who do not desire surgery or who are unable to perform self-catheterization.

Treatment of DSD by transperineal injection into the external urethral sphincter was further evaluated in five tetraplegic patients (20). Single injections of 100 U of BOTOX through the perineum were used. All cases noticed improved bladder function, with a significant decrease in residual urine volume. Autonomic dysreflexia dramatically decreased in four cases. The improvement was observed approximately 15 days after the injection. The results of the urodynamic studies showed a significant increase of the functional detrusor capacity and a decrease of the maximal detrusor pressure during voiding. Good clinical results persisted for an average of 3 months. Four of the five patients asked for a new injection when the benefits of the first one had disappeared. A total of 15 injections were performed without any adverse effect. Two patients were treated for more than 1 year. The authors concluded that this treatment has to be considered in cases of failure of more traditional conservative treatment. It is reversible and therefore should definitely be considered before surgery or use of stents.

Recently, a study was done to evaluate the effects of two types of BoNT-A (BOTOX vs DYSPORT) on the external urethral sphincter in patients with neurogenic voiding disorders (21). Ten male spinal cord injury patients with DSD were clinically assessed before and 4 to 6 weeks after, transurethral or transperineal BoNT-A injections (BOTOX 100 U or DYSPORT 250 U) into the external urethral sphincter. Patients with persistent difficulties in voiding or high postvoid residual volumes were reinjected with the same product up to three times. All patients were urodynamically examined within 120 days of injection. In total, 30 BoNT-A injection cycles (one to three injections) were administered. Significant ($p < 0.05$) reductions in the DSD duration postinjection, the time interval between the start of bladder contractions and voiding and DSD severity posttreatment were observed. All patients who presented with a residual volume pretreatment showed a marked decrease posttreatment. These effects lasted about 6 months. Improvements in urodynamic parameters were significantly better following BOTOX than DYSPORT treatment ($p < 0.05$), although the DYSPORT dose used is now considered less potent than that of BOTOX.

DETRUSOR HYPERREFLEXIA

Detrusor hyperreflexia denotes involuntary detrusor contractions that result from a neurologic condition such as spinal cord injury, stroke, Parkinson's disease, or multiple sclerosis. Current treatment relies on anticholinergic medication to partially block the efferent parasympathetic innervation to the detrusor. However, these drugs have troublesome side effects and may be ineffective to restore continence in patients with severe detrusor hyperreflexia. The use of BoNT-A in smooth as well as skeletal muscle has been found to be effective and safe in the treatment of muscle overactivity (22). For these reasons, injections of BoNT-A into the overactive detrusor muscle may result in improved bladder continence.

Use of Botulinum Toxin

Recently, the use of BoNT-A in the treatment of smooth muscle overactivity in spinal cord injured patients with detrusor hyperreflexia was studied (23). The purpose of this treatment was to suppress incontinence episodes and to increase functional bladder capacity. Traumatic spinal cord injury patients were evaluated in a prospective nonrandomized study. These patients had severe detrusor hyperreflexia and incontinence despite a high dose of anticholinergic medication. Under cystoscopic control, a total of 200 to 300 U of BOTOX were injected into the detrusor muscle at 20 to 30 sites sparing the trigone. At the 6-week follow-up, complete continence was restored in 17 of 19 cases in which anticholinergic medication was markedly decreased or withdrawn. Less satisfactory results in two cases were associated with an insufficient dose of 200 U of toxin. Satisfaction was high in all successfully treated patients and no side effects were observed. The duration of bladder paresis induced by the toxin is at least 9 months, at which point repeat injections may be required.

CONCLUSIONS

Botulinum neurotoxin type A has proved useful in spinal cord injury patients with DSD and detrusor hyperreflexia. Future studies are needed to evaluate the effects of other types of botulinum toxins such as botulinum neurotoxin type B on these patients. Research also needs to be done on patients with multiple sclerosis, Parkinson's disease, and stroke to determine whether botulinum toxin can help with their overactive bladder problems.

REFERENCES

1. Wein AJ, Raezer DM. Physiology of micturition. In: Krane FJ, Siroky MD, eds. *Clinical neuro-urology.* Boston: Little Brown, 1997:26–29.
2. Bates P, Bradley WE, Glen E, et al. Standardization of

terminology of lower urinary tract function. *Urology* 1977;9:237–241.

3. Lapides J. Neuromuscular vesical and ureteral dysfunction. In: Campbell MF, Harrison JH, eds. *Urology.* Philadelphia, PA: WB Saunders, 1976.

4. Krane FJ, Siroky MD. Classification of neuro-urologic disorders. In: Krane FJ, Siroky MD, eds. *Clinical neurourology.* Boston: Little Brown, 1976:144–147.

5. Barrington FJF. The nervous mechanism of micturition. *Q J Exp Physiol* 1941;8:7–71.

6. Barrington FJF. The component reflexes of micturition in the cat: part III. *Brain* 1941;64:239–243.

7. DeGroat NC. Nervous control of the urinary bladder of the cat. *Brain Res* 1975;87:201–211.

8. Anderson JT. Detrusor hyperreflexia in benign intravesical obstruction: A cystometric study. *J Urol* 1976; 115:532–534.

9. Liu CN, Chambers WW. Intraspinal sprouting of dorsal root axons. *Arch Neurol Psychiatry* 1958;79:46–61.

10. Diokno AC, Doff SA, Bender LF. Periurethral striated muscle activity in neurogenic bladder dysfunction. *J Urol* 1974;112:743–749.

11. Gary RC, Roberts TDM, Todd JK. Reflexes involving the external urethral sphincter in the cat. *J Physiol* 1959; 149:653–665.

12. Kuru M. Nervous control of micturition. *Physiol Rev* 1965;45:426–484.

13. Yalla SV, Rossier AB, Fam B. Dyssynergic vesicourethral responses during bladder rehabilitation in spinal cord patients: effects of suprapubic percussion, Crede method and bethanechol chloride. *J Urol* 1976; 115:575–579.

14. Scott M, Marrow JW. Phenoxy-benzamine in neuro-

genic bladder dysfunction after spinal cord injury: I. Voiding dysfunction. *J Urol* 1978;119:480–482.

15. Scott M, Morrow JW. Phenoxy-benzamine in neurogenic bladder dysfunction after spinal cord injury: II. Automatic dysreflexia. *J Urol* 1978;119:483–484.

16. Thomas, DG: Spinal cord injury. In: Mundy AR, Stephenson TP, Wein AJ, eds. *Urodynamics: principles, practice and application.* New York: Churchill Livingstone, 1984:259–272.

17. Dykstra DD, Sidi AA, Scot AB, et al. Effects of botulinum A toxin on detrusor-sphincter dyssynergia in spinal cord injury patients. *J Urol* 1988;139:919–922.

18. Dykstra DD, Sidi AA. Treatment of detrusor-sphincter dyssynergia with botulinum A toxin: a double-blind study. *Arch Phys Med Rehabil* 1990;71:24–26.

19. Schurch B, Hauri D, Rodic B, et al. Botulinum-A toxin as a treatment of detrusor-sphincter dyssynergia: a prospective study in 24 spinal cord injury patients. *J Urol* 1996;155:1023–1029.

20. Gallien P, Robineau S, Verin M, et al. Treatment of detrusor sphincter dyssynergia by transperineal injection of botulinum toxin. *Arch Phys Med Rehabil* 1998; 79:715–717.

21. Schurch B, Schmid DM, Knapp PA. An update on the treatment of detrusor-sphincter dyssynergia with botulinum toxin type A. *Eur J Neurol* 1999;6(Suppl 4): S83–S89.

22. Pasricha PJ, Ravich WJ, Kalloo AN. Effects of intrasphincteric botulinum toxin of the lower esophageal sphincter in piglets. *Gastroenterology* 1993;105: 1045–1049.

23. Schurch B, Stohrer M, Kramer G, et al. Botulinum-A toxin for treating detrusor hyperreflexia in spinal cord injured patients: a new alternative to anticholinergic drugs? Preliminary results. *J Urol* 2000;164:692–697.

CLINICAL TRIALS

Scientific and Therapeutic Aspects of Botulinum Toxin
edited by M.F. Brin, J. Jankovic, and M. Hallett
Lippincott Williams & Wilkins, Philadelphia, © 2002.

35

Cervical Dystonia: Treatment with Botulinum Toxin Serotype A as BOTOX® or Dysport®

Cynthia L. Comella

CERVICAL DYSTONIA

Cervical dystonia (CD), originally called spasmodic torticollis, was thought by many to be a psychiatric disorder and the term "torticollis mentalis" was the original term used to describe this condition (1). Subsequently, the neurologic origin of the disorder was recognized and spasmodic torticollis was redefined as a subtype of dystonia and renamed cervical dystonia. Dystonia refers to a syndrome of sustained muscle contractions usually producing twisting and repetitive movements or abnormal postures (2). CD is defined as a focal dystonia involving the cervical musculature causing abnormal postures of the head, neck and shoulders. There may be overlying muscle spasms causing quick, repetitive, jerking movements that may be mistaken for tremor. The feature of CD that sets it apart from tremor is the directional preponderance of the movements. The symptoms of focal CD usually begin in adulthood in the fifth decade and affect women one-half to three times as often as men (3,4).

BOTULINUM TOXIN AND THE TREATMENT OF CERVICAL DYSTONIA

Botulinum toxin (BTX) has been widely accepted as a safe and effective treatment for CD (5–8). In particular, pain associated with CD may improve (9). Many view BTX as the treatment of choice for CD, largely replacing oral pharmacologic agents. A controlled, randomized study comparing BTX type A to trihexyphenidyl in 66 CD patients showed that chemodenervation with BTX-A was markedly superior with greater benefit and fewer side effects (10).

Studies assessing BTX treatment for CD are largely open-label trials, uncontrolled studies, or controlled studies composed of a small number of patients (7). The initial report of BTX-A in 12 patients was single blinded using electromyography guidance and a total maximum dose of 200 U of BTX-A as Oculinum (Smith-Kettlewell). Improvement occurred in 92% of the patients and lasted at least 4 to 8 weeks, with the most common side effect being transient neck weakness that was reported by 25% (11). A double-blinded, placebo-controlled, crossover study of 21 patients using 100 U confirmed these early results (12). Subsequent studies showed that from 65% to 90% of CD patients improved with BTX-A. Improvement occurred for head posture and CD-related pain (13–25). Benefit was enhanced for patients injected in multiple sites in each muscle (26).

A large, randomized, double-blind, placebo-controlled study of 170 CD patients presented in abstract form and included in the package insert for BOTOX verified the benefits of chemodenervation. This study consisted of two study periods: an open-label period in which all patients received BOTOX, and a double-blind treatment period in which patients who benefited from the open-label period injection were randomized to receive either BOTOX or placebo. Patients were assessed at peak effect (week 6 after injection) and at 2-week intervals up to 10 weeks after treatment. BOTOX was superior to placebo as measured by the Cervical Dystonia Severity Scale at all evaluation visits (8). The termination of the study at week 10 did not allow for a measure of the duration of effect. Adverse reactions included dysphagia, upper respiratory tract infection, neck pain, and headache (27).

DYSPORT is another brand of BTX serotype A. Comparison of DYSPORT to BOTOX showed that in the 73 patients randomized to either BTX-A brand, a dosing ratio of 1U of BOTOX to 3 U of DYSPORT provided equivalent treatment efficacy and similar side effect frequency (28). This study emphasizes that dosing may vary in different brands of the same serotype. A dose-response study using DYSPORT at doses up to 1,000 U in CD patients showed that increasing the dose of DYSPORT provided a greater magnitude and duration of improvement but also increased the adverse events, especially neck weakness and voice change (29).

Patients most improved by injections are those with muscle involvement that moves the head in one direction (ipsilateral splenius and contralateral sternocleidomastoid) (14). However, CD is often a complex movement, with a combination of rotation, anterior flexion or extension, lateral flexion, and shifting of the neck on the shoulders. One study of 30 patients with CD in whom the same muscles were injected with a fixed total dose of 150 U of BOTOX did not find an objective improvement, and highlighted the need to individually assess each patient for dose and muscle involvement (30). CD severity may also fluctuate as a part of the natural history of the disorder. In addition, there may be changes in the pattern of activation following BTX treatment (31). This highlights the need to reevaluate patients at every injection visit, and not to simply administer the same pattern of injection repetitively.

The duration of benefit from BTX-A treatment has been assessed both prospectively and retrospectively. A prospective assessment of 37 CD patients treated with DYSPORT found that duration of effect lasted a mean of 95 days (24). A chart review from two treatment sites with 60 CD patients treated for at least 1 year showed a mean clinical response lasting 15.6 weeks, with a range of 12.2 to 24.3 weeks. Duration of benefit tended to be most prolonged in patients experiencing moderate symptoms (32).

Another study of 303 patients treated with six or more injection series using DYSPORT showed that the greatest magnitude of improvement was found after the first injection series, but significant improvement continued over subsequent injections. This was likely because there were patients returning for repeat treatment prior to reaching baseline severity who were still experiencing residual benefit from the previous injection (33). In this study, approximately 20% of the 616 patients treated at least once chose not to continue long-term treatment with BTX. The most common reason for discontinuation was an unsatisfactory outcome or absence of effect. The occurrence of adverse events, most frequently dysphagia, was the second most common reason for discontinuation. Fifteen percent reported complete relief of symptoms, suggesting a coincident partial or complete remission of symptoms, although the possibility that BTX treatment may increase the chances of remission in CD has been suggested (34).

In a similar survey study, 155 CD patients lost to follow-up were asked to complete a questionnaire. Surveys were returned by 86.6%. Of those returning surveys, 21.8% discontinued treatment because treatment was not effective or too expensive, or equal benefit was obtained using oral medications (35). The occurrence of adverse events was not a frequent cause of treatment cessation in this study.

BOTOX has been shown in a prospective study to have benefit over the course of prolonged repeated treatment. A prospective study of 115 CD patients treated over 2 years found that similar benefit was achieved following repeated injections with a reduction of complications with successive injections (36). Assessment of the effect of BTX on muscle in patients chronically treated with BOTOX compared to those never treated previously demonstrates that there is no reduction in paralyzing effect with repeated toxin exposure (37).

IMMUNOGENICITY OF BTX SEROTYPE A

Antibodies may form that render the toxin clinically ineffective. A prospective study of 115 patients found such blocking antibodies to BTX-A in approximately 4.4% of the patients (36). Patients who have previously done well with injections of BOTOX but who now experience a secondary loss of benefit or BOTOX resistance likely have immunologically mediated resistance and the development of BTX serotype-specific antibodies. The estimated frequency of secondary nonresponse varies widely. In one study, 9.9% reported a secondary nonresponse (33), having lost the benefit initially obtained. A second study of 242 patients with adequate follow-up showed that 16% were nonresponders, and that of these nonresponders, 35.7% had antibodies to BTX-A by the Mouse Neutralization Assay (38). Possible risk factors for the development of resistance include a short interval between injection series (less than 3 months), and large doses of BTX-A (39). The prescribing information included on the package insert for BOTOX revealed that of CD patients who considered themselves responsive, 17% had neutralizing antibodies and did not show benefit on clinical measures following treatment (27). These observations are now being further evaluated for BOTOX in prospective studies.

In patients who are resistant to serotype A, other serotypes have been used successfully. Serotype F improves CD symptoms in CD patients with secondary nonresponse. The duration of benefit using serotype F was shorter than with serotype A, with clinical benefit lasting only 1 month (40,41). Increasing the dose of serotype F prolonged the duration but at the price of increased adverse effects (42). Patients who had never benefited from injections of serotype A (primary nonresponders) did not improve with serotype F (41,43). With repeated injections, however, approximately one-third of these patients also developed resistance to serotype F (43).

Similar findings of efficacy in serotype A-resistant patients have been found using serotype B (44). A randomized, placebo-controlled study evaluated 77 serotype A-resistant CD patients treated with either 10,000 U of serotype B or with placebo. The active drug group had significant improvement following a single treatment. The continued response of these patients following repeated injections of serotype B has not yet been published.

ELECTROMYOGRAPHY GUIDANCE FOR BTX TREATMENT OF CD

Several studies have evaluated the technique of BTX treatment, specifically the role of electromyography (EMG). EMG has been used to evaluate the pattern of muscle activation in CD, the effective dose of BTX, and the electrophysiologic consequences following BTX injection. EMG has also been proposed as a technique that, when used in conjunction with clinical evaluation, may optimize clinical effect and lower the BTX dosage required for benefit.

EMG studies have shown that in CD there are long-duration EMG bursts often with cocontraction of agonist and antagonist muscles. Most patients have complicated CD, with involvement of multiple muscles (1,45). Quantitative EMG has been used to evaluate the effect of varying doses of BTX into a single dystonic muscle, the sternocleidomastoid, in CD patients. The dose-ranging effect of single doses of BTX-A (either BOTOX or DYSPORT) into dystonic sternocleidomastoid muscle showed that doses as low as 20 U of BOTOX or 100 U of DYSPORT causes a marked reduction in turns per second, with minimal additional reductions at higher doses (46,47). Application of quantitative EMG to assess the duration of BTX showed a reduction of turns per second, mean amplitude, and turns per amplitude ratio to nearly zero by 6 weeks after injection. Over subsequent weeks, each parameter gradually returned toward baseline with turns per second reaching pretreatment values at 30 weeks (48). Repeated injections of BTX did not show a cumulative effect on the muscle (49).

The utility of EMG guidance in identifying dystonic muscles in CD and targeting muscles for injection has been tested (50–52). A study of 52 consecutive CD patients randomized to injection with or without EMG assistance showed that the addition of EMG increased the magnitude of improvement following BTX injection (51). The role of EMG in conjunction with clinical examination in improving outcome could arise from either correct identification of dystonic muscle (52–54) or the ability to accurately target injections into overactive muscle (55–57). The deep posterior cervical muscles, including the semispinalis capitis, longissimus capitis, and muscles of the suboccipital triangle, are not easily examined or injected from the surface. These muscles were spontaneously overactive in 68% of consecutive CD patients (52). Without EMG identification of involvement, these muscles may be omitted during injection.

Speelman and Brans showed that clinical placement of a needle into dystonic muscle is frequently inaccurate. Needle placement by clinical examination was accurate 83% of the time in the superficial sternocleidomastoid, and only 47% of the time in the levator scapulae (55). An additional advantage of EMG assistance may be in limiting the dose needed for improvement. This may be attributed in part to the limited diffusion of BTX following injection. In animals, the diffusion gradient of a single-site injection in the rabbit model showed a marked reduction in BTX effect at a distance between 30 to 45 mm from the injection (58). By using EMG, the dose of BTX was substantially reduced without loss of clinical benefit (59) in an open study of CD patients injected with DYSPORT. Although there are some advantages to EMG-guided injections, there are many disadvantages. Indeed, many clinicians believe that even if EMG-guided injections provide additional benefit, because about 90% of treated patients obtain satisfactory results whether the BTX is administered with EMG guidance or not, the use of EMG does not justify the extra cost, time, effort, and discomfort associated with the procedure (60).

ADVERSE EFFECTS OF BTX SEROTYPE A IN THE TREATMENT OF CD

The adverse effects of botulinum injection for CD included pain at injection site, neck weakness, a flu-like syndrome, hoarseness, dry mouth, and dysphagia (33). Dysphagia was the most frequent complication following injection, reported in 25% to 90% of patients injected with either BOTOX or DYSPORT (8,15–17, 19,22,25). Women were more likely than men to experience dysphagia, as were patients receiving injections into the sternocleidomastoid muscle (38). Although usually mild and transient, in some patients, the severity may be sufficient to require a change in diet to soft or pureed foods; rarely, nasogastric feedings are necessary (33). Radiologic evaluations assessing BTX-related dysphagia show paralysis of vocal cords and pharyngeal paralysis (61). Although 22% of CD patients may have radiologic evidence of pharyngeal peristaltic abnormalities prior to treatment, up to 50% develop new abnormalities following treatment, and 33% have new dysphagia symptoms (62). Doses of 100 U into the sternocleidomastoid muscle were found to be associated with posttreatment dysphagia (58), although a dose relationship has not been found in other studies (17). Dysphagia existing prior to injections of BTX does not predict an increased susceptibility to complications following treatment (62).

Other rare complications of BTX injections for treatment of CD include cervical radiculopathy, polyradiculoneuritis, and brachial plexopathy (63–67). Idiosyncratic adverse reactions, including a rash at the site of injection, ptosis, and a localized anaphylactic reaction, have been rarely observed (68).

BTX FOR CD: OTHER CONSIDERATIONS

The annual cost per patient of BTX as a treatment for CD is high, with estimates based on a study conducted in Germany ranging from $800 to $1,600 (69). This is somewhat variable depending on the severity of CD, the dose of BTX needed, the number of treatment sessions per year and the additional cost of electromyography. However, measurement of emotional, social, and pain-related domains of quality of life shows significant improvement as does depression and disability following BTX. These improvements in functional health measures following BTX treatment may offset the cost of treatment (70,71).

REFERENCES

1. Podivinsky F. Torticollis. In: Vinken PJ, Bruyn GW. *Handbook of clinical neurology.* New York: North Holland Publishing Co., 1968:567–603.
2. Fahn S, Bressman SB, Marsden CD. Classification of dystonia. *Adv Neurol* 1998;78:1–10.
3. Chan J, Brin MF, Fahn S. Idiopathic cervical dystonia: clinical characteristics. *Mov Disord* 1991;6:119–126.
4. Epidemiologic study of Dystonia in Europe (EDSE) Collaborative Group. Sex-related influences on the frequency and age of onset of primary dystonia. *Neurology* 1999;53:1871–1872.
5. Therapeutics and Technology Assessment Subcommittee of the American Academy of Neurology. Assessment: the clinical usefulness of BTX-A in treating neurologic disorders. *Neurology* 1990;40:1332–1336.
6. Jankovic J, Brin MF. Therapeutic uses of BTX. *N Engl J Med* 1991;324:1186–1194.
7. Ceballos-Baumann AO. Evidence-based medicine in BTX therapy for cervical dystonia. *J Neurol* 2001; 248(Suppl 1):I14–I20.
8. Brashear A. The BTXs in the treatment of cervical dystonia. *Semin Neurol* 2001;21:85–90.
9. Tarsy D, First ER. Painful cervical dystonia: clinical features and response to treatment with BTX. *Mov Disord* 1999;14:1043–1045.
10. Brans JWM, Lindeboom R, Snoek JW, et al. BTX versus trihexyphenidyl in cervical dystonia: a prospective, randomized, double-blind controlled trial. *Neurology* 1996; 46:1066–1072.
11. Tsui JK, Eisen A, Mak E, et al. A pilot study on the use of BTX in spasmodic torticollis. *Can J Neurol Sci* 1985;12:314–316.
12. Tsui JK, Eisen A, Stoessl AJ, et al. Double-blind study of BTX in spasmodic torticollis. *Lancet* 1986;2: 245–246.
13. Tsui JKC, Fross RD, Calne S, et al. Local treatment of spasmodic torticollis with BTX. *Can J Neurol Sci* 1987; 14:533–535.
14. Tsui JK, Calne DB. BTX in cervical dystonia. *Adv Neurol* 1988;49:473–478.
15. Gelb DJ, Lowenstein DH, Aminoff MJ. Controlled trial of BTX injections in the treatment of spasmodic torticollis. *Neurology* 1989;39:80–84.
16. Greene P, Kang U, Fahn S, et al. Double-blind, placebo-controlled trial of BTX injections for the treatment of spasmodic torticollis. *Neurology* 1990;40:1213–1218.
17. Jankovic J, Schwartz K. BTX injections for cervical dystonia. *Neurology* 1990;40:277–280.
18. Jankovic J, Orman J. Botulinum A toxin for cranial-cervical dystonia: a double-blind, placebo-controlled study. *Neurology* 1987;37:616–623.
19. Moore AP, Blumhardt LD. A double-blind trial of BTX "A" in torticollis, with one-year follow-up. *J Neurol Neurosurg Psychiatry* 1991;54:813–816.
20. Lorentz IT, Subramaniam SS, Yiannikas C. Treatment of idiopathic spasmodic torticollis with botulinum-A toxin: a pilot study of 19 patients. *Med J Aust* 1990; 152:528–530.
21. Lorentz IT, Subramaniam SS, Yiannikas C. Treatment of idiopathic spasmodic torticollis with BTX A: a double-blind study on twenty-three patients. *Mov Disord* 1991;6:145–150.
22. Blackie JD, Lees AJ. BTX treatment in spasmodic torticollis. *J Neurol Neurosurg Psychiatry* 1990;53: 640–643.
23. Borodic GE, Mills L, Joseph M. Botulinum A toxin for the treatment of adult-onset spasmodic torticollis. *Plast Reconstr Surg* 1991;87:285–289.
24. Poewe W, Schelosky L, Kleedorfer B, et al. Treatment of spasmodic torticollis with local injections of BTX. *J Neurol* 1992;239:21–25.
25. Stell R, Thompson PD, Marsden CD. BTX in spasmodic torticollis. *J Neurol Neurosurg Psychiatry* 1988;51: 920–923.
26. Borodic GE, Pearce B, Smith K, et al. Botulinum A toxin for spasmodic torticollis: multiple vs single injection points per muscle. *Head Neck* 1992;14:33–37.
27. Package insert, BOTOX. Allergan Pharmaceuticals, Dec. 2000.
28. Odergren T, Hjaltason H, Kaakkola S, et al. A double blind, randomized, parallel group study to investigate the dose equivalence of Dysport and Botox in the treatment of cervical dystonia. *J Neurol Neurosurg Psychiatry* 1998;64:6–12.
29. Poewe W, Deuschl G, Nebe A, et al. What is the optimal dose of botulinum toxin A in the treatment of cervical dystonia? Results of a double blind, placebo controlled dose ranging study using Dysport. *J Neurol Neurosurg Psychiatry* 1998;64:13–17.
30. Koller W, Vetere-Overfield B, Gray C, et al. Failure of fixed-dose, fixed muscle injection of BTX in torticolllis. *Clin Neuropharmacol* 1990;13:355–358.
31. Gelb DJ, Yoshimura DM, Olney RK, et al. Change in pattern of muscle activity following BTX injections for torticollis. *Ann Neurol* 1991;29:370–376.
32. Brashear A, Watts MW, Marchetti A, et al. Duration of effect of BTX type A in adult patients with cervical dystonia: a retrospective chart review. *Clin Ther* 2000; 22:1516–1524.
33. Kessler KR, Skutta M, Benecke R. Long-term treatment of cervical dystonia with BTX A: efficacy, safety, and antibody frequency. German Dystonia Study Group. *J Neurol* 1999;246:265–274.
34. Giladi N, Meer J, Kidan H, et al. Long-term remission of idiopathic cervical dystonia after treatment with BTX. *Eur Neurol* 2000;44:144–146.
35. Brashear A, Bergan K, Wojcieszek J, et al. Patients' perception of stopping or continuing treatment of cervical dystonia with BTX type A. *Mov Disord* 2000;15: 150–153.
36. Jankovic J, Schwartz KS. Longitudinal experience with BTX injections for treatment of blepharospasm and cervical dystonia. *Neurology* 1993;43:834–836.
37. Sloop RR, Cole D, Patel MC. Muscle paralysis produced by BTX type A injection in treated torticollis patients compared with toxin naive individuals. *Mov Disord* 2001;16:100–105.
38. Jankovic J, Schwartz KS. Clinical correlates of response to BTX injections. *Arch Neurol* 1991;48:1253–1256.
39. Greene P, Fahn S, Diamond B. Development of resistance to BTX type A in patients with torticollis. *Mov Disord* 1994;9:213–217.
40. Greene PE, Fahn S. Use of BTX type F injections to

treat torticollis in patients with immunity to BTX type A. *Mov Disord* 1993;8:479–483.

41. Sheean GL, Lees AJ. BTX F in the treatment of torticollis clinically resistant to BTX A. *J Neurol Neurosurg Psychiatry* 1995;59:601–607.

42. Houser MK, Sheean GL, Lees AJ. Further studies using higher doses of BTX type F for torticollis resistant to BTX type A. *J Neurol Neurosurg Psychiatry* 1998;64: 577–580.

43. Chen R, Karp BI, Jallett M. BTX serotype F for treatment of dystonia: long-term experience. *Neurology* 1998;51:1494–1496.

44. Brin MF, Lew MF, Adler CH, et al. Safety and efficacy of NeuroBloc (BTX type B) in type A-resistant cervical dystonia. *Neurology* 1999;53:1431–8.

45. Dauer WT, Burke RE, Greene P, et al. Current concepts on the clinical features, aetiology, and management of idiopathic cervical dystonia. *Brain* 1998;121:547–560.

46. Buchman AS, Comella CL, Stebbins GT, et al. Determining a dose-effect curve for BTX in the sternocleidomastoid muscle in cervical dystonia. *Clin Neuropharmacol* 1994;17:188–195.

47. Dressler D, Rothwell JC. Electromyographic quantification of the paralyzing effect of BTX in the sternocleidomastoid muscle. *Eur Neurol* 2000;43:13–16.

48. Fuglsang-Frederiksen A, Ostergaard L, Sjo O, et al. Quantitative electromyographical changes in cervical dystonia after treatment with BTX. *Electromyogr Clin Neurophysiol* 1998;38:75–79.

49. Erdal J, Ostergaard L, Fuglsang-Frederiksen A, et al. Long-term BTX treatment of cervical dystonia—EMG changes in injected and noninjected muscles. *Clin Neurophysiol* 1999;110:1650–1654.

50. Dubinsky RM, Gray CS, Vetere-Overfield B, et al. Electromyographic guidance of BTX treatment in cervical dystonia. *Clin Neuropharmacol* 1991;14:262–267.

51. Comella CL, Buchman AS, Tanner CM, et al. BTX injection for spasmodic torticollis: increased magnitude of benefit with electromyographic assistance. *Neurology* 1992;42:878–882.

52. Ostergaard L, Fuglsang-Frederiksen A, Sjo O, et al. Quantitative EMG in cervical dystonia. *Electromyogr Clin Neurophysiol* 1996;36:179–185.

53. Dressler D. Electromyographic evaluation of cervical dystonia for planning of BTX therapy. *Eur J Neurol* 2000;7:713–718.

54. Van Gerpen JA, Matsumoto JY, Ahlskog JE, et al. Utility of an EMG mapping study in treating cervical dystonia. *Muscle Nerve* 2000;23:1752–1756.

55. Speelman JD, Brans JW. Cervical dystonia and botulinum treatment: is electromyographic guidance necessary? *Mov Disord* 1995;10:802.

56. Finsterer J, Fuchs I, Mamoli B. Quantitative electromyography-guided BTX treatment of cervical dystonia. *Clin Neuropharmacol* 1997;20:42–48.

57. Ajax T, Ross MA, Rodnitzky RL. The role of electromyography in guiding BTX injections for focal dystonia and spasticity. *J Neurol Rehabil* 1998;12:1–4.

58. Borodic GE, Joseph M, Fay L, et al. Botulinum A toxin for the treatment of spasmodic torticollis: dysphagia and regional toxin spread. *Head Neck* 1990;12:392–398.

59. Brans JWM, deBoer IP, Aramideh M, et al. BTX in cervical dystonia: low dosage with electromyographic guidance. *J Neurol* 1995;242:529–534.

60. Jankovic J. Needle EMG guidance is rarely required. *Muscle Nerve* 2001;24:1568–1570.

61. Koay CE, Allun-Jones T. Pharyngeal paralysis due to BTX injection. *J Laryngol Otol* 1989;103:698–699.

62. Comella CL, Tanner CM, Defoor L, Smith C. Dysphagia following BTX injections for spasmodic torticollis. *Neurology* 1992;42:1307–1310.

63. Defazio G, Lepore V, Melpignano C, et al. Cervical radiculopathy following BTX therapy for cervical dystonia. *Funct Neurol* 1993;8:193–196.

64. Huag BA, Dresslet D, Prange HW. Polyradiculoneuritis following BTX therapy. *J Neurol* 1990;237:62–63.

65. Glanzman RL, Gelb DJ, Drury I, et al. Brachial plexopathy after BTX injections. *Neurology* 1990;40:1143.

66. Tarsy D. Brachial plexus neuropathy after BTX injection. *Neurology* 1997;49:1176–1177.

67. Sampaio C, Castro-Caldas A, Sales-Luis ML, et al. Brachial plexopathy after BTX administration for cervical dystonia. *J Neurol Neurosurg Psychiatry* 1993;56: 220–221.

68. LeWitt PA, Trosch RM. Idiosyncratic adverse reactions to intramuscular BTX type A injection. *Mov Disord* 1997;12:1064–1067.

69. Dodel RC, Kirchner A, Koehne-Volland R, et al. Costs of treating dystonias and hemifacial spasm with BTX A. *Pharmacoeconomics* 1997;12:695–706.

70. Jahanshahi M, Marsden. Psychological functioning before and after treatment of torticollis with BTX. *J Neurol Neurosurg Psychiatry* 1992;55:229–231.

71. Brefel-Courbon C, Simonetta-Moreau M, More C, et al. A pharmacoeconomic evaluation of BTX in the treatment of spasmodic torticollis. *Clin Neuropharmacol* 2000;23:203–207.

Scientific and Therapeutic Aspects of Botulinum Toxin
edited by M.F. Brin, J. Jankovic, and M. Hallett
Lippincott Williams & Wilkins, Philadelphia, © 2002.

36

Studies with Dysport® in Cervical Dystonia

Werner Poewe and Tanja Entner

Over the past 15 years two preparations of botulinum neurotoxin type A (BTX-A), BOTOX and DYSPORT, have been clinically used to treat patients with cervical dystonia (CD). This indication was approved by US and European drug regulatory authorities between 1991 and 2000. Most European studies on BTX-A for CD have used DYSPORT; BOTOX reports mainly originate from US centers. Very recently botulinum neurotoxin type B (BTX-B) has also been approved for use in this type of dystonia patient (1,2). This chapter focuses on the use of the DYSPORT preparation of BTX-A in CD. Studies are reviewed with respect to short- and long-term efficacy and to safety and dose-response relationships. The issues of dose-equivalence of DYSPORT versus BOTOX and secondary resistance are also discussed.

SHORT-TERM STUDIES WITH DYSPORT IN CD PATIENTS

Early studies with DYSPORT in patients with cervical dystonia date back to the 1980s. Most of them were open-label trials in small numbers of patients (Table 36.1). Doses employed varied over a wide range between 240 and 1,200 U per session. Injection patterns and methods of identification of target muscles also were largely unstandardized. Practically all studies used the Tsui score as primary efficacy criterion. Despite the variations in dose and injection schedule, 70% to 90% of patients noted improvement in postural deformity and pain (Table 36.1). The reported degrees of improvement, however, when quantified, showed some variation between 20% and more than 50% improvement in Tsui scores. Latencies to onset of clinical effects

were most often in the order of 3 to 7 days and reported durations of injection-induced improvement clustered around 12 weeks (2 to 28 weeks). Durations of follow-up were generally short, between 3 and 19 months (mean 8.3 months). One study involving 37 patients over 12 months found reproducible responder rates and degrees of improvement of posture and pain over a mean of 138 injection sessions. Recurrences did not seem to reach baseline severity and doses for reinjection were 24% lower on average as compared to the first treatment session (3).

Local DYSPORT injections are generally well tolerated and side-effects are usually mild and transient. The most common adverse events include dysphagia, followed by neck muscle weakness, local pain at injection sites, hoarseness, and dry mouth. The rates of DYSPORT-related side-effects show marked variation between the reports (Table 36.2) as did the total doses employed in each study. For example, the single study (4) that reported very high dysphagia rates of 90% used doses of DYSPORT above 1000 U, which is about double the dose now commonly employed for initial treatment (see below). In addition, injections into the sterno-mastoid muscle were more likely to produce swallowing problems than was administration of the toxin into posterior neck muscles. Overall, there is a tendency for later studies to use lower doses than reported in earlier series.

Only two studies (5,6) were double-blind trials. Moore and Blumhardt (6) performed a double-blind placebo-controlled crossover trial in 20 CD patients. Tsui score changes from baseline to week 4 as the primary outcome revealed

TABLE 36.1. *Short-term trials with DYSPORT in cervical dystonia*

Study	Design	Number of patients	Mean dose/session	Response rate (%) Posture	Response rate (%) Pain	Improvement % Tsui scores
Stell et al., 1988 (4)	o.t.	10	1200	90	100	47
Blackie and Lees, 1990 (5)	d.b.	19	960	84	75	22
Blackie and Lees, 1990 (5)	o.t.	50	875	83	77	22
Ceballos-Baumann et al., 1990 (15)	o.t.	45	692	73	78	25
Moore and Blumhardt, 1991 (6)	d.b.	20	1000	n.r.	?	35*
Lees et al., 1992 (16)	o.t.	89	666	62	68	>50
D'Costa and Abbott, 1991 (17)	o.t.	12	520	91	91	>40
Poewe et al., 1992 (3)	o.t.	37	632	86	84	>50
Wissel and Poewe, 1992 (11)	o.t.	108	594	85	85	>50
Brans et al., 1995	o.t.	60	240	80	90	n.r.

o.t., open trial; d.b., double-blind trial; n.r., not reported; * estimated from figure

significantly greater improvement with DYS-PORT. Blackie and Lees (5) included 19 patients in a double-blind placebo controlled trial and again found significantly better improvement and duration of effect with DYSPORT.

In summary, those early, mostly short-term studies suggest that local injections with DYS-PORT in cervical dystonia are effective in usually more than 80% of patients, onset of clinical effects will appear within 5 to 7 days, and will usually last between 10 and 12 weeks. Follow-up injections induce similar improvements as

TABLE 36.2. *Frequency of dysphagia and neck muscle weakness in short-term studies of DYSPORT in cervical dystonia*

Study	Frequency of side effects % Dysphagia	Frequency of side effects % Neck muscle weakness
Stell et al., 1988 (4)	90	n.r.
Blackie and Lees, 1990 (5)	16	10
Blackie and Lees, 1990 (5)	28	5
Ceballos-Baumann et al., 1990 (15)	6	31
Moore and Blumhardt, 1991 (6)	35	25
Lees et al., 1992 (16)	22	2
D'Costa and Abbott, 1991 (17)	25	n.r.
Poewe et al., 1992 (3)	22	10
Wissel and Poewe, 1992 (11)	32	17
Brans et al., 1995	9	3

n.r., not reported

first treatment and dose requirements seem to decrease. The incidence of side-effects, in particular dysphagia, shows wide variations most likely reflecting differences in total daily doses with earlier studies employing the highest total doses.

DOSE-RESPONSE RELATIONSHIPS

Although results from open-label studies suggest that adverse events, in particular dysphagia and neck weakness, tend to become more frequent with higher doses, dose-response relationships were formally assessed in only one study. The German Dystonia Study Group (7) included 75 (39 men, 36 women) previously untreated patients with rotational torticollis and clinical hyperactivity confined to one splenius capitis and the contralateral sternomastoid muscle. The patients were randomized to four groups receiving total DYSPORT doses of 250, 500, and 1,000 U or placebo. Doses injected into the splenius capitis were fixed at 0, 175, 350, or 700 U and those to the contralateral sternomastoid muscle at 0, 75, 150, or 300 U. Assessments were made at 0, 2, 4, and 8 weeks after treatment, and comprised the Modified Tsui Score, a 4-point pain scale assessment of swallowing difficulties and a global assessment of improvement by the patient and the physician. Tsui scores remained virtually unchanged in the placebo group and showed similar reductions (20% to 25%) for all active groups at week 2. At week 4, pronounced and statistically significant changes

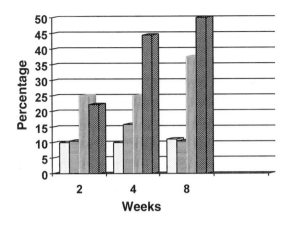

FIG. 36.1. Percentage of patients in the different treatment groups experiencing greater than 50% global subjective improvement following DYSPORT injections. (Modified from Poewe W, Deuschl G, Nebe A, et al. What is the optimal dose of botulinum toxin A in the treatment of cervical dystonia? Results of a double-blind, placebo-controlled, dose-ranging study using DYSPORT. German Dystonia Study Group. *J Neurol Neurosurg Psychiatry* 1998;64: 13–17, with permission.)

were seen for the 500- and 1,000-U arms only. The 1,000-U arm continued to show marked effects by week 8 (Fig. 36.1). Similarly, the number of patients reporting greater than 50% global improvement grew in a dose-dependent fashion with significantly more patients in the 500- and 1,000-U arms reaching this criterion in weeks 4 and 8. While the latency of onset to clinical benefit was 8 to 9 days for all active groups, the duration of effect seemed to be dose-dependent, and longer in the 1,000-U group as compared to the 250- and 500-U groups. Pain was reduced to a significantly greater degree in all active groups as compared to placebo at week 4, but there was no clear dose-response relationship.

Adverse events were mostly mild and transient with a duration of 1 to 4 weeks. The difference of the incidence of side-effects was significant between the 1,000-U group and the placebo ($p = 0.004$) and between the 1,000-U group and the 250-U group ($p = 0.05$). The most common adverse event was dysphagia followed by neck muscle weakness and voice changes.

In summary, 1,000 U of DYSPORT seems to produce greater and longer benefit at the expense of more dysphagia and neck muscle weakness and 500 U of DYSPORT appears to be the "optimal" starting dose in cervical dystonia. In addition, this study failed to show superiority of 250 U over placebo after the 4 weeks assessment.

DOSE EQUIVALENCE DYSPORT VERSUS BOTOX

Although theoretically mouse units of the two available type A toxin preparations should be identical, doses of DYSPORT and BOTOX as reported in open-label and double-blind studies vary by a factor of 3 to 5. To clarify the issue of relative potency, a single double-blind trial tried to assess the dose equivalence of DYSPORT versus BOTOX preparations of botulinum toxin A in patients with cervical dystonia.

Odergren et al. (8) studied 73 patients with predominantly rotational cervical dystonia, who had received at least four previous injections with BOTOX and who had experienced a satisfactory response. They were then randomized to receive either the clinically indicated dose of BOTOX as evident from their previous response or a dose of DYSPORT set three times the number of BOTOX units. The DYSPORT group (38 patients) received a mean dose of 477 (240 to 720) U, and the BOTOX group (35 patients) received a mean dose of 152 (70 to 240) U.

Posttreatment assessments were made at 2, 4, 8, and 12 weeks with Tsui score as primary efficacy criterion. Pain scores, a global assessment of improvement, and adverse events were also recorded. Both groups showed marked improvements in Tsui scores by week 2 with a peak effect at week 4. Improvements were in the order of 40% to 50% and not significantly different between the groups. The duration of effect as assessed by time to reinjection was also similar: 84 days for DYSPORT versus 81 days for BOTOX.

Thirty-nine adverse effects were recorded in 58% of DYSPORT patients; 56 adverse effects were recorded in 69% of BOTOX patients. There was no statistically significant difference between the groups. Dysphagia was most common (six DYSPORT patients; four BOTOX patients), followed by fatigue (three DYSPORT; four BOTOX), neck pain (three DYSPORT; one BOTOX), dry mouth (zero DYSPORT; three BOTOX), muscle weakness (three DYSPORT; zero BOTOX), and dysphonia (zero DYSPORT; two BOTOX). The authors concluded that a ratio of 3:1 of DYSPORT versus BOTOX units will produce equivalent efficacy and safety in CD patients.

The reasons for these differences in potency between the two preparations are not entirely clear. Recent studies suggest that albumin content dilution volume may play a role (9).

LONG-TERM OUTCOME

While all of the studies cited in the prior section had short follow-up times and only few reported results up to 12 months after the first injection, Kessler et al. (10), with the German Dystonia Study Group, reported on the outcome of 303 patients with CD followed for a mean of 3 years or 10 injection sessions. These 303 patients had received a total of 3,088 injections with a mean dose of 778 U. Of these patients, 40% had a pure rotational cervical dystonia, 29% had a combination of rotational and tilt (laterocollis), 10% had pure laterocollis, and 8% had pure ante- or retrocollis; 13% suffered from complex forms of cervical dystonia.

A modified Tsui score used to assess efficacy and severity of symptoms, was found to decrease by about 60% from baseline to assessments made before the fifteenth injection, indicating reduced baseline or preinjection severity over time. Accordingly, baseline versus posttreatment differences were greatest following the initial injection. At the same time, there was a progressive decrease of DYSPORT doses from an average of 1,072 U at first to about 720 U by the sixth injection. Total duration of effect averaged 11 weeks without significant change over time.

Of 3,088 injection sessions, 685 (22%) were complicated by adverse events, while 25% of these patients remained free of any side-effect. Dysphagia was most frequent adverse event and occurred in 77% of all injections that had produced side-effects; neck weakness and dry mouth were seen in 17% and 10% of these sessions, respectively. The incidence of side-effects was dose-related and virtually all injection sessions with doses above 1,200 U elicited some adverse event.

Overall similar results were also reported by Wissel and Poewe (11) in a smaller series of 108 patients followed for up to nine injection sessions.

SECONDARY NONRESPONSIVENESS AND IMMUNOGENICITY

Up to 15% of CD patients have been reported as failing to respond in a meaningful way to the first and follow-up injections of botulinum toxin type A (5,11). The reasons for this primary unresponsiveness are incompletely understood and probably heterogeneous, including incorrect targeting of muscles, failure to identify deep muscles causing dystonia, and dosing issues, as well as the possibility of low titers of neutralizing antibodies (Ab). Secondary nonresponsiveness, on the other hand, is characterized by a loss of an initially satisfactory and reproducible response to injections. It is frequently, but not always, associated with detectable serum-antibodies to the toxin (6,7).

There is limited information on the rate of development of secondary nonresponsiveness during long-term treatment of CD patients with DYSPORT. In their series of 303 patients with ongoing therapy and 162 dropouts, Kessler et al. (10) identified 17 secondary nonresponders in the latter group. Fifty percent of non-responders had neutralizing Ab as assessed by diverse techniques (mouse bioassay, phrenic nerve-hemidiaphragm preparation), while the other 50% did not show antibodies. From this, Kessler et al.

calculated a minimum antibody frequency of 2.5% of patients receiving at least six injections. None of their patients had developed antibodies with fewer injections. Main predictors for antibody formation on their study included high dose (875 U in Ab$^+$ nonresponders vs 750 U in responders), shorter injection intervals (91 vs 105 days), and number of booster sessions (4.2% vs 1.3% of sessions). Similar figures were reported by Zuber and colleagues (12). They reported 3% of secondary nonresponders with antibodies using DYSPORT in 96 patients with different dystonic syndromes. The three patients who became secondary nonresponders suffered from cervical dystonia for several years, had received a high cumulative dose (55 to 90 ng), and had a shorter interval (4 to 5 weeks) between two injections.

Reduction of neutralizing antibodies with plasma exchange and immunoadsorption on a protein A column below the detection limit temporarily restores BTX-A responsiveness, which is in contrast to treatment with i.v. immunoglobulins (13,14). However, BTX-A resistant patients with CD do respond to injections with type B toxin, which is now available in the United States and Europe (1,2).

REFERENCES

1. Brin MF, Lew MF, Adler CH, et al. Safety and efficacy of NeuroBloc (botulinum toxin type B) in type A-resistant cervical dystonia. *Neurology* 1999;53:1431–1438.
2. Brashear A, Lew MF, Dykstra DD, et al. Safety and efficacy of NeuroBloc (botulinum toxin type B) in type A-responsive cervical dystonia. *Neurology* 1999;53: 1439–1446.
3. Poewe W, Schelosky L, Kleedorfer B, et al. Treatment of spasmodic torticollis with local injection of botulinum toxin—one-year follow-up in 37 patients. *J Neurol* 1992;1:21–26.
4. Stell R, Thompson PD, Marsden CD. Botulinum toxin in spasmodic torticollis. *J Neurol Neurosurg Psychiatry* 1988;51:920–923.
5. Blackie JD, Lees AJ. Botulinum toxin treatment in spasmodic torticollis. *J Neurol Neurosurg Psychiatry* 1990; 53:640–643.
6. Moore AP, Blumhardt LD. A double-blind trial of botulinum toxin "A" in torticollis, with one-year follow-up. *J Neurol Neurosurg Psychiatry* 1991;54:813–816.
7. Poewe W, Deuschl G, Nebe A, et al. What is the optimal dose of botulinum toxin A in the treatment of cervical dystonia? Results of a double-blind, placebo-controlled, dose-ranging study using DYSPORT. German Dystonia Study Group. *J Neurol Neurosurg Psychiatry* 1998;64: 13–17.
8. Odergren T, Hjaltason H, Kaakkola S, et al. A double-blind, randomised, parallel group study to investigate the dose equivalence of DYSPORT and BOTOX in the treatment of cervical dystonia. *J Neurol Neurosurg Psychiatry* 1998;64:6–12.
9. Bigalke H, Wohlfarth K, Irmer A, et al. Botulinum A toxin: DYSPORT improvement of biological availability. *Exp Neurol* 2001;168:162–170.
10. Kessler KR, Skutta M, Benecke R for the German Dystonia Study Group. Long-term treatment of cervical dystonia with botulinum toxin A: efficacy, safety, and antibody frequency. *J Neurol* 1999;246:265–274.
11. Wissel J, Poewe W. Dystonia—clinical, neuropathological and therapeutic review. *J Neural Transm Suppl* 1992;38:91–104.
12. Zuber M, Sebald M, Bathien N, et al. Botulinum antibodies in dystonic patients treated with type A botulinum toxin: frequency and significance. *Neurology* 1993; 43:1715–1718.
13. Naumann M, Toyka KV, Mansouri Taleghani B, et al. Depletion of neutralising antibodies resensitises a secondary non-responder to botulinum A neurotoxin. *J Neurol Neurosurg Psychiatry* 1998;65:924–927.
14. Dressler D, Zettl U, Benecke R, et al. Can intravenous immunoglobulin improve antibody-mediated botulinum toxin therapy failure? *Mov Disord* 2000;15:1279–1281.
15. Ceballos-Baumann AO, Gasser T, Dengler R, et al. Lokale botulinum toxin A injektionen bei blepharospasmus, meige syndrom und hemifacialem spasmus. Beobachtungen an 106 patienten. *Nervenarzt* 1990;61: 604–610.
16. Lees AJ, Turjanski N, Rivest J, et al. Treatment of cervical dystonia hand spasms and laryngeal dystonia with botulinum toxin. *J Neurol* 1992;239:1–4.
17. D'Costa DF, Abbott RJ. Low-dose botulinum toxin in spasmodic torticollis. *J R Soc Med* 1991;84:650–651.

Scientific and Therapeutic Aspects of Botulinum Toxin
edited by M.F. Brin, J. Jankovic, and M. Hallett
Lippincott Williams & Wilkins, Philadelphia, © 2002.

37

Review of Clinical Efficacy Studies with Botulinum Toxin Type B (MYOBLOC™) for Cervical Dystonia

Stewart A. Factor

INTRODUCTION

Cervical dystonia is the most common form of adult-onset focal dystonia (1). It occurs more often in women and has a mean age of onset of about 40 years (2). The disorder is characterized by intermittent or sustained muscle contractions in the neck and/or shoulder muscles, resulting in involuntary twisting and turning, and abnormal postures of the head and neck (3). Rotational torticollis is the most common type of deviation observed, but any direction of movement is possible. Progression of dystonia to other anatomic sites, particularly the arms and face, and a tremor similar to essential tremor in the hands are reported in up to 25% of patients (2,4,5). Muscle hypertrophy and head tremor are also prominent features; spasmodic movements of the neck are not as common as previously thought (2).

In addition to motor dysfunction, other clinical symptoms are commonly associated with cervical dystonia. Nearly all patients develop a repertoire of maneuvers such as touching the chin, face, or the back of the head to correct the abnormal movements and posturing (2,6). These ''sensory tricks'' are usually effective early in the disorder, but tend to lose effectiveness as the disease progresses. The presence of musculoskeletal pain is another very prominent feature of cervical dystonia, occurring in about 80% of patients (2,7–9). The pain is typically diffuse and widespread around the neck and shoulders, and is strongly associated with the constant head turning and muscle spasms (7). Although cervi-

cal dystonia is not a life-threatening disease, it substantially affects the patient's ability to lead a normal life. In a recent study, approximately 35% of patients needed to change or cease employment as a result of the disability from their dystonia (10). In addition, cervical dystonia has been shown to have a negative impact on psychological well-being (11,12).

The goals of treatment are to alleviate symptoms, improve quality of life, and prevent secondary complications of the disorder, such as cervical spondylosis with radiculopathy or myelopathy (13). For many years, oral medications including anticholinergics, benzodiazepines, dopamine depletors, and muscle relaxants were the cornerstone of therapy for moderate to severe cervical dystonia. However, use of these agents was generally inadequate, benefiting less than half of all treated patients (14–16) and having little effect on regaining employment status (10).

In the early 1980s, the introduction of chemodenervation therapy using botulinum toxin type A (BTX-A; BOTOX) radically changed the treatment of cervical dystonia and other types of focal dystonias. Botulinum toxins act by blocking the release of acetylcholine from presynaptic nerve terminals at the neuromuscular junction. Local intramuscular injection of minute doses into affected muscles produces a temporary and dose-dependent degree of muscle paralysis and atrophy. The effectiveness of BTX-A in cervical dystonia has been demonstrated in a number of clinical studies (17–22). With this therapy, nearly 60% of patients are able to return to work

(10). Despite the success of BTX-A, however, approximately 10% of treated patients develop resistance to the toxin after one or more injections, which limits its usefulness (23–25). This incidence may be even higher because these data were collected from retrospective reviews of studies. The cause for secondary resistance has been attributed to the formation of neutralizing antibodies that block the clinical effects of the toxin (26,27).

Other serotypes of botulinum toxin—types B, C, and F—have also been studied as possible treatments for dystonia (28–30). Types C and F are currently under investigational development. The type B serotype (BTX-B; MYOBLOC; NeuroBloc) was recently approved in the United States and in the European Union for the treatment of cervical dystonia. During its development, BTX-B was referred to as NeuroBloc. Although it retains this name in Europe, it is now called MYOBLOC in the United States. BTX-B is antigenically distinct from the type A toxin, such that antibodies produced against BTX-A do not inhibit the clinical effects of BTX-B and vice versa (31). In addition, BTX-B has unique mechanistic features as compared with the type A toxin. It catalyzes the cleavage of the intracellular target protein synaptobrevin in the vesicle docking and fusion complex to inhibit acetylcholine release (32). In contrast, BTX-A cleaves synaptosomal-associated protein 25 kDa (SNAP-25) (33).

The research program for BTX-B has included several studies. Preliminary double-blind and open-label studies (29,34–36) have shown that BTX-B is safe and effective for the treatment of cervical dystonia, and ultimately led to the doses used in the pivotal phase III trials. Three key randomized, double-blind, placebo-controlled clinical trials were used as the basis of approval of BTX-B in the United States and in European Union member countries. The results of these studies, herein referred to as Studies 1 (37), 2 (38), and 3 (39), are reviewed in this chapter.

STUDY DESIGNS

Each of the three studies was a multicenter, 16-week, single-treatment, randomized, double-blind, and placebo-controlled trial (Table 37.1) (37–39). Patients in these studies were 18 years of age or older and had cervical dystonia for at least 1 year in duration, involving two or more of the following muscles: levator scapulae, scalene complex, semispinalis capitis, splenius capitis, sternocleidomastoid, or trapezius. In Study 1, a total of 122 patients, including type A responsive (79%) and type A resistant (21%) patients, were enrolled and randomly assigned to one of four dose groups: placebo, 2,500 U, 5,000 U, or 10,000 U of BTX-B (37). Patients were considered "type A resistant" if they had previously responded to the type A toxin but failed to respond to the last two successive treatments, including a higher dose in the last dosing session. In Study 2, only patients who were responsive to BTX-A were included (38). These patients (n = 109) were stratified to treatment with placebo, 5,000 U, or 10,000 U of BTX-B.

In Study 3, only type A-resistant patients were included (39). Resistance was determined by one of two definitions: (a) prior response to BTX-A, followed by loss of response in two consecutive treatments with at least one of these treatments using a dose higher than that which the patient responded to previously; or (b) prior response to BTX-A, followed by loss of response in the last treatment and either a positive mouse neutralizing assay or a failed response to an appropriate injection of BTX-A in a selected muscle (using electromyography or clinical findings to assess that response). Secondary nonresponse was confirmed by using a frontalis type A test (F-TAT) (39). The F-TAT consisted of an injection of 15 U of BTX-A, divided into two 7.5-U doses, administered in the right frontalis muscle. Patients were considered type A-resistant if they could wrinkle their right frontalis muscle 2 weeks after the F-TAT injection, indicating no weakness of that muscle. Patients were considered type A-responsive if they could not wrinkle their forehead. In Study 3, 77 type A-resistant patients were randomized to either placebo or 10,000 U of BTX-B.

For all three studies, study drug was provided in 3.5-mL vials that contained 5,000 U of BTX-B or placebo in 1.0-mL sterile solution, buffered to a pH of 5.6. On day 1, all patients received

TABLE 37.1. *Study designs and efficacy assessments*

Parameter	Study 1 [Lew et al. (37)]	Study 2 [Brashear et al. (38)]	Study 3 [Brin et al. (39)]
Design	Multicenter (12), double-blind, placebo-controlled	Multicenter (9), double-blind, placebo-controlled	Multicenter (7), double-blind, placebo-controlled
Study duration	16 weeks	16 weeks	16 weeks
Population	Type A responsive; type A resistant	Type A responsive only	Type A resistant only
Enrolled (n)	122	109	77
Treatment groups (n)			
Placebo	30	36	38
2,500 U	31	—	—
5,000 U	31	36	—
10,000 U	30	37	39
Primary efficacy assessment	TWSTRS-Total score at week 4	TWSTRS-Total score at week 4	TWSTRS-Total score at week 4
Other efficacy assessments	TWSTRS-Subscale scores (Severity, Disability, Pain); Patient and Physician Global Assessments; Patient Analog Pain	TWSTRS-Subscale scores (Severity, Disability, Pain); Patient and Physician Global Assessments; Patient Analog Pain	TWSTRS-Subscale scores (Severity, Disability, Pain); Patient and Physician Global Assessments; Patient Analog Pain

TWSTRS, Toronto Western Spasmodic Torticollis Rating Scale (range, 0 to 87); composed of three subscales: Severity (range, 0 to 35), Disability (range, 0 to 32), Pain (range, 0 to 20).

a single dose of study drug. It was injected into two to four affected neck and/or shoulder muscles based on the treating investigator's clinical findings. The proportionate volume per muscle was divided and injected in up to five sites, with each site receiving 0.1 to 1.0 mL. Study drug was injected with or without use of electromyography at the principal investigator's discretion. Patients returned for a visit at weeks 2 and 4, and then every 4 weeks thereafter up to 16 weeks. Each patient received only one treatment. In Studies 2 and 3, two investigators—principal and administrative—were involved at each study site to maintain blinding as best as possible. The principal investigator conducted all screening assessments, selected muscles for injection, performed injections, and completed efficacy assessments. The administrative investigator was responsible for all other activities at each study visit, including collection and assessment of adverse events.

In all studies, the primary efficacy assessment was the change in Toronto Western Spasmodic Torticollis Rating Scale (TWSTRS)-Total score at week 4. The TWSTRS-Total score (range, 0 to 87) consists of three subscale scores, including Severity (range, 0 to 35), Disability (range, 0 to 32), and Pain (range, 0 to 20). A higher score denotes a more severe clinical manifestation. Importantly, the TWSTRS is a validated outcome measurement for cervical dystonia (6). To be eligible for any of the three studies, patients had to have a baseline TWSTRS-Total score of 20 or higher, with a TWSTRS-Severity score of 10 or higher, a TWSTRS-Disability score of 3 or higher, and a TWSTRS-Pain score of 1 or higher. Analyses also included change in subscale scores at week 4 and TWSTRS-Total scores at weeks 8, 12, and 16. In Studies 2 and 3, Kaplan–Meier survival analyses were conducted to provide an estimate of the duration of treatment effect. The event of interest was the time to return to the baseline TWSTRS-Total score. The median time until return to baseline was estimated for each treatment group.

Other efficacy assessments included the Patient and Physician Global Assessments of Change, and Patient Analog Pain. All three assessments were completed using a 100-mm visual analog scale. For the Patient Global Assessment of Change, patients indicated how they felt at the time of evaluation as compared with preinjection baseline by marking the 100-mm scale, with 0 mm (on the left end) representing "much worse" and 100 mm (on the right end) representing "much better." A score of 50 was defined as no change. Similarly, principal investigators completed the Physician Global Assessment of Change. Investigators and patients completed their Global Assessments independently, and results of the Patient Global Assessments remained blinded to the investigator throughout the study. For the Patient Analog Pain assessment, patients were asked to indicate their current impression of pain again using the 100-mm visual analog scale, with 0 mm representing "worst ever pain" and 100 mm representing "no pain." Scores were obtained at baseline and each visit after treatment injection.

The safety of BTX-B was assessed by collecting adverse event data at each visit during the studies. In addition, vital signs and clinical laboratory assessments were performed on each patient at each visit.

RESULTS

Demographics and Baseline Characteristics

Table 37.2 summarizes patient characteristics for each study. In general, patients were in their mid-50s and had mean TWSTRS-Total scores that ranged between 40 and 55 at study entry, signifying moderate to severe cervical dystonia. Patients in Study 3 (type A-resistant patients) had slightly higher baseline TWSTRS-Total scores, suggesting worse disease at baseline. There were no statistically significant differences among the studies and across treatment groups in baseline values.

Efficacy Assessments

In the three studies, mean improvements in TWSTRS-Total scores at week 4 were significantly better in all dose groups as compared with placebo (Fig. 37.1). In Study 1, at week 4, improvements were 3.3 points for the placebo

TABLE 37.2. *Baseline and demographic characteristics of patients by study*

Characteristic	Study 1 [Lew et al. (37)]				Study 2 [Brashear et al. (38)]			Study 3 [Brin et al. (39)]	
	Placebo ($n = 30$)	2,500 U ($n = 31$)	5,000 U ($n = 31$)	10,000 U ($n = 30$)	Placebo ($n = 36$)	5,000 U ($n = 36$)	10,000 U ($n = 37$)	Placebo ($n = 38$)	10,000 U ($n = 39$)
Age, mean (y)	57.0	54.1	52.4	56.5	54.3	57.6	56.2	52.6	56.6
Gender, % female	70.0	67.7	71.0	60.0	58.3	50.0	75.7	68.4	69.2
Height, mean (cm)	168.4	166.8	168.5	168.3	169.5	169.2	167.0	169.6	166.5
Weight, mean (kg)	73.7	75.1	75.4	71.0	74.5	77.0	74.5	74.7	74.9
TWSTRS-Total score (mean)	45.5	45.6	45.2	47.5	43.6	46.4	46.9	51.2	52.8
Severity	20.3	18.9	19.7	19.4	18.4	20.2	20.2	22.1	22.6
Disability	14.2	15.8	15.1	15.7	14.3	14.4	14.4	16.9	18.3
Pain	11.0	10.9	10.5	12.4	10.9	11.8	12.4	12.2	11.9

TWSTRS, Toronto Western Spasmodic Torticollis Rating Scale.

group, 11.6 points for the 2,500-U group, 12.5 points for the 5,000-U group, and 16.4 points for the 10,000-U group. In Study 2, mean improvements were 4.3 points for the placebo group, 9.3 points for the 5,000-U group, and 11.7 points for the 10,000-U group. In Study 3, mean improvements were 2.0 points for the placebo group and 11.1 points for the 10,000-U group. A significant dose-response relationship that favored the 10,000-U dose was observed in TWSTRS-Total scores.

In Study 2, mean improvement in TWSTRS-Total score at week 8 was significantly better

for both 5,000-U and 10,000-U treatment groups as compared with placebo ($p < 0.02$). However, the difference in scores was not significant at week 12. In Study 3, mean improvement of the TWSTRS-Total score was significantly greater with 10,000 U as compared with placebo at weeks 8 ($p < 0.002$) and 12 ($p < 0.02$). In Studies 2 and 3, Kaplan–Meier analyses showed that the median duration of BTX-B treatment effect was 12 to 16 weeks for both doses tested (Fig. 37.2). In Study 2, the estimated median time until return to baseline TWSTRS-Total score was 63 days for placebo, 114 days for the 5,000-

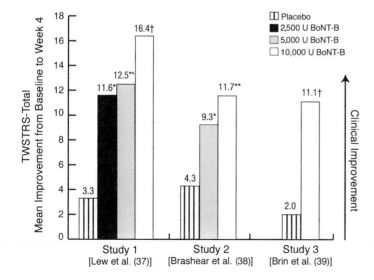

FIG. 37.1. TWSTRS-Total score: mean improvement from baseline to week 4 after treatment injection. At all doses evaluated, BTX-B was significantly more effective than placebo. Within-study comparisons against placebo: *$p = 0.05$; **$p = 0.0005$; †$p = 0.0001$.

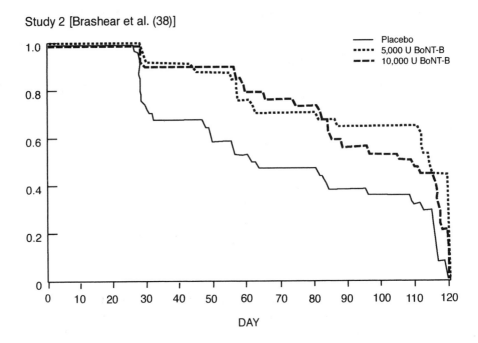

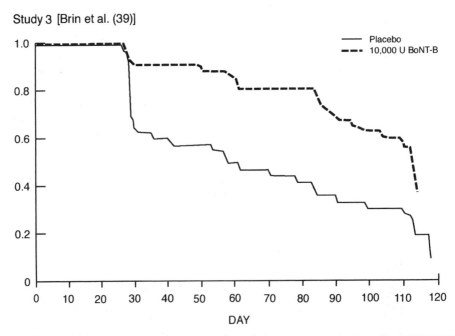

FIG. 37.2. Kaplan–Meier survival analyses: number of days to return to baseline TWSTRS-Total score. **A:** In Study 2, median time was 63 days with placebo, 114 days with 5,000 U, and 111 days with 10,000 U; $p = 0.0008$ for both dose groups versus placebo using the Cox proportional hazard regression model. **B:** In Study 3, median time was 59 days with placebo and 112 days with 10,000 U; $p = 0.004$ using Log-Rank statistic.

TABLE 37.3. *Results of TWSTRS-Subscale scores from baseline to week 4 by study**

TWSTRS-Subscale	Study 1 [Lew et al. (37)]				Study 2 [Brashear et al. (38)]			Study 3 [Brin et al. (39)]	
	Placebo ($n = 30$)	2,500 U ($n = 31$)	5,000 U ($n = 31$)	10,000 U ($n = 30$)	Placebo ($n = 36$)	5,000 U ($n = 36$)	10,000 U ($n = 37$)	Placebo ($n = 38$)	10,000 U ($n = 39$)
Severity	1.6	3.5	4.5**	4.7†	2.3	3.2	4.8**	1.1	3.7**
Disability	0.7	3.8*	3.6*	5.4‡	1.6	2.5	2.7	0.8	3.8**
Pain	1.0	4.4**	4.3**	6.4‡	0.5	3.6**	4.2†	0.1	3.5‡

* Within study comparison with placebo: *$p < 0.05$, **$p < 0.01$, †$p < 0.001$, ‡$p \leq 0.0001$.
TWSTRS, Toronto Western Spasmodic Torticollis Rating Scale.

U group, and 111 days for the 10,000-U group. In Study 3, the median duration was 59 days for placebo and 112 days for the 10,000-U group. Study 1 was not designed to demonstrate duration of treatment effect; however, in general, effects were sustained for at least 12 weeks.

Results of other efficacy assessments generally correlated with that of the TWSTRS-Total scores; i.e., improvements were noted within each BTX-B treatment group as compared with placebo, and improvements tended to increase as the BTX-B dose increased. Results from the change in the three TWSTRS-Subscale scores (Severity, Disability, and Pain) at week 4 are shown in Table 37.3. Overall, scores improved from baseline to week 4 for all BTX-B treatment groups as compared with placebo, with better response observed in the higher dose group. Values for the Patient and Physician Global Assessments of Change and for the Patient Analog Pain Assessment are shown in Figs. 37.3 and 37.4,

respectively. Again, scores were more improved in patients who received BTX-B treatment as compared to those who received placebo, and a dose-response relationship was observed.

Safety

BTX-B was safe and well-tolerated. Table 37.4 summarizes the most commonly reported adverse events in each study. In each study, dry mouth and dysphagia were the most common treatment-related adverse effects, and the only effects that occurred at a significantly greater frequency in the treatment groups compared with placebo. A higher incidence occurred in the higher dose groups. These events were generally mild or moderate in severity and self-resolving. None required intervention, and no patients discontinued from the studies because of these events. In addition, no systemic toxicity was reported, and no clinically significant changes in

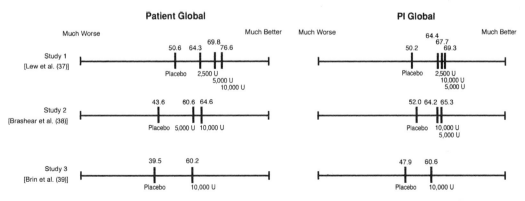

FIG. 37.3. Patient and Physician Global visual analog scale assessments at week 4. Score of 50 equals no change in status; greater than 50 equals improvement in status; less than 50 equals worsened status. All BTX-B treatment scores significantly different from placebo within study ($p < 0.05$).

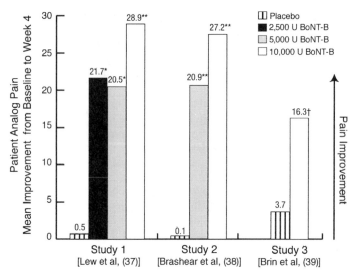

FIG. 37.4. Patient Analog Pain Assessment mean improvement from baseline to week 4 after treatment injection. At all doses evaluated, BTX-B was significantly more effective than placebo. Within-study comparisons against placebo: *$p < 0.05$; **$p = 0.001$; †$p = 0.0001$.

TABLE 37.4. *Adverse events reported with a frequency of 10% or greater* by study*

	Patients (%)								
	Study 1 [Lew et al. (37)]				Study 2 [Brashear et al. (38)]			Study 3 [Brin et al. (39)]	
Adverse event	Placebo ($n = 30$)	2,500 U ($n = 31$)	5,000 U ($n = 31$)	10,000 U ($n = 30$)	Placebo ($n = 36$)	5,000 U ($n = 36$)	10,000 U ($n = 37$)	Placebo ($n = 38$)	10,000 U ($n = 39$)
Dry mouth	3	3	10	33	3	14	24	3	44
Dysphagia	0	16	10	27	3	11	22	5	28
Pain secondary to CD	13	10	10	23	25	31	27	21	21
Infection	0	13	13	17	28	25	8	16	21
Injection-site pain	10	16	19	17	8	6	11	8	18
Headache	7	10	6	13	8	25	14	—	—
Flu syndrome	0	6	10	10	—	—	—	—	—
Nausea	3	10	3	10	—	—	—	8	15
Pain	7	6	10	10	14	6	24	—	—
Dyspepsia	—	—	—	—	8	3	11	—	—

*Percentage data based on within-group determinations.

laboratory values or vital signs were observed in any of the studies.

CONCLUSIONS

The introduction of BTX-B represents an important therapeutic breakthrough because it is the first effective alternative to BTX-B to become available in more than 10 years. Local injection of BTX-B into skeletal muscles can relieve symptoms caused by involuntary muscle spasms associated with cervical dystonia and potentially a variety of other neurologic disorders. Like the type A toxin, the basis for its effectiveness resides in its ability to cause a chemical denervation related to prevention of acetylcholine release in the neuromuscular junction, ultimately resulting in long-term muscle weakness and atrophy (40). It is important to recognize, however, that although the clinical effects of the two toxins are similar, BTX-B is antigenically distinct (41,42), and different structurally and mechanistically from BTX-A (43,44). The well-controlled studies of BTX-B described here substantiate its efficacy in patients with cervical dystonia, including in those patients who no longer respond to therapy with BTX-A. Importantly, as with the type A toxin, secondary immunoresistance to BTX-B following long-term therapy may be a potential concern. The studies described here involve only a single treatment and therefore do not provide any data on this issue. Information on the frequency of immunoresistance to BTX-B can be obtained only through the results of studies examining long-term treatment with repeat dosing.

In the three controlled clinical trials reported here (37–39), BTX-B was shown to improve the severity, disability, and pain associated with cervical dystonia. The benefit extended even to those patients with secondary resistance to BTX-A. Efficacy was based on the validated TWSTRS, as well as on subjective measurements (visual analog scales) of patient well-being and control of pain. Overall, treatment with BTX-B was consistently superior to placebo, with statistically significant improvements observed for most efficacy assessments at the doses evaluated (i.e., 2,500 U, 5,000 U, and 10,000 U). Results also support a significant dose-dependent response, such that the highest dose evaluated (10,000 U) resulted in the most dramatic improvements. The duration of treatment effect was 12 to 16 weeks.

Based on these studies, BTX-B can be used safely at doses up to 10,000 U in the treatment of cervical dystonia. Dry mouth and dysphagia were the most commonly reported treatment-related adverse events, and the incidence of these events also tended to be dose-related. Most cases were mild or moderate and self-resolving. In a large well-controlled trial of the type A toxin DYSPORT, dry mouth was reported with similar frequency as in studies with BTX-B (45). In this same study, dysphagia occurred in nearly 75% of patients. The other available type A toxin, BOTOX, is also associated with dysphagia in addition to significant neck weakness (17,22,46), the latter of which has not been seen with BTX-B therapy. However, because no trials that directly compare the two serotypes have been conducted to date, such comparisons of adverse events should be made with caution.

BTX-B (MYOBLOC) is available as a sterile injectable solution in three dosing volumes: 2,500 U, 5,000 U, and 10,000 U. The previously described controlled clinical trials have demonstrated its efficacy and safety at doses up to 10,000 U in the treatment of patients with cervical dystonia (37–39). In addition, the safety of doses higher than 1,000 U has been shown in several open-label studies (29). With its proven efficacy in reducing the severity, disability, and pain associated with cervical dystonia, BTX-B is likely to become an important therapeutic tool for primary treatment in patients with this disorder as well as in those patients who no longer respond to the type A toxin. In addition, given its mechanism of action, the potential use of BTX-B in the treatment of other conditions involving involuntary muscle contractions (e.g., spasticity, pain) may be beneficial, and clinical trials are warranted in these areas.

ACKNOWLEDGMENTS

This work was supported by the AMC Parkinson's Research Fund and the Riley Family Chair in Parkinson's Disease. Special thanks to Tina Lin for her assistance in the writing of this manuscript.

REFERENCES

1. Nutt JG, Muenter MD, Aronson A, et al. Epidemiology of focal and generalized dystonia in Rochester, Minnesota. *Mov Disord* 1988;3:188–194.
2. Molho ES, Feustel PJ, Factor SA. Clinical comparison of tardive and idiopathic cervical dystonia. *Mov Disord* 1998;13:486–489.
3. Fahn S, Marsden CD, Calne DB. Classification and investigation of dystonia. In: Marsden CD, Fahn S, eds. *Movement disorders 2*. London: Butterworths; 1987: 332–358.
4. Jankovic J, Leder S, Warner D, et al. Cervical dystonia: clinical findings and associated movement disorders. *Neurology* 1991;41:1088–1091.
5. Lowenstein D, Aminoff MJ. The clinical course of spasmodic torticollis. *Neurology* 1988;38:530–532.
6. Consky ES, Lang AE. Assessment of cervical dystonia: the Toronto Western Spasmodic Torticollis Rating Scale (TWSTRS). In: Jankovic J, Hallet M, eds. *Therapy with botulinum toxin*. New York: Marcel Dekker, 1994: 224–237.
7. Chan J, Brin MF, Fahn S. Idiopathic cervical dystonia: clinical characteristics. *Mov Disord* 1991;6:119–126.
8. Kutvonen O, Dastidar P, Nurmikko T. Pain in spasmodic torticollis. *Pain* 1997;69:279–286.
9. Lobbezoo F, Tanguay R, Thu Thon M, et al. Pain perception in idiopathic cervical dystonia (spasmodic torticollis). *Pain* 1996;67:483–491.
10. Molho ES, Factor SA. Employment in cervical dystonia patients. *Mov Disord* 2000;15:1043.
11. Comella CL, Stebbins GT, Miller S. Specific dystonic factors contributing to work limitation and disability in cervical dystonia. *Neurology* 1996;46(2 Suppl): A295(abstr).
12. Jahanshahi M, Marsden CD. Psychological functioning before and after treatment of torticollis with botulinum toxin. *J Neurol Neurosurg Psychiatry* 1992;55: 229–231.
13. Dauer WT, Burke RE, Greene P, et al. Current concepts on the clinical features, aetiology and management of idiopathic cervical dystonia. *Brain* 1998;121:547–560.
14. Adler CH, Kumar R. Pharmacological and surgical options for the treatment of cervical dystonia. *Neurology* 2000;55(Suppl 5):S9–S14.
15. Greene P, Shale H, Fahn S. Analysis of open-label trials in torsion dystonia using high dosages of anticholinergics and other drugs. *Mov Disord* 1988;3:46–60.
16. Lal S. Pathophysiology and pharmacotherapy of spasmodic torticollis: a review. *Can J Neurol Sci* 1979;6: 427–435.
17. Greene P, Kang U, Fahn S, et al. Double-blind, placebo-controlled trial of botulinum toxin injections for the treatment of spasmodic torticollis. *Neurology* 1990;40: 878–882.
18. Jankovic J, Schwartz K. Botulinum toxin injections for cervical dystonia. *Neurology* 1990;40:277–280.
19. Lorentz IT, Subramaniam SS, Yiannikas C. Treatment of idiopathic spasmodic torticollis with botulinum toxin

20. A: a double-blind study on twenty-three patients. *Mov Disord* 1991;6:145–150.
20. Perlmutter JS, Tempel LW, Burde R. Double-blind placebo-controlled, crossover trial of botulinum-A toxin injections for torticollis. *Neurology* 1989;39:352–356.
21. Stell R, Thompson PD, Marsden CD. Botulinum toxin in spasmodic torticollis. *J Neurol Neurosurg Psychiatry* 1988;51:920–923.
22. Tsui JK, Eisen A, Stoessl AJ, et al. Double-blind study of botulinum toxin-A in spasmodic torticollis. *Lancet* 1986;2:245–246.
23. Greene P, Fahn S, Diamond B. Development of resistance to botulinum toxin type A in patients with torticollis. *Mov Disord* 1994;9:213–217.
24. Jankovic J, Schwartz KS. Clinical correlates of response to botulinum toxin injections. *Arch Neurol* 1991;48: 1253–1256.
25. Zuber M, Sebald M, Bathien N, et al. Botulinum antibodies in dystonic patients treated with type A botulinum toxin: frequency and significance. *Neurology* 1993; 43:1715–1718.
26. Borodic G, Johnson E, Goodnough M, et al. Botulinum toxin therapy, immunological resistance, and problems with available materials. *Neurology* 1996;46:26–29.
27. Jankovic J, Schwartz K. Response and immunoresistance to botulinum toxin injections. *Neurology* 1995;45: 1743–1746.
28. Eleopra R, Tugnoli V, Rossetto O, et al. Botulinum neurotoxin serotype C: a novel effect botulinum toxin in human. *Neurosci Lett* 1997;24:91–94.
29. Cullis PA, O'Brien CF, Truong DD, et al. Botulinum toxin type B: an open-label, dose-escalation, safety and preliminary efficacy study in cervical dystonia patients. In: Fahn S, Marsden CD, DeLong M, eds. *Dystonia 3—advances in neurology. Vol 78*. Philadelphia, PA: Lippincott-Raven Publishers, 1998:227–230.
30. Greene P, Fahn S. Use of botulinum toxin type F injections to treat torticollis in patients with immunity to botulinum toxin type A. *Mov Disord* 1993;8:479–483.
31. Halpern JL, Smith LA, Seamon KB, et al. Sequence homology between tetanus and botulinum toxins detected by an antipeptide antibody. *Infect Immun* 1989; 57:18–22.
32. Schiavo G, Benfenati F, Poulain B, et al. Tetanus and botulinum-B neurotoxins block neurotransmitter release by proteolytic cleavage of synaptobrevin. *Nature* 1992; 359:832–835.
33. Blasi J, Chapman ER, Link E, et al. Botulinum neurotoxin A selectively cleaves the synaptic protein SNAP-25. *Nature* 1993;365:160–163.
34. American BotB Cervical Dystonia Study Group. BotB (botulinum toxin type B) in the treatment of cervical dystonia (CD)—protocol AN072–008: an interim analysis. *Mov Disord* 1995;10:2874(abstr).
35. Truong DD, Cullis PA, O'Brien CF, et al. BotB (botulinum toxin type B): Evaluation of safety and tolerability in botulinum toxin type A-resistant cervical dystonia patients (preliminary study). *Mov Disord* 1997;12: 772–775.
36. Tsui JKC, Hayward M, Mak EKM, et al. Botulinum toxin type B in the treatment of cervical dystonia: a pilot study. *Neurology* 1995;45:2109–2110.
37. Lew MF, Albanese A, Duane DD, et al. Botulinum toxin type B: A double-blind, placebo-controlled safety and

efficacy study in cervical dystonia. *Neurology* 1997;49: 701–707.

38. Brashear A, Lew MF, Dykstra DD, et al. Safety and efficacy of NeuroBloc (botulinum toxin type B) in type A-responsive cervical dystonia. *Neurology* 1999;53: 1439–1446.

39. Brin MF, Lew MF, Adler CH, et al. Safety and efficacy of NeuroBloc (botulinum type B) in type A-resistant cervical dystonia. *Neurology* 1999;53:1431–1438.

40. Tsui JC. Botulinum toxin as a therapeutic agent. *Pharmacol Ther* 1996;72:13–24.

41. Black JD, Dolly JO. Interaction of ^{125}I-labeled botulinum neurotoxins with nerve terminals. I. Ultrastructural autoradiographic localization and quantification of distinct membrane acceptors for type A and B on motor nerves. *J Cell Biol* 1986;103:521–534.

42. Simpson LL. The origin, structure, and pharmacological activity of botulinum toxin. *Pharmacol Rev* 1981;33: 155–188.

43. Sakaguchi G. *Clostridium botulinum* toxins. *Pharmacol Ther* 1983;19:165–194.

44. Setler P. The biochemistry of botulinum toxin type B. *Neurology* 2000;55(Suppl 5):S22–S28.

45. Anderson TJ, Rivest J, Stell R, et al. Botulinum toxin treatment of spasmodic torticollis. *J R Soc Med* 1992; 67:48–53.

46. Jankovic J, Schwartz K, Donovan DT. Botulinum toxin treatment of cranial-cervical dystonia, spasmodic dysphonia, other focal dystonias and hemifacial spasm. *J Neurol Neurosurg Psychiatry* 1990;53: 633–639.

IMMUNOLOGY OF
BOTULINUM TOXIN

Scientific and Therapeutic Aspects of Botulinum Toxin
edited by M.F. Brin, J. Jankovic, and M. Hallett
Lippincott Williams & Wilkins, Philadelphia, © 2002.

38

Immune Recognition and Cross-Reactivity of Botulinum Neurotoxins

M. Zouhair Atassi

The biologic actions of botulinum neurotoxins (BoNTs), which result in their ability to block neurotransmitter release, have been exploited in therapeutic applications to reduce muscle hyperactivity for the treatment of a variety of clinical conditions associated with involuntary muscle spasm and contractions. These applications lead to the appearance of immune responses against the immunizing toxin, which cause nonresponsiveness to further treatment (see Chapter 39 for a discussion of immunoresistance).

Investigations of the immune recognition of BoNTs have, until recently, employed mainly the BoNT subunits or relatively large peptide fragments (50 kDa) (1–3), perhaps primarily because of the lack of structural information on the neurotoxins. More recent studies (4) have aimed at identifying with synthetic peptides recognition regions on the L chain that are recognized by monoclonal antibodies. On the other hand, the immune recognition of tetanus neurotoxin (TeNT) has been extensively investigated (5–9), perhaps because of the earlier availability of its primary structure and of human test samples. However, recent elucidation of the primary structures of BoNTs has allowed the mapping of the T- and B-cell Ab recognition regions on the BoNT-A molecule.

Antibodies (Abs) against the receptor-binding regions on related bacterial toxins are very effective at neutralization of the correlate toxin. For example, immunization with the H_C-fragment of TeNT was reported to protect mice against double the minimal lethal dose of TeNT (9–11). In contrast, recombinant H_C (C-terminal fragment corresponding to residues 855–1296 of the

heavy chain of BoNT-A) of BoNT-A afforded, as an immunogen, protection of mice against a higher challenge dose (10^5 LD_{50}) of BoNT-A (12–14). Immunization of mice with a recombinant H_C fragment microencapsulated in biodegradable poly-DL-lactide-coglycoside microspheres, provided 71% protection against aerosol challenge with BoNT-A (15). Overlapping BoNT-A gene fragments were expressed in *Escherichia coli* to prepare ten overlapping proteins (16). Only two of these (H455–661 and H1150–1289) were found to confer protection against BoNT-A poisoning (16). Other reports also indicate that two receptor-binding sites may be present on H_C that are involved in BoNT internalization and toxicity (17). Blockage of these sites by monoclonal antibodies might provide protection against BoNT-A toxicity (17). BoNT-E–neutralizing activity of five monoclonal antibodies against BoNT-E has been reported in mice (18). Three of these monoclonal antibodies recognized regions around residues 663–668, 731–787, and 811–897. Region 663–668 is close to the ion channel-forming domain. The fourth monoclonal antibody, which recognized a region around the C-terminal of H_C, might have interfered with BoNT-binding to the target cell receptor (18).

A recombinant BoNT-C variant with three amino acids replacements (His229 → Gly, Glu230 → Thr, His233 → Asn) in the zinc-binding motif, which was nontoxic to mice and did not cleave syntaxin in synaptosome preparations (19), stimulated high antibody (Ab) levels and provided protective immunity when administered orally or subcutaneously (18).

The ability of H_C of BoNT-A, when used as an immunogen in mice, to provide excellent protection against BoNT-A poisoning (13,14), indicated that mapping of the regions that are recognized by Abs and T cells on this domain of BoNT-A would be extremely valuable for formulating a design for a synthetic peptide vaccine against BoNT. In recent studies, therefore, we have mapped the continuous regions of molecular and cellular immune recognition on H_C of BoNT-A (continuous regions are sites constructed of residues that are directly linked by peptide bonds; discontinuous regions are sites comprising residues that are distant in sequence but come in close spatial proximity through folding of the polypeptide chain (20). For the localization of Ab and T-cell epitopes recognized by anti–BoNT-A and anti–H_C T- and B-cell responses, we employed a comprehensive synthetic overlapping peptide strategy, previously introduced and developed in this laboratory (21–24). In addition, we determined the peptides that, when used as immunogens, elicited Ab and/or T-cell responses that cross-reacted with H_C and/or with intact BoNT-A, because these peptides would most likely evoke protective active or passive (by Ab transfer) immunity against BoNT-A poisoning. Furthermore, after the protective regions on the H_C of BoNT-A are localized it is then possible to design synthetic peptides that correspond to the structural counterparts of the protective BoNT-A peptides on the other BoNT serotypes known to infect humans (most frequently types A, B, and E; rarely type F). It is well known that the regions of immune recognition on a set of homologous proteins occur on structurally equivalent locations (25–28). Peptide immunization, although it has not generally provided useful protection against viral infections, has proved to be quite effective for protection against protein toxins (29–32). We recently showed (32) that appropriate synthetic regions of α-bungarotoxin when used as immunogens in mice protected the mice against a high α-bungarotoxin challenge dose ($LD_{50} > 58$ μg, as compared to an $LD_{50} = 2.6$ μg for nonimmunized mice). The protection afforded by the peptides was in fact higher than

the protection obtained by immunization with the whole toxin ($LD_{50} = 9.69$ μg).

MAPPING OF THE MOLECULAR AND CELLULAR IMMUNE RECOGNITION OF H_C

To map the T- and B-cell epitopes on the H_C of BoNT-A, we synthesized a panel of 31 consecutive overlapping peptides that encompassed the entire H_C polypeptide chain (residues 855–1296) and had uniform size and overlaps. The peptides were 19 residues each (except for peptide 31, which was 22 residues) and overlapped by five residues (Fig. 38.1). It should be noted that this strategy is not designed to define the boundaries of the sites of immune recognition, but rather to obtain the locations within which these sites reside (21–24).

H_C Regions Recognized by Anti–BoNT-A Antibodies from Three Outbred Host Species

Initially, we conducted the mapping of the epitopes of immune recognition on the highly protective H_C domain of BoNT-A with anti–BoNT-A Abs that were prepared in three outbred species (33): horse, human, and mouse. Horse antisera were prepared by subcutaneous immunization with a formaldehyde-inactivated BoNT-A in Ribi adjuvant, in multiple sites every 2 weeks for a year. The binding studies were done with antisera that were obtained after four injections (33). Human antisera against the pentavalent toxoid (BoNTs A, B, C, D, and E) that were prepared in human volunteers (34) were obtained from Dr. John L. Middlebrook (Fort Detrick, Frederick, MD). The binding assays were done with the IgG fractions of these antisera (33). Mouse anti-BoNT antisera were prepared in outbred ICR mice by subcutaneous immunization with toxoid (33) and were obtained 91 days after the first injection (33). Controls included nonimmune horse and mouse sera that were obtained from the animals before immunization and a nonimmune human IgG fraction from preimmune human sera.

Horse, human and mouse anti-BoNT-A Abs

Peptide	Residue Nos.	Amino acid sequence
1	855–873	K Y V D N Q R L L S T F T E **Y I K N I**
2	869–887	**Y I K N I** I N T S I L N L R **Y E S N H**
3	883–901	**Y E S N H** L I D L S R Y A S **K I N I G**
4	897–915	**K I N I G** S K V N F D P I D **K N Q I Q**
5	911–929	**K N Q I Q** L F N L E S S K I E **V I L K**
6	925–943	**E V I L K** N A I V Y N S M Y **E N F S T**
7	939–957	**E N F S T** S F W I R I P K Y **F N S I S**
8	953–971	**F N S I S** L N N E Y T I I N **C M E N N**
9	967–985	**C M E N N** S G W K V S L N Y **G E I I W**
10	981–999	**G E I I W** T L Q D T Q E I K **Q R V V F**
11	995–1013	**Q R V V F** K Y S Q M I N I S **D Y I N R**
12	1009–1027	**D Y I N R** W I F V T I T N N **R L N N S**
13	1023–1041	**R L N N S** K I Y I N G R L I **D Q K P I**
14	1037–1055	**D Q K P I** S N L G N I H A S **N N I M F**
15	1051–1069	**N N I M F** K L D G C R D T H **R Y I W I**
16	1065–1083	**R Y I W I** K Y F N L F D K E **L N E K E**
17	1079–1097	**L N E K E** I K D L Y D N Q S **N S G I L**
18	1093–1111	**N S G I L** K D F W G D Y L Q **Y D K P Y**
19	1107–1125	**Y D K P Y** Y M L N L Y D P N **K Y V D V**
20	1121–1139	**K Y V D V** N N V G I R G Y M **Y L K G P**
21	1135–1153	**Y L K G P** R G S V M T T N I **Y L N S S**
22	1149–1167	**Y L N S S** L Y R G T K F I I **K K Y A S**
23	1163–1181	**K K Y A S** G N K D N I V R N **N D R V Y**
24	1177–1195	**N D R V Y** I N V V V K N K E **Y R L A T**
25	1191–1209	**Y R L A T** N A S Q A G V E K **I L S A L**
26	1205–1223	**I L S A L** E I P D V G N L S **Q V V V M**
27	1219–1237	**Q V V V M** K S K N D Q G I T **N K C K M**
28	1233–1251	**N K C K M** N L Q D N N G N D **I G F I G**
29	1247–1265	**I G F I G** F H Q F N N I A K **L V A S N**
30	1261–1279	**L V A S N** W Y N R Q I E R S **S R T L G**
31	1275–1296	**S R T L G** C S W E F I P V D D G W G E R P L

FIG. 38.1. Synthetic overlapping peptides of the protective H_C region of BoNT-A. The 31 peptides shown started at residue 855 and covered the entire sequence of H_C (residues 860–1296 of the H chain). Each peptide overlapped by five residues with each of its adjacent neighbors; the regions of overlap are shown in bold type. (From Atassi MZ, Dolimbek BZ, Hayakari M, et al. Mapping of the antibody-binding regions on botulinum neurotoxin H-chain domain 855–1296 with anti-toxin antibodies from three host species. *J Prot Chem* 1996;15:691–700, with permission.)

recognized several regions of H_C and the peptide-binding profiles (33) for these antibodies showed considerable similarities (Figs. 38.2, 38.3, and 38.4, and the summary in Table 38.1). Peptides 2 (residues 869–887), 15 (1051–1069), and 24 (1177–1195) were recognized by both human and mouse antisera. With horse antiserum, both the epitopes on peptides 2 and 15 were shifted to the left and resided within peptides 1 (855–873) and 13/14 (1023–1041/ 1037–1055), respectively, while the epitope on peptide 24 shifted to the right and resided within the 25/26 (1191–1209/1205–1223) overlap. A region localized by the human antisera to be within the overlap of peptides 5/6/7 (911–929/ 925–943/939–957) was recognized more weakly by the mouse antisera and shifted to the right in favor of peptide 7 (939–957). Horse antiserum recognized both peptides 5 (911–929)

and 7 (939–957), but not 6 (925–943). The absence of Abs toward peptide 6 (925–943) suggested that this region contains two epitopes that can be distinctly resolved with the present panel of peptides by the horse antiserum, but not by the human and mouse antisera. A region residing within the overlap 10/11 (981–999/995–1013) was recognized by human and more weakly by horse antisera. Mouse antisera also recognized this region, but more weakly, and it was shifted to the right toward peptide 11 (995–1013). Peptide 18 (1093–1111) was recognized by horse, weakly by mouse, and not by human antisera. The three antisera recognized a very weak region around the overlap 20/21 (1121–1139/ 1135–1153) (human and mouse) or 20/21/22 (1121–1139/1135–1153/1149–1167) (horse). A broad region located within peptides 29/30/ 31 (1247–1265/1261–1279/1275–1296) was

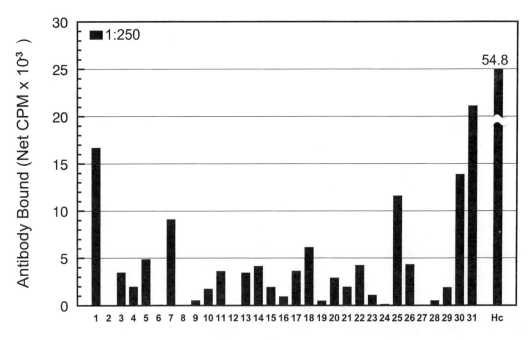

FIG. 38.2. Binding of horse anti–BoNT-A antibodies to the overlapping BoNT-A peptides and to H_C. Binding was determined by solid-phase plate radioimmunoassay using the antiserum at a dilution of 1:250 (vol/vol). The results were corrected for nonspecific binding of the antibodies to unrelated protein (bovine serum albumin [BSA]) and of preimmune sera to the peptides and to H_C. The data are expressed in net cpm and represent the average of triplicate analyses which varied ±2.0% or less. (From Atassi MZ, Dolimbek BZ, Hayakari M, et al. Mapping of the antibody-binding regions on botulinum neurotoxin H-chain domain 855–1296 with anti-toxin antibodies from three host species. *J Prot Chem* 1996;15:691–700, with permission.)

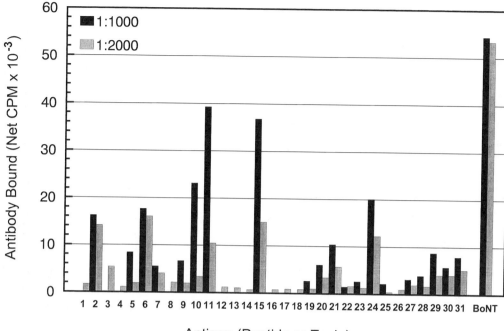

FIG. 38.3. Binding of human antitoxoid antibodies to toxoid and to the overlapping peptides of the H_C domain of BoNT-A. Binding was done by solid phase plate radioimmunoassay at dilutions of 1: 1000 and 1:2000 (vol/vol) of a 1.05 mg/mL solution of the IgG fraction of the antibody and has been corrected for nonspecific binding of the antibodies to an unrelated protein (BSA) and of nonimmune human IgG to the peptides and to BoNT-A. The results are given in net cpm of bound antibody and represent the average of triplicate analyses which varied ±2.0% or less. For details see the text. (From Atassi MZ, Dolimbek BZ, Hayakari M, et al. Mapping of the antibody-binding regions on botulinum neurotoxin H-chain domain 855–1296 with anti-toxin antibodies from three host species. *J Prot Chem* 1996;15:691–700, with permission.)

recognized by human antisera and within 30/31 (1261–1279/1275–1296) by horse antisera and more sharply within peptide 31 (1275–1296) by mouse antisera. In addition to the shifts that have been described, antisera of the three species displayed differences in immunodominance of the peptides that they recognized. Antigenic sites on a given protein are known to display boundary frame shifts and variation in immunodominance, depending on the host species in which the Abs are raised; in fact, such variations may even occur among individual animals of the same host species (28,35,36). These observations are consistent with genetic control operating at the antigenic site level. It is well established that H-2–linked genes (37–39) control the immune responses to proteins and, furthermore, both B- (i.e., Ab) and T-cell responses to individual epi-

topes on a multideterminant protein antigen are each under separate genetic control (28,40–42).

The H_C Regions Recognized by Mouse Anti–BoNT-A Antibodies and T Cells

Regions that Bind Antitoxoid Antibodies

The Ab-binding profile to the peptides was determined with mouse antisera that were prepared against the pentavalent toxoid (BoNTs A, B, C, D, and E) in BALB/c ($H-2^d$) and SJL (H-2^s) mice (43). The binding profiles of BALB/c and SJL antitoxoid Abs were quite similar (Fig. 38.5). With antitoxoid Abs of BALB/c, peptide 24 (1177–1195) was strongly immunodominant. These Abs also bound to peptides 2/3 (869–887/883–901) overlap, 21 (1135–1153), and 31

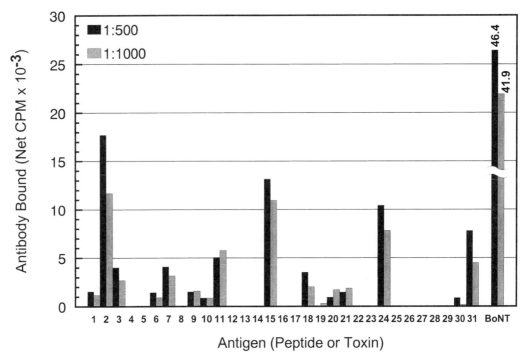

FIG. 38.4. Binding of outbred (ICR) mouse antisera to the overlapping synthetic H_C peptides of BoNT-A. Binding was determined at two dilutions (1:500 and 1:1000, vol/vol) of the antisera and the results, which are expressed in net cpm, have been corrected for nonspecific binding of the antisera to unrelated protein (BSA) and by the preimmune sera to the toxoid and to each of the synthetic peptides. For details, see the text. (From Atassi MZ, Dolimbek BZ, Hayakari M, et al. Mapping of the antibody-binding regions on botulinum neurotoxin H-chain domain 855–1296 with anti-toxin antibodies from three host species. *J Prot Chem* 1996;15:691–700, with permission.)

(1275–1296) and, in addition, lower but significant amounts of Abs were bound by peptides 11 (995–1013) and 15 (1051–1069). The other peptides bound very little or no Abs. Antitoxoid Abs of SJL bound to five antigenic regions within peptides 2/3 (869–887/883–901) overlap, 11 (995–1013), 15 (1051–1069), 24 (1177–1195), and 31 (1275–1296). But in contrast to BALB/c Abs [which exhibited low binding to peptides 11 (995–1013) and 15 (1051–1069)], the Abs of SJL possessed high binding to both peptides and lower binding to peptide 21 (1135–1153).

Mapping of the T-Cell Recognition Profiles

T cells of BALB/c and SJL mice that had been primed with various doses of toxoid gave similar profiles of *in vitro* proliferative responses to tox-

oid and gave the highest response at a priming dose of 1 μg/mouse (43). BALB/c T cells, primed with one injection of toxoid, responded *in vitro* to two major regions within peptides 4 (residues 897–915) and 7 (939–957) (Fig. 38.6). After multiple inoculations with toxoid (i.e., at the time the hyperimmune antisera were obtained from the mice), BALB/c T cells showed an expanded recognition profile and responded very well to challenge with peptide 30 (1261–1279) and moderately to stimulation with peptide 22 (1149–1167). In contrast to BALB/c T cells, toxoid-primed SJL T cells responded *in vitro,* with a more complex profile, to challenge with a large number of overlapping peptides. After one toxoid injection, however, SJL T cells were stimulated strongly *in vitro* by three regions within peptides 4 (897–915), 7/8 overlap (939–957/953–971), and 15 (1051–1069)

TABLE 38.1. *Summary of peptides recognized by horse Abs against BoNT-A and human and mouse Abs against pentavalent toxoid*[a]

Peptide no.	Sequence position	Horse	Human	Mouse
1	855–873	+++	−	±
2	869–887	−	+++	+++
3	883–901	+	−	+
4	897–915	±	−	−
5	911–929	+	++	−
6	925–943	−	+++	−
7	939–957	++	+	+
8	953–971	−	−	−
9	967–985	−	+	±
10	981–999	±	+++	−
11	995–1013	+	+++++	+
12	1009–1027	−	−	−
13	1023–1041	+	−	−
14	1037–1055	+	−	−
15	1051–1069	±	+++++	++
16	1065–1083	−	−	−
17	1079–1097	+	−	−
18	1093–1111	+	−	+
19	1107–1125	−	±	−
20	1121–1139	+	+	±
21	1135–1153	±	++	±
22	1149–1167	+	−	−
23	1163–1181	−	±	−
24	1177–1195	−	+++	++
25	1191–1209	++	±	−
26	1205–1223	+	−	−
27	1219–1237	−	+	−
28	1233–1251	−	+	−
29	1247–1265	±	++	−
30	1261–1279	++	+	−
31	1275–1296	+++	++	++

[a] For the purpose of this table, (+) or (−) assignments were based on net cpm values which, for human and mouse, were derived from the dilution that gave the highest binding. The symbols denote the following: (−), less than 1,500 cpm; (±), 1,500 to 3,000 cpm; (+), 3,000 to 7,000 cpm; (++), 7,000 to 15,000 cpm; (+++), 15,000 to 25,000 cpm; (++++), 25,000 to 35,000 cpm; (+++++), greater than 35,000 cpm. (From Atassi MZ, Dolimbek BZ, Hayakari M, et al. Mapping of the antibody-binding regions on botulinum neurotoxin H-chain domain 855–1296 with anti-toxin antibodies from three host species. *J Prot Chem* 1996;15:691–700, with permission.)

(Fig. 38.6). After three toxoid injections (i.e., at the time the hyperimmune antitoxoid antisera were obtained from the SJL mice), immunodominance of peptides 4 (897–915) and 15 (1051–1069) persisted while the third region exhibited a shift upstream and resided within the 6/7 (925–943/939–957) overlap. As mentioned above, BALB/c T cell also recognized peptides 4 (897–915) and 7 (939–957) (Fig. 38.6). Table 38.2 compares the recognition profiles of antitoxoid Abs and T cells from the two strains (43). It should be noted that no Abs were detected against the immunodominant T cell epitope within peptide 4 (897–915).

Examination of the results summarized in Table 38.2 shows that (a) in a given strain, certain H_C regions were recognized by both Abs and T cells. Such T/B regions were identified within peptide 7 (939–957) in both strains. Additionally, SJL recognized three T/B regions located within peptides 15 (1051–1069), 24 (1177–1195), and 31 (1275–1296). (b) H_C contained regions that were recognized only by T cell and no Abs were detectable against these sites. One such exclusive T cell epitope, recognized in both mouse strains but particularly prominent in SJL mice, resided within peptide 4 (897–915). (c) Finally, H_C possessed regions

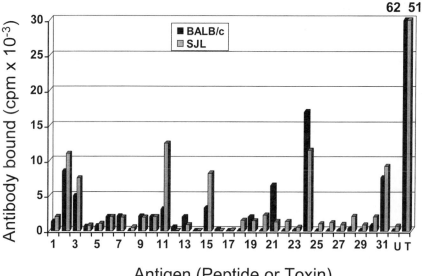

FIG. 38.5. Binding of BALB/c antitoxoid Abs to toxoid (T), to the synthetic overlapping peptides of BoNT-A, and to the unrelated synthetic peptide (U) used as a negative control. For radioimmunoassay, the antiserum was diluted 1:500 (vol/vol). Results are given in net cpm ± SD of triplicate analyses and have been corrected for nonspecific binding of the Abs to unrelated protein (BSA) and of the preimmune sera to the toxoid and to each of the synthetic peptides. The value on the top of bar designated T shows the amount of Abs (61,957 ± 778 net cpm) bound to the toxoid. (From Rosenberg JS, Middlebrook JL, Atassi MZ. Localization of the regions on the C-terminal domain of the heavy chain of botulinum toxin A recognized by T lymphocytes and by antibodies after immunization of mice with pentavalent toxoid. *Immunol Invest* 1997;26:491–504, with permission.)

that were recognized only by Abs and for which no T cell responses were detected. Two exclusively B cell determinants, common for both strains, were found within regions 869–887/ 883–901 and 995–1013. These findings (Table 38.2) show (44) that, in a given strain, the regions recognized by antitoxoid Abs and T cells may coincide or may be uniquely B or T cells determinants.

Comparison of the T-cell recognition profiles of toxoid-primed lymph node cells (LNC) from BALB/c and SJL revealed that H_C has two distinct types of T-cell epitopes. Some epitopes were unique for a given strain, while the others were recognized by toxoid-primed mice of both strains, irrespective of their major histocompatibility complex (MHC) haplotype. In contrast to the T cell profiles, the differences between the B-cell recognition profiles of the two mouse strains were less pronounced. Abs recognized several regions that were similar, although the

Ab levels against a given region varied with the strain (Fig. 38.5 and Table 38.2). Peptides that are recognized across MHC haplotypes would be advantageous for a universal synthetic vaccine as they would be functional in many individuals. It is important to note that the aforementioned results, which were obtained with toxoid-primed LNC (i.e., unselected Th cells) (43), should be more useful for the design of a synthetic vaccine than those derived from the best-growing T cell clones (28,44–46).

Regions Recognized by Antibodies and/or by T Cells When H_C is Used as an Immunogen

Responses to H_C were determined *in vitro* with H_C-primed T cells of H-2^b, H-2^d, H-2^k, and H-2^s mouse haplotypes (47). The results showed that SJL (H-2^s) and BALB/c (H-2^d) mouse strains are very high and high responders, respectively, to H_C. Therefore, SJL and BALB/c

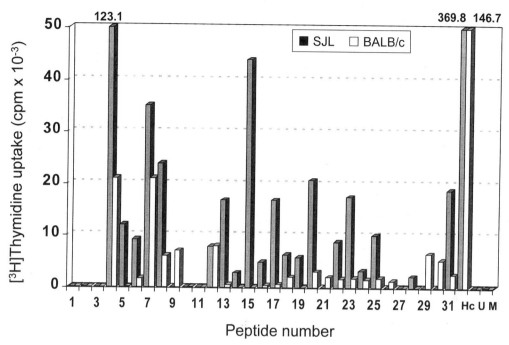

FIG. 38.6. Proliferative response of lymph node cells from toxoid-primed BALB/c and SJL mice to *in vitro* challenge with the synthetic overlapping BoNT-A peptides. Numbers 1–31 under the abscissa refer to the peptide numbers shown in Fig. 38.1. Controls included H_C, unrelated synthetic peptide (U), and myoglobin (M). Results are expressed in net cpm ± SD of triplicate cultures at the optimal stimulation dose of each challenge antigen. The values on top of the bars show the strong response of T cells to the challenge with peptide 4 (SJL 123,120 ± 1,219 cpm), and H_C (SJL 369,801 ± 1,800 cpm; BALB/c 146,684 ± 1,801 cpm). The amounts of [H^3]TdR incorporated by unstimulated cells were SJL 12,331 ± 97 cpm; BALB/c 6,166 ± 53 cpm. (Figure is redrawn from Rosenberg JS, Middlebrook JL, Atassi MZ. Localization of the regions on the C-terminal domain of the heavy chain of botulinum toxin A recognized by T-lymphocytes and by antibodies after immunization of mice with pentavalent toxoid. *Immunol Invest* 1997;26:491–504, with permission.)

were used, with the synthetic overlapping peptides of the entire H_C (residues 855–1296, Fig. 38.1), to map the continuous T- and B-cell (Ab) recognition regions on H_C (47).

Regions Recognized by Anti-H_C T Cells

The immunodominance in T-cell recognition of various H_C regions varied with the haplotype (Fig. 38.7) (47), which is consistent with genetic control operating at the antigenic site level (36–42,47). H_C-primed BALB/c T cells recognized three regions within peptides 7 (residues 939–957), 12 (1009–1027), and 21 (1135–1153). Peptide 21 was immunodominant

at 1 week (Fig. 38.7) and its immunodominance persisted in long-term immunization (47). H_C-primed SJL T cells recognized strongly regions that clustered in a large area within the first N-terminal third of H_C (residues 897–985, comprising the overlapping peptides 4, 5, 6, 7, 8, and 9). An additional region within peptide 15 (1051–1069) stimulated a moderate response in these T cells (47). This cluster around peptides 4, 5, 6, 7, 8, and 9 might consist of at least two immunodominant epitopes around peptides 4 (897–915) and 7 (939–957) (47). The immunodominance of region 939–957 persisted in hyperimmune T cells (long-term immunization). Both SJL and BALB/c T cells recognized region

TABLE 38.2. *The regions on the H_C domain of BoNT-A that are recognized by Abs and/or T cells after immunization of BALB/c and SJL mouse strains with toxoid*[a]

Peptide	Position in sequence (residue numbers)	BALB/c (H-2^d) Ab	BALB/c (H-2^d) T cells	SJL (H-2^s) Ab	SJL (H-2^s) T cells
1	855–873	−	−	+	−
2	869–887	+ +	−	+ + +	−
3	883–901	+ +	−	+ +	−
4	897–915	−	+ +	−	+ + + +
5	911–929	−	−	±	+
6	925–943	+	−	+	+
7	939–957	+	+ +	+	+ + +
8	953–971	−	−	−	+ +
9	967–985	+	−	+	−
10	981–999	+	−	+	−
11	995–1013	+	−	+ + +	−
12	1009–1027	−	+	−	+
13	1023–1041	±	−	−	+ +
14	1037–1055	−	−	−	+
15	1051–1069	+	−	+ +	+ + +
16	1065–1083	−	−	−	+
17	1079–1097	−	−	−	+ +
18	1093–1111	−	−	+	+
19	1107–1125	±	−	+	+
20	1121–1139	−	−	+	+ +
21	1135–1153	+ +	−	±	+
22	1149–1167	−	−	±	+
23	1163–1181	−	−	−	+ +
24	1177–1195	+ + +	−	+ + +	+
25	1191–1209	−	−	±	+
26	1205–1223	−	−	±	−
27	1219–1237	−	−	−	−
28	1233–1251	−	−	+	+
29	1247–1265	−	−	−	+
30	1261–1279	−	−	+	−
31	1275–1296	+ +	−	+ +	+ +

[a] For the purpose of this table, (+) and (−) assignments were based on net cpm values for Ab binding and stimulation index (SI) values for T cell proliferation. For Ab binding, the symbols denote the following values: (−), less than 1,000 cpm; (+), 1,001 to 1,500 cpm; (+), 1,501 to 4,000 cpm; (++), 4,001 to 10,000 cpm; (+++), greater than 10,000. For T cell proliferation, the symbols indicate the following: (−), SI value less than 2.0; (+), SI 2.0 to 3.5; (++), SI 3.6 to 4.5; (+++), SI 4.6 to 10.0; (++++), SI greater than 10.0. Results of T and B cell-mapping studies were obtained with mice that received single and multiple injections, respectively. (From Rosenberg JS, Middlebrook JL, Atassi MZ. Localization of the regions on the C-terminal domain of the heavy chain of botulinum toxin A recognized by T lymphocytes and by antibodies after immunization of mice with pentavalent toxoid. *Immunol Invest* 1997;26:491–504, with permission.)

939–957 (peptide 7) (Fig. 38.7), indicating that this H_C region can bind different MHC class II alleles. Promiscuous T-cell epitopes that can be recognized by different MHC class II molecules might be beneficial for a universal vaccine, because human vaccine recipients possess different MHC class II haplotypes.

BoNT-A region 938–958 within peptide 7 (residues 939–957), which is recognized by SJL and BALB/c T cells, is homologous to region 947–967 of TeNT. The latter has been reported (5) to be recognized by human peripheral blood lymphocytes. Region 916–932 of TeNT, which is equivalent to BoNT-A region 907–923 within the overlap of peptides 4 (residues 897–915) and 5 (residues 911–929) recognized by SJL T cells (47), is also recognized by human T cells (7). Clearly, the two clostridial toxins—BoNT and TeNT—share some T-cell recognition features, along with a number of structural and functional similarities. As already mentioned, in closely related proteins, the sites of immune recognition

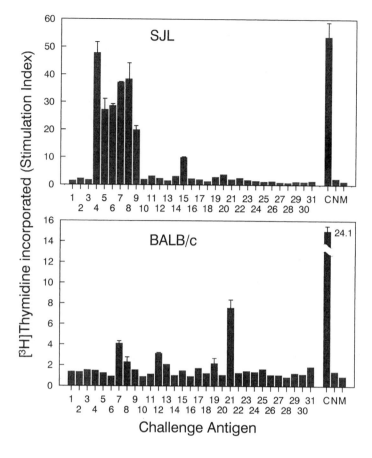

FIG. 38.7. Presentation showing the *in vitro* proliferative response to the BoNT-A peptides 1–31 of LNC from SJL mice and from BALB/c mice primed with 0.25 μg/mouse of H_C. The diagram shows SI at the optimum challenge doses of each peptide and H_C. Unstimulated cells gave 2,330 ± 168 cpm for SJL and 3,534 ± 141 cpm for BALB/c. Numbers 1 to 31 refer to the peptides shown in Table 38.1. Additional antigen letter symbols are: C, H_C; M, myoglobin; N, unrelated synthetic peptide. (From Oshima M, Hayakari M, Middlebrook JL, et al. Immune recognition of botulinum neurotoxin type A: regions recognized by T cells and antibodies against the protective H_C fragment (residues 855–1296) of the toxin. *Mol Immunol* 1997; 34:1031–1040, with permission.)

often occur at structurally equivalent locations (25,28).

The Regions Recognized by Anti-H_C Antibodies

In contrast to H_C-primed SJL and BALB/c LNC, which recognized both common and different epitope regions on H_C, Ab-recognition regions of the two mouse strains essentially overlapped (47). There were seven common or similar regions (four common; three similar) of recognition in the two strains. However, in a given antiserum different amounts of Abs were bound by the active peptides (Figs. 38.8 and 38.9 and Table 38.3). Similar observations were recently made in acetylcholine receptor-primed SJL and C57BL/6 mice, which reported (48) that major Ab recognition regions for both strains were clustered into three similar regions within 1–210

of the acetylcholine receptor chain, whereas T cells of the two strains recognized different regions.

As discussed earlier with the anti-BoNT-A responses, the profiles of the anti-H_C Ab and T-cell responses in a given mouse strain revealed that, in a given mouse strain, certain regions are recognized by both Abs and T cells. But H_C also has regions that are predominantly recognized only by Abs or only by T cells. It was previously shown (23,28,30,48) that in a given mouse strain, the regions on a protein that are recognized by Abs and by T cells may coincide, but the protein may also have regions that are recognized only by Abs and for which no T-cell responses are detectable, and/or conversely, regions recognized only by T-cells and for which Ab responses are not detectable.

Abs and/or T cells from either strain recognized well (≥ + +, see Table 38.3) peptides

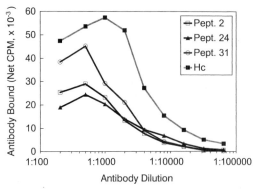

FIG. 38.8. Binding of anti-H_C Abs (BALB/c, at 12 weeks) to H_C and three selected BoNT-A peptides. Different dilutions (from 1:200 to 1:64000; vol/vol) of anti-H_C antisera were assayed by solid-phase radioimmunoassay. Preimmune sera were used as a negative control, and their values were subtracted to obtain the net cpm. (From Oshima M, Hayakari M, Middlebrook JL, et al. Immune recognition of botulinum neurotoxin type A: regions recognized by T cells and antibodies against the protective H_C fragment (residues 855–1296) of the toxin. *Mol Immunol* 1997;34: 1031–1040, with permission.)

2–11 (869–1013), 15 (1051–1069), 17 (1079–1097), 18 (1093–1111), 21 (1135–1153), 24 (1177–1195), and 31 (1275–1296) (47). Alignment of the primary structures of these 16 peptide regions in BoNTs A through G and TeNT revealed (47) that 11 of the peptides have five or more contiguous residues that are identical or similar to BoNT-A in one or more of these BoNTs (Fig. 38.10). A five-residue homology (or similarity) is often sufficient for cross-reaction (28,35).

Cross-Reactions of the BoNT Serotypes and Consequences to Therapeutic Applications

The ability of BoNTs to block neurotransmitter release has been employed in minute doses (less than 1 ng), in symptoms where it is desirable to obtain reduction of muscle hyperactivity, to produce a reversible partial paralysis at the neuromuscular junction. BoNTs have been applied, often with good results, in the treatment of a variety of clinical conditions associated with involuntary muscle spasm and contractions

(49–59). These have included various forms of dystonia (60–64); disorders of the alimentary tract (65–67); amyotrophic lateral sclerosis (68); dermatologic and cosmetic uses (69–76); various types of tremors and neuromyotonia (77–83); spasticity (54,84–86); clinical ophthalmology (87–92); cerebral palsy (52,93–95); disorders of anal sphincter (96–100); urethral dilatation (101); otorhinolaryngology (102,103); tardive dyskinesia (104); stiff-person syndrome (105); adult strabismus (106); gustatory sweating of the neck (Frey's syndrome) (107–111); focal hyperhidrosis (112); and esophageal motor disorders (113).

Results obtained with the injection of BoNT are not permanent and require periodic injections of the neurotoxin. Furthermore, the treatment leads to the appearance in some patients of Ab responses against the toxin, which reduce the patient's responsiveness to further treatment (114). This immunoresistance has been overcome by using another BoNT serotype that will not be neutralized by the Abs against the first BoNT that was employed in the therapy. For example, when BoNT-A was used in patients with focal dystonia some patients mounted Ab responses against BoNT-A and became unresponsive to further treatment with BoNT-A, but showed improvement that was sustained for three additional injections of BoNT-F (115). Clearly, this strategy would not resolve the problem and the recipient did in fact mount immune responses against the second BoNT. Increasing the BoNT dose is risky and obviously it will not resolve the problem either, because it would simply boost the Ab titer. In these treatments, lowering the BoNT dose has been recommended (116). Studies have screened only for Ab responses (114–116), but the results could not be explained on the basis of Ab titer only, most likely because of the presence of anti-BoNT T-cell responses, which were not investigated.

Our mapping of the epitopes on the C-terminal H_C domain BoNT-A showed that 13 peptides contain regions that are recognized by Abs and/ or by T cells (Fig. 38.10). At least 11 of these peptide regions are highly conserved in three or more BoNT serotypes, including type B.

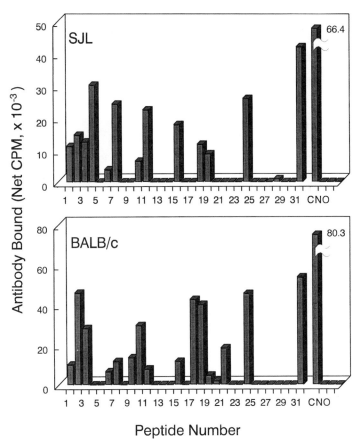

FIG. 38.9. Ab binding to the synthetic BoNT-A peptides of antisera from SJL and BALB/c after four immunizations (12 weeks after initial injection) with H_C (SJL, 0.5 mg/mouse; BALB/c, 0.25 mg/mouse). The diagram shows the net cpm in which the average binding value of the same antigen to the preimmune sera was subtracted. Numbers 1 to 31 refer to the peptides shown in Table 38.1. Additional antigen letter symbols are: C, H_C; N, unrelated synthetic peptide; O, ovalbumin. (From Oshima M, Hayakari M, Middlebrook JL, et al. Immune recognition of botulinum neurotoxin type A: regions recognized by T cells and antibodies against the protective H_C fragment (residues 855–1296) of the toxin. *Mol Immunol* 1997;34:1031–1040, with permission.)

It is evident from Fig. 38.10, which shows the structural alignment of regions recognized as H_C, that five amino residues or as many as 12 or 13 residues in some regions are conserved among certain toxin serotypes. A five-residue identity within an epitope on a related protein is sufficient to permit a cross-reaction of that region on the related protein (28,35). Of course, when the number of identical residues is larger than five, the cross-reaction becomes stronger. Even situations in which a residue is similar but not identical (for example, replacements of the type Asp-Glu, Val-Ile, Lys-Arg, and even sometimes Trp-Phe) might allow cross-reactivity. So from this figure, a number of cross-reacting epitopes and the BoNT serotype that carry these epitopes can be identified. Based on the structural similarities of these three toxins, Table 38.4 summarizes the expected cross-reactions of H_C domain epitopes of BoNTs B and F with anti-

bodies against BoNT-A, and Table 38.5 shows the number of these cross-reacting epitopes in the H_C domain of these three toxins. In BoNT-B 7 of 13 epitopes are potentially cross-reactive with anti–BoNT-A Abs, while BoNT-F has 8 of 13 potentially cross-reactive epitopes. The cross-reaction depends, of course, on which of the epitopes of a maximum of 13 on the H_C domain are recognized by a given patient upon initial treatment with the first toxin (usually BoNT-A). The epitopes that are so recognized initially will be dependent on the patient's HLA haplotype, on the toxin dose, and on the toxin preparation.

It is important to take these considerations into account because no single BoNT serotype carries completely unique epitopes that would not cross-react with other BoNT serotypes. Therefore, one would expect that cycling of BoNT serotypes to avoid immune responses will

TABLE 38.3. *Summary of peptides recognized by Abs and by T lymphocytes when H_C is used as an immunogen in SJL and BALB/c mouse strains*[a]

Peptide number	Sequence position	SJL (H-2^s)		BALB/c (H-2^d)	
		Ab	T Cells	Ab	T Cells
1	855–873	+	−	+	−
2	869–887	++	−	++++	−
3	883–901	++	−	+++	−
4	897–915	+++	++++	−	−
5	911–929	−	+++	−	−
6	925–943	±	+++	+	−
7	939–957	+++	++++	+	+
8	953–971	−	++++	−	±
9	967–985	−	+++	++	−
10	981–999	+	−	+++	−
11	995–1013	+++	+	+	−
12	1009–1027	−	±	−	+
13	1023–1041	−	−	−	±
14	1037–1055	−	+	−	−
15	1051–1069	++	++	+	−
16	1065–1083	−	±	−	−
17	1079–1097	−	−	++++	−
18	1093–1111	+	−	++++	−
19	1107–1125	+	±	±	±
20	1121–1139	−	+	−	−
21	1135–1153	−	−	++	++
22	1149–1167	−	±	−	−
23	1163–1181	−	−	−	−
24	1177–1195	+++	−	++++	−
25	1191–1209	−	−	−	−
26	1205–1223	−	−	−	−
27	1219–1237	−	−	−	−
28	1233–1251	−	−	−	−
29	1247–1265	−	−	−	−
30	1261–1279	−	−	−	−
31	1275–1296	++++	−	++++	−

[a] Assignment of positive and negative responses for the purpose of this table was based on net cpm values for Ab study and of SI values for T-cell study. For Ab binding, the symbols denote the following values: (−), less than 2,000 cpm; (±), 2,000 to 5,000 cpm; (+), 5,000 to 12,000 cpm; (++), 12,000 to 22,000 cpm; (+++), 22,000 to 40,000 cpm; (++++), greater than 40,000 cpm. For T cell recognition, the symbols denote the following: (−), SI value less than 2.0; (±), SI 2.0 to 2.9; (+), SI 3.0 to 4.9; (++), SI 5.0 to 9.9; (+++), SI 10.0 to 29.9; (++++), SI ≥30.0. (From Oshima M, Hayakari M, Middlebrook JL, et al. Immune recognition of botulinum neurotoxin type A: regions recognized by T cells and antibodies against the protective H_C fragment (residues 855–1296) of the toxin. *Mol Immunol* 1997;34:1031–1040, with permission and with modification.)

FIG. 38.10. Comparative alignment of BoNT types A through G and TeNT within 13 peptide regions that are recognized by Abs and/or by T cells when H_C is used as immunogen. Alignment is from Whelan et al. (125). Bold letters in BoNT-A signify residues that are identical or similar to the amino acid in one or more of the toxin types listed. In BoNTs B through G, residues identical to those of BoNT-A are in boldface type. Bold and italic letters represent the residues in which conservative replacements have occurred. Regions that have five or more continuous residues identical or similar to BoNT-A sequence are underlined. (Adapted with expansion from Oshima M, Hayakari M, Middlebrook JL, et al. Immune recognition of botulinum neurotoxin type A: regions recognized by T cells and antibodies against the protective H_C fragment (residues 855–1296) of the toxin. *Mol Immunol* 1997;34:1031–1040, with permission.)

Sequence position	Toxin type	Structure		Sequence position	Toxin type	Structure
869–887 (peptide 2)	A	YIKNIINTSILNLRYESNH		995–1013 (peptide 11)	A	QRVVFKYSQMINISDYI-NR
	B	YNSEILNNIILNLRYKDNN			B	KSVFFEYNIREDISEYI-NR
	C	YFNNINDSKILSLQNRKNT			C	QSINFSYDISNNAPGY--NK
	D	YFNSINDSKILSLQNKKNA			D	KSLIFDYSESLSHTGYT-NK
	E	FFKRIKSSSVLNMRYKNDK			E	QKLAFNYGNANGISDYI-NK
	F	LYKKIKDSSILDMRYENNK			F	ENLIFRYEELNRISNYI-NK
	G	YISNISSNAILSLSYRGGR			G	KSIFFEYSIKDNISDYI-NK
	Te	IDVILKKSTILNLDINNDI			Te	RQITFR-DLPDKFNAYLANK
883–901 (peptide 3)	A	YESNHLIDLSRYASKINIG		1009–1027 (peptide 12)	A	DYI-NRWIFVTITNNRLNNS
	B	YKDNNLIDLSGYGAKVEVY			B	EYI-NRWFFVTITNN-LNKA
	C	NRKNTLVDTSGYNAEVSEE			C	GY--NKWFFVTVTNNMMGNM
	D	NKKNALVDTSGYNAEVRVG			D	GYT-NKWFFVTITNNIMGYM
	E	YKNDKYVDTSGYDSNININ			E	DYI-NKWIFVTITNDRLGDS
	F	YENNKFIDISGYGSNISIN			F	NYI-NKWIFVTITNNRLGNS
	G	YRGGRLIDSSGYGATMNVG			G	DYI-NKWFSITITNDRLGNA
	Te	IMNDIISDISGFNSSVITY			Te	AYLANKWVFITITNDRLSSA
925–943 (peptide 6)	A	EVILKNAIVYNSMYENFST		1051–1069 (peptide 15)	A	NNIMFKLDG--------CRDTHRYIWI
	B	RVTQNQNIIFNSVFLDFSV			B	GEIIFKLDGDIDR--------TQFIWM
	C	IVTQNENIVYNSMYESFSI			C	KTITFEINKIPDTGLITSDSDNINMWI
	D	IVNLNNNILYSAIYENSSV			D	KTIVFGIDENID--------ENQMLWI
	E	NISQNDYIIYDNKYKNFSI			E	DNILFKIVN--------CSYT-RYIGI
	F	NIAQNNDIIYNSRYQNFSI			F	DNILFKIVG--------CDDE-TYVGI
	G	TAHQSKFVVYDSMFDNFSI			G	NDIDFKLIN--------CTDTTKFVWI
	Te	IVHKAMDIEYNDMFNNFTV			Te	NNITLKLDR--------CNNNNQYVSI
939–57 (peptide 7)	A	ENFSTSFWIRIPKYFNSIS		1093–111 (peptide 18)	A	NSGILKDFWGDYLQYDKPY
	B	LDFSVSFWIRIPNIRMMVY			B	YSEYLKDFWGNPLMYNKEY
	C	ESFSISFWIRINK-WVSNL			C	YTNVVKDYWGNDLRYNKEY
	D	ENSSVSFWIKISKDLTNSH			D	LRNVIKDYWGNPLKFDTEY
	E	KNFSISFWVRIPNYDNKIV			E	NTNILKDFWGNYLLYDKEY
	F	QNFSISFWIRIPKHYKPMN			F	DPSILKNYWGNYLLYNKKY
	G	DNFSINFWVRTPKYNNNDI			G	STNTLKDFWGNPLRYDTQY
	Te	NNFTVSFWLRVPKVSASHL			Te	SITFLRDFWGNPLRYDTEY
953–971 (peptide 8)	A	FNSISL---NNEYTIINCM-ENN		1177–1195 (peptide 24)	A	NDRVYIN-VVVKNKEYRL-AT
	B	RMMVYKIIFIMNIQIINCM-KNN			B	EDYIYLD-FFNLNQEWRV---
	C	WVSNLP-----GYTIIDSV-KNN			C	GDILYFD-MTINNKAYNL-FM
	D	LTNSH-----NEYTIINSI-EQN			D	GDNIILH-MLYNSRKYMI-IR
	E	DNKIVNV-NNEYTIINCMRDNN			E	NDQVYINFVASKTHLFPL-YA
	F	YKPMNH-NREYTIINCMGNNN			F	NDLAYIN-VVDRGVEYRL-YA
	G	NNNDIQTYLQNEYTIISCI-KND			G	GDYIYLNIDNISDESYRV-YV
	Te	SASHLEQYGTNEYSIISSMKKHS			Te	GDFIKLY-VSYNNNEHIVGYP
967–985 (peptide 9)	A	CM-ENN----SGWKVSLNYG---EIIW		1275–1296 (peptide 31)	A	SRT-----LGCSWEFIPVDDGWGERPI
	B	CM-KNN----SGWKISIRGN---RIIW			B	PYNLK---LGCNWQFIPKDEGWTE
	C	SV-KNN----SGWSIGIISN---FLVF			C	NYASLLESTSTHWGFVPVSE
	D	SI-EQN----SGWKLCIRNG---NIEW			D	NYETKLLSTSSFWKFISRDPGWVE
	E	CMRDNN----SGWKVSLNHN---EIIW			E	TNS-----NGCFWNFISEEHGWQEK
	F	CMGNNN----SGWKISLRTVRDCEIIW			F	TSS-----NGCFWSSISKENGWKE
	G	CI-KND----SGWKVSIKGN---RIIW			G	KLR-----LGCNWQFIPVDEGWTE
	Te	SMKKHSLSIGSGWSVSLKGN---NLIW			Te	I-------LGCDWYFVPTDEGWTND
981–999 (peptide 10)	A	G---EIIWTLQDTQEIKQRVVF				
	B	N---RIIWTLIDINGKTKSVFF				
	C	N---FLVFTLKQNEDSEQSINF				
	D	G---NIEWILQDVNRKYKSLIF				
	E	N---EIIWTLQDNAGINQKLAF				
	F	VRDCEIIWTLQDTSGNKENLIF				
	G	N---RIIWTLIDVNAKSKSIFF				
	Te	N---NLIWTLKDSAGEVRQITF				

TABLE 38.4. *Expected (predicted) cross-reaction of HC domain epitopes of BoNTs B and F with Abs against BoNT-A[a]*

Peptide no.	2	3	6	7	8	9	10	11	12	15	18	24	31
BoNT/B	+	+	−	+	−	+	±	+	+	−	+	−	±
BoNT/F	±	±	+	+	+	+	+	±	+	−	+	+	−

[a] Predictions are based on the expectation that a five-residue identity within an epitope on a related protein is sufficient to permit a cross-reaction of that region on the related protein (28,35). Of course, when the number of identical residues is larger, the cross-reaction becomes stronger.

not be an effective strategy to overcome immunoresistance to treatment because the cross-reacting epitopes on the first BoNT would simply prime the recipient for a higher response to the next botulinum neurotoxin serotype.

Reaction with H_C of Antibodies and T Cells Obtained After Immunization with Peptides

Ab and T-cell responses against individual peptides and against mixtures of selected peptides were also studied in order to understand the role of T cell and Ab recognition in cross-reaction with H_C and to devise an effective design for a synthetic peptide vaccine. To complement the work described in the foregoing sections (which determined the immunodominant peptide regions on H_C that are recognized by T and/or B cells when either BoNT-A or H_C is used as an immunogen) and to determine the peptides that stimulate immune responses that recognize intact H_C, we used these peptide regions as immunogens (117). The following three different mixtures of peptides were used as immunogens in

TABLE 38.5. *Number of expected crossreacting epitopes on H_C of BoNTs B and F with Abs against BoNT-A*

BoNT/B	7/13
BoNT/F	8/13

13 is the total number of epitopes on the C-terminal domain of the heavy chain (H_C) of botulinum neurotoxin type A.

7 and 8 are the number of regions on H_C of BoNT-B and BoNT-F that have five or more contiguous residues that are identical or functionally similar to the corresponding regions on BoNT-A.

BALB/c and SJL mice (Table 38.6): (a) peptides recognized by anti-H_C T cells; (b) peptides recognized by anti-H_C B cells Abs; or (c) peptides containing T cell plus B cell epitopes (117).

For BALB/c, all peptides that contained Ab and/or T-cell epitopes [when H_C was used as the immunogen (47)] elicited Ab responses against the immunizing peptide that cross-reacted with H_C. Peptides 2, 3, 10, and 31 that contain epitopes recognized by anti-H_C Abs (47) stimulated strong H_C-cross-reactive Abs (117) (Table 38.7). However, the amounts of Abs bound by the immunizing peptides and by H_C varied. Of these, Abs against peptide 31 (residues 1275–1296) exhibited the highest binding to H_C. In the case of SJL, most of the peptides that contain Ab and T cell epitopes elicited antipeptide Abs. Although Ab responses were elicited, in decreasing order, by peptides 10, 4, 6, 7, 5, 8, 11, 24, 31, and 15 (117), very strong H_C-reactive antipeptide Abs were elicited only by peptide 4 (897–915) followed by peptide 10 (981–999). The greater immunogenicity in SJL of peptide 4 might be because this peptide contains both T and B cell epitopes (47,117). Thus, peptide 4 in SJL and peptide 31 in BALB/c elicited Abs that possessed the highest cross-reactivity with H_C.

We also studied T cell responses against the individual peptides (117). In BALB/c, the antipeptide T cells that were H_C-cross reactive were those elicited by peptides 7 (939–957), 12 (1009–1027), and 17 (1079–1097). Each of these peptide-primed T cells, except for peptide 17, showed moderate to very strong proliferative response to the immunizing peptide. In SJL, H_C-cross-reactive T cell responses were elicited by peptides 4–8 and 10 (981–999). T cells against

TABLE 38.6. *Constituent peptides of peptide mixtures containing T cell and/or Ab epitopes*

Peptide mixture	SJL	BALB/c
T Cell	peptides 4–9 and 15	peptides 7, 12, and 21
Ab	peptides 2–4, 7, 10, 11, 15, 24, and 31	peptides 2, 3, 10, 17, 18, 21, 24, and 31
T Cell +Ab	peptides 2–11, 15, 24, and 31	peptides 2, 3, 7, 10, 12, 17, 18, 21, 24, and 31

From Oshima M, Middlebrook JL, Atassi MZ. Antibodies and T cells against synthetic peptides of the C-terminal domain (H$_C$) of botulinum neurotoxin type A and their cross-reaction with H$_C$. *Immunol Lett* 1998;60:7–12, with permission.

peptides 2, 21, 24, and 31 in BALB/c, and 15 and 31 in SJL, showed negligible response to challenge *in vitro* with H$_C$ (Table 38.7). This laboratory (44,118,119) and others (120) have reported similar observations with antipeptide T cells that failed to recognize the parent protein.

Selected peptides were also employed in equimolar mixtures as immunogens to stimulate Ab and T cell responses. We determined the cross-reactivity of these antimixture responses with H$_C$ and with each of the peptides present in the immunizing mixture (117). A mixture of peptides that contained both Ab and T cell epitopes usually elicited most effectively in both mouse strains T cells and Abs that were cross-reactive with intact H$_C$ (Fig. 38.11). The peptide recognition profiles obtained after immunization with this peptide mixture were qualitatively and quantitatively different from those obtained by individual peptide immunization (Tables 38.7 and 38.8). Significantly, immunization with this mixture caused production of Ab responses to some peptides that were otherwise unable to stimulate Ab responses when each was used individually as an immunogen (peptides 2, 3, and 9 in SJL). Mixture immunization also suppressed Ab responses to certain peptides that could otherwise elicit Abs when injected individually (peptides 12, 17, and 21 in BALB/c). It is evident that Ab production to these regions in the peptide mixture is modulated by intersite influences of the cellular responses against the constituent peptides. It is known that intersite T-T and T-B cell interactions modulate and regulate the immune responses to various epitopes on an antigen (118,119,121–124). These cell–cell interactions among the responses to the individ-

ual sites and coimmunization effects (118,119) contribute to the complex responses of T cells and Abs obtained after immunization with peptide mixture.

We obtained a quicker rise (after two injections, at 4 weeks) in Ab titer that cross-reacted with H$_C$ compared to the other mixtures or to individual peptides (117) by immunization with the peptide mixture that contained Ab and T-cell epitope peptides [when H$_C$ is the immunogen (47)]. Also, in the case of BALB/c, the mixture sustained a high titer of H$_C$-cross-reacting Abs (Fig. 38.11). Thus, immunization with a peptide mixture containing all the T- and B-cell epitopes was particularly effective in BALB/c mice. The results suggest that when the vaccine formula includes peptides containing T-cell epitopes, that these will help to activate B cells that make H$_C$-cross-reactive Abs and will enhance the production of such Abs. Recent work from this laboratory (32) has shown that a mixture of three α-bungarotoxin peptides was a more protective immunogen against toxin poisoning than when any of the peptides present in the mixture was used individually.

Alignment of primary structures of BoNT serotypes A through G and TeNT in the 17 peptide regions used as immunogens revealed (117) that in one or more of these clostridial toxins, 13 peptides have 5 or more contiguous residues that are identical or similar to BoNT-A (Fig. 38.10). Of these, peptides 2, 3, 7, 10, 12, 15, 18, 24, and 31 generate H$_C$ cross-reactive Abs in either strain (Table 38.6). Production of H$_C$ cross-reactive Abs was augmented in BALB/c (Fig. 38.11) when peptides 7 (residues 939–957) and 12 (1009–1027) (which contain T-cell epitopes and

TABLE 38.7. Summary of reaction with immunizing peptide and H_C of immune responses elicited when individual BoNT-A peptides, including T and/or Ab epitope, are used as immunogens in SJL and BALB/c mouse strains[a]

Peptide immunogen		SJL (H-2^s)					BALB/c (H-2^d)				
			Ab		T Cell			Ab		T Cell	
Pept. No.	Sequence Position	Epitope for[b]	pept.	H_C	pept.	H_C	Epitope for[b]	pept.	H_C	pept.	H_C
2	869–887	Ab	±	−	−	−	Ab	++++	++++	+++	−
3	883–901	Ab	−	−	±	−	Ab	++	++++	±	−
4	897–915	T, Ab	+++++	++++++	+++++	++++	n/e[c]	n/e	n/e	n/e	n/e
5	911–929	T	++++	+	++++	++++	n/e	n/e	n/e	n/e	n/e
6	925–943	T	+++++	−	+++	+++	n/e	n/e	n/e	+++	+++
7	939–957	T, Ab	+++++	+	+++++	++++	T	+++++	++	+++	+++
8	953–971	T	+++	−	++++	++++	n/e	n/e	n/e	n/e	n/e
9	967–985	T	−	−	±	−	n/e	n/e	n/e	n/e	n/e
10	981–999	Ab	+++++	++	+++	+	Ab	++++	++++	−	−
11	995–1013	Ab	++	±	−	+	n/e	n/e	n/e	n/e	n/e
12	1009–1027	n/e	n/e	n/e	n/e	n/e	T	+++++	++	+++	+
15	1051–1069	T, Ab	+	+	+++	±	n/e	n/e	n/e	n/e	n/e
17	1079–1097	n/e	n/e	n/e	n/e	n/e	Ab	+++	+++	±	+
18	1093–1111	n/e	n/e	n/e	n/e	n/e	Ab	++	++	−	−
21	1135–1153	n/e	n/e	n/e	±	−	T, Ab	+++	+++	+++	−
24	1177–1195	Ab	++	+	++	−	Ab	+++	+++	++	−
31	1275–1296	Ab	+	+	+	−	Ab	++++	++++	++	−

[a] Assignment of positive and negative responses for the purpose of this table was based on net cpm values for Ab study and of SI values for T-cell study. For Ab binding, the symbols denote the following values: (−), less than 2,000 cpm; (±), 2,000 to 5,000 cpm; (+), 5,000 to 12,000 cpm; (++), 12,000 to 22,000 cpm; (+++), 22,000 to 40,000 cpm; (++++), 40,000 to 60,000 cpm; (+++++), greater than 60,000 cpm. For T-cell recognition, the symbols denote the following: (−), SI value less than 2.0; (±), SI 2.0 to 2.9; (+), SI 3.0 to 5.0; (++), SI 5.1 to 10.0; (+++), SI 10.1 to 30.0; (++++), SI 30.1 to 60.0; (+++++), SI ≥60.1. All the antipeptide antisera were unresponsive to protein and peptide controls used. The LNC of all experiments were unresponsive to unrelated proteins or peptide but responded appropriately to concanavalin A (Con A) and lipopolysaccharide (LPS).

[b] When H_C is used as the immunogen.

[c] n/e indicates that the peptide is neither an Ab nor a T-cell epitope in this mouse strain when it is immunized with H_C, thus the peptide was not used as an immunogen in this mouse strain.

Results in this table are summarized from the data reported by Oshima et al. (117).

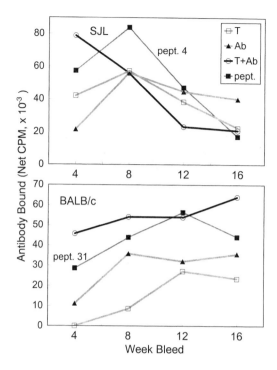

FIG. 38.11. Binding to H_C of Abs against three peptide mixtures or against peptide 4 (SJL) and peptide 31 (BALB/c) obtained at 4, 8, 12, and 16 weeks. SJL and BALB/c mice were immunized with an equimolar mixture of peptides containing T cell and/or Ab epitopes [when H_C is the immunogen (47)] or with individual peptides at 0, 3, 7, 11, and 15 weeks. Preimmune sera were used as negative controls, and their values were subtracted to obtain the net cpm. For details see text. *T, Ab,* and *T + Ab* represent mixture of peptides containing T-cell epitopes, mixture of peptides containing Ab epitopes, and mixture of peptides containing both T-cell and Ab epitopes, respectively. For the constituent peptides of each T-cell and/or Ab epitope peptide mixtures, see Table 38.3. (From Oshima M, Middlebrook JL, Atassi MZ. Antibodies and T cells against synthetic peptides of the C-terminal domain (H_C) of botulinum neurotoxin type A and their cross-reaction with H_C. *Immunol Lett* 1998;60:7–12, with permission.)

TABLE 38.8. *Summary of immune responses elicited when an equimolar mixture of peptides containing T and B cell epitopes was used as an immunogen in SJL and BALB/c*[a]

Peptide no.	SJL (H-2^s)		BALB/c (H-2^d)	
	Ab	T Cell	Ab	T Cell
2	+ +	−	+ + +	±
3	+ + +	+ + +	+ + +	−
4	+ + + + +	+ + + +	n/e[b]	n/e
5	±	+ +	n/e	n/e
6	+	+ + +	n/e	n/e
7	+ + +	+ + + +	+ + +	+ + +
8	+ + +	+ +	n/e	n/e
9	+ + +	+ + +	n/e	n/e
10	+ + + +	+ + +	+ + +	−
11	+	−	n/e	n/e
12	n/e	n/e	−	+ + +
15	±	+ + +	n/e	n/e
17	n/e	n/e	−	−
18	n/e	n/e	+ +	−
21	n/e	n/e	−	+ +
24	+ +	+ +	+ + +	±
31	+ + +	+ + +	+ + + +	−
H_C	+ + + + +	+ + + + +	+ + + + +	+ + +

[a,b] See footnotes for Table 38.7. Results in this table are summarized from the data reported by Oshima et al. (117).

have identical or similar regions in most of the clostridial toxins) were added to the mixture that consisted of peptides containing Ab epitopes. These results suggest that one or more of the synthetic peptides provide help that might contribute to cross-protection against those toxins. Peptide 7 (939–957), a T and/or Ab epitope containing peptide for both BALB/c and SJL strains, stimulates T- and B-cell responses in each strain when used as immunogen either individually or in a mixture (Tables 38.7 and 38.8). Peptide 7 also elicited H_C cross-reactive T cell and Ab responses (Table 38.7). It is noteworthy that region 947–967 of TeNT, a similar region to peptide 7 (residues 939–957), is also an epitope on TeNT for human T cells (124). The effectiveness of peptide 7 in both mouse strains suggests that it should be included in a synthetic vaccine design that will be active across MHC haplotypes.

CONCLUSIONS

The advantages, limitations, and potential risks of the therapeutic applications are discussed in the context of the mapping of the T- and B-cell epitopes that has been completed in this laboratory on the binding domain of the toxin.

We have mapped the epitopes on the protective H_C region of BoNT-A (residues 855–1296) that are recognized by anti–BoNT-A Abs raised in horse, human, and outbred mouse. We also mapped, in two mouse strains [BALB/c (H–2^d) and SJL (H–2^s)], the epitopes on H_C that are recognized by anti-H_C Abs and by H_C-primed T lymphocytes. The mapping of the epitopes on H_C revealed the molecular bases for the cross-reaction of the various BoNT serotypes and this information should be useful in explaining the development immunoresistance of some patients after therapeutic treatment with one BoNT serotype before switching to another serotype and the limited usefulness of such a switch. We also used the peptides that contain Ab or T-cell epitopes (or both) on the H_C domain as immunogens in BALB/c and SJL mice and identified those peptides whose Ab and/or T-cell responses cross-react with intact H_C. Localization of these peptides constitutes an important first step in the

requirements for the design of a synthetic vaccine.

ACKNOWLEDGMENTS

The immunologic studies reviewed here were supported by the Department of the Army Contract No. DAMD 17–93-C-3159. The support of the Welch Foundation with the award to the author of the Robert A. Welch Chair of Chemistry is also gratefully acknowledged.

REFERENCES

1. Kozaki S, Kamata Y, Nagai, T, et al. The use of monoclonal antibodies to analyze the structure of *Clostridium botulinum* type E derivative toxin. *Infect Immun* 1986;52:786–791.
2. Tsuzuki K, Yokosawa N, Syuto B, et al. Establishment of a monoclonal antibody recognizing an antigenic site common to *Clostridium botulinum* types B, C1, D, and E toxins and tetanus toxin. *Infect Immun* 1988;56:898–902.
3. Chan WL, Sesardic D, Shone CC. Proliferative T-cell response to botulinum toxin type A in mice. In: Das-Gupta BR, ed. *Botulinum and tetanus neurotoxins: neurotransmission and biomedical aspects.* New York: Plenum Press, 1993:337–339.
4. Cenci di Bello I, Poulain B, Shone CC, et al. Antagonism of the intracellular action of botulinum neurotoxin type A by monoclonal antibodies that map to light chain epitopes. *Eur J Biochem* 1994;219:161–169.
5. Demotz S, Matricardi PM, Irle C, et al. Processing of tetanus toxin by human antigen–presenting cells: evidence for donor- and epitope-specific processing pathways. *J Immunol* 1989;143:3881–3886.
6. Demotz S, Lanzavecchia A, Eisel U, et al. Delineation of several DR-restricted tetanus toxin T cell epitopes. *J Immunol* 1989;142:394–402.
7. Ho PC, Mutch DA, Winkel KD, et al. Identification of two promiscuous T-cell epitopes from tetanus toxin. *Eur J Immunol* 1990;20:477–483.
8. Reece JC, Geysen HM, Rodda SJ. Mapping the major human T-helper epitopes of tetanus toxin: the emerging picture. *J Immunol* 1993;151:6175–6184.
9. Fischer PM, Howden MEH. Synthetic peptide antigens of tetanus toxin. *Mol Immunol* 1994;31:1141–1148.
10. Makoff AJ, Ballantine SP, Smallwood AE, et al. Expression of tetanus toxin fragment C in *E. coli*: its purification and potential use as a vaccine. *Biotechnology* 1989;7:1043–1046.
11. Clare JJ, Rayment FB, Ballantine SP, et al. High-level expression of tetanus toxin fragment C in *Pichia pastoris* strains containing multiple tandem integrations of the gene. *Biotechnology* 1991;9:455–460.
12. LaPenotiere HF, Clayton MA, Middlebrook JL. Expression of a large, nontoxic fragment of botulinum neurotoxin serotype A and its use as an immunogen. *Toxicon* 1995;33:1383–1386.

13. Clayton MA, Clayton JM, Brown DR, et al. Protective vaccination with a recombinant fragment of *Clostridium botulinum* neurotoxin serotype A expressed from a synthetic gene in *Escherichia coli*. *Infect Immun* 1995;63:2738–2742.

14. Middlebrook JL. Protection strategies against botulinum toxin. *Adv Exp Med Biol* 1995;383:93–98.

15. Whalen RL, Dempsey DJ, Thompson LM, et al. Microencapsulated vaccines to provide prolonged immunity with a single administration. *ASAIO J* 1996;42:M649–M654.

16. Dertzbaugh MT, West MW. Mapping of protective and cross-reactive domains of the type A neurotoxin of *Clostridium botulinum*. *Vaccine* 1996;14:1538–1544.

17. Amersdorfer P, Wong C, Chen S, et al. Molecular characterization of murine humoral immune response to botulinum neurotoxin type A binding domain as assessed by using phage Ab libraries. *Infect Immun* 1997;65:3743–3752.

18. Kubota T, Watanabe T, Yokosawa N, et al. Epitope regions in the heavy chain of *Clostridium botulinum* type E neurotoxin recognized by monoclonal antibodies. *Appl Environ Microbiol* 1997;63:1214–1218.

19. Kiyatkin N, Maksymowych AB, Simpson LL. Induction of an immune response by oral administration of recombinant botulinum toxin. *Infect Immun* 1997;65:4586–4591.

20. Atassi MZ, Smith JA. A proposal for the nomenclature of antigen sites in peptides and proteins. *Immunochemistry* 1978;15:609–610.

21. Kazim AL, Atassi MZ. A novel and comprehensive synthetic approach for the elucidation of protein antigenic structures: determination of the full antigenic profile of the α-chain of human haemoglobin. *Biochem J* 1980;191:261–264.

22. Kazim AL, Atassi MZ. Structurally inherent antigenic sites: localization of the antigenic sites of the α-chain of human haemoglobin in three host species by a comprehensive synthetic approach. *Biochem J* 1982;203:201–208.

23. Bixler GS, Atassi MZ. Molecular localization of the full profile of the continuous regions recognized by myoglobin primed T cells using synthetic overlapping peptides encompassing the entire molecule. *Immunol Commun* 1983;12:593–603.

24. Bixler GS, Atassi MZ. T-Cell recognition of myoglobin: localization of the sites stimulating T-cell proliferative responses by synthetic overlapping peptides encompassing the entire molecule. *J Immunogen* 1984;11:339–353.

25. Kazim AL, Atassi MZ. Prediction and confirmation by synthesis of two antigenic sites in human haemoglobin by extrapolation from the known antigenic structure of sperm whale myoglobin. *Biochem J* 1977;167:275–278.

26. Kazim AL, Atassi MZ. First consequences of the determination of the entire antigenic structure of sperm whale myoglobin. *Adv Exp Med Biol* 1978;98:19–40.

27. Yoshioka N, Atassi MZ. Antigenic structure of human haemoglobin: localization of the antigenic sites of the α-chain in three host species by synthetic overlapping peptides representing the entire chain. *Biochem J* 1986;234:441–447.

28. Atassi MZ. Antigenic structures of proteins: their determination has revealed important aspects of immune recognition and generated strategies for synthetic mimicking of protein binding sites. *Eur J Biochem* 1984;145:1–20.

29. Dolimbek BZ, Atassi MZ. α-Bungarotoxin peptides afford a synthetic vaccine against toxin poisoning. *J Prot Chem* 1994;13:490–493.

30. Atassi MZ, Dolimbek BZ, Manshouri T. Antibody and T-cell recognition of α-bungarotoxin and its synthetic loop peptides. *Mol Immunol* 1995;13:927–932.

31. Atassi MZ, Dolimbek BZ. Regions of interaction between nicotinic acetylcholine receptor and α-neurotoxins and development of a synthetic vaccine against toxin poisoning. In: Atassi MZ, Appella E, eds. *Methods of protein structure analysis*. New York: Plenum Press, 1995:311–326.

32. Dolimbek BZ, Atassi MZ. Protection against α-bungarotoxin poisoning by immunization with synthetic toxin peptides. *Mol Immunol* 1996;33:681–689.

33. Atassi MZ, Dolimbek BZ, Hayakari M, et al. Mapping of the antibody-binding regions on botulinum neurotoxin H-chain domain 855–1296 with anti-toxin antibodies from three host species. *J Prot Chem* 1996;15:691–700.

34. Metzger JF, Lewis GE Jr. Human-derived immune globulins for the treatment of botulism. *Rev Infect Dis* 1979;1:689–690.

35. Atassi MZ. Antigenic structure of myoglobin. The complete immunochemical anatomy of a protein and conclusions relating to antigenic structures of proteins. *Immunochemistry* 1975;12:423–438.

36. Atassi MZ. Precise determination of protein antigenic structures has unraveled the molecular immune recognition of proteins and provided a prototype for synthetic mimicking of other protein binding sites. *Mol Cell Biochem* 1980;32:21–44.

37. Okuda K, Twining SS, Atassi MZ, et al. Genetic control of T-lymphocyte proliferative responses to sperm whale myoglobin and its synthetic antigenic sites in mice. *J Immunol* 1978;121:866–868.

38. Rosenwasser LJ, Barcinski MA, Schwartz RH, et al. Immune response gene control of determinant selection. II. Genetic control of the murine T lymphocyte proliferative response to insulin. *J Immunol* 1979;123:471–476.

39. Krco CJ, David CS. Genetics of immune response: a survey. *Crit Rev Immunol* 1981;1:211–257.

40. Okuda K, Twining SS, David CS, et al. Genetic control of immune response to sperm whale myoglobin in mice. II. T lymphocyte proliferative response to the synthetic antigenic sites. *J Immunol* 1979;123:182–188.

41. Atassi MZ, Twining SS, Lehmann H, et al. Genetic control of the immune response to myoglobin. V. Analysis of the cross-reactivity of 12 myoglobins with sperm whale myoglobin antisera of inbred mouse strains in terms of substitutions in the antigenic sites and in the environmental residues of the sites. *Immunol Commun* 1981;10:359–365.

42. David CS, Atassi MZ. Genetic control and intersite influences on the immune response to sperm whale myoglobin. *Adv Exp Med Biol* 1982;150:97–126.

43. Rosenberg JS, Middlebrook JL, Atassi MZ. Localiza-

tion of the regions on the C-terminal domain of the heavy chain of botulinum toxin A recognized by T lymphocytes and by antibodies after immunization of mice with pentavalent toxoid. *Immunol Invest* 1997; 26:491–504.

44. Atassi MZ, Bixler GS Jr. Comparison of the submolecular recognition of proteins by T and B cells. In: Kohler H, LoVerde PT, eds. *Vaccines: new concepts and developments.* Harlow, England: Longman Scientific and Technical, 1988:58–70.

45. Atassi MZ, Torres JV, Wyde PR. Cytotoxic and helper T-lymphocyte responses to antibody recognition regions on influenza virus hemagglutinin. *Adv Exp Med Biol* 1989;251:49–63.

46. Gammon G, Klotz J, Ando D, et al. The T cell repertoire to a multideterminant antigen: clonal heterogeneity of the T cell response, variation between syngeneic individuals, and *in vitro* selection of T cell specificities. *J Imunol* 1990;144:1571–1577.

47. Oshima M, Hayakari M, Middlebrook JL, et al. Immune recognition of botulinum neurotoxin type A: regions recognized by T cells and antibodies against the protective H_C fragment (residues 855–1296) of the toxin. *Mol Immunol* 1997;34:1031–1040.

48. Oshima M, Pachner AR, Atassi MZ. Profile of the regions of acetylcholine receptor α chain recognized by T lymphocytes and by antibodies in EAMG-susceptible and non-susceptible mouse strains after different periods of immunization with the receptor. *Mol Immunol* 1994;31:833–843.

49. Cardoso F, Jankovic J. Clinical use of botulinum neurotoxins. *Curr Top Microbiol Immunol* 1995;195: 123–141.

50. Borodic G, Johnson E, Goodnough M, et al. Botulinum toxin therapy, immunologic resistance, and problems with available materials. *Neurology* 1996;46:26–29.

51. Erbguth FJ. Historical note on the therapeutic use of botulinum toxin in neurological disorders. *J Neurol Neurosurg Psychiatry* 1996;60:151.

52. Lagueny A, Burbaud P. Mechanism of action, clinical indication and results of treatment of botulinum toxin. *Neurophysiol Clin* 1996;26:216–226.

53. Montecucco C, Schiavo G, Tugnoli V, et al. Botulinum neurotoxins: mechanism of action and therapeutic applications. *Mol Med Today* 1996;2:418–424.

54. Tsui JK. Botulinum toxin as a therapeutic agent. *Pharmacol Ther* 1996;72:13–24.

55. Schantz EJ, Johnson EA. Botulinum toxin: the story of its development for the treatment of human disease. *Perspect Biol Med* 1997;40:317–327.

56. Wheeler AH. Therapeutic uses of botulinum toxin. *Am Fam Physician* 1997;55:541–545, 548.

57. Kessler KR, Benecke R. Botulinum toxin: from poison to remedy. *Neurotoxicology* 1997;18:761–770.

58. Pearce LB, First ER, MacCallum RD, et al. Pharmacologic characterization of botulinum toxin for basic science and medicine. *Toxicon* 1997;35:1373–1412.

59. Berardelli A, Abbruzzese G, Bertolasi L, et al. Guidelines for the therapeutic use of botulinum toxin in movement disorders. *Ital J Neurol Sci* 1997;18: 261–269.

60. Cuevas C, Madrazo I, Magallon E, et al. Botulinum toxin-A for the treatment of hemifacial spasm. *Arch Med Res* 1995;26:405–408.

61. Sloop RR, Cole BA, Escutin RO. Human response to

botulinum toxin injection: type B compared with type A. *Neurology* 1997;49:189–194.

62. Eleopra R, Tugnoli V, Rossetto O, et al. Botulinum neurotoxin serotype C: a novel effective botulinum toxin therapy in human. *Neurosci Lett* 1997;224: 91–94.

63. Poewe W, Deuschl G, Nebe A, et al. What is the optimal dose of botulinum toxin A in the treatment of cervical dystonia? Results of a double-blind, placebo-controlled, dose-ranging study using DYSPORT. *J Neurol Neurosurg Psychiatry* 1998;64:13–17.

64. Zwirner P, Murry T, Woodson GE. Effects of botulinum toxin on vocal tract steadiness in patients with spasmodic dysphonia. *Eur Arch Otorhinolaryngol* 1997;254:391–395.

65. Albanese A, Bentivoglio AR, Cassetta E, et al. The use of botulinum toxin in the alimentary tract. *Aliment Pharmacol Ther* 1995;9:599–604.

66. Bhutani MS. Gastrointestinal uses of botulinum toxin. *Am J Gastroenterol* 1997;92:929–933.

67. Albanese A, Maria G, Bentivoglio AR, et al. Severe constipation in Parkinson's disease relieved by botulinum toxin. *Mov Disord* 1997;12:764–766.

68. Mezaki T, Kaji R, Kohara N, et al. Development of general weakness in a patient with amyotrophic lateral sclerosis after focal botulinum toxin injection. *Neurology* 1996;46:845–846.

69. Carruthers A, Kiene K, Carruthers J. Botulinum A exotoxin use in clinical dermatology. *J Am Acad Dermatol* 1996;34:788–797.

70. Ellis DA, Tan AK. Cosmetic upper-facial rejuvenation with botulinum. *J Otolaryngol* 1997;26:92–96.

71. Carter SR, Seiff SR. Cosmetic botulinum toxin injections. *Int Ophthalmol Clin* 1997;37:69–79.

72. Carruthers A, Carruthers J. Cosmetic uses of botulinum A exotoxin. *Adv Dermatol* 1997;12:325–348.

73. Bikhazi NB, Maas CS. Refinement in the rehabilitation of the paralyzed face using botulinum toxin. *Otolaryngol Head Neck Surg* 1997;117:303–307.

74. Ellis DA, Chi PL, Tan AK. Facial rejuvenation with botulinum. *Dermatol Nurs* 1997;9:329–333, 365.

75. Spencer RF, Tucker MG, Choi RY, et al. Botulinum toxin management of childhood intermittent exotropia. *Ophthalmology* 1997;104:1762–1767.

76. Diels HJ, Combs D. Neuromuscular retraining for facial paralysis. *Otolaryngol Clin North Am* 1997;30: 727–743.

77. Marchand L. Treatment of essential tremor. *Union Medicale du Canada* 1995;124:32–34.

78. Henderson JM, Ghika JA, Van Melle G, et al. Botulinum toxin A in non-dystonic tremors. *Eur Neurol* 1996;36:29–35.

79. Jankovic J, Schwartz K, Clemence W, et al. A randomized, double-blind, placebo-controlled study to evaluate botulinum toxin type A in essential hand tremor. *Mov Disord* 1996;11:250–256.

80. Brennan HG, Koch RJ. Management of aging neck. *Facial Plast Surg* 1996;12:241–255.

81. Sampaio C, Ferreira JJ, Pinto AA, et al. Botulinum toxin type A for the treatment of arm and hand spasticity in stroke patients. *Clin Rehabil* 1997;11:3–7.

82. Wissel J, Masuhr F, Schelosky L, et al. Quantitative assessment of botulinum toxin treatment in 43 patients with head tremor. *Mov Disord* 1997;12:722–726.

83. Deymeer F, Oge AE, Serdaroglu P, et al. The use of

botulinum toxin in localizing neuromyotonia to the terminal branches of the peripheral nerve. *Muscle Nerve* 1998;21:643–646.

84. Kerty E, Stien R. Treatment of spasticity with botulinum toxin. *Tidsskr Nor Laegeforen* 1997;117:2022–2024.

85. Hesse S, Mauritz KH. Management of spasticity. *Curr Opin Neurol* 1997;10:498–501.

86. Ko CK, Ward AB. Management of spasticity. *Br J Hosp Med* 1997;58:400–405.

87. Bentley C. Botulinum neurotoxin A in ophthalmology. *Ophthal Physiol Optics* 1997;16(Suppl 1):S9–S14.

88. Carruthers JD, Carruthers A. Botulinum A exotoxin in clinical ophthalmology. *Can J Ophthalmol* 1996;31:389–400.

89. Kikkawa DO, Kim JW. Lower-eyelid blepharoplasty. *Int Ophthalmol Clin* 1997;37:163–178.

90. Huber A. Use of botulinum toxin in ophthalmology. *Klin Monatsbl Augenheilkd* 1997;210:289–292.

91. Tapiero B, Robert PY, Adenis JP, et al. Use of botulinum toxin in ophthalmology: Current concepts and problems. *J Fr Ophtalmol* 1997;20:134–145.

92. Acheson JF, Bentley CR, Shallo-Hoffmann J, et al. Dissociated effects of botulinum toxin chemodenervation on ocular deviation and saccade dynamics in chronic lateral rectus palsy. *Br J Ophthalmol* 1998;82:67–71.

93. Papazian O, Alfonso I. Cerebral palsy therapy. *Rev Neurol* 1997;25:728–739.

94. Arens LJ, Leary PM, Goldschmidt RB. Experience with botulinum toxin in the treatment of cerebral palsy. *S Afr Med J* 1997;87:1001–1003.

95. Pascual-Pascual SI, Sanchez de Muniain P, Roche MC, et al. Botulinum toxin as a treatment for infantile cerebral palsy. *Rev Neurol* 1997;25:1369–1375.

96. Jost WH, Schimrigk K. Botulinum toxin in therapy of anal fissure. *Lancet* 1995;345:188–189.

97. Goel AK, Seenu V. Botulinum toxin in the management of anal fissure: innovative use of a familiar agent. *Trop Gastroenterol* 1995;16:68–69.

98. Jost WH. One hundred cases of anal fissure treated with botulin toxin: early and long-term results. *Dis Colon Rectum* 1997;40:1029–1032.

99. Maria G, Cassetta E, Gui Det, al. A comparison of botulinum toxin and saline for the treatment of chronic anal fissure. *N Engl J Med* 1998;338:257–259.

100. Jost WH, Muller-Lobeck H, Merkle W. Involuntary contractions of the striated anal sphincters as a cause of constipation: report of a case. *Dis Colon Rectum* 1998;41:258–260.

101. Steinhardt GF, Naseer S, Cruz OA. Botulinum toxin: novel treatment for dramatic urethral dilatation associated with dysfunctional voiding. *J Urol* 1997;158:190–191.

102. Werner JA, Gottschlich S. Recent advances: otorhinolaryngology. *BMJ* 1997;315:354–357.

103. Laskawi R. [The use of botulinum toxin in otorhinolaryngology: experiences and outlook.] *Laryngorhinootologie* 1997;76:656–659.

104. Egan MF, Apud J, Wyatt RJ. Treatment of tardive dyskinesia. *Schizophr Bull* 1997;23:583–609.

105. Liguori R, Cordivari C, Lugaresi E, et al. Botulinum toxin A improves muscle spasms and rigidity in stiff-person syndrome. *Mov Disord* 1997;12:1060–1063.

106. Horgan SE, Lee JP, Bunce C. The long-term use of botulinum toxin for adult strabismus. *J Pediatr Ophthalmol Strabismus* 1998;35:9–16.

107. Drobik C, Laskawi R. Frey's syndrome: Treatment with botulinum toxin. *Acta Otolaryngol* 1995;115:459–461.

108. Schulze-Bonhage A, Schroder M, Ferbert A. Botulinum toxin in the therapy of gustatory sweating. *J Neurol* 1996;243:143–146.

109. Bjerkhoel A, Trobbe O. Frey's syndrome: treatment with botulinum toxin. *J Laryngol Otol* 1997;111:839–844.

110. Laccourreye O, Muscatelo L, Naude C, et al. Botulinum toxin type A for Frey's syndrome: a preliminary prospective study. *Ann Otol Rhino Laryngol* 1998;107:52–55.

111. Laskawi R, Drobik C, Schonebeck C. Up-to-date report of botulinum toxin type A treatment in patients with gustatory sweating (Frey's syndrome). *Laryngoscope* 1998;108:381–384.

112. Naumann M, Hofmann U, Bergmann I, et al. Focal hyperhidrosis: effective treatment with intracutaneous botulinum toxin. *Arch Dermatol* 1998;134:301–304.

113. Schiano TD, Parkman HP, Miller LS, et al. Use of botulinum toxin in the treatment of achalasia. *Dig Dis* 1998;16:14–22.

114. Doellgast GJ, Brown JE, Koufman JA, et al. Sensitive assay for measurement of Abs to *Clostridium botulinum* neurotoxins A, B, and E: use of hapten-labeled Ab elution to isolate specific complexes. *J Clin Microbiol* 1997;35:578–583.

115. Greene PE, Fahn S. Response to botulinum toxin F in seronegative botulinum toxin A-resistant patients. *Mov Disord* 1996;11:181–184.

116. Goschel H, Wohlfarth K, Frevert J, et al. Botulinum A toxin therapy: neutralizing and nonneutralizing Abs—therapeutic consequences. *Exp Neurol* 1997;147:96–102.

117. Oshima M, Middlebrook JL, Atassi MZ. Antibodies and T cells against synthetic peptides of the C-terminal domain (H$_C$) of botulinum neurotoxin type A and their cross-reaction with H$_C$. *Immunol Lett* 1998;60:7–12.

118. Bixler GS Jr, Atassi MZ. Antigen presentation of myoglobin: profiles of T-cell proliferative responses following priming with synthetic overlapping peptides encompassing the entire protein molecule. *Eur J Immunol* 1985;15:917–922.

119. Bixler GS Jr, Yoshida T, Atassi MZ. Antigen presentation of lysozyme: T-cell recognition of peptide and intact protein after priming with synthetic overlapping peptides comprising the entire protein chain. *Immunology* 1985;56:103–112.

120. Bhardwaj V, Kumar V, Grewal IS, et al. T-cell determinant structure of myelin basic protein in B10.PL, SJL/J and their F$_1$s. *J Immunol* 1994;152:3711–3719.

121. Atassi MZ, Yokota S, Twining SS, et al. Genetic control of the immune response to myoglobin. VI. Intersite influences in T-lymphocyte proliferative response from analysis of cross-reactions of ten myoglobins in terms of substitutions in the antigenic sites and in environmental residues of the sites. *Mol Immunol* 1981;18:961–967.

122. Rosenberg JS, Oshima M, Atassi MZ. B-Cell activation in vitro by helper T cells specific to region α146–162 of Torpedo californica acetylcholine receptor. *J Immunol* 1996;157:3192–3299.

123. Hamajima S, Atassi MZ. B-Cell activation *in vitro* by helper T cells specific to a protein region that is recognized both T cells and by antibodies. *Immunol Invest* 1998;27:121–134.

124. Panina-Bordignon P, Tan A, Termijtelen A, et al. Universally immunogenic T cell epitopes: promiscuous binding to human MHC class II and promiscuous rec-ognition by T cells. *Eur J Immunol* 1989;19: 2237–2242.

125. Whelan SM, Elmore MJ, Bodsworth NJ, et al. Molecular cloning of the *Clostridium botulinum* structural gene encoding the type B neurotoxin and determination of its entire nucleotide sequence. *Appl Env Microbiol* 1992;58:2345–2354.

Scientific and Therapeutic Aspects of Botulinum Toxin
edited by M.F. Brin, J. Jankovic, and M. Hallett
Lippincott Williams & Wilkins, Philadelphia, © 2002.

39

Botulinum Toxin: Clinical Implications of Antigenicity and Immunoresistance

Joseph Jankovic

Since the first report of clinical application of botulinum neurotoxin type A (BTX-A) in 1984 (1), BTX, the most potent biologic toxin, has become a powerful therapeutic tool in a variety of neurologic and other disorders. Although its widest application is still in the treatment of disorders manifested by abnormal, excessive, or inappropriate muscle contractions (2), its use is rapidly expanding to include treatment of a variety of ophthalmologic, gastrointestinal, urologic, orthopedic, and dermatologic disorders (3–6). BTX is also increasingly used in the management of various musculoskeletal, painful, and cosmetic conditions. Initially approved in 1989 by the Food and Drug Administration for the treatment of blepharospasm and other facial spasms, BTX-A (BOTOX) was also approved in 2000 for the treatment of cervical dystonia. The same year BTX-B (MYOBLOC, formerly known as NeuroBloc) was also approved for the treatment of cervical dystonia.

With the expanding use of BTX, there is growing concern about the antigenicity of BTX and development of immunoresistance as a result of blocking antibodies. A certain percentage of patients receiving repeated injections develop antibodies (immunoresistance) against BTX causing them to be completely resistant to the effects of subsequent BTX injections (7–13). Studies show that the H_C fragment of the heavy chain contains epitopes that are recognized by anti-H_C antibodies (Ab) and by H_C-primed T lymphocytes (14).

There are several methods used to detect BTX antibodies, but the mouse protection assay (MPA) is considered clinically most relevant be-

cause it detects neutralizing (blocking) antibodies (15). Four Swiss Webster mice are injected intraperitoneally with a mixture of a lethal dose of BTX and the patient's test serum. If at least three of the four mice die, this indicates absence of blocking antibodies. The presence of antibodies in the test serum is indicated if there are no deaths or only one mouse dies, suggesting that the mice were protected by blocking antibodies in the patient's serum. This assay may be refined by providing titers, by evaluating the ability of increasing dilutions of a patient's serum to protect experimental mice from lethal test doses of BTX. Other *in vivo* assays for BTX Ab include the mouse protection assay of the diaphragm (MPDA), also referred to as the mouse diaphragm assay (MDA) (16). In contrast to the MPA in which a positive response correlates essentially 100% with complete therapeutic failure (10), only 62% of patients with positive BTX Ab determined by the MDA had complete therapy failure and 38% had partial failure (16). Furthermore, Dressler et al. (17) found that a reduction of maximal voluntary contraction as measured by electromyograph (EMG) of the sternocleidomastoid muscle more than two standard deviations below nondisease control values correlated well with BTX-A Ab status as measured by the MDA assay.

Using the MPA assays, we compared 22 randomly selected BTX antibody-negative (Ab−) patients with 20 patients who were immunoresistant (Ab+) and found that the BTX Ab+ patients had an earlier age at onset (mean age: 31.8 ± 16.7 vs 43.4 ± 10.5; $p < 0.05$), higher mean dose per visit (249.2 ± 32.5 vs

180.8 ± 68.7, $p < 0.0005$), and higher total cumulative dose (mean dose, 1709 ± 638 vs 1066 ± 938; $p < 0.01$) (12). Four of five Ab+ patients later responded to BTX type F injections. In another study, 24 of 559 (4.3%) patients treated for cervical dystonia developed secondary nonresponsiveness, presumably caused by BTX antibodies (18). In addition, the authors found that BTX-resistant patients had a shorter interval between injections, more "boosters," and a higher dose at the "nonbooster" injection as compared to nonresistant patients treated during the same period. As a result of this experience clinicians are warned against using booster injections and are encouraged to extend the interval between treatment as long as possible, certainly at least 2 months, and to use the smallest possible doses. We, and others, have observed that if immunoresistance does develop, it tends to occur within the first 4 years of treatment, and Ab formation seems less likely after this treatment period.

In some patients who become Ab+, their immunologic status reverts to Ab– after an average 30 months (range, 10–78) (19). When these Ab– patients are reinjected with BTX-A, they usually benefit with a response comparable to their earlier experience. Most, however, lose their clinical response to subsequent injections and when retested are found to be Ab+ again. Another study, using MDA (16), estimated the onset of decrease in Ab titer to occur about 2 to 5 years after the last injection, with the average estimated latency to nondetectable levels of 2,000 days (5.6 years) (Dressler, personal communication). This is substantially longer than the estimated duration found in the study by Sankhla et al. (19) and the 1-year latency estimated from immunization experiments with pentavalent botulinum toxoid (20). The difference could be possibly because of the higher doses of BTX per session (546 U) used by Dressler (personal communication), and high sensitivity of the MDA. Otherwise, the MPA and MDA are comparable (21).

Although the MPA assay is currently used most extensively, other assays are being developed to detect Abs against BTX. These other assays appear to have an advantage over the MPA in that they use *in vitro* rather than *in vivo* methods and they appear to be more sensitive than the MPA. We compared the MPA assay to the Western blot assay (WBA) in detecting Ab against BTX-A and correlated the assay results with clinical responses to BTX-A injections (10). MPA and WBA were compared in 51 patients (34 nonresponders and 17 responders) who received BTX-A injections, most commonly for cervical dystonia. A subset of patients received a test injection into either the right brow (14) or right frontalis, the frontalis type A test (F-TAT) (12). In this test, 15 U of BTX-A is administered as 2 doses of 7.5 U each into the right frontalis muscle. The patient is considered to be type A resistant if they are able to wrinkle both right and left frontalis muscles symmetrically (type A-responsive patient cannot wrinkle the injected right frontalis muscle). Alternatively, patients who are resistant to BTX and are injected into the right brow frown symmetrically, whereas responsive patients frown asymmetrically by contracting only the left corrugator/procerus muscle. We prefer injecting the right brow (unilateral brow injection or UBI) rather than the frontalis muscle (F-TAT) because some patients have difficulty voluntarily raising their brows, making their response to a frontalis injection difficult to determine. Furthermore, the brow injections are more cosmetically acceptable in that the asymmetric responses are present only during voluntary contractions, whereas unilateral disappearance of frontal wrinkles may not be desirable. In the UBI test, 20 U of BOTOX or 1,000 U of MYOBLOC is injected, by convention, into the right eyebrow. One or 2 weeks later, the patient is instructed to look in the mirror and frown. If the medial eyebrows contract symmetrically, then the right medial eyebrow muscles (procerus and corrugator) is not active, suggesting immunoresistance. On the other hand, an asymmetrical frown indicates unilateral medial brow paralysis, hence no blocking antibodies (Fig. 39.1).

Specificity of the MPA was 100% on all three parameters (clinical, eyebrow, and frontalis injections), whereas the WBA specificity was only 71% for clinical response but 100% for both eyebrow and frontalis responses. Sensitivities for

Unilateral Brow Injection (UBI)

Baylor College of Medicine

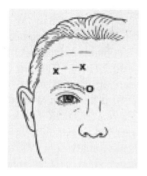

O = 20 U BOTOX®

or

1,000 U MYOBLOC™

FIG. 39.1. Clinical test for BTX responsiveness. Unilateral brow injection (UBI) or frontalis type A toxin or (F-TAT) injection. O, 20 U of BOTOX or 1,000 U of MYOBLOC(UBI); X, 10 U of BOTOX or 500 U of MYOBLOC (F-TAT).

both assays were low (33% to 53%). Of the 16 patients previously Ab+ by MPA, seven became negative on retesting after a mean interval of 33 months (range, 6 to 93 months). We concluded that UBI and F-TAT correlated well with MPA results and with clinical responses and may be useful in the evaluation of BTX nonresponders.

An immunoprecipitation assay (IPA), which quantitatively assesses the degree of immunoresistance (22), is more sensitive than MPA and may have a predictive value in determining impending or future unresponsiveness (11). After the iodination reaction, the ^{125}I-BTX is microfiltered and stored at 4°C (39.2°F) in phosphate-buffered saline (PBS). It is then diluted in PBS and centrifuged to remove any aggregates immediately before use. The supernatant, containing 30,000 to 50,000 cpm, is then incubated with 2.5 μL of each serum in a total volume of 50 μL PTX buffer (0.02 M phosphate, pH 7.4, 0.1% Triton X100) PBS. After 2 hours at room temperature, or overnight at 4°C (39.2°F), excess goat antihuman IgG is added. When a precipitate is formed, 600 μL of PTX is added before centrifuging. The pellets are washed twice briefly in PTX and counted on a Cobra Packard gamma counter. Results are expressed as pM (picomoles of ^{125}I-BTX precipitated/L serum). All patients who are Ab+ by MPA were also Ab+ by IPA, while an additional 19 patients (17 with reduced or no clinical response) who were MPA Ab− were Ab+, with low titers, by IPA. Two of these 19 patients (nonresponders) were initially MPA Ab− but later became MPA Ab+. Similar to previous studies, the sensitivity for the MPA was low: 50% for clinical, 38% for eyebrow, and 30% for frontalis responses, while the IPA sensitivity was much higher at 84% for clinical ($p < 0.001$), 77% for eyebrow ($p = 0.111$, NS), and 90% for frontalis responses ($p < 0.02$). The IPA specificity was 89% for clinical, 81% for eyebrow, and 89% for frontalis responses, while the MPA specificity was 100% for all three response types, which were all nonsignificant differences. Both assays had high specificity, but the sensitivity of the IPA was higher than that of the MPA. In addition, the IPA appeared to display positivity earlier than the MPA, and as such, it could prognosticate future nonresponsiveness. Eyebrow (UBI) and frontalis test injections correlated well with clinical and immunologic results and are useful in the assessment of BTX nonresponders.

Another useful test for detection of blocking Ab is the MDA (16). In this assay, the left phrenic nerve and the left hemidiaphragm are excised from a mouse and placed in an organ bath. The phrenic nerve is then stimulated at a frequency of 1 Hz, pulse duration of 0.1 ms and supramaximal amplitude of 3mV. Isometric contractions are recorded with a force transducer and the time required for reduction of the twitch amplitude by 50% after local application of BTX is called "paralysis time." If the paralysis time is outside of two standard deviations of the mean paralysis time of the control population, the test result is considered positive. The MDA has a potential advantage over the MPA in that it requires only one mouse per sample tested, and the results can be available within hours. The concordance between the MPA and the MDA, however, is only 63% and further studies are needed to determine the relative sensitivity and specificity of the MDA assay. Another way to test for BTX immunoresistance is by taking advantage of the observation that BTX inhibits sweating. Using iodine starch staining and capacitance hygrometry, this sudometric technique shows that sweating persists in BTX nonresponders after subcutaneous injection of 12.5 U of BTX-A, whereas this dose quite reliably inhibits sweating in control responders (23).

Besides WBA and IPA, there are other *in vitro* assays, including the sphere-linked immunodiagnostic assay (SLIDA) (24), enzyme-linked immunosorbent assay (ELISA) (25), and a monoclonal antibody-based immunoassay (26), that have been reported to detect BTX Ab, but the presence or absence of Ab measured by these assays do not correlate well with the observed clinical response. Dot blot is another *in vitro* assay that evaluates patient serum sample for its ability to bind to nondenatured BTX immobilized on a nitrocellulose membrane in a 96 well format (27). Strips of nitrocellulose membrane containing duplicate "dots" of BTX and appropriate controls are incubated overnight with the diluted sera at 4°C (39.2°F). Standard immunochemical methods are used to visualize captured human immunoglobulins on the nitrocellulose membrane. Positive samples (color develop-

ment) are then tested with serial dilutions beginning from 1/300 to estimate an Ab titer.

It has been suggested that the antigenicity of BTX is related to the amount of neurotoxin complex protein. In contrast to the original BOTOX (lot 79–11), which contained 25 ng of neurotoxin complex protein per 100 U, the current BOTOX preparation, approved by the FDA in 1997, contains only 5 ng of the complex protein per 100 U (27). The two preparations have a similar efficacy and adverse effect profile (28,29). It has been shown in rabbits (27) that the current BOTOX has less antigenicity than the original preparation. In one multicenter, retrospective analysis of 191 randomly selected patients who had received at least two consecutive treatments with original BOTOX, followed by at least three consecutive treatments with current BOTOX for the treatment of cervical dystonia, the mean doses of original and current BOTOX were comparable (245 and 250 U, respectively). With current BOTOX, patients were exposed to less neurotoxin complex protein (~12 ng/250 U) than with original (~61 ng/245 U). Response rate per period averaged 90% for both original and current BOTOX. Adverse events of any type were reported by an average of 14.4% of patients per period receiving original BOTOX as compared to an average of 19.4% of patients per period receiving current BOTOX. The mean percentage of patients reporting dysphagia was slightly higher with current BOTOX (4.2%) than with original (1.9%). The conclusion of the study was that the efficacy and safety of current BOTOX is comparable to original BOTOX in the treatment of cervical dystonia and that the treatment with current BOTOX results in lower exposure to neurotoxin complex protein and may, therefore, result in reduced antigenicity compared to treatment with original BOTOX. In a comparison of the usual doses used in patients with cervical dystonia, the following are estimated protein loads from injections of the various toxins: BOTOX (20 U/ng), Dysport (40 U/ng), and MYOBLOC/NeuroBloc 100 U/ng using reported doses of 187 U (9 ng), 732 U (18 ng), and 10,000 U (100 ng), respectively (Dr. R. Aoki, personal communication).

Unnicked or "nonactivated," single-chain

neurotoxin may also contribute to the overall neurotoxin protein load without contributing to the therapeutic efficacy of the BTX. In this regard, it is notable that BTX-A and BTX-F are released in the nicked form, whereas the nicking in BTX-B is more variable depending on the strain and preparation.

Besides overall protein load, another factor that may contribute to the development of antibodies is serum cross-reactivity between different BTX serotypes. Although traditionally considered immunologically distinct, the different BTX serotypes share a remarkable homology in the various epitopes (14). Epitopes are small (six to eight amino acid residues) components of the protein that have distinct boundaries, occupy surface locations, and are limited in number. The Ab response to each epitope is under separate genetic control and therefore varies with the host. T cells, under HLA-2 gene control, also recognize the epitopes recognized by Ab, but may also recognize other sites to which antibody response has not been mounted. Because of the marked homology (in some cases involving up to 13 residues), there is a strong possibility that Ab directed against one type of BTX can also cross-react and cross-neutralize another BTX serotype. In addition, the epitopes can stimulate or prime the second response for the second serotype. For example, certain serotypes of BTX, such as A, B, C1, and E, can cross-react with tetanus toxin (30). This may account for the detection of BTX-B antibodies in some individuals even without exposure to BTX-B (31,32). Mice treated with BTX-A fragments developed antibodies that cross-reacted with other serotypes (33). In one study, patients with spasticity who received BTX-A produced measurable titers of antibodies against several other serotypes (31). Further studies are needed to determine whether immunoresistance to one type of BTX increases the risk of developing blocking antibodies to another type of BTX, but the immunologic studies raise the concern that alternating between two different BTX serotypes increases the risk of immunoresistance to both. Finally, it should be noted that there are many other factors besides protein antigenicity and protein load that play a role in determining whether or not a patient develops blocking antibodies, including the patient's own immunologic status.

The frequency of neutralizing or blocking antibodies (immunoresistance) against BTX is unknown because no long-term prospective studies have been designed to specifically address this issue. Although the initial studies suggested that less than 10% of patients become immunoresistant after chronic treatment with BTX, more recent studies suggest that the frequency may be higher. Using the original 79–11 lot of BOTOX, 33 of 192 (17%) patients previously treated with BOTOX for cervical dystonia were Ab+, but only 2 of 96 (2%) who were Ab− at baseline became Ab+ after at least two BOTOX treatments (package insert, 2000). None of the Ab+ patients responded to BOTOX treatments. In another study involving 446 patients treated with BTX-B (MYOBLOC), 18% were estimated to be Ab+ after 18 months of treatment (package insert, 2000). Based on our long-term experience with the current BOTOX preparation 2024, it appears that the risk of immunoresistance is considerably lower than with the original preparation.

BTX-A–resistant patients usually benefit from injections with other serotypes of BTX, such as BTX-B, BTX-C, or BTX-F (18,34–40). A combination of BTX-A and BTX-F used in double-blind controlled trial of blepharospasm produced no prolongation of the beneficial effect (41). Other than using a different serotype, some investigators suggest that plasma exchange and immunoabsorption on a protein A column provide an alternative therapy for these secondary nonresponders (42). Furthermore, intravenous immunoglobulin and other methods have been used, largely unsuccessfully, to deplete the BTX-A antibodies (43). Finally, mycophenolate, an immunosuppressant commonly used to prevent transplant organ rejection, at 750 mg twice a day starting 48 hours before BTX treatment and continuing for 10 days, has been reported anecdotally to possibly prevent BTX antibody formation (44).

Prevention of immunoresistance, by using preparations of BTX with the lowest possible antigenicity and by keeping the dose per treatment session as low as possible and the interdose interval as long as possible (particularly in young women), is of paramount importance in maintaining the beneficial response to this most effective treatment.

REFERENCES

1. Frueh BR, Felt DP, Wojno TH, et al. Treatment of blepharospasm with botulinum toxin. A preliminary report. *Arch Ophthalmol* 1984;102:1464–1468.
2. Comella CL, Jankovic J, Brin MF. Use of botulinum toxin type A in the treatment of cervical dystonia. *Neurology* 2000;55(Suppl 5):S15–S21.
3. Jankovic J, Hallett M, eds. *Therapy with botulinum toxin.* New York: Marcel Dekker, 1994:1–608.
4. Jankovic J, Brin M. Botulinum toxin: historical perspective and potential new indications. *Muscle Nerve* 1997; 20(Suppl 6):S129–S145.
5. Hallett M. One man's poison—clinical applications of botulinum toxin. *N Engl J Med* 1999;341:118–120.
6. Gracies J-M, Simpson DM. Botulinum toxin therapy. *Neurologist* 2000;6:98–115.
7. Zuber M, Sebald M, Bathien N, et al. Botulinum antibodies in dystonic patients treated with type A botulinum toxin: frequency and significance. *Neurology* 1993; 43:1715–1718.
8. Göschel H, Wolhfart K, Frevert J, et al. Botulinum A toxin therapy: neutralizing and non-neutralizing antibodies-therapeutic consequences. *Exp Neurol* 1997;147: 96–102.
9. Greene P, Fahn S, Diamond B. Development of resistance to botulinum toxin type A in patients with torticollis. *Mov Disord* 1994;9:213–217.
10. Hanna PA, Jankovic J. Mouse bioassay versus Western blot assay for botulinum toxin antibodies: correlation with clinical response. *Neurology* 1998;50:1624–1629.
11. Hanna PA, Jankovic J, Vincent A. Comparison of mouse bioassay and immunoprecipitation assay for botulinum toxin antibodies. *J Neurol Neurosurg Psychiatry* 1999; 66:612–616 (correction: *J Neurol Neurosurg Psychiatry* 1999;67:133).
12. Jankovic J, Schwartz K. Response and immunoresistance to botulinum toxin injections. *Neurology* 1995;45: 1743–1746.
13. Borodic G, Johnson E, Goodenough M, et al. Botulinum toxin therapy, immunologic resistance, and problems with available materials. *Neurology* 1996;46:26–29.
14. Atassi MZ, Oshima M. Structure, activity, and immune (T and B cell) recognition of botulinum neurotoxins. *Crit Rev Immunol* 1999;19:219–260.
15. Hatheway CL, Dang C. Immunogenicity of the neurotoxins of *Clostridium botulinum.* In: Jankovic J, Hallett M, eds. *Therapy with botulinum toxin.* New York: Marcel Dekker, 1994:93–108.
16. Dressler D, Dirnberger G, Bhatia K, et al. Botulinum toxin antibody testing: comparison between the mouse diaphragm assay and the mouse lethality assay. *Mov Disord* 2000;15:973–976.
17. Dressler D, Bigalke H, Rothwell JC. The sternocleidomastoid test: an *in vivo* assay to investigate botulinum toxin antibody formation in humans. *J Neurol* 2000;247: 630–632.

18. Greene PE, Fahn S. Response to botulinum toxin F in seronegative botulinum toxin A-resistant patients. *Mov Disord* 1996;11:181–184.
19. Sankhla C, Jankovic J, Duane D. Variability of the immunologic and clinical response in dystonic patients immunoresistant to botulinum toxin injections. *Mov Disord* 1998;13:150–154.
20. Siegel LS. Human immune response to botulinum pentavalent (ABCDE) toxoid determined by a neutralizing test and by an enzyme-linked immunoabsorbent assay. *J Clin Microbiol* 1988;26:2351–2356.
21. Dressler D, Dirnberger G, Bhatia KP, et al. Botulinum toxin antibody testing: comparison between the mouse protection assay and the mouse lethality assay. *Mov Disord* 2000;15:973–976.
22. Palace J, Nairne A, Hyman N, et al. A radioimmunoprecipitation assay for antibodies to botulinum A. *Neurology* 1998;50:1463–1466.
23. Birklein F, Erbguth F. Sudomotor testing discriminates between subjects with and without antibodies against botulinum toxin A—a preliminary observation. *Mov Disord* 2000;15:146–149.
24. Siatkowski RM, Tyutyunikov A, Biglan AW, et al. Serum antibody production to botulinum A toxin. *Ophthalmology* 1993;100:1861–1866.
25. Notermans S, Nagel J. Assays for botulinum and tetanus toxins. In: Simpson LL, eds. *Botulinum neurotoxin and tetanus toxin.* San Diego, CA: Academic Press, 1989: 319–331.
26. Shone C, Wilton-Smith P, Appleton N, et al. Monoclonal antibody-based immunoassay for type A *Clostridium botulinum* toxin is comparable to the mouse bioassay. *Appl Environ Microbiol* 1985;50:63–67.
27. Aoki KR, Merlino G, Spanoyannis AF, et al. BOTOX (botulinum toxin type A) purified neurotoxin complex prepared from the new bulk toxin retains the same preclinical efficacy as the original but with reduced antigenicity. *Neurology* 1999;52(Suppl 2):A521–A522.
28. Benabou R, Brin MF, Doucette JT. Cervical dystonia: a retrospective study on safety and efficacy of BOTOX lots 79–11 and 2024. *Neurology* 1999;52(Suppl 2): A117–A118.
29. Jankovic J, Davis T, Wooten-Watts M, et al. The Safety of BOTOX (botulinum toxin type A) prepared from new US bulk toxin is comparable to the original in cervical dystonia treatment: a retrospective analysis. *Mov Disord* 2000;15(Suppl 2):31.
30. Halpern JL, Smith LA, Seamon KB, et al. Sequence homology between tetanus and botulinum toxins detected by an antipeptide antibody. *Infect Immun* 1989; 57:13–22.
31. Doellgast GJ, Brown JE, Koufman JA, et al. Sensitive assay for measurement of antibodies to *Clostridium botulinum* toxins A, B, and E: use of hapten-labeled antibody elution to isolate specific complexes. *J Clin Microbiol* 1997;35:578–583.
32. Aoki KR. Preclinical update on BOTOX (botulinum toxin-A)-purified neurotoxin complex relative to other botulinum toxin preparations. *Eur J Neurol* 1999; 6(Suppl 4):S3–S10.
33. Dertzbaugh MT, West MW. Mapping of protective and cross-reactive domains of the type A neurotoxin of *Clostridium botulinum. Vaccine* 1996;14:1538–1544.
34. Brashear A, Lew MF, Dykstra DD, et al. Safety and efficacy of NeuroBloc (botulinum toxin type B) in type

A-responsive cervical dystonia. *Neurology* 1999;53: 1439–1446.

35. Brin MF, Lew MF, Adler CH, et al. Safety and efficacy of NeuroBloc (botulinum toxin type B) in type A-resistant cervical dystonia. *Neurology* 1999;53:1431–1438.

36. Chen R, Karp BI, Hallett M. Botulinum toxin type F for treatment of dystonia: long-term experience. *Neurology* 1998;51:1494–1496.

37. Eleopra R, Tugnoli V, Rossetto O, et al. Botulinum neurotoxin serotype C: a novel effective botulinum toxin therapy in human. *Neurosci Lett* 1997;224:91–94.

38. Houser MK, Sheean GL, Lees AJ. Further studies using higher doses of botulinum toxin type F for torticollis resistant to botulinum toxin type A. *J Neurol Neurosurg Psychiatry* 1998;64:577–580.

39. Lew MF, Adomato BT, Duane DD, et al. Botulinum toxin type B (BotB): a double-blind, placebo-controlled, safety and efficacy study in cervical dystonia. *Neurology* 1997;49:701–707.

40. Truong DD, Cullis PA, O'Brien CF, et al. BotB (botulinum toxin type B): evaluations of safety and tolerability in botulinum toxin type A-resistant cervical dystonia patients (preliminary study). *Mov Disord* 1997;12: 772–775.

41. Mezaki T, Kaji R, Brin MF, et al. Combined use of type A and F botulinum toxins for blepharospasm: a double-blind controlled trial. *Mov Disord* 1999;14:1017–1020.

42. Naumann M, Toyka KV, Taleghani M, et al. Depletion of neutralizing antibodies resensitizes a secondary nonresponder to botulinum A neurotoxin. *J Neurol Neurosurg Psychiatry* 1998;65:924–927.

43. Dressler D, Zettl U, Bigalke H, et al. Can intravenous immunoglobulin improve antibody mediated botulinum toxin therapy failure? *Mov Disord* 2000;15:1279–1281.

44. Duane D, Monroe J, Morris RE. Mycophenolate in the prevention of recurrent neutralizing botulinum toxin A antibodies in cervical dystonia. *Mov Disord* 2000;15: 365–366.

Scientific and Therapeutic Aspects of Botulinum Toxin
edited by M.F. Brin, J. Jankovic, and M. Hallett
Lippincott Williams & Wilkins, Philadelphia, © 2002.

40

Managing Patients with Botulinum Toxin Antibodies

Dirk Dressler

Botulinum toxin (BTX) has been used since 1984 to treat dystonia (1) and various other muscle hyperactivity syndromes (2,3). Generally, results of BTX therapy are so impressive that it is considered the treatment of choice for most of its indications. With BTX consisting of a complex mixture of various proteins, concerns about immune reactions against BTX have been brought up from the very beginning of its therapeutic use. After mouse protection assays (MPA) failed to demonstrate antibodies against BTX in patients receiving BTX therapy for blepharospasm (4,5), it was believed that BTX doses applied, immunoreactivity of target tissues, and other therapy parameters were such that formation of BTX antibodies would not be stimulated. Shortly afterwards, however, the first reports of BTX therapy failure in the presence of BTX antibodies detected by MPA occurred (6). With BTX antibodies potentially blocking BTX's action completely and permanently, thus depriving patients from their most effective therapeutic option, investigations into this problem seem warranted.

Immunologic aspects of BTX treatment have been presented in the preceding two chapters. In this chapter, we review the basic properties of BTX antibodies, as well as methods for their detection. We then investigate the relevance of BTX antibodies with respect to BTX therapy and discuss five possible strategies for managing patients with BTX antibody formation.

WHAT ARE ANTIBODIES AGAINST BOTULINUM TOXIN?

BTX consists of neurotoxin, the protein responsible for BTX's toxic or therapeutic effect, and of a large number of nontoxic proteins (7). All of those proteins are antigens and all of them can trigger formation of corresponding antibodies. For the purpose of this presentation, we concentrate on antibodies against BTX-neurotoxin (BTX-AB) that reduce BTX's toxic and therapeutic action. Thus they are called blocking or neutralizing antibodies. BTX-AB are acting specifically against the different BTX types. We can therefore distinguish antibodies against BTX type A neurotoxin (BTX-A-AB), antibodies against BTX type B neurotoxin (BTX-B-AB), and antibodies against all other BTX neurotoxin types. Whether there are BTX-AB which are not interfering with BTX's toxic and therapeutic action is unknown. It is believed that formation of antibodies against non-toxic proteins can occur. Effects of those antibodies, however, remain unclear at this moment. Distinction between antibodies against BTX neurotoxin and those against non-toxic BTX proteins is crucial for understanding their role in BTX therapy failure.

How can Antibodies Against Botulinum Toxin be Detetcted?

BTX-AB are most frequently detected by animal-based tests. Conventionally, the MPA is used for this purpose (8). The MPA monitors BTX's toxic effect in a mouse population. If a serum sample containing BTX-AB is added to the test system, BTX's toxic effect is reduced, thus increasing the mouse population's survival rate. Up to now, the MPA has been considered the "gold standard" for BTX-AB detection. BTX-AB detected by the MPA are neutralizing, thus false-positive results caused by antibodies directed against nontoxic BTX proteins are unlikely. The MPA requires large quantities of test animals and exposes them to prolonged agony. It takes days before results can be obtained. The parameters of the assay are difficult to control and its results are semiquantitative only. Consequently, the mouse diaphragm assay (MDA) was introduced (9). The MDA monitors BTX's paralyzing effect in a mouse hemidiaphragm preparation by measuring the time between the BTX application and the reduction of the electrically induced twitch force to its half-maximal level. It was demonstrated that there is a linear relationship between the amount of BTX-AB added to the assay and the reduction of the time to reach half-maximal paralysis (9). The MDA reduces mouse consumption substantially and avoids their prolonged agony. Results are quantitative and linear. They become available within a few hours and control of the assay parameters is easier than in the MPA. The MDA has been thoroughly assessed with respect to its quality. Its sensitivity is superior to that of the MPA (10). With these properties the MDA is able to replace the MPA as the gold standard for BTX-AB detection.

BTX-AB can also be detected by immunologic tests. For years, enzyme-linked immunosorbent assays (ELISA) have been tried (11). Because ELISA techniques cannot distinguish between antibodies against BTX-neurotoxin and those directed against nontoxic BTX proteins, low specificity and false-positive results remain a major problem. Additional application of Western blot techniques can solve this problem only partly, as this assay has been shown to be less specific than the MPA (12). ELISA's low sensitivity is an equally unsolved problem. Consequently, ELISA techniques have not been used to study BTX-AB in BTX-therapy failure. Recently, an immunoprecipitation assay (IPA) was introduced (13). Comparison between the MDA and the IPA indicates almost equal sensitivity and specificity of the IPA (14). With the MDA being more sensitive than the MPA and equally specific as the MPA (10), the IPA has advantages over the MPA. This finding was recently confirmed by a direct comparison between the IPA and the MPA (15). Additionally, the IPA

does not employ animals, its results are quantitative, and they become available within a few hours. Its parameters are relatively easy to control. Its costs are moderate, thus allowing large-scale epidemiologic studies.

Another method for BTX-AB detection is patient-based testing. Most of these tests are monitoring motor functions. For the extensor digitorum brevis test (EDB test) (16), electric stimulation of the peroneal nerve and surface electromyographic measurement of the EDB compound muscle action potential before and after BTX application is performed. Unfortunately, this test was not tested in a control population and the optimal BTX doses to produce maximal sensitivity and specificity have not been studied, so that false-positive results occur, especially when higher BTX test doses are applied. The sternocleidomastoid test (SCM test) (17) measures surface electromyographic activity under maximal isometric activation before and after BTX application. This test was assessed in a control population and found to produce quantitative results. Figure 40.1 shows results of the SCM-test in a group of six patients with secondary BTX therapy failure in whom BTX-AB were detected by MPA and MDA. The frowning test or the unilateral brow injection test (UBI test) monitors the function of the frontalis muscle before and after BTX application (15). Although it is qualitative only and its sensitivity and specificity have never been assessed, it has the advantage of being simple and reproducible. This test is described in more detail in Chapter 39. Patient-based tests can also monitor sudomotor functions such as sweating in skin areas injected with BTX, but these tests have not yet been standardized (18). Precise and quantitative BTX-AB detection is complicated and prone to errors. We recommend using BTX-AB tests only when their quality parameters, such as quantification, sensitivity, reproducibility, specificity, and linearity, are assessed properly.

HOW CAN TITERS OF ANTIBODIES AGAINST BOTULINUM TOXIN BE INTERPRETED?

Until recently it was believed that BTX-AB are either present or absent, and that when they are

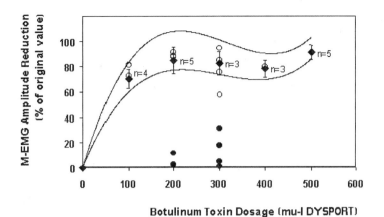

FIG. 40.1. Results of the sternocleidomastoid test in patients with secondary botulinum toxin therapy failure. The diagram shows the relationship between botulinum toxin type A dose and induced reduction of the mean maximal electromyographic amplitude (M-EMG) in the sternocleidomastoid muscle in a group of controls as published before. Diamonds represent the mean values; bars give the doubled standard deviations. Curves are polynomial trend curves ($n = 3$) of the doubled standard deviations. The BTX dose is given in Ipsen mouse units (mu-I). Filled circles show the results of six patients with BTX antibodies on the MDA and MPA. All of their M-EMG reductions fall below the mean value minus the doubled standard deviation of their corresponding controls. Open circles give the results of 11 patients with no BTX antibodies by the MDA and the MPA. Ten of their M-EMG reductions are within the range of the mean value minus the doubled standard deviation of their corresponding controls. The result with a reduced M-EMG reduction is discussed in the text. (From Dressler D, Rothwell JC, Bigalke H. The sternocleidomastoid test: an *in vivo* assay to investigate botulinum toxin antibody formation in man. *J Neurol* 2000;247:630–632, with permission.)

present, they completely abolish BTX's action. About 30% of patients receiving BTX for cervical dystonia with continuing subjective response have evidence of BTX-AB formation when determined by MDA (19). With these results, an all-or-nothing rule for BTX-AB formation and induction of therapy failure seems unlikely. We suggest that the therapeutic effect of BTX depends on a balance between the amount of BTX applied and the amount of BTX-AB blocking it. Interpretation of the relevance of BTX-AB titers with respect to BTX therapy, therefore, becomes necessary. Unfortunately, not much data is available on this topic.

Table 40.1 shows the results of MPA testing and MDA testing in a group of 43 patients with BTX therapy failure. Ten of 11 patients with low-positive, low to intermediate-positive, intermediate to high-positive, and high-positive BTX-AB titers by the MPA had complete therapy failure; one had partial therapy failure. Conversely, 11 of 43 patients with therapy failure tested positive in the MPA. Ten of 24 patients

with complete therapy failure tested positive in the MPA; 12 tested negative. One of 19 patients with partial secondary therapy failure tested positive in the MPA and 18 tested negative. In summary, positive MPA testing is usually associated with complete therapy failure, whereas fewer than half of the patients with complete therapy failure test positive in the MPA. Low sensitivity of the MPA seems to be a likely explanation for this finding.

In the same group, 27 of 43 patients with BTX therapy failure tested positive in the MDA. Of eight patients with MDA titers below 0.0007 U, six had partial and two had complete therapy failure. Of six patients with MDA titers between 0.0008 and 0.002 U, four had complete and two had partial therapy failure. Of nine patients with MDA titers above 0.002 U, eight had complete and one had partial therapy failure. In another group of 33 patients with continued sensitivity to long-term BTX therapy (19), 12 tested positive on MDA. Seven had MDA titers below 0.0007 U, four had MDA titers between 0.008

TABLE 40.1. *Comparison of the titers of antibodies against botulinum toxin as measured by the mouse diaphragm assay (MDA) and the mouse protection assay (MPA). MDA results are reported in U*

Case	MDA	MPA	CO
A. Concordant results: MDA-positive, MPA-positive			
1a	0.01	hp	cstf
1b	0.01	hp	cstf
2	0.01	hp	cstf
3	0.01	hp	cstf
4	0.01	i/hp	cstf
5	0.01	i/hp	cstf
6	0.01	lp	cstf
7	0.0065	hp	pstf
4	0.0036	i/hp	cstf
8	0.001	l/ip	cstf
9	0.0009	lp	cstf
B. Discordant results: MDA-positive, MPA-negative			
6	0.01	n	cstf
9	0.006	n	cstf
10	0.006	n	cstf
11	0.0025	n	pstf
12	0.002	n	cstf
13	0.0017	n	pstf
14	0.0015	n	cstf
15	0.0015	n	pstf
16	0.0007	n	pstf
17	0.0006	n	pstf
18	0.0004	n	pstf
19	0.0004	n	pstf
20	0.0004	n	pptf
21	0.0003	n	cstf
22	0.0003	n	cstf
23	0.0003	n	pstf
C. Concordant results: MDA-negative, MPA-negative			
24	n	n	pstf
24	n	n	pstf
25	n	n	cstf
26	n	n	cstf
27	n	n	cstf
28	n	n	cstf
29	n	n	cstf
30	n	n	pstf
31	n	n	pstf
32	n	n	cstf
33	n	n	pstf
34	n	n	pstf
35	n	n	pstf
36	n	n	pptf
37	n	n	cstf
38	n	n	pstf

CO, clinical outcome of botulinum toxin therapy; cstf, complete secondary botulinum toxin therapy failure; hp, high-positive; i/hp, intermediate to high-positive; l/ip, low to intermediate-positive; lp, low-positive; n, negative; pptf, partial primary botulinum toxin therapy failure; pstf, partial secondary botulinum toxin therapy failure.

From Dressler D, Dirnberger G, Bhatia K, et al. Botulinum toxin antibody testing: comparison between the mouse diaphragm bioassay and the mouse lethality bioassay. *Mov Disord* 2000;15:973–976, with permission.

and 0.002 U, and one had MDA titers above 0.002 U. In summary, the MDA is more sensitive than the MPA. MDA titers above 0.002 U are likely to produce BTX therapy failure, MDA titers below 0.0007 U are unlikely to produce BTX therapy failure, and if so, BTX therapy failure is usually partial. MDA titers between 0.008 and 0.002 U may or may not produce BTX therapy failure.

For practical purposes we suggest the following guidelines: positive MPA testing is indicative of BTX-AB induced therapy failure, negative MPA testing does not exclude it. MDA titers above 0.002 U are indicative of BTX-AB induced therapy failure. MDA titers below 0.0007 U are unlikely to produce therapy failure and MDA titers in between are not contributory. High MPA and MDA titers should be repeated for confirmation before patients are excluded from further BTX therapy. Low and intermediate MDA titers should be repeated for titer movements during the further course of the treatment. Where possible, more than one BTX-AB test system should be applied. From our experience, a combination of MDA and SCM tests seems helpful. It is hoped that inexpensive and properly validated tests will soon be available for clinical practice.

Another approach to correlate BTX-AB with secondary therapy failure is analysis of its clinical presentation. We examined 27 patients with BTX-AB associated complete secondary therapy failure (20). In 81% of patients, complete secondary therapy failure was preceded by partial therapy failure equally affecting the extent and the duration of the therapeutic effect. Partial therapy failure became evident on average 2.5 treatment visits before complete therapy failure occurred. Complete therapy failure was seen after latencies between the first and last treatment of around 320 days; the longest period was 2,341 days.

Before deciding whether secondary therapy failure is caused by BTX-AB formation, it is important to exclude other causes of BTX therapy failure (21). Although marked exacerbation of previously stable dystonia is unlikely, there can be exogenous fluctuations caused by psychological or physical stress, or by drug interactions. Psychological factors influencing the patient's perception of the therapy outcome include "honeymoon" effects and high expectation. Occasionally, technical problems, especially changes of the injecting physician or difficulties with the injection technique, can cause therapy failure.

CAN ANTIBODIES AGAINST BOTULINUM TOXIN DISAPPEAR SPONTANEOUSLY?

When BTX-AB titers were first detected, it was hoped that after cessation of BTX application BTX-AB titers would gradually decrease and patients would become sensitive again to BTX therapy in a foreseeable period of time. The hope that a short "drug holiday" might be sufficient to regain sensitivity mainly stemmed from observations made during military immunization programs when BTX-AB titers provoked by attenuated pentavalent botulinum toxoid vanished in about half of the subjects after 1 year (22).

In an initial study, seven patients with BTX-AB in the MPA were retested with the MDA at random intervals. In all seven patients, no BTX-AB could be detected after intervals of 10 to 78 months (23). In a recently published study, the time course of BTX-AB titers after cessation of BTX therapy was followed by MDA in 12 patients (24). Figure 40.2 shows the results of this study. Eight of 12 BTX-AB titers tested decreased. In three of the eight, a decrease could be detected after about 500 to 1,000 days, and in five, it could be detected after about 1,500 to 1,750 days. After 1,250 to 2,250 days, all of the decreasing BTX-AB titers fell below 0.002 U, where complete therapy failure is unlikely. Five BTX-AB titers did not decrease. Their monitoring periods were 761, 1,409, 1,533, 2,423, and 2,427 days. These results indicate that about two-thirds of BTX-AB titers decrease. However, it will take at least around 3 years before BTX-AB titers decrease to levels where sensitivity to BTX therapy may be regained. About one-third of the BTX-AB titers do not decrease despite prolonged cessation of BTX therapy. Whether

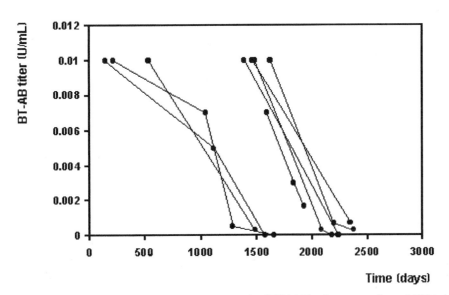

FIG. 40.2. Titers of antibodies against botulinum toxin (BTX-AB) after cessation of BTX therapy. Eight BTX-AB titers decreased. Their decrease could be detected in three cases after about 500 to 1,000 days and in five cases after about 1,500 to 1,750 days. After between 1,250 and 2,250 days, all of the decreasing BTX-AB titers fell below a level of 0.002 U where complete secondary therapy failure is unlikely. Five BTX-AB did not decrease. Their monitoring periods were 761, 1,409, 1,533, 2,423 and 2,427 days. (From Dressler D, Bigalke H. Botulinum toxin antibody titres after cessation of botulinum toxin therapy. *Mov Disord* 2002;17:170–173, with permission.)

and when those BTX-AB titers will eventually decrease remains open.

With these prolonged latencies, a useful BTX therapy cannot be maintained. Whether re-initiation of BTX therapy after decrease of BTX-AB titers will induce reincrease of BTX-AB titers has not been studied with sensitive BTX-AB tests. Re-initiation of BTX therapy using an alternative serotype or using improved BTX preparations with lower antigenicity might offer a second chance to those patients.

CAN ANTIBODIES AGAINST BOTULINUM TOXIN BE OVERCOME BY INCREASED BOTULINUM TOXIN DOSES?

Assuming a functional balance between BTX-AB and BTX applied, one possible strategy to overcome antibody induced therapy failure could be the application of increased BTX doses. This hypothesis was recently tested (25). Eight patients with cervical dystonia and antibody-induced therapy failure, as indicated by appropriate BTX-AB titers in the MDA, received various BTX test doses of DYDPORT injected into one of their sternocleidomastoid muscles. Test doses were increased in three steps at three monthly intervals, and their effect on the amplitude of the electromyographic activity of the sternocleidomastoid muscle under maximal isometric activation (M-EMG) was measured and compared to a control group. In step 1 [200 or 300 mouse units (mu)], the M-EMG reduction was $12 \pm 13\%$ compared to $85 \pm 10\%$ (200 mu) and $83 \pm 9\%$ (300 mu) in the control group. In step 2 (400, 600, or 800 mu), the M-EMG reduction was $25 \pm 21\%$ compared to $78 \pm 7\%$ (400 mu) in the control group. In step 3 (1,600 or 1,800 mu), the M-EMG reduction was $24 \pm 10\%$. Side effects were not observed in any of the patients studied. In one patient with partial secondary therapy failure, with a low BTX-AB titer (0.0015 U) and with a moderately pathologic M-EMG reduction (40% with 200 mu), a normal M-EMG reduction of 71% could be regained with 800 mu. In three subsequent therapeutic injection series with quadrupled BTX doses in all target muscles, the original therapy outcome could be regained and maintained. Side effects or increasing BTX-AB titers were not observed. Figure 40.3 summarizes the M-EMG

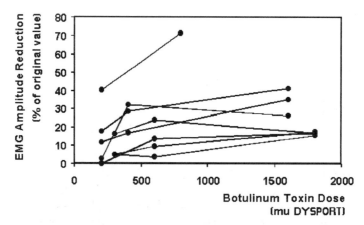

FIG. 40.3. Botulinum toxin (BTX)-induced reduction of the electromyographic amplitude produced by maximal isometric sternocleidomastoid activation (M-EMG amplitude reduction) (35). All M-EMG amplitude reductions induced by 200 and 300 mu DYSPORT were at least two standard deviations below the mean M-EMG amplitude reductions induced by the same BTX dose in a control group. All M-EMG amplitude reductions induced by more than 300 mu DYSPORT were—with one exception—less than those seen with average therapeutic BTX doses in a control group. In the exceptional patient, a BTX dose of 800 mu DYSPORT induced an M-EMG reduction of 71%, which is similar to those induced by average therapeutic BTX doses in a control group. (From Dressler D, Muenchau A, Bigalke H. Antibody-induced botulinum toxin therapy failure: can it be overcome by increased botulinum toxin doses? *Eur Neurol* 2002;47:118–121, with permission.)

reductions after the different BTX dosages for all subjects tested.

Even massively increased BTX doses cannot overcome BTX-AB-induced complete secondary therapy failure. However, in patients with partial secondary therapy failure, low BTX-AB titers and a moderately pathologic M-EMG reduction, increased BTX doses might regain and maintain normal BTX efficacy without induction of side effects or increasing BTX-AB titers.

CAN ANTIBODIES AGAINST BOTULINUM TOXIN BE OVERCOME BY USING DIFFERENT BOTULINUM TOXIN SEROTYPES OR BY USING DIFFERENT BOTULINUM TOXIN PREPARATIONS?

BTX for therapeutic purposes is commercially available as BOTOX, DYSPORT, and MYOBLOC or NeuroBloc. Although both BOTOX and DYSPORT are based on BTX type A (BTX-A) they differ slightly in their stabilizing compounds. Because of different manufacturing processes, the proportion of biologically active to biologically inactive BTX differs between both preparations. With recent changes in the manufacturing process of BOTOX, those differences became marginal. No formal study is available at the moment to test whether BTX-A-AB might affect BOTOX and DYSPORT differently. With both preparations using BTX-A, BTX-A-AB should affect both preparations in the same way. In five patients with BTX-A-AB induced therapy failure, exchange between BOTOX and DYSPORT did not produce different therapeutic effects (Dressler, unpublished observations).

MYOBLOC or NeuroBloc is based on BTX type B (BTX-B). Initial studies indicate that BTX-A-AB do not interfere with the therapeutic action of this preparation (26). However, because of high structural similarity to BTX-A, BTX-B can also be expected to stimulate BTX-AB formation. With therapeutic doses of BTX-B being substantially higher than those of BTX-A, the amount of potentially antigenic proteins, and therefore the intrinsic risk of BTX-AB formation, might be higher for BTX-B than for BTX-A. Studies testing this hypothesis, however, have not yet been performed. Additionally, patients whose immune system is already sensitized to produce BTX-A-AB, might be more prone to produce BTX-B-AB. Some years ago, BTX type F (BTX-F) was successfully tried in patients with BTX-A-AB (27,28). Again, some patients developed BTX-F-AB during further treatment (28).

CAN ANTIBODIES AGAINST BOTULINUM TOXIN BE DEPLETED OR INACTIVATED?

Depletion of BTX-AB by plasma exchange and subsequent IgG immunoadsorption on a protein A column was recently tried successfully in a single case (29). After MDA testing could no longer detect BTX-AB, BTX therapy was re-administered and produced its original therapeutic benefit. Over a period of 15 months this procedure remained successful. Whether the repeated BTX applications will eventually stimulate BTX-AB formation to the point that this procedure will no longer be able to successfully deplete BTX-AB needs further studying. In addition, the procedure described is complicated, potentially risky, and expensive so that it will remain reserved for severe cases only.

Another possible method for depletion or inactivation of BTX-AB is the application of intravenous immunoglobulin (IVIg). However, when it was given in five single doses of 35 g, equivalent to 4.5 g/kg body weight every second day, no BTX-AB reduction in the MDA and no BTX-AB inactivation was detected (30).

Another possible strategy to reduce BTX-AB titers is application of immunosuppressants. No formal study has been performed for this purpose yet. Six patients with BTX-AB–induced complete secondary therapy failure received oral steroids 5 days before BTX application but did not improve their therapeutic response as monitored by quantitative electromyography (Dressler, unpublished observation). Recently, mycophenolate was used to suppress re-occurrence of BTX-AB formation (31). Whether this compound can also be used to reduce BTX-AB titers needs to be studied.

CAN FORMATION OF ANTIBODIES AGAINST BOTULINUM TOXIN BE PREVENTED?

Because management of BTX-AB formation is apparently difficult, prevention of BTX-AB formation is of paramount importance. To prevent BTX-AB formation, its risk factors need to be identified. In an initial study, treatment parameters of eight patients with secondary therapy failure were compared to a control group (32). Although it did not become clear how many of those patients actually had BTX-AB formation, group comparison suggested a shorter interinjection interval, a larger number of booster injections, and higher BTX doses per injection series in patients with BTX therapy failure. In another study, 20 patients with evidence of BTX-AB formation in the MPA were compared to a control group (33). There were significant differences between both groups for age of onset of dystonia, BTX dose per injection series, and cumulative BTX dose. Number of injection series and treatment time were not different. Demographic parameters, such as gender, age at onset of therapy, and duration of symptoms, were not different. Using a multivariate analysis as an improved statistical method, dose per injection series and interinjection intervals were confirmed as independent risk factors (34). Number of booster injections, cumulative BTX dose, and age at onset of dystonia, however, were excluded as independent risk factors. Additional factors, such as gender, age at onset of therapy, duration of symptoms, and treatment time were studied, but could not be identified as independent risk factors. Other possible risk factors, especially the reactivity of the individual patient's immune system, might play an important role, but needs further studying.

Avoidance of BTX-AB formation is of paramount importance. BTX therapy should, therefore, only be applied with long inter-injection intervals and the lowest BTX dose possible. The exact relationship between those risk factors and the actual risk of an individual patient as well as other possible risk factors need to determined.

Managing patients with BTX-AB is a highly complex task. It takes special expertise and leaves the physician with a high responsibility. Further studies are needed to develop the most efficient strategy.

ACKNOWLEDGMENTS

The author is grateful for financial support from The Dystonia Society, London, UK.

REFERENCES

1. Frueh BR, Felt DP, Wojno TH, et al. Treatment of blepharospasm with botulinum toxin. A preliminary report. *Arch Ophthalmol* 1984;102:1464–1468.
2. Jankovic J, Hallett M, eds. *Therapy with botulinum toxin.* New York: Marcel Dekker, 1994.
3. Dressler D. *Botulinum toxin Therapy.* Stuttgart: Thieme-Verlag, 2000.
4. Biglan AW, Gonnering R, Lockhart LB, et al. Absence of antibody production in patients treated with botulinum A toxin. *Am J Ophthalmol* 1986;101:232–235.
5. Gonnering RS. Negative antibody response to long-term treatment of facial spasm with botulinum toxin. *Am J Ophthalmol* 1988;105:313–315.
6. Zuber M, Sebald M, Bathien N, et al. Botulinum antibodies in dystonic patients treated with type A botulinum toxin: frequency and significance. *Neurology* 1993; 43:1715–1718.
7. DasGupta BR. Structures of botulinum neurotoxin, its functional domains, and perspectives on the crystalline type A toxin. In: Jankovic J, Hallett M, eds. *Therapy with botulinum toxin.* New York: Marcel Dekker, 1994: 15–40.
8. Pearce LB, Borodic GE, First ER, et al. Measurement of botulinum toxin activity: evaluation of the lethality assay. *Toxicol Appl Pharmacol* 1994;128:69–77.
9. Goeschel H, Wohlfahrt K, Frevert J, et al. Botulinum A toxin: neutralizing and nonneutralizing antibodies—therapeutic consequences. *Exp Neurol* 1997;147: 96–102.
10. Dressler D, Dirnberger G, Bhatia K, et al. Botulinum toxin antibody testing: comparison between the mouse diaphragm bioassay and the mouse lethality bioassay. *Mov Disord* 2000;15:973–976.
11. Notermans S, Nagel J. Assays for botulinum and tetanus toxins. In: Simpson LL, ed. *Botulinum neurotoxin and tetanus toxin.* San Diego, CA: Academic Press, 2000: 319–331.
12. Hanna PA, Jankovic J. Mouse bioassay versus Western blot assay for botulinum toxin antibodies: correlation with clinical response. *Neurology* 1998;50:1624–1629.
13. Palace J, Nairne A, Hyman N, et al. A radioimmunoprecipitation assay for antibodies to botulinum A. *Neurology* 1998;50:1463–1466.
14. Dressler D, Dirnberger G. Botulinum toxin antibody testing: comparison between an immunoprecipitation assay and the mouse diaphragm assay. *Eur Neurol* 2001; 45:257–260.
15. Hanna PA, Jankovic J, Vincent A. Comparison of mouse bioassay and immunoprecipitation assay for botulinum toxin antibodies. *J Neurol Neurosurg Psychiatry* 1998;

66:612–616 (correction: *J Neurol Neurosurg Psychiatry* 1999;67:133).

16. Kessler KR, Benecke R. The EBD test—a clinical test for the detection of antibodies to botulinum toxin type A. *Mov Disord* 1997;12:95–99.

17. Dressler D, Rothwell JC, Bigalke H. The sternocleidomastoid test: an *in vivo* assay to investigate botulinum toxin antibody formation in man. *J Neurol* 2000;247: 630–632.

18. Braune C, Erbguth F, Birklein F. Dose thresholds and duration of the local anhidrotic effect of botulinum toxin injections: measured by sudometry. *Br J Dermatol* 2001; 144:111–117.

19. Wittstock M, Benecke R, Bigalke H, et al. Quantitative antibody status of patients with continued sensitivity to long-term botulinum toxin therapy. *Neurology* 2001; 56(Suppl 3):A347.

20. Dressler D. Clinical features of secondary failure of botulinum toxin therapy. *Eur Neurol* (*In press*).

21. Dressler D. Botulinum toxin therapy failure: causes, evaluation procedures and management strategies. *Eur J Neurol* 1997;4(Suppl 2):S67–S70.

22. Siegel LS. Human immune response to botulinum pentavalent (ABCDE) toxoid determined by a neutralization test and by an enzyme-linked immunosorbent assay. *J Clin Microbiol* 1988;26:2351–2356.

23. Sankhla C, Jankovic J, Duane D. Variability of the immunologic and clinical response in dystonic patients immunoresistant to botulinum toxin injections. *Mov Disord* 1998;13:150–154.

24. Dressler D, Bigalke H. Botulinum toxin antibody titres after cessation of botulinum toxin therapy. *Mov Disord* 2002;17:170–173.

25. Dressler D, Muenchau A, Bigalke H. Antibody-induced botulinum toxin therapy failure: can it be overcome by increased botulinum toxin doses? *Eur Neurol* 2002;47: 118–121.

26. Brin MF, Lew MF, Adler CH, et al. Safety and efficacy of NeuroBloc (botulinum toxin type B) in type A-resistant cervical dystonia. *Neurology* 1999;53:1431–1438.

27. Chen R, Karp BI, Hallett M. Botulinum toxin type F for treatment of dystonia: long-term experience. *Neurology* 1998;51:1494–1496.

28. Houser MK, Sheean GL, Lees AJ. Further studies using higher doses of botulinum toxin type F for torticollis resistant to botulinum toxin type A. *J Neurol Neurosurg Psychiatry* 1998;64:577–580.

29. Naumann M, Toyka KV, Mansouri Taleghani B, et al. Depletion of neutralising antibodies resensitises a secondary non-responder to botulinum A neurotoxin. *J Neurol Neurosurg Psychiatry* 1998;65:924–927.

30. Dressler D, Zettl U, Benecke R, et al. Can intravenous immunoglobulin improve antibody-mediated botulinum toxin therapy failure? *Mov Disord* 2000;15:1279–1281.

31. Duane DD, Monroe J, Morris RE. Mycophenolate in the prevention of recurrent neutralizing botulinum toxin A antibodies in cervical dystonia. *Mov Disord* 2000;15: 365–366.

32. Greene P, Fahn S, Diamond B. Development of resistance to botulinum toxin type A in patients with torticollis. *Mov Disord* 1994;9:213–217.

33. Jankovic J, Schwartz K. Response and immunoresistance to botulinum toxin injections. *Neurology* 1995;45: 1743–1746.

34. Dressler D, Dirnberger G. Antibody induced botulinum toxin therapy failure: Analysis of risk factors. *Neurology* (*In press*).

35. Dressler D, Rothwell JC. Electromyographic quantification of the paralysing effect of botulinum toxin. *Eur Neurol* 2000;43:13–16.

Scientific and Therapeutic Aspects of Botulinum Toxin
edited by M.F. Brin, J. Jankovic, and M. Hallett
Lippincott Williams & Wilkins, Philadelphia, © 2002.

41

Vaccines for Preventing Botulism

Leonard A. Smith and Michael P. Byrne

Botulism is a severe and often-fatal disease marked by flaccid paralysis prior to respiratory failure and/or cardiac arrest. The term "botulism," derived from the Latin *botulus* (sausage), was first introduced in 1870 to describe a fatal food-poisoning syndrome associated with consumption of sausage. In 1895, van Ermengem (University of Ghent) isolated an obligatory anaerobic, endospore-forming bacillus from a ham implicated in the historic outbreak of botulism in Ellezelles, Belgium. The same microbe was also isolated from the spleen of a victim that succumbed to the disease. Culture filtrates of the bacterium induced characteristic and often-fatal paralysis when injected into laboratory animals (1). The substance in the culture filtrates was subsequently shown to be a protein toxin (type A). In 1904, another outbreak of botulism occurred in Darmstadt (2), resulting in 11 fatalities. In this case, contaminated wax beans, rather than meat, were implicated in the outbreak, and the toxin was immunologically distinct from that isolated previously in Ellezelles (3). It soon became apparent that a host of different foods (fish, meat, vegetables, fruit) when improperly preserved afforded a suitable environment for the gram-positive Eubacterium *Clostridium botulinum* to grow and produce potent neurotoxin(s). Today, we know that *C. botulinum* is widely distributed in soil and aquatic environments throughout the world. The various strains of *C. botulinum* produce seven antigenically distinct exotoxins, the sole causative agents of botulism. With an estimated human lethal dose as low as 1 ng/kg body weight (4,5), the botulinum toxins are the most potent of all known substances. The toxins (designated A through G) can be distin-

guished serologically by neutralizing antitoxin (6).

Four classes of botulism are now recognized according to the site of toxin production: (a) Classic foodborne botulism is the most prevalent and results from ingestion of preformed toxin in improperly preserved foodstuffs. (b) Infant botulism (7) most frequently occurs in infants 2 to 3 months old, and originates from the ingestion of *C. botulinum* spores, colonization in the gut lumen, and subsequent *in vivo* production of toxin. (c) Wound botulism (8) emerges from local tissue infection and *in situ* toxin production of the bacterium. (d) The fourth category of botulism reflects those incidents emanating from an undetermined origin, or not easily categorized, or resulting from the use of the toxin(s) in a biowarfare or bioterrorist action.

Botulinum neurotoxins (BoNT) are initially synthesized as 150-kDa, single-polypeptide chain, precursor proteins that are posttranslationally nicked forming a di-chain consisting of a C-terminal 100-kDa heavy chain and a N-terminal 50-kDa light chain. The di-chain remains covalently attached by a disulfide link (9,10) but the extent of nicking varies from completely nicked (serotype A) to completely unnicked (serotype E) (Fig. 41.1). The mechanism of nerve intoxication is accomplished through the interplay of three key events, each of which is performed by a separate portion of the neurotoxin molecule (see references 11–13 for reviews). First, the carboxy half of the heavy chain (fragment C or H_C) is required for receptor-specific binding to cholinergic nerve cells (14–16). After binding, the toxin is internalized into an endosome through receptor-mediated endocyto-

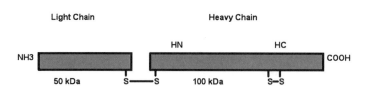

FIG. 41.1. Diagram of BoNT primary structures. Protease nicking site distinguishes between the light and heavy chains, which remain covalently associated by a disulfide link.

sis (17,18). The amino-terminal half of the heavy chain (H_N) presumably participates in translocation of the light chain across the endosomal membrane (19–23). The final event of intoxication involves catalytic hydrolysis of key synaptic vesicle proteins (24–27) by the light chain (24,28). The light chains are zinc-dependent endoproteases that selectively inactivate three essential proteins involved in the docking and fusion of acetylcholine-containing synaptic vesicles to the plasma membrane. The light chains of BoNT serotypes A, C1, and E cleave SNAP-25 (synaptosomal-associated protein of 25 kDa) (29–32); serotypes B, D, F, and G cleave vesicle-associated membrane protein (VAMP, also known as synaptobrevin) (33); and serotype C1 cleaves syntaxin (34). Inactivation of SNAP-25, VAMP, or syntaxin by BoNT prevents the nerve cells from releasing acetylcholine, resulting in neuromuscular paralysis.

Incubation periods for foodborne botulism are reportedly as short as 6 hours or as long as 10 days (35). Generally, the time between toxin ingestion and onset of symptoms ranges from 18 to 36 hours (36). Among those intoxicated by foodborne botulism, incubation periods are shorter for those with illness caused by type E (36). The incubation periods for wound botulism are longer (about 4 to 14 days) than those normally seen in cases of foodborne botulism, and probably reflect the time required for multiplication of *C. botulinum* in the wound and release of toxin. In general, the rapidity of onset and severity of botulism depends upon the amount of toxin entering the circulatory system, locating its target site, and arresting the release of neurotransmitter at motor endplates.

Clinical manifestations of botulism reflect the functional disturbance and blockade of the voluntary motor and autonomic cholinergic junctions. Symmetric cranial nerve palsies affecting the bulbar musculature frequently mark the onset of symptoms such as ptosis, amblyopia and/or blurred vision, dysphonia, and a dry, sore throat. Flaccid paralysis of the pharyngeal and laryngeal muscles gives rise to dysphagia and dysarthria. If botulism is a consequence of ingesting improperly preserved foodstuffs contaminated with bacteria and their preformed toxins, nausea, abdominal pain, vomiting, and diarrhea may often precede or accompany the neurologic indications. As the disease progresses, a descending paralysis ensues in which muscles of the neck, extremities, trunk and respiratory mechanism are affected. Paralysis of the respiratory muscles, leading to dyspnea and asphyxiation, is usually the cause of death in botulism.

BONT TOXOID VACCINES

The development of vaccines to protect against botulism has been investigated since the late 1930s. Similar to the case with diphtheria and tetanus toxins, a toxoid vaccine produces an immune response capable of neutralizing the biologic activity of botulinum toxins (37). The potential use of botulinum toxin(s) as biologic warfare agents has necessitated the development of protective modalities against this potential weapon of mass destruction. Research initially conducted on a toxoid vaccine against serotypes A and B toxins at the US Army's installation at Fort Detrick, Maryland, during the early 1940s led to the development of a pentavalent botulinum toxoid (PBT). Currently, this toxoid, protective against serotypes A through E (38–41), is used to vaccinate specific populations of at-risk individuals, i.e., scientists and health care providers who handle BoNT, and members of the armed forces, who may be subjected to weaponized forms of the toxin. The manufacture of PBT by the Michigan Department of Public Health (MDPH) took place in stages and over many years. The fermentation conditions, purification of toxins, and detoxification steps for each serotype took place in the late 1960s and early 1970s. The toxoid was manufactured by initially culturing *C. botulinum* serotypes A to E to produce crude neurotoxin preparations. Toxins were separated from the culture fluid by acid precipitation overnight in the cold, and then separated from the supernatant fluid by filtration and/or centrifugation. The precipitated toxin was washed, extracted, and filtered to remove any particulate material. Toxins were again precipitated, filter sterilized, and detoxified by adding formalin. Residual formalin was left in the vaccine products to ensure that the neurotoxins remained nontoxic. Monovalent vaccines were then adsorbed to aluminum hydroxide and blended into a pentavalent vaccine. The monovalent bulks were completed in 1971, and first packaged in 1978. Investigational new drug (IND) status was granted for the PBT under the Centers for Disease Control's IND 161 (at-risk workers) and under the US Army's Office of Surgeon General IND 3723 (for military deployment). The MDPH product was studied and used as an investigational vaccine from 1979 until the present time.

Since 1996, there has been an ongoing effort on the part of the US Army to obtain Food and Drug Administration (FDA) licensure for the PBT lots PBP003 and PBP004. For licensure of the PBT, FDA required (a) that a clinical trial be performed to reevaluate safety and assess immunogenicity of the toxoid, and (b) that a new lot of toxoid be manufactured to demonstrate reproducibility and robustness of the manufacturing process, and consistency of the manufactured product. From 1970–1994, more than 14,000 doses of the PBT vaccine were administered to at-risk persons who were subsequently observed for adverse reactions. Data gathered during that period demonstrated an acceptable level of reactogenicity. However, immunogenicity data in humans have been limited. Most human immunogenicity data had been for serotype A. In compliance with FDA requirements, MDS Harris, Inc., under contract with the US

Army, conducted a clinical trial (360 participants) to evaluate the efficacy of the vaccine for all five toxin serotypes represented in the PBT. Efficacy was demonstrated by correlating toxin-neutralizing antibody titers in humans vaccinated with PBT with titers of passively vaccinated guinea pigs protected against lethal aerosol challenge with each of five BoNT serotypes. It was hoped that 80% of the study group would have titers indicating protection from an aerosol challenge of 25 LCt_{50} for all five serotypes of toxin. Results from the clinical study demonstrated that PBT vaccine under the tested vaccination schedule of 1, 15, 85, and 183 days (primary series) did not produce the aspired protection levels for all serotypes.

We raise two concerns regarding this clinical trial. First, the study was conducted with vaccine that was manufactured in the 1970s. Perhaps the potency of the vaccine would have been higher if the vaccine had been manufactured more recently. The second concern relates to the level of protection required from the participants in the clinical study. The question to ask was whether the target level for protection was too high to be achieved by this, or any, vaccine. Presumably, the exposure levels for an ''at-risk'' worker is expected to be much lower than for a soldier imperiled from a battlefield assault with BoNT. What level of protection is required for the soldier is very difficult to ascertain and a continuing question. Future development of the PBT will depend on the status of a new-generation recombinant vaccine.

Although serotypes A, B, and E are most associated with botulism outbreaks in humans, type F has also been reported (42–44). A separate monovalent toxoid vaccine against BoNT-F (45) was manufactured for the US Army by Porton Products Limited in cooperation with the United Kingdom Governments Center for Applied Microbiology and Research (CAMR) in 1990. The vaccine batch #002/90 was derived from pooling three production lots of *C. botulinum* F toxin. The harvested toxin (i.e., by acid precipitation, tangential flow filtration, and centrifugation) from each of three fermentation runs was pooled, and the type F toxin extracted with sodium phosphate buffer. After ribonuclease treatment, the toxin was further purified by ammonium sulfate precipitation, and repeated fractionation on fast liquid-column chromatography on a fast-flow Q Sepharose column. Unlike the toxoid (estimated toxoid purity of 10%) (41), the purity of the type F botulinum toxoid Lot #002/90 was greater than 60% pure (IND 5077). The partially purified F toxin was formalin-detoxified and adsorbed to aluminum hydroxide.

In April 1993, an IND application to conduct a phase I clinical trial to evaluate the safety of the botulinum F toxoid vaccine was filed with the FDA. The clinical study was conducted by the Medical Division at the US Army Medical Research Institute of Infectious Diseases under IND 5077. The toxoid was well-tolerated in all of the 35 participants receiving the vaccine. Immunogenicity data gathered on sera from vaccine recipients demonstrated that two doses (10 μg per dose) produced an antibody response considered protective by the CDC guidelines (a titer greater than 0.02 IU/mL). Ninety percent (18/20) of the volunteers seroconverted after two vaccinations and 100% (10/10) after three vaccinations (46).

A phase II clinical trial was conducted under IND 5077 at the University of Maryland Medical School (Baltimore, MD) over 3 years (1995–1998) in 144 healthy adult volunteers. The phase II trial was conducted to expand the limited Army phase I trial and to identify a vaccination schedule that was safe and maximally immunogenic for volunteers. All participants in the study groups received 10 μg per dose of vaccine. Study group A received vaccine by subcutaneous (SC) administration on 0, 7, and 28 days; group B SC on 0, 14, and 42 days; and groups C, D, and E on 0, 21, and 42 days. The CDE groups were divided into three groups: (a) those receiving the F toxoid vaccine intramuscularly (IM), (b) vaccination with toxoid F vaccine by SC route, and (c) a hepatitis B vaccine (HBV) IM control. The clinical protocol included a booster injection 12 months postprimary series if titers fell below 0.10 IU/mL after 6 months. The SC and IM routes of vaccine administration were similarly immunogenic. The longer primary vaccination schedules (0, 14, 42 vs 0, 21,

42) were also similarly immunogenic. Both 42-day schedules were more immunogenic than the 28-day schedule. The *C. botulinum* type F toxoid was generally well-tolerated and safe whether injected SC or IM. The *C. botulinum* type F toxoid induced significantly more immediate pain on injection than did the licensed hepatitis B vaccine control, although the pain was transient and tolerated (Dr. Robert Edelman, personal communication).

Immunologic response indicated that 61% to 83% of the study subjects met the criteria for a booster dose at 1 year because of their low antitoxin levels (i.e., less than 0.10 IU/mL) at 6 months. One hundred percent of the subjects boosted at 1 year developed high concentrations of protective antitoxin by day 56 postboost, and protective levels (greater than 0.02 IU/mL) persisted for at least 360 days in all subjects (Dr. Robert Edelman, personal communication).

Even though toxoid vaccines are available, there are numerous shortcomings with their current use and ease of production. First, because *C. botulinum* is a spore-former, a dedicated facility is required to manufacture a toxin-based product. The requirement for a dedicated manufacturing facility is not trivial. It is extremely costly to renovate and upgrade an existing facility or to build a new one and then to maintain the facility in accordance with current good manufacturing practices to manufacture one vaccine. Second, the yields of toxin production from *C. botulinum* are relatively low. Third, the toxoiding process involves handling large quantities of toxin and thus is dangerous. Added safety precautions increase the cost of manufacturing. Fourth, the toxoid product for types A to E consists of a crude extract of clostridial proteins that may influence immunogenicity or reactivity of the vaccine, and the type F toxoid is only partially purified (IND 5077). Fifth, because the toxoiding process involves formaldehyde, which inactivates the toxin, and residual levels of formaldehyde (not to exceed 0.02%) are part of the product formulation to prevent reactivation of the toxin, the vaccine is reactogenic. An additional component of the toxoid vaccine is a thimerosal (0.01%) preservative, which also increases product reactogenicity.

Development of a new-generation, recombinant vaccine could alleviate many of the associated toxoid problems. A recombinant vaccine would eliminate the need for a dedicated manufacturing facility. There are many current good manufacturing practices facilities in existence and available that could manufacture a recombinant product. There would be no need to culture large quantities of hazardous, toxin-producing bacteria. Production yields from a genetically engineered product are expected to be high. Presumably, there would be no need for formalin if the recombinant vaccine candidate represented a nontoxic fragment of the toxin. A fragment would not possess all three functional domains (i.e., binding, internalization, catalytic) which are all required for biologic action. Recombinant products would be purer, less reactogenic, and more fully characterized. Thus, the cost of a recombinant product would be expected to be much lower than a toxoid because there would be no expenditures required to support a dedicated facility, and the higher production yields would reduce product cost.

RECOMBINANT VACCINES AGAINST BONT

In 1984, Helting and Nau (47) demonstrated that protein fragments generated from papain-digested tetanus neurotoxin (TeNT) elicited protective immunity in mice. A few years later, Fairweather and coworkers (48) showed that partially purified recombinant C fragment from tetanus toxin [rTeNT(H_C)] protected mice when challenged with 10 LD_{50} of tetanus toxin. Because of the high sequence and structural homology that exists between the clostridial neurotoxins produced by *C. tetani* and *C. botulinum*, we applied this strategy to developing a vaccine to protect against botulism.

We demonstrated early on that we could subclone segments of the BoNT-A gene and express these nontoxic fragments in *Escherichia coli* (49). We were then able to vaccinate mice with the nontoxic recombinants and test their ability to elicit protective immunity *in vivo*. Clones pCBA2, pCBA3, and pCBA4 (gift from Nigel Minton) containing overlapping gene fragments

of the BoNT-A gene (50) were the templates used to produce the various antigens. Smaller versions of the gene fragments were constructed via restriction enzyme cleavage. Specific gene segments were produced by polymerase chain reactions (PCR). Expressed products were identified by sodium dodecyl sulfate-polyacrylamide gel electrophoresis (SDS-PAGE) and Western blot analyses, partially purified, and used to vaccinate mice. Antigens representing various regions from the three functional domains of the toxin were analyzed for their ability to elicit protective antibodies in mice. Of all the fragments we and others (51–53) tested, only one was able to completely protect mice. This was the fragment located at the carboxy-terminus of the toxin (~50 kDa) designated as the fragment C region. Our subsequent efforts to develop vaccine candidates to protect against BoNT forthwith focused exclusively on the H_C region.

DESIGN OF SYNTHETIC BONT(H_C) GENES AND PRODUCTION IN PICHIA PASTORIS

The yeast strain *Pichia pastoris,* originally developed by the Phillips Petroleum Company (Bartlesville, OK), was chosen as a host because of the high level of recombinant expression exhibited by this system with other proteins (54–57). Clare and coworkers (58) reported yields of 12 g/L of TeNT(H_C) when expressed in *P. pastoris.* Using *P. pastoris* would also eliminate the potential problems associated with inclusion bodies formed during expression in *E. coli,* as well as the need to remove endotoxin.

Because of rare codons (59) and high adenine and thymine (A + T)-rich base compositions (60) found in the naturally occurring clostridial DNA, it was necessary to construct synthetic genes (56,58,60) to eliminate these impediments to optimal expression in heterologous expression systems such as *E. coli* and yeast. We prepared synthetic genes for the H_C of BoNT with codon usage specified by highly expressed genes in *E. coli* and yeast. Genes designed and constructed with *E. coli* codon usage (61) expressed full-length products in both *E. coli* and *P. pastoris,* while genes designed and constructed with

P. pastoris codon usage (62) likewise expressed proteins with the expected molecular mass in both hosts.

Synthetic genes were inserted into the yeast expression vector pHILD4 (Phillips Petroleum Company) for intracellular expression. The expression cassette was integrated into the alcohol oxidase gene of *P. pastoris* strain GS115 (58). Yeast transformants expressing the selectable markers, histidine dehydrogenase (63) and aminoglycoside phosphotransferase 3′ I (64), were isolated. Clones were assessed by their ability to express recombinant proteins with expected molecular masses as judged by SDS-PAGE and Western blot analysis. Positive clones were selected for growth in a fermentation reactor under the control of methanol induction. The fermentation process consisted of three phases: a batch phase in which *Pichia* cells grew exclusively on glycerol, followed by a fed-batch phase of decreasing glycerol, and, finally, a fed-batch phase of increasing methanol. Typically, the methanol induction phase was 10 to 70 hours depending on the antigen, yielding a final cell mass of approximately 60 g dry cell weight per liter of fermentation broth.

Manufacturing processes to include fermentation, cell harvesting, cell lysis, product capture, and downstream purification streams were developed for rBoNT-A(H_C) (65–67), rBoNT-B(H_C) (68), rBoNT-C1(H_C) (69), and rBoNT-F(H_C) (70). Purification strategies relied on scalable ionic exchange and hydrophobic chromatographic techniques to produce highly purified vaccine products. Because C-fragments lack catalytic activity and any distinguishing chromophores, purity and identity of the H_C throughout the process development were monitored by SDS-PAGE and immunologic [Western blot and enzyme-linked immunoassay (ELISA)] detection methods. Recombinant products were judged to be greater than 98% pure as detected by SDS-PAGE and their yields were generally 200 to 500 mg/kg of cells wet weight. A typical cell yield (i.e., wet cell weight) from a 30-L bioreactor was 6 kg of wet cell mass. Currently, recombinant (H_C) vaccines are being developed for serotypes E, D, and G toxins.

POTENCY, EFFICACY, AND ELISA OF BONT (H_C)

With any vaccine, the most important question is, how safe and efficacious is the product? In our laboratory and others, many studies have been performed addressing this question, primarily using mice as the animal model, but studies have been performed in nonhuman primates as well (71). In general, the BoNT(H_C) are remarkably efficacious antigens. For example, mice vaccinated with as little as 1 μg of BoNT(H_C) were fully protected when challenged with as much as 10^6 mouse LD_{50} of BoNT-B (49). Mice vaccinated with three doses of vaccine remain protected against a challenge of 10^6 mouse LD_{50} of BoNT-B 12 months postvaccination. Similar long-term protection was also observed in mice for the A serotype vaccine (unpublished data).

One of the most important analyses of a drug product is a potency test. Potency is the specific ability or capacity of the product, as indicated by appropriate laboratory tests or by adequately controlled clinical data obtained through the administration of the product in the manner intended, to effect the given result. The potency assay should be relevant to its intended use, which for a vaccine, is the ability to elicit protective immunity against disease. The potency assay (65,68) developed to measure the strength of rBoNT(H_c) vaccines employs a mouse bioassay. Vaccine adsorbed to an aluminum hydroxide (0.2% Alhydrogel) adjuvant was administered as a single IM injection to seven groups of mice (ten mice per group for statistical relevance), at doses varying from submicrogram (2.4 ng) to microgram (10 μg) amounts. Three weeks postvaccination, the mice were actively challenged with 10^3 mouse LD_{50} of neurotoxin by intraperitoneal (IP) injection. Figure 41.2 summarizes the potency results for H_C serotypes A, B, C1, and F. Each antigen yielded a dose-response curve liberating ED_{50} values ranging from 0.089 to 0.25 μg/mouse. Full protection was realized at a single vaccine dose of 2 μg/mouse with each serotype except F, where nine of ten survived a 10^3 LD_{50} toxin challenge.

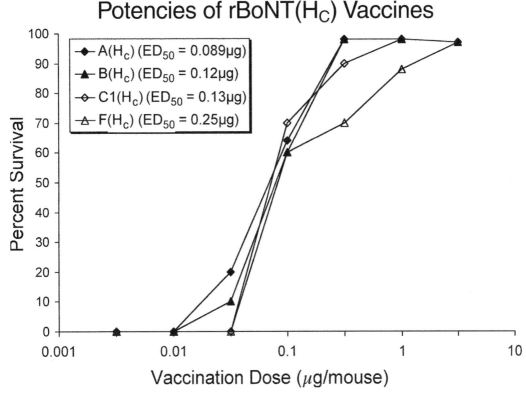

Potencies of rBoNT(H$_C$) Vaccines

Legend:
- ◆ A(H$_C$) (ED$_{50}$ = 0.089µg)
- ▲ B(H$_C$) (ED$_{50}$ = 0.12µg)
- ◇ C1(H$_C$) (ED$_{50}$ = 0.13µg)
- △ F(H$_C$) (ED$_{50}$ = 0.25µg)

X-axis: Vaccination Dose (µg/mouse)
Y-axis: Percent Survival

FIG. 41.2. Dependence of mouse survival on a single dose of purified H$_C$. Mice [10 Cr1:CD-(ICR) per group] were challenged with 10^3 IP LD$_{50}$ of BoNT toxin 21 days after vaccination.

An efficacy study provides a thorough analysis of the protective effectiveness of an antigen and can be performed in a variety of manners. Antigen dose, number of vaccinations, and challenge levels are the three primary parameters that can be investigated individually in an efficacy study. Generally, any two of these parameters can vary in a given study. For example, animals can be offered a range of antigen doses and then challenged with increasing amounts of toxin (e.g., 10^3, 10^4, and 10^5 LD$_{50}$), keeping the number of vaccinations constant. Our procedure usually varied antigen dose and number of vaccinations while subjecting the animals to a con-

TABLE 41.1. *Efficacy of rBoNT(H$_C$) vaccines*

Vaccination dose (µg)	% Survival[a] A(H$_C$) Number of vaccinations			% Survival[b] B(H$_C$) Number of vaccinations		
	1X	2X	3X	1X	2X	3X
0.01	0	60	50	0	17	58
0.1	20	50	90	33	83	100
0.5	40	90	100	ND	ND	ND
1.0	70	100	100	67	100	100
2.0	80	100	100	ND	ND	ND
5.0	ND[c]	ND	ND	100	100	100

[a]Each group consisted of ten mice [Cr1:CD-1(ICR)], which were all challenged with 10^5 mouse LD$_{50}$ BoNT-A.
[b]Each group consisted of 12 mice [Cr1:CD-1(ICR)], which were all challenged with 10^5 mouse LD$_{50}$ BoNT-B.
[c]ND, value not determined.

stant high level challenge. Table 41.1 presents the protective efficacy results for H_C serotypes A and B. The data clearly reveal that protection increases with increasing number of vaccinations. With three vaccinations of only 0.1 μg, 9 of 10 mice (serotype A) and 12 out of 12 mice (serotype B) survived a challenge of 10^5 LD_{50} of toxin. Standardized efficacy protocols to provide information on short- and long-term immunity elicited by the $C1(H_C)$ and $F(H_C)$ vaccines are currently in progress.

Human vaccine efficacy is normally addressed by performing clinical trials in locations where the incidence of disease is predictable and is sufficient to measure a statistically significant reduction in the number of cases of disease. However, the limited and unpredictable appearance of botulism cases does not allow for the identification of a candidate study population to evaluate the efficacy of a BoNT vaccine by any route of exposure. There is no possibility of a clinical trial where controlled challenge studies could be conducted with a lethal substance in an ethical manner. The ethical and practical obstacles to obtaining direct evidence of human efficacy of a BoNT vaccine led to the development of a human correlate of clinical efficacy for the PBT. An FDA advisory panel, in addressing efficacy issues for bacterial vaccines and toxoids, made the following statement (Federal Register, 1985 [72]): "For diseases in which immunity depends upon specific antibodies which either neutralize toxin or which opsonize bacteria and lead to their prompt destruction within phago-

cytes, induction of such antibodies correlates well with protection, and the measurement of such antibodies may reflect efficacy quite faithfully."

For a BoNT vaccine, it is necessary that a correlation be made between the antibodies elicited by the vaccine and their ability to neutralize active toxin. This is accomplished by taking serial dilutions of sera from vaccinated animals, mixing the sera with a constant amount of toxin, and injecting the mixture back into other animals (e.g., mice). The number of neutralizing antibodies can be determined by the survival rate of the animals used in the test. By definition, 1 international unit (IU) of antitoxin neutralizes 10^4 mouse IP LD_{50} of toxin. There are variations to this neutralization assay that can be more tedious but more indicative of protective efficacy. After antibodies are purified from the sera of vaccinated animals and assayed, they are administered passively to other animals, those animals are then challenged with a known quantity of active toxin by a specified route of delivery (e.g., by aerosol), and the survival rate observed.

We routinely performed mouse neutralization assays on serum samples derived from the recombinant BoNT vaccine efficacy studies to show the correlation between antibody production and toxin neutralization (Table 41.2). Additionally, we have assay development studies ongoing to determine the correlation between an immunologic response detected by ELISA as compared to the mouse neutralization assay. ELISA is, in most cases, an effective and suita-

TABLE 41.2. *Antibody ELISA titers and serum neutralization titers of mice after vaccination with rBoNT(H_C)*

Vaccination dose (μg)	BoNT serotype A(H_C)						BoNT serotype B(H_C)					
	Antibody ELISA titers[a] No. vaccinations			Serum neutralization titers[b] No. vaccinations			Antibody ELISA titers[a] No. vaccinations			Serum neutralization titers[b] No. vaccinations		
	1X	2X	3X	1X	2X	3X	1X	2X	3X	1X	2X	3X
0.01	400	1600	1600	<0.16	<0.16	0.49	100	1600	25600	<0.10	<0.10	0.76
0.1	400	1600	25600	<0.16	0.40	26.62	1600	25600	100000	0.18	0.62	4.23
0.5	400	640	25600	<0.21	1.28	13.31	ND	ND	ND	ND	ND	ND
1.0	1600	6400	25600	<0.16	1.28	33.55	6400	25600	100000	0.48	1.52	13.66
2.0	1600	25600	102400	<0.16	13.31	33.55	ND	ND	ND	ND	ND	ND
5.0	ND[c]	ND	ND	ND	ND	ND	25600	100000	100000	0.99	3.69	12.50

[a] Pooled mouse serum (50 μL per mouse) from each group was initially diluted 1:100, then fourfold for serum ELISA titers. Titer is reciprocal of the highest dilution having an OD_{405} greater than 0.2 AU after correcting for background. [b] Pooled mouse serum (50 μL per mouse) from each group was initially diluted 1:8, then fourfold for serum neutralization titers in units of IU/mL. [c] ND, value not determined.

ble means to analyze immunologic responses to antigens. We have developed a host of ELISAs aimed at detecting BoNT and BoNT fragments for determining serum and neutralization titers of vaccinated animals, for identifying which purification fractions contain product, and for measuring product at various stages of a purification process. Perhaps the greatest benefit an ELISA can provide, however, is the reduced use of animals during product development and evaluation. If there exists a high correlation between protection and serum titer, then titers can be used as an alternative to actively challenging mice with toxin. Serum ELISA titers measure the total antibody response to a given antigen. It does not measure the antibodies responsible for toxin neutralization.

Table 41.2 summarizes the serum ELISA titers and serum-neutralizing antibody results of the same mice that were used in the efficacy study described above for H_C serotypes A and B. The data depicted in Table 41.2 represent pooled serum from each animal within the group. Although we observed a correlation between survival and group ELISA titer data, a significantly higher correlation between survival and individual serum ELISA titers existed. For serotype A(H_C), 82 of 83 mice with titers =1,600 (65) survived toxin challenge; similarly, for serotype F(H_C), all 34 mice with titers =100 (70) survived toxin challenge.

REGULATORY ISSUES AND REQUIREMENTS

The time and cost in developing prophylactic and therapeutic drugs destined for human use are substantial. For this reason, it is critical to know and understand the guidance documents and regulatory issues put forth from one's regulatory agency early in the discovery phase of the product. Title 21 of US Code of Federal Regulations (73) states the purpose of good manufacturing practices is "to assure that all pharmaceutical, biologic, diagnostic, and medical device products meet all of the requirements of the Federal Food, Drug, and Cosmetic Act as to safety, and efficacy and have the identity and strength to meet the quality and purity characteristics which

they purport to have." The expectation from FDA is that a recombinant vaccine shall be well-characterized in terms of its purity, identity, efficacy, potency, consistency, stability, and, most importantly, its safety.

The goal of a manufacturing process is to produce an adequate predetermined quantity of product at a predetermined level of quality (i.e., a product that meets rigorous acceptance criteria for purity, identity, efficacy, potency, consistency, stability, and safety). Because traditional biologic products (including vaccines) are prepared from biologic sources that exhibit inherent biologic variability, the ability of a manufacturer to prepare a safe product consistently and reproducibly is a concern. In-line processing data or in-process testing provide information that the manufacturing process is consistent and reproducible. If the process is consistent and reproducible, there is a high probability the product will be of the same high quality each time it is manufactured.

Much of our work over the past 4 years has been devoted to developing scaled-up manufacturing processes for each H_C vaccine, and the in-process and lot release testing to validate the product's quality. Detail information on assay development and assay validation, genetic characterization of clones, in-process and lot release testing, product stability testing (e.g., real-time, reconstituted, and accelerated stability), and formulation studies on the vaccine candidates are beyond the scope of this review and are not provided. However, it should be realized that extensive testing must be performed on the products if the products are to be well-characterized and allowed into clinical trials.

ACKNOWLEDGMENTS

The authors thank Theresa Smith, Vickie Montgomery, and Matthew Hinz for performing potency, efficacy, and ELISA experiments.

REFERENCES

1. van Ermengen E. Ueber eainen neuren anaeroben Bacillus und seine Beziehungen zum Botilismus. *Z Hyg Infektionskrankh* 1897;26:1–56.

2. Landmann G. Ueber die Ursache der Darmstadter Boh-nenvergiftung. *Hyg Rundschau* 1904;14:449–452.

3. Leuchs J.Beitrage zur Kenntnis des Toxins and Antitox-ins des Bacillus botulinus. *Z Hyg Infektionskrankh* 1910; 65:55–84.

4. Lamanna C. The most poisonous poison. *Science* 1959; 130:763–772.

5. Gill DM. Bacterial toxins: a table of lethal amounts. *Microbiol Rev* 1982;46:86–94.

6. Hatheway CL. *Clostridium botulinum* and other clos-tridia that produce botulinum neurotoxins. In: Hauschild AHW, Dodds KL, eds. *Clostridium botulinum—ecol-ogy and control in foods.* New York: Marcel Dekker, 1992:3–10.

7. Midura TF, Arnon SS. Infant botulism: identification of *Clostridium botulinum* and its toxin in faeces. *Lancet* 1976;2:934–936.

8. Davis JB, Mattman LH, Wiley M. *Clostridium botuli-num* in a fatal wound infection. *JAMA* 1951;146: 646–648.

9. DasGupta BR, Sugiyama H. A common subunit struc-ture in *Clostridium botulinum* type A, B, and E toxins. *Biochem Biophys Res Commun* 1972;48:108–112.

10. DasGupta BR. The structure of botulinum neurotoxins. In: Simpson LL, ed. *Botulinum neurotoxin and tetanus toxin.* New York: Academic Press, 1989:53–67.

11. Montecucco C, Schiavo G. Mechanism of action of teta-nus and botulinum neurotoxins. *Mol Microbiol* 1994; 13:1–8.

12. Montecucco C, Papini E, Schiavo G. Bacterial protein toxins penetrate cells via a four-step mechanism. *FEBS Lett* 1994;346:92–98.

13. Halpern JL, Neale EA. Neurospecific binding, internali-zation, and retrograde axonal transport. In: Montecucco C, ed. *Current topics in microbiology and immunology, clostridial neurotoxins: the molecular pathogenesis of tetanus and botulism.* Berlin: Springer, 1995:221–241.

14. Black JD, Dolly O. Interaction of ^{125}I-botulinum neuro-toxins with nerve terminals. I. Ultrastructural autoradio-graphic localization and quantitation of distinct mem-brane acceptors for types A and B on motor nerves. *J Cell Biol* 1986;103:521–534.

15. Nishiki T-I, Kamata Y, Nemoto Y, et al. Identification of protein receptor for *Clostridium botulinum* type B neurotoxin in rat brain synaptosomes. *J Biol Chem* 1994; 269:10498–10503.

16. Shone CC, Hambleton P, Melling J. Inactivation of *Clostridium botulinum* type A neurotoxin by trypsin and purification of two tryptic fragments. Proteolytic action near the COOH-terminus of the heavy subunit destroys toxin-binding activity. *Eur J Biochem* 1985;151:75–82.

17. Shone CC, Hambleton P, Melling J. A 50-kDa fragment from the NH$_2$-terminus of the heavy subunit of *Clostrid-ium botulinum* type A neurotoxin forms channels in lipid vesicles. *Eur J Biochem* 1987;167:175–180.

18. Black JD, Dolly JO. Interaction of ^{125}I-labelled botuli-num neurotoxins with nerve terminals. II. Autoradio-graphic evidence for its uptake into motor nerves by acceptor-mediated endocytosis. *J Cell Biol* 1986;103: 535–544.

19. Simpson LL. Molecular pharmacology of botulinum toxin and tetanus toxin. *Ann Rev Pharmacol Toxicol* 1986;26:427–453.

20. Poulain B, Mochida S, Weller U, et al. Heterologous combinations of heavy and light chains from botulinum

21. neurotoxin A and tetanus toxin inhibit neurotransmitter release in aplysia. *J Biol Chem* 1991;266:9580–9585.

21. Montal MS, Blewitt R, Tomich JM, et al. Identification of an ion channel-forming motif in the primary structure of tetanus and botulinum neurotoxins. *FEBS Lett* 1992; 313:12–18.

22. Schmid MF, Robinson JP, DasGupta BR. Direct visual-ization of botulinum neurotoxin-induced channels in phospholipid vesicles. *Nature* 1993;364:827–830.

23. Lebeda FJ, Singh BR. Membrane channel activity and translocation of botulinum and tetanus neurotoxins. *J Toxicol Toxin Revs* 1999;18:45–76.

24. Schiavo G, Benfenati F, Poulain B, et al. Tetanus and botulinum-B neurotoxins block neurotransmitter release by proteolytic cleavage of synaptobrevin. *Nature* 1992; 359:832–835.

25. Oguma K, Fujinaga Y, Inoue K. Structure and function of *Clostridium botulinum* toxins. *Microbiol Immunol* 1995;39:161–168.

26. Schiavo G, Rossetto O, Catsicas S, et al. Identification of the nerve terminal targets of botulinum neurotoxin serotypes A, D, and E. *J Biol Chem* 1993;268: 23784–23787.

27. Shone CC, Quinn CP, Wait R, et al. Proteolytic cleavage of synthetic fragments of vesicle-associated membrane protein, isoform-2 by botulinum type B neurotoxin. *Eur J Biochem* 1993;217:965–971.

28. Schiavo G, Poulain B, Rossetto O, et al. Tetanus toxin is a zinc protein and its inhibition of neurotransmitter release and protease activity depend on zinc. *EMBO J* 1992;11:3577–3583.

29. Blasi J, Chapman ER, Link E, et al. Botulinum neuro-toxin A selectively cleaves the synaptic protein SNAP-25. *Nature* 1993;365:160–163.

30. Schiavo G, Sabtucci A, DasGupta BR, et al. Botulinum neurotoxin serotypes A and E cleave SNAP-25 at dis-tinct COOH-terminal peptide bonds. *FEBS Lett* 1993; 335:99–103.

31. Binz T, Blasi J, Yamasaki S, et al. Proteolysis of SNAP-25 by types E and A botulinal neurotoxins. *J Biol Chem* 1994;269:1617–1620.

32. Foran P, Lawrence GW, Shone CC, et al. Botulinum neurotoxin C1 cleaves both syntaxin and SNAP-25 in intact and permeabilized chromaffin cells: correlation with its blockade of catecholamine release. *Biochemis-try* 1996;35:2630–2636.

33. Niemann H, Blasi J, Jahn R. Clostridial neurotoxins: new tools for dissecting exocytosis. *Trends Cell Biol* 1994;4:179–185.

34. Blasi J, Chapman ER, Yamaski S, et al. Botulinum neu-rotoxin C1 blocks neurotransmitter release by means of cleaving HPC1/syntaxin. *EMBO J* 1993;12:4821–4828.

35. St. Louis ME, Peck SH, Bowering D, et al. Botulism from chopped garlic: delayed recognition of a major outbreak. *Ann Intern Med* 1988;108:363–368.

36. Woodruff BA, Griffin PM, McCroskey LM, et al. Clini-cal and laboratory comparison of botulism from toxin types A, B, and E in the United States 1978–1988. *J Infect Dis* 1992;166:1281–1286.

37. Reames HR, Kadull PJ, Housewright RD, et al. Studies on botulinum toxoids, types A and B III. Immunization in man. *J Immunol* 1947;55:309–324.

38. Anderson JH, Lewis GE. Clinical evaluation of botuli-num toxoids. In: Lewis GE, ed. *Biomedical aspects of botulism.* New York: Academic Press, 1981:233–246.

39. Ellis RJ. *Immunobiologic agents and drugs available from the Centers for Disease Control. Descriptions, recommendations, adverse reactions, and serologic response, 3rd ed.* Atlanta, GA: Centers for Disease Control, 1982.

40. Fiock MA, Cardella MA, Gearinger NF. Studies of immunities to toxins of *Clostridium botulinum*. IX. Immunologic response of man to purified pentavalent ABCDE botulinum toxoid. *J Immunol* 1963;90:697–702.

41. Siegel LS. Human immune response to botulinum pentavalent (ABCDE) toxoid determined by a neutralization test and by an enzyme-linked immunosorbent assay. *J Clin Microbiol* 1988;26:2351–2356.

42. Midura TF, Nygaard GS, Wood RM, et al. *Clostridium botulinum* type F: isolation from venison jerky. *Appl Microbiol* 1972;24:165–167.

43. Green J, Spear H, Brinson RR. Human botulism (type F)—a rare type. *Am J Med* 1983;75:893–895.

44. Sonnabend WF, Sonnabend OA, Grundler P, et al. Intestinal toxicoinfection by *Clostridium botulinum* type F in an adult. Case associated with Guillain-Barré syndrome. *Lancet* 1987;1:357–361.

45. Hatheway CL. Toxoid of *Clostridium botulinum* type F: purification and immunogenicity studies. *Appl Environ Microbiol* 1976;31:234–242.

46. Montgomery VA, Makuch RS, Brown JE, et al. The immunogenicity in humans of a botulinum type F vaccine. *Vaccine* 2000;18:728–735.

47. Helting TB, Nau HH. Analysis of the immune response to papain digestion products of tetanus toxin. *Acta Pathol Microbiol Scand Section C* 1984;92:59–63.

48. Fairweather NF, Lyness VA, Maskell DJ. Immunization of mice against tetanus with fragments of tetanus toxin synthesized in Escherichia coli. *Infect Immun* 1987;55:2541–2545.

49. Smith LA. Development of recombinant vaccines for botulinum neurotoxin. *Toxicon* 1998;36:1539–1548.

50. Thompson DE, Brehm JK, Oultram JD, et al. The complete amino acid sequence of the *Clostridium botulinum* type A neurotoxin, deduced by nucleotide sequence analysis of the encoding gene. *Eur J Biochem* 1990;189:73–81.

51. LaPenotiere HF, Clayton MA, Middlebrook JL. Expression of a large, nontoxic fragment of botulinum neurotoxin serotype A and its use as an immunogen. *Toxicon* 1995;33:1383–1386.

52. Clayton MA, Clayton JM, Brown DR, et al. Protective vaccination with a recombinant fragment of *Clostridium botulinum* neurotoxin serotype A expressed from a synthetic gene in *Escherichia coli*. *Infect Immun* 1995;63:2738–2742.

53. Dertzbaugh MT, West MW. Mapping of protective and cross-reactive domains of the type A neurotoxin of *Clostridium botulinum*. *Vaccine* 1996;14:1538–1544.

54. Cregg JM, Tschopp JF, Stillman C, et al. High-level expression and efficient assembly of hepatitis B surface antigen in the methylotrophic yeast, *Pichia pastoris*. *Biotechnology* 1987;5:479–485.

55. Sreekrishna K, Potenz RHB, Cruze JA, et al. High-level expression of heterologous proteins in methylotrophic yeast *Pichia pastoris*. *J Bas Microbiol* 1988;28:265–278.

56. Romanos MA, Scorer CA, Clare JJ. Foreign gene expression in yeast: a review. *Yeast* 1992;8:423:488.

57. Cregg JM, Vedvick TS, Raschke WC. Recent advances in the expression of foreign genes in *Pichia pastoris*. *Biotechnology* 1993;11:905–909.

58. Clare JJ, Rayment FB, Ballantine SP, et al. High-level expression of tetanus toxin fragment C in *Pichia pastoris* strains containing multiple tandem integrations of the gene. *Biotechnology* 1991;9:455–460.

59. Makoff AJ, Oxer MD, Romanos MA, et al. Expression of tetanus toxin fragment C in *E. coli*: high-level expression by removing rare codons. *Nucleic Acids Res* 1989;17:10191–10202.

60. Romanos MA, Makoff AJ, Fairweather NF, et al. Expression of tetanus toxin fragment C in yeast: gene synthesis is required to eliminate fortuitous polyadenylation sites in AT-rich DNA. *Nucleic Acids Res* 1991;19:1461–1467.

61. Anderson SGE, Kurland CG. Codon preferences in free-living microorganisms. *Microbiol Rev* 1990;54:198–210.

62. Sreekrishna K. Strategies for optimizing protein expression and secretion I the methylotrophic yeast *Pichia pastoris*. In: Baltz RH, Hegeman GD, Skatrud PL, eds. *Industrial microorganisms: basic and applied molecular genetics*. Washington, DC: American Society for Microbiology, 1993:119–126.

63. Cregg JM, Barringer KJ, Hessler AY, et al. *Pichia pastoris* as a host system for transformations. *Mol Cell Biol* 1985;5:3376–3385.

64. Scorer CA, Clare JJ, McCombie WR, et al. Rapid selection using G418 of high copy number transformants of *Pichia pastoris* for high-level foreign gene expression. *Biotechnology* 1994;12:181–184.

65. Byrne MP, Smith TJ, Montgomery VA, et al. Purification, potency, and efficacy of the botulinum neurotoxin type A binding domain from *Pichia pastoris* as a recombinant vaccine candidate. *Infect Immun* 1998;66:4817–4822 .

66. Zhang W, Bevins MA, Plantz BA, et al. Modeling *Pichia pastoris* growth on methanol and optimizing the production of a recombinant protein, the heavy-chain fragment C of botulinum neurotoxin, serotype A. *Biotechnol Bioeng* 2000;70:1–8.

67. Potter KA, Zhang W, Smith LA, et al. Production and purification of the heavy chain fragment C of botulinum neurotoxin, serotype A, expressed in the methylotrophic yeast *Pichia pastoris*. *Prot Exp Purif* 2000;19:393–402.

68. Potter KJ, Bevins MA, Vassilieva EV, et al. Production and purification of heavy chain fragment C of botulinum neurotoxin, serotype B, expressed in the methylotropic yeast *Pichia pastoris*. *J Prot Expr Purif* 1998;13:357–365.

69. Byrne MP, Smith LA. Development of vaccines for prevention of botulism. *Biochimie* 2000;82:955–966.

70. Byrne MP, Holley J, Titball R, et al. Expression, purification and efficacy of a recombinant vaccine candidate against botulinum neurotoxin type F from *Pichia pastoris*. *J Prot Expr Purif* 2000;18:327–337.

71. Boles JW, West MW, Montgomery VA, et al. Efficacy of recombinant C fragment of heavy chain botulinum neurotoxin serotype B against lethal aerosol challenge of botulinum B toxin in rhesus monkeys. *Toxicologist* 2000;54:174(abstr 817A).

72. Biologic Products; Bacterial Vaccines and Toxoids; Implementation of Efficacy Review. Proposed Rules. p. 51006–51007.

73. Title 21, USCFR, Part 210.1. Status of current goal manufacturing practice regulations.

OTHER SEROTYPES AND CHEMODENERVATING AGENTS

Scientific and Therapeutic Aspects of Botulinum Toxin
edited by M.F. Brin, J. Jankovic, and M. Hallett
Lippincott Williams & Wilkins, Philadelphia, © 2002.

42

Botulinum Neurotoxin Serotypes C and E: Clinical Trials

Roberto Eleopra, Valeria Tugnoli, Rocco Quatrale, Ornella Rossetto,
Cesare Montecucco, and Domenico De Grandis

Botulinum neurotoxins (BoNTs) are metalloproteases specific for protein components of the neuroexocytosis machinery. They act by inducing a neuromuscular block of cholinergic fibers of the peripheral nervous system (1,2). Seven serotypes of BoNT have been identified so far, and are indicated with the letters from A to G. The large majority of outbreaks of human botulism are caused by intoxication with botulinum toxin type A, B, or E (BoNT-A, BoNT-B, BoNT-E) (3). BoNTs act in the neuronal cytosol by preventing the synaptosomal vesicles fusion: in particular, BoNT-A, BoNT-C, and BoNT-E cleave the same protein, synaptosomal-associated protein of 25 kDa (SNAP-25); BoNT-C additionally cleaves syntaxin (1,2).

The injection of BoNT-A in muscles of subjects affected by focal dystonia is now considered a useful therapy (4–12). Selected neuromuscular junctions are blocked for many weeks, followed by a progressive and slow recovery of function, which can again be paralyzed by a second injection. However, an increasing number of patients not responsive to this treatment are being identified in clinical practice. The absence of clinical response after the first treatment (primary nonresponders) or after the following injections (secondary nonresponders) could be the consequence of an immune response mechanism caused by the production of specific anti–BoNT-A antibodies (13–18). In both cases, the problem can be overcome by using different BoNT serotypes (19–22).

Botulinum toxins type F and B have been tested in humans. The beneficial effects of type F are of rather short time duration with respect to BoNT-A, lasting 5 to 8 weeks (23,24). The duration of action of BoNT-B is 12 to 16 weeks at doses normally used for cervical dystonia (25–28).

Botulinum toxin type C is unique among the various BoNTs because it cleaves two different intracytoplasmic SNARE proteins: SNAP-25 and syntaxin. [SNARE is an acronym for soluble NSF (N-ethylmaleimide–sensitive factor) attachment receptor.] Moreover, BoNT-E and BoNT-A share their intracellular target protein. Both cleave SNAP-25 and remove nine amino acid residues (BoNT-A) or 26 amino acid residues (BoNT-E) from the carboxyl-terminus (1,2).

Hence, BoNT-E and BoNT-C are expected to cause an inhibition of acetylcholine release, followed by recovery of function with a time course closely similar to that caused by BoNT-A, because they act upon the same cytosolic target protein (SNAP-25).

Therefore, we decided to test BoNT-E and BoNT-C in humans in order to find valuable alternatives to BoNT-A when an immune resistance was proved. Our study was divided into three different parts, although a successful result of the first study was considered necessary to start with the subsequent ones.

Study A: At the beginning, a population of voluntary normal subjects was tested for BoNT-A, BoNT-E, and BoNT-C ''sensitivity'' using a simple electrophysiologic measure (CMAP amplitude variation) in the extensor digitorum brevis (EDB) muscle of the foot, in order to verify in humans the extent of the neuromuscular blockade induced and the temporal profile of the functional recovery.

Study B: After the selection of the best BoNT serotype with a temporal profile similar to that of BoNT-A, we tested its safety in humans on motor neuron (MN) cell survival by quantification using the Motor Unit Number Estimate (MUNE) technique.

Study C: Finally, we injected the best alternative BoNT serotype in nonresponder subjects affected by focal dystonia to evaluate the clinical response. We also evaluated the effect of repetitive treatments.

STUDY A

To address the issue of human sensitivity to BoNT-C and BoNT-E with respect to that of BoNT-A, we used the CMAP amplitude variation after BoNT injection in EDB muscle, because standard needle electrode investigation, such as concentric-needle or single-fiber electromyogram, although confirming the effect of the BoNTs, are unable to quantify the extent of its action in an absolute mode. With this experimental technique, an objective quantification and comparison of the blockade induced by the different BoNT types can be obtained. Moreover, there is general consensus that this electrophysiologic analysis provides a reliable evaluation of neuromuscular function (29–33).

All patients examined entered the study voluntarily and provided their informed consent to the present research, which was previously approved by the local ethics committee. The results of these preliminary studies were published in 1997 and 1998 (34,35).

In our studies, 26 voluntary subjects affected by facial dystonia and never treated before with any kind of BoNTs were examined. Fifteen subjects were evaluated by comparing BoNT-A with BoNT-C. Another 11 patients were compared for their response to BoNT-A and BoNT-E.

In each subject, we injected 3 IU of BoNT-A (BOTOX) in 0.1 mL of saline solution in one EDB muscle of the foot and 3 IU of BoNT-C or BoNT-E in the contralateral one.

BoNT-C and BoNT-E were obtained from WAKO (Japan); in addition, they were trypsin activated, purified, and tested as previously described (36). The BoNTs were prepared for injections in a 0.1-mL of phosphate-buffered saline (PBS) containing 2% human serum albumin.

In both groups, the neuromuscular blockade induced in the EDB muscles was quantified by the electrophysiologic evaluation of the CMAP peak-to-peak amplitude elicited by the supramaximal electrical stimulation of the peroneal nerve at the ankle before and after 7, 15, 30, 45, 60, and 90 days from injections.

Electrical stimulation was performed with a single pulse of 0.5 msec, delivered in a random pattern, at low frequency, with supramaximal intensity. The recording electrode placement was the same for each patient, using similar environmental conditions, at the same time of the day and after control of the skin temperature. Moreover, the CMAP percentage variation (%CMAP) by a comparison of the value with the CMAP at baseline was analyzed. Therefore, a %CMAP mean value (%CMAPm) for all the subjects injected with the same BoNT serotype was calculated on the different days.

In all the subjects studied, the maximal neuromuscular blockade was detected after 7 days from injection for all the serotypes analyzed. Figure 42.1 shows that, surprisingly, the muscles blocked with BoNT-E recovered faster than those poisoned with BoNT-A. On the contrary, the recovery following BoNT-C intoxication had a time course similar to that of BoNT-A.

To understand the unexpected differences in the extent of neuromuscular paralysis caused by BoNT-A and BoNT-E, evident from the thirtieth day onward, we examined another group of seven voluntary subjects by injecting a mixture of the two BoNT serotypes (4 IU of BoNT-A plus 2 IU of BoNT-E in one EDB muscle of the foot and 2 IU of BoNT-A plus 4 IU of BoNT-E in the contralateral one). Also in these cases, a fast BoNT-E-type of recovery of function from the initial paralysis was observed (see Fig. 42.2).

Several conclusions can be drawn from this study: First, that BoNT-E cannot be considered

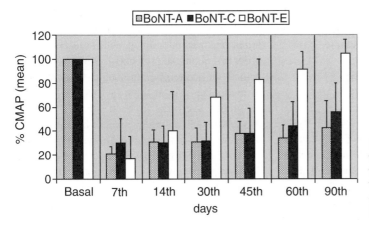

FIG. 42.1. Percentage trend variation of the CMAP amplitude of the EDB muscle of the feet over time, after injections of BoNT-A, BoNT-E, and BoNT-C.

a valid alternative to BoNT-A in nonresponder patients; second, that the different time-course of recovery of function with BoNT-E or BoNT-A is not a result of different strengths of action of the units used, because they cause a similar and maximal neuromuscular block at the seventh day; and third, that the different BoNT-E or BoNT-A recovery of function is a cytosol effect. In fact, if the longer-lasting activity of BoNT-A is a result of its longer lifetime, then in the doubly poisoned neuromuscular junction, the paralytic effect has to be that caused by the BoNT-A molecules, which survive the already inactivated BoNT-E molecules. We would like to interpret these results in terms of an interference with neuroexocytosis caused by the BoNT-A–cleaved SNAP-25, which preserves more

than 95% of its sequence, as suggested by recent experiments on the frog and mouse neuromuscular junction (37,38). This C-terminally truncated SNAP-25 is nonfunctional in neuroexocytosis, but is not altered to such an extent as to be removed from the terminal. On the contrary, the BoNT-E–cleaved SNAP-25, which has lost more than 13% of its sequence, is removed and replaced by newly synthesized molecules, with an ensuing more-rapid recovery of function. The BoNT-A type of recovery following BoNT-C injection may be similarly interpreted by assuming that the grossly altered syntaxin is rapidly replaced, while the BoNT-C–cleaved SNAP-25 (which is one amino acid residue longer than the BoNT-A–cleaved one) remains at the poisoned synapse and interferes with function.

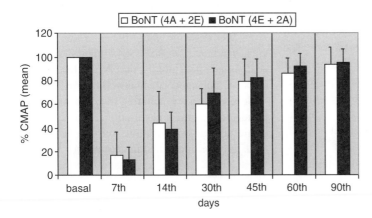

FIG. 42.2. Percentage trend variation of the CMAP amplitude of the EDB muscle of the feet over time, after injections of double poisoning drug (4 IU of BoNT-A + 2 IU of BoNT-E and 2 IU of BoNT-A + 4 IU of BoNT-E). There is no statistical difference at each day of the follow-up.

Because of this similarity with BoNT-A, BoNT-C was chosen for further studies on the treatment of focal dystonia in humans.

STUDY B

Before treating patients affected by focal dystonia and who were resistant to BoNT-A, we tested the effect of BoNT-C on MN survival, because BoNT-C has been reported to cause cell death *in vitro* of cultured neurons (39,40). Moreover, an influence of the different BoNT serotypes on MNs has not previously been reported for human muscles.

Accordingly, in a population of voluntary health subjects, we injected low dosages of BoNT-C and BoNT-A and monitored the effect with the electrophysiologic technique of MUNE. Eight subjects affected by facial dystonia or idiopathic hemifacial spasm and never treated before with any kind of BoNT, voluntarily participated in this study. In each individual, 3 IU of BoNT-C were injected in the central part of the EDB muscle of one foot and, similarly, in the contralateral EDB muscle with 3 IU of BoNT-A (BOTOX). Our local committee approved the study and all the subjects gave us their informed consent. Before and after the injections (4 months), a MUNE analysis was performed in both feet of each subject using the "multiple point nerve stimulation" technique, as previously described (41,42).

Superficial electrocardiogram (EKG) electrodes were applied on the EDB muscle of the foot: the "active electrode" on the belly of the EDB muscle and the "reference electrode" on the lateral and distal part of the dorsal foot. The peroneal nerve was stimulated at more than four different sites, situated at more than 5 cm one from the other, in order to collect a single motor-action potential (S-MAP) sample by using an electrical square shock with short duration (0.05 sec) and delivered at liminal intensity. At the first S-MAP, we accepted the "all-or-nothing" waveform obtained at liminal intensity. The following variation in waveform, obtained by a manual step increase of the voltage output stimulator, was considered as the addition of new S-MAP. From the new waveform evoked, the previous one was subtracted with an algorithm in order to obtain a "second" S-MAP. We repeated the same operation until we were able to recognize at least three or four well-defined different waveforms for each site. We repeated this analysis in a similar manner by stimulating different parts of the peroneal nerve (proximally, at least 5 to 6 cm) until we collected 15 different S-MAPs. Moreover, we calculated the mean value of the "peak-to-peak" amplitude (S-Amp) and the mean value of the "area" (S-Area) to obtain the value of the S-MAP sample. Finally, we recorded the maximal C-MAP (M-MAP) of the peroneal nerve elicited by a supramaximal electrical shock applied at the ankle, and we calculated the "peak-to-peak" amplitude (M-Amp) and area (M-Area). The MUNE value estimated by considering the Amplitude parameter (Amp-MUNE) was calculated by the ratio between M-Amp and S-Amp. Similarly, the ratio between M-Area and S-Area was the MUNE value for the Area parameter (Area-MUNE). (For more explanation and details see references 41 and 42.)

In normal subjects, among different controls, the variation in the Amp-MUNE or Area-MUNE was considered significant when the difference was more than 30% as compared to the baseline (our normal intraindividual variability, unpublished data).

Figure 42.3 shows that none of the injected persons revealed a significant Amp-MUNE ($p = 0.10$) or Area-MUNE ($p = 0.20$) variation after 4 months from BoNT-A injections, nor from BoNT-C treatment (Amp-MUNE with $p = 0.25$; Area-MUNE with $p = 0.29$). These results clearly indicate that BoNT-C, similarly to BoNT-A, does not affect motor unit survival. In addition, BoNT-C appeared safe and well tolerated.

Several factors, including the orders of magnitude, different concentrations, and the anatomic and trophic relations only preserved *in vivo*, may be implicated in determining this difference between the *in vivo* and *in vitro* effects of BoNT-C on neuron survival.

Building on these encouraging observations, we decided to proceed in treating patients af-

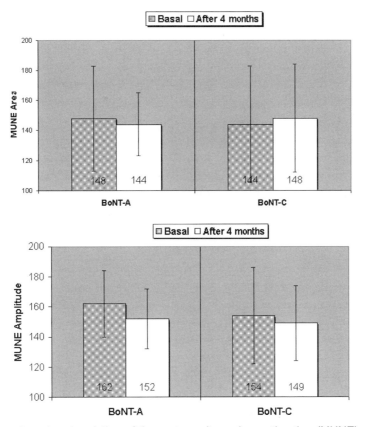

FIG. 42.3. Percentage trend variation of the motor unit number estimation (MUNE) after injections of BoNT-A and BoNT-C in the EDB muscle of the feet. There is no statistical difference after 4 months from poisoning by considering the Area (*top*) or the Amplitude value (*bottom half*).

fected by focal dystonia and resistant to BoNT-A with BoNT-C.

STUDY C

Preliminary results were presented at the American Academy of Neurology meeting in 1998 (43).

We examined a population of four subjects with cervical dystonia (CD) and two with blepharospasm who were nonresponders to BoNT-A injections (see Table 42.1). Our local ethics committee approved the study and all the subjects gave us their informed consent. Each individual had previously been treated at least five times with high doses of BoNT-A without any evidence of clinical improvement. In all subjects, the resistance was proven to be caused by

TABLE 42.1. *Characteristics of the subjects affected by blepharospasm and cervical dystonia resistant to BoNT-A and selected for the clinical trials with BoNT-C*

	Cervical dystonia		
Patient	Sex	Age	Disease
FC	Male	65 yr	T + L
RG	Female	56 yr	T
GM	Male	28 yr	R + T
BC	Male	61 yr	T
	Blepharospasm		
Patient	Sex	Age	Disease
BD	Male	75 yr	Clonic blephospasm
CG	Male	29 yr	Clonic blephospasm

specific antibodies by ELISA and Western blot, by an immunobioassay test in mice, by the absence of atrophy after the injection of 20 IU of BOTOX in the frontalis muscle and by detecting the absence of the CMAP block in the EDB muscle of the foot after injections of 10 IU of BoNT-A. We used BoNT-C obtained from WAKO (Japan); in addition, it was trypsin activated, purified, and tested as previously described (36). Accordingly, it did not contain accessory proteins. The BoNTs were prepared for injections in 0.1 mL of PBS containing 2% human serum albumin. The mean dosage used was 40 IU for the sternocleidomastoid (SCM) muscle, 120 IU for trapezius or splenius muscles, and 25 IU for orbicularis oculi muscle.

Indeed, the sensitivity to BoNT-C was tested by injecting 3 IU of the drug in an EDB muscle and was evaluated by the analysis of the CMAP peak-to-peak amplitude decrement (more than 50%). Before treatment, 2 weeks, and 4 weeks after the treatments an objective quantification of the involuntary movement was performed using the Toronto Western Spasmodic Torticollis Rating Scale (TWSTRS) for CD (44) and the Blepharospasm Grading Scale (BGS) of Elston for subjects with blepharospasm (11). A specialist in movement disorders performed the evaluation in a blind manner using videotapes of the subjects.

In addition, a subjective evaluation was accomplished by considering the Global Rating Score (GRS) of Jankovic obtained by the diary compiled from each individual patient during a period of 3 months (45). The "latency of the clinical effect" (onset effect), the "maximal period of clinical benefit" (peak effect) and the "total duration of the clinical benefit" (time effect) were analyzed. Finally, each subject was reinjected at least five times at 3-month intervals in order to detect the efficacy of repetitive injections.

All the subjects examined revealed a clinical improvement according to our previous CMAP test. The results of the objective evaluation (TWSTRS and BGS) before and after the treatment are summarized in Table 42.2. GRS results monitored over a 3-month period are reported in Fig. 42.4. For the subjects with blepharospasm, the "onset effect" was at the third day, the "peak effect" at the twentieth day, and the "time effect" was 11 weeks. For CD patients the "onset effect" was at the seventh day, the "peak effect" at the thirtieth day, and the "time effect" was 7 weeks. None of the persons enrolled in the present study revealed a significant

TABLE 42.2. *Results of the "objective clinical evaluation" in subjects with blepharospasm or cervical dystonia resistant to BoNT-A by considering the Toronto Western Spasmodic Torticollis Rating Scale (TWSTRS) for cervical dystonia or Elston's Blepharospasm Grading Scale (BGS) for blepharospasm, before BoNT-C injections and 2 and 4 weeks after BoNT-C injections. For BGS, the grading is from 0 (blind) to 6 (normal); for TWSTRS, the grading is different in relation to the pattern of involuntary movement, from 0 (normal movement) to 24 (severe dystonic movement by considering different items)*

Patient	Age/Sex	Blepharospasm (BGS)		
		Before BoNT-C	After 2 weeks	After 4 weeks
BD	72/male	2	5	6
CG	29/male	3	6	6

Patient	Age/Sex	Cervical dystonia (TWSTRS)		
		Before BoNT-C	After 2 weeks	After 4 weeks
FC	65/male	11	7	8
RG	56/female	9	6	6
GM	28/male	13	5	8
BC	61/male	10	7	8

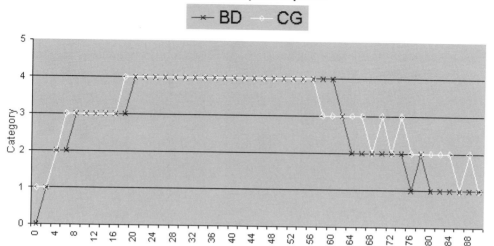

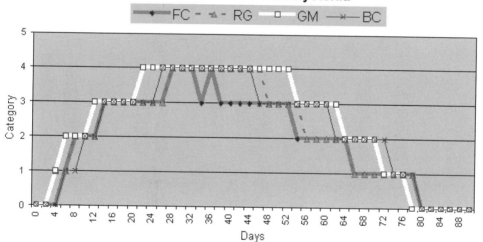

FIG. 42.4. Jankovic's Global Rating Score (GRS) over a period of 19 days after BoNT-C injections in nonresponder subjects affected by blepharospasm (*top*) or cervical dystonia (*bottom*). The category expressed is from 0 (no effect) to 4 (relevant clinical improvement).

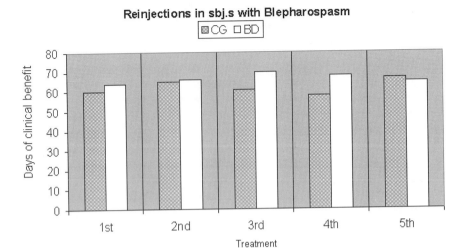

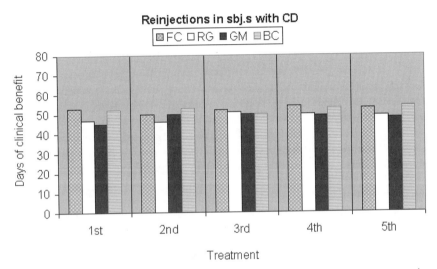

FIG. 42.5. Evaluation of repetitive treatments (five times) with BoNT-C in nonresponder subjects affected by blepharospasm (*top*) or cervical dystonia (*bottom*). The analysis was done by considering the "time effect" (period of clinical benefit) of the patients.

variation in clinical improvement after repetitive injections (see Fig. 42.5). All these observations indicate that BoNT-C has a clinical profile similar to BoNT-A.

CONCLUSIONS

BoNT-C is a serotype prevalently associated with botulism in birds. Only one case of infant human botulism caused by BoNT-C has been reported (46). The present results document that BoNT-C is very effective in humans; its lack of association to human botulism is probably related to ecologic and/or growth conditions. The present results also show that BoNT-C is a novel and effective botulinum neurotoxin serotype for the therapy of focal dystonia, with a general profile of action similar to that of BoNT-A. BoNT-C clearly has longer duration of action than BoNT-E and BoNT-F. Thus, BoNT-C is a valid alternative to BoNT-A that could be particularly useful in the treatment of nonresponders to

BoNT-A. We would like to suggest that BoNT-C be tested for efficacy in the treatment of other diseases where it may be found even more useful than BoNT-A.

REFERENCES

1. Schiavo G, Matteoli M, Montecucco C. Neurotoxins affecting neuroexocytosis. *Physiol Rev* 2000;80:717–766.
2. Humeau Y, Doussau F, Grant NJ, et al. How botulinum and tetanus neurotoxins block neurotransmitter release. *Biochimie* 2000;82:427–446.
3. Cherington, M. Clinical spectrum of botulism. *Muscle Nerve* 1998;21:701–710.
4. Elston JS. Botulinum toxin A in clinical medicine. *J Physiol (Paris)* 1990;84:285–289.
5. Greene P, Kang U, Fahn S, et al. Double-blind, placebo-controlled trial of botulinum toxin injections for the treatment of spasmodic torticollis. *Neurology* 1990;40:1213–1218.
6. Jankovic J, Schwartz K. Botulinum toxin injection for cervical dystonia. *Neurology* 1990;40:277–280.
7. Lees AJ, Turjanski N, Rivest J, et al. Treatment of cervical dystonia hand spasm and laryngeal dystonia with botulinum toxin. *J Neurol* 1992;239:1–4.
8. Poewe W, Schelosky L, Kleedorfer B, et al. Treatment of spasmodic torticollis with local injections of botulinum toxin: one-year follow-up in 37 patients. *J Neurol* 1992;239:21–25.
9. Blackie JD, Lees AJ. Botulinum toxin treatment in spasmodic torticollis. *J Neurol Neurosurg Psychiatry* 1990;53:640–643.
10. Grandas F, Elston J, Quinn N, et al. Blepharospasm: a review of 264 patients. *J Neurol Neurosurg Psychiatry* 1991;51:767–772.
11. Elston JS. The management of blepharospasm and hemifacial spasm. *J Neurol* 1992;239:5–8.
12. Jankovic J, Hallett M, eds. *Therapy with botulinum toxin.* New York: Marcel Dekker, 1994.
13. Borodic G, Johnson E, Goodnough M, et al. Botulinum toxin therapy, immunologic resistance, and problem with available materials. *Neurology* 1996;46:26–29.
14. Jankovic J, Schwartz K. Response and immunoresistance to botulinum toxin injections. *Neurology* 1995;45:1743–1746.
15. Brin M. Botulinum toxin: chemistry, pharmacology, toxicity, and immunology. *Muscle Nerve* 1997;6(Suppl):S146–Sl65.
16. Zuber M, Sebald M, Bathien N, et al. Botulinum antibodies in dystonic patients treated with type A botulinum toxin: frequency and significance. *Neurology* 1993;43:1715–1718.
17. Sankhla C, Jankovic J, Duane D. Variability of the immunologic and clinical response in dystonic patients immunoresistant to botulinum toxin injections. *Mov Disord* 1998;13:150–154.
18. Hanna PA, Jankovic J. Mouse bioassay versus Western blot assay for botulinum toxin antibodies: correlation with clinical response. *Neurology* 1998;50:1624–1629.
19. Ludlow CL, Hallett M, Rhew K, et al. Therapeutic use of type F botulinum toxin. *N Engl J Med* 1992;326:349–350.

20. Greene PE, Fahn S. Use of botulinum toxin type F injections to treat torticollis in patients with immunity to botulinum toxin type A. *Mov Disord* 1993;8:479–483.
21. Tsui JKC, Hayward M, Ming Mak EK, et al. Botulinum toxin type B in the treatment of cervical dystonia: a pilot study. *Neurology* 1995;45:2109–2110.
22. Greene PE, Fahn S. Response to botulinum toxin F in seronegative botulinum toxin A-resistant patients. *Mov Disord* 1996;11:181–184.
23. Mezaki T, Kaji R, Kohara N, et al. Comparison of therapeutic efficacies of type A and F botulinum toxins for blepharospasm: a double-blind, controlled study. *Neurology* 1995;45:506–508.
24. Chen R, Karp BI, Hallett M. Botulinum toxin type F for treatment of dystonia: long-term experience. *Neurology* 1998;51:1494–1496.
25. Lew MF, Adornato BT, Duane DD, et al. Botulinum toxin type B: a double-blind, placebo-controlled, safety and efficacy study in cervical dystonia. *Neurology* 1997;49:701–707.
26. Sloop RR, Cole BA, Escutin RO. Human response to botulinum toxin injection: type B compared with type A. *Neurology* 1997;49:189–194.
27. Brin MF, Lew MF, Adler CH, et al. Safety and efficacy of NeuroBloc (botulinum toxin type B) in type A-resistant cervical dystonia. *Neurology* 1999;53:1431–1438.
28. Brashear A, Lew MF, Dykstra DD, et al. Safety and efficacy of NeuroBloc (botulinum toxin type B) in type A-responsive cervical dystonia. *Neurology* 1999;53:1439–1446.
29. Hamjian JA, Walker FO. Serial neurophysiological studies of intramuscular botulinum A toxin in humans. *Muscle Nerve* 1994;17:1385–1392.
30. Sloop RR, Escutin RO, Matus JA, et al. Dose-response curve of human extensor digitorum brevis muscle function to i.m. injected botulinum toxin type A. *Neurology* 1996;46:1382–1386.
31. Kessler KR, Benecke R. The EBD test: a clinical test for the detection of antibodies to botulinum toxin type A. *Mov Disord* 1997;12:95–99.
32. Eleopra R, Tugnoli V, De Grandis D. The variability in the clinical effect induced by botulinum toxin type A: the role of muscle activity in humans. *Mov Disord* 1997;12:89–94.
33. Eleopra R, Tugnoli V, Rossetto O, et al. Botulinum neurotoxin serotype C: a novel effective botulinum toxin therapy in human. *Neurosci Lett* 1997;224:91–94.
34. Eleopra R, Tugnoli V, Rossetto O, et al. Different time courses of recovery after poisoning with botulinum neurotoxin serotypes A and E in humans. *Neurosci Lett* 1998;256:135–138.
35. Montecucco C, Schiavo G. Tetanus and botulinum neurotoxins: isolation and assay. *Methods Enzymol* 1995;248:643–652.
36. Raciborska DA, Charlton MP. Retention of cleaved synaptosome-associated protein of 25 kDa (SNAP-25) in neuromuscular junctions: a new hypothesis to explain persistence of botulinum A poisoning. *Can J Physiol Pharmacol* 1999;77:679–688.
37. De Paiva A, Meunier FA, Molgo J, et al. Functional repair of motor endplates after botulinum neurotoxin type A poisoning: biphasic switch of synaptic activity between nerve sprouts and their parents terminals. *Proc Natl Acad Sci U S A* 1999;96:3200–3205.
38. Leist M, Fava E, Montecucco C, et al. Peroxynitrite

and NO-donors induce neuronal apoptosis by eliciting autocrine excitotoxicity. *Eur J Neurosci* 1997;9: 1488–1498.

39. Williamson LC, Neale EA. Syntaxin and 25-kDa synaptosomal-associated protein: differential effects of botulinum neurotoxins C1 and A on neuronal survival. *J Neurosci Res* 1998;52:569–583.

40. Doherty TJ, Stashuk DW, Brown WF. Determinants of mean motor unit size: impact on estimates of motor unit number. *Muscle Nerve* 1993;16:1326–1331.

41. Wang FC, Delwaide PJ. Number and relative size of thenar motor units estimated by an adapted multiple point stimulation method. *Muscle Nerve* 1995;18: 969–979.

42. Eleopra R, Tugnoli V, De Grandis D, et al. Botulinum toxin serotype C treatment in subjects affected by focal dystonia and resistant to botulinum toxin serotype A. *Neurology* 1998;50(Suppl 4):A72.

43. Comella CL, Stebbins GT, Goetz CG, et al. Teaching tape for the motor section of the Toronto Western Spasmodic Torticollis Scale. *Mov Disord* 1997;12:570–575.

44. Jankovic J, Schwartz K. Botulinum toxin injections for cervical dystonia. *Neurology* 1990;40:277–280.

45. Oguma K, Yokota K, Hayashi S, et al. Infant botulism due to *Clostridium botulinum* type C toxin. *Lancet* 1990; 336:1449–1450.

43

Long-Term Use of Botulinum Toxin Type F to Treat Patients Resistant to Botulinum Toxin Type A

Paul E. Greene

Botulinum toxin type A (BTX-A) injections are now recognized as the most useful treatment for many focal symptoms in patients with dystonia (1–11). Serious side effects from BTX-A injections are uncommon. However, patients have now been recognized with antibodies to BTX-A in sufficient titers to block all clinical effect (12,13). The prevalence of antibodies to BTX-A is not known with certainty. Nonetheless, immunity to BTX-A is a major therapeutic problem for some patients.

There are seven known antigenically distinct botulinum toxins, all acting at presynaptic sites to block cholinergic neuromuscular transmission. Human antibodies to type A toxoid (inactivated BTX-A) do not have significant neutralizing effect against botulinum toxin type F (BTX-F) (14), suggesting that BTX-F might be an alternative therapy for patients who have developed antibodies to BTX-A. BTX-F is less lethal in animals than BTX-A per unit protein (15). When injected intramuscularly in rats, BTX-F causes less muscle weakness and has a shorter duration of action than an equivalent LD_{50} of type A (16). The first use of BTX-F in patients with antibodies to BTX-A was reported in two patients with torticollis, one patient with oromandibular dystonia, and one patient with stuttering (17). Since then, there have been at least five other reports of the use of BTX-F to treat patients resistant to BTX-A (18–22). This chapter discusses the results of long-term follow-up on patients treated with BTX-F at the Movement Disorder Center at Columbia-Presbyterian Medical Center.

METHODS

BTX-F was supplied by Dr. Genji Sakaguchi in vials containing either 2,000 or 2,500 U and was diluted with normal saline without preservative to a concentration of 50 U/mL. Injection doses were calculated assuming equivalence between 1 U of BTX-A and 1 U of BTX-F. In patients receiving all their BTX-A injections at Columbia, BTX-F was given initially in the same doses and sites as the last successful BTX-A injection series.

Our original BTX-F study started in 1991 and enrolled 15 patients with serologically documented antibodies to BTX-A (18). Subsequently, we accepted any patient who had benefited from BTX-A injection followed by loss of benefit. This included some patients who had improvement after only one injection session with BTX-A and who actually may have had primary resistance to BTX-A, possibly followed by development of secondary resistance as a result of repeated unsuccessful injections. Although we continue to see patients injected at our center who develop resistance to BTX-A, this study also includes patients who were injected at other centers at the time they lost benefit from BTX-A. Most of the patients who became resistant at our center had resistance documented by lack of atrophy of the sternocleidomastoid muscle (SCM) after injection of 50 to 75 U of BTX-A. Some had serologic documentation by mouse neutralization assay. This was not always the case for patients from other centers, so that the methods for determining resistance were not uniform. Many patients did not live within easy traveling distance of the Movement Disorder Center. Therefore, patients without subjective benefit from BTX-F were not always examined after BTX-F injection. Patients rated the results of each injection series at the subsequent visit or by phone. They were not routinely examined after each BTX-F injection series to determine objective benefit. All patients were encouraged to have at least two injection series with BTX-F before considering the BTX-F injections a failure.

Because these subjective ratings are difficult to interpret, I have arbitrarily used greater than five injection visits as indicative of benefit from BTX-F injections.

RESULTS

Patient Population

Eighty-eight patients with torticollis were injected over 482 injection series with 122,765 U of BTX-F. Thirty-two patients had serologic assay for antibodies to BTX-A, and 16 of 32 (50%) were positive. There were 56 women and 32 men. Eighty-two of the 88 patients (93.2%) had idiopathic dystonia. The rest had dystonia after birth injury, tardive dystonia, or dystonia after trauma or head injury, and one had suspected secondary dystonia without a specific diagnosis. Dystonia was limited to the neck in 50 of 88 patients (56.8%). Nine had neck and arm involvement, eight had neck and upper or lower face involvement and the rest had the neck and various other body parts involved, including four patients with generalized dystonia.

The injection histories prior to the development were known in 53 patients. The rest were either referred to our center because of resistance, or had at least some of their injections at other centers. Because it was often difficult to precisely determine when resistance developed, I have used the beginning of BTX-F injections as a surrogate for the development of resistance. These patients had a mean 9.6 injection series before requiring BTX-F (range, 4 to 24 sessions). The mean total dose of BTX-A per patient before starting BTX-F was 1,964 U (range, 750 to 5210 U). The mean dose per session per patient was 205 U (range, 130 to 266 U). The mean time elapsed between the beginning of BTX-A injections and the beginning of BTX-F injections was 29.3 months (range, 10 to 96 months).

Only nine patients with blepharospasm were injected over 50 sessions with 4,450 U of BTX-F. There were four women and five men. Eight of the nine patients had idiopathic dystonia and one had tardive dystonia. Seven of the patients had lower face involvement in addition to blepharospasm, and six had involvement of muscles not innervated by cranial nerve VII, including five with cervical involvement. Because of the small number of patients, no comparison was made with other patients injected for blepharospasm. Four of these patients had been injected in the past for torticollis. Of the five patients developing resistance after injections for blepharospasm only, two patients required BTX-F after fewer than five injection sessions with BTX-A. Three patients required BTX-F after 9 to 13 years of continuous injections approximately every 3 months with BTX-A.

Outcome

Patients with torticollis were injected with BTX-F for a mean 20.8 months between March 1991 and September 1999. The mean dose per session per patient was 258 U (range, 100 to 438 U; median dose, 250 U). As in the previous study (18), the duration of benefit was approximately 4 weeks. Excluding patients who were seen for only one or two visits, patients had a mean 8.8 injection sessions (range, 3 to 29 sessions; median, 7 sessions). The mean duration of treatment in this group was 36 months (range, 4 to 97 months; median, 31 months). Of the 88 patients, 46 (52.3%) reported subjective benefit on at least one occasion. Most reported improvement in pain, head turning or muscle tension. Only rarely did patients report improvement in head tremor. Of the 88 patients, 31 (35.2%) had successful BTX-F treatment in that they had more than five injection series. Six of these 31 patients (19.4%) stopped receiving BTX-F injections because they experienced substantial loss of benefit. At least three of the six patients no longer developed atrophy after SCM injections, and one had a positive mouse paralysis assay by Dr. Douglas Brown, USAMRIID (23). Two patients stopped receiving BTX-F injections because they went into remission (after two and four injection sessions).

Seven of the nine patients with blepharospasm had at least one apparently successful injection series with BTX-F. The mean duration of subjective benefit was about 4 weeks in these patients, approximately the same duration of action as in patients with torticollis. However, three patients lost benefit. One patient lost benefit to both BTX-A and BTX-F after several injection series. At least one patient stopped developing lid weakness from BTX-F injections at the time benefit disappeared.

CONCLUSIONS

Eighty-eight patients with torticollis and possible resistance to BTX-A injections underwent BTX-F injections in this open-label study. Some of these patients may have been primary BTX-A failures, but many had antibodies to BTX-A as indicated by mouse neutralization assay or by lack of muscle atrophy after BTX-A injection. Although some seemed to develop resistance to BTX-A after as few as 4 injection sessions, the mean number of injection sessions before requiring BTX-F was between 9 and 10, representing about 29 months of injections. Patients could develop resistance after as many as 24 injection sessions, representing over 6 years of BTX-A injections. Although the risk of becoming resistant to BTX-A may decline with continuing treatment, it appears that the risk does not entirely disappear.

There were also nine patients with blepharospasm who had developed resistance to BTX-A. Four of these may have developed resistance after injections for torticollis. However, three of the remaining five patients developed resistance after 9 to 13 years of BTX-A injections. This raises the possibility that, as more patients with blepharospasm approach a decade or more of continuous BTX-A injections, we will see more resistant blepharospasm patients.

In this open-label study, subjective patient reports of benefit cannot be convincing evidence for the efficacy of BTX-F. Nonetheless, it is likely that most of the patients receiving injections approximately every 3 months for more than five injection cycles had some useful benefit. These patients went to trouble and expense to receive the injections, knowing that any benefit would only last for approximately 1 month. By patient report, BTX-F injections resulted in either pain reduction or improvement in head turning. Patients who stopped receiving BTX-F injections after a small number of sessions could have been receiving minimal benefit, or could have decided that the degree of benefit lasting only approximately 4 weeks did not justify the trouble and expense. Without a controlled study, it was impossible to quantify the results of the BTX-F injections in this population. Patients who lose benefit from BTX-A exclusively because of antibodies to BTX-A should benefit from BTX-F injections. However, given the many uncertainties in this kind of study, the low apparent success rate of approximately 35% is not surprising.

Almost 20% of patients receiving chronic BTX-F injections seemed to eventually lose benefit from BTX-F. At least some of these patients developed antibodies to BTX-F, as indicated by loss of muscle atrophy after injection or abnormal mouse paralysis assay. The actual prevalence of antibodies to BTX-F is difficult to estimate without a reliable assay for antibodies to BTX-F. However, this prevalence is higher than most reports of prevalence for resistance to BTX-A, suggesting the possibility that BTX-F is more likely to stimulate neutralizing antibodies than BTX-A, or that patients who become resistant to BTX-A are more likely to develop resistance to BTX-F.

REFERENCES

1. Jankovic J, Orman J. Botulinum A toxin for cranial-cervical dystonia: a double-blind, placebo-controlled study. *Neurology* 1987;37:616–623.
2. Fahn S, List T, Moskowitz C, et al. Double-blind con-

trolled study of botulinum toxin for blepharospasm. *Neurology* 1985;35(Suppl 1):271.

3. Tsui JKC, Eisen A, Stoessl AJ, et al. Double-blind study of botulinum toxin in spasmodic torticollis. *Lancet* 1986;2:245–247.

4. Jankovic J, Schwartz K. Longitudinal follow-up of botulinum toxin injections for treatment of blepharospasm and cervical dystonia. *Neurology* 1993;43:834–836.

5. Gelb DJ, Lowenstein DH, Aminoff MJ. Controlled trial of botulinum toxin injections in the treatment of spasmodic torticollis. *Neurology* 1989;39:80–84.

6. Greene P, Kang U, Fahn S, et al. Double-blind, placebo-controlled trial of botulinum toxin injections for the treatment of spasmodic torticollis. *Neurology* 1990;40:1213–1218.

7. Blackie JD, Lees AJ. Botulinum toxin treatment in spasmodic torticollis. *J Neurol Neurosurg Psychiatry* 1990;53:640–643.

8. Lorentz IT, Subramanian SS, Yiannikas. Treatment of idiopathic spasmodic torticollis with botulinum toxin A double-blind study on twenty-three patients. *Mov Disord* 1991;6:145–150.

9. Moore AP, Blumhardt LD. A double-blind trial of botulinum toxin-A in torticollis, with one-year follow up. *J Neurol Neurosurg Psychiatry* 1991;54:813–816.

10. Truong DD, Rontal M, Rolnick M, et al. Double-blind controlled study of botulinum toxin in adductor spasmodic dysphonia. *Laryngoscope* 1991;101:630–634.

11. Tsui JK, Bhatt M, Calne S, et al. Botulinum toxin in the treatment of writer's cramp: a double-blind study. *Neurology* 1993;43:183–185.

12. Greene PE, Fahn S, Diamond B. Development of resistance to botulinum toxin type A in patients with torticollis treated with injections of botulinum toxin type A. *Mov Disord* 1994;9:213–217.

13. Tsui JK, Wong NLM, Wong E, et al. Production of circulating antibodies to botulinum-A toxin in patients receiving repeated injections for dystonia. *Ann Neurol* 1988;23:181.

14. Siegel LS. Evaluation of neutralizing antibodies to type A, B, E, and F botulinum toxins in sera from human recipients of botulinum pentavalent (ABCDE) toxoid. *J Clin Microbiol* 1989;27:1906–1908.

15. Yang KH, Sugiyama H. Purification and properties of *Clostridium botulinum* type F toxin. *Appl Microbiol* 1975;29:598–603.

16. Kaufman JA, Way JF, Siegel LS, et al. Comparison of the action of types A and F botulinum toxin at the rat neuromuscular junction. *Toxicol Appl Pharmacol* 1985;79:211–217.

17. Ludlow CL, Hallett M, Rhew K, et al. Therapeutic use of type F botulinum toxin. *N Engl J Med* 1992;326:349–350.

18. Greene PE, Fahn S. Use of botulinum toxin type F injections to treat torticollis in patients with immunity to botulinum toxin type A. *Mov Disord* 1993;8:479–484.

19. Sheean GL, Lees AJ. Botulinum toxin F in the treatment of torticollis clinically resistant to botulinum toxin A. *J Neurol Neurosurg Psychiatry* 1995;59:601–607.

20. Greene PE, Fahn S. Response to botulinum toxin F in seronegative botulinum toxin A-resistant patients. *Mov Disord* 1996;11:181–184.

21. Chen R, Karp BI, Hallett M. Botulinum toxin type F for treatment of dystonia: long-term experience. *Neurology* 1998;51:1494–1496.

22. Houser MK, Sheean GL, Lees AJ. Further studies using higher doses of botulinum toxin type F for torticollis resistant to botulinum toxin type A. *J Neurol Neurosurg Psychiatry* 1998;64:577–580.

23. Brown DR, Lloyd JP, Schmidt JJ. Identification and characterization of a neutralizing monoclonal antibody against botulinum neurotoxin serotype F, following vaccination with active toxin. *Hybridoma* 1997;16:447–456.

Scientific and Therapeutic Aspects of Botulinum Toxin
edited by M.F. Brin, J. Jankovic, and M. Hallett
Lippincott Williams & Wilkins, Philadelphia, © 2002.

44

Muscle Afferent Block for Dystonia: Implications for the Physiologic Mechanism of Action of Botulinum Toxin

Ryuji Kaji

Botulinum toxin injection has been widely used for treating patients with dystonia and spasticity. Despite its popularity, its physiologic mechanism of action still remains obscure because the clinical benefit frequently outlasts muscle weakness in many patients (1,2). Dystonia has a peculiar characteristic of sensory trick, in which tactile or proprioceptive sensory input ameliorates symptoms: patients with cervical dystonia try to correct torticollis by placing their hand on a certain area of the skin over the head or neck. Those with blepharospasm wear dark sunglasses to relieve involuntary contractions of orbicularis oculi muscles. Activation of muscle afferents was found to reproduce dystonic contractions in writer's cramp (3). These clinical observations suggest sensory-motor disintegration as a pathophysiologic mechanism in dystonia.

In 1924, Walshe (4) reported a method of treating akinesia and rigidity in a boy with postencephalitic parkinsonism. He used an intramuscular injection of diluted procaine into the biceps brachii muscle to instantly correct reduced excursion and speed of elbow flexion and extension. There was no gross muscle weakness in the biceps, and he ascribed the effect to muscle deafferentation because the biceps' jerk was significantly attenuated. This phenomenon is now thought to reflect gamma-efferent blockage with intact alpha fibers, because diluted local anesthetics are known to preferentially affect thin fibers. Desensitization of the muscle spindles by the gamma-efferent blockage, and thus improves motor function in parkinsonism, a disorder of basal ganglia.

In our previous studies, diluted lidocaine (0.5%) was injected into muscles showing dystonic contractions in writer's cramp (5). Dystonic symptoms were almost abolished by this method. A large volume of lidocaine solution (5 to 25 mL/muscle) was needed to accomplish this, because a small amount targeted to the motor point was not successful. It was concluded therefore that the effect of this method was not through blocking the innervation of extrafusal muscles fibers but through affecting muscle spindles distributed widely within a muscle (Fig. 44.1), and that selective gamma efferent blockage by the diluted local anesthetic was likely the mechanism (Fig. 44.2). This method of desensitizing muscle afferents was also used for treating spasticity (6).

METHODS

The major drawback of this muscle afferent block (MAB) was its short duration of action. The beneficial effect lasted only for a few hours. Ethanol in 5% to 10% concentration is known to work as a local anesthetic with a longer duration of action, because it blocks sodium channels similar to lidocaine or procaine. However, ethanol causes intense pain before it attains an anesthetic effect. We therefore combined these two anesthetics to achieve longer-lasting effects (Fig. 44.3). A large syringe (5 to 25 mL) is attached to a small one (1 to 5 mL) with a tripolar connector. Selection of the muscle to be injected is similar to that in botulinum toxin injection.

Phenol Block

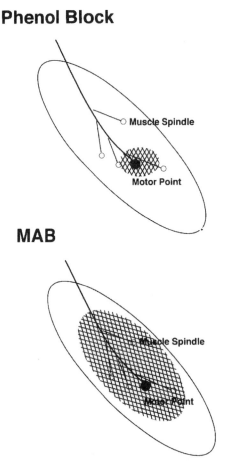

MAB

FIG. 44.1. Comparison of muscle afferent block (MAB) and conventional phenol block for treating dystonia. Note that MAB is designed to infiltrate a large part of the muscle by using a large volume of diluted local anesthetic.

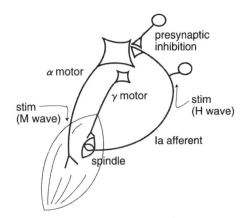

FIG. 44.2. A diagram of alpha and gamma motoneurons and Ia afferent fibers. Note that the H wave (reflex) is evoked by stimulating the group Ia fibers directly, bypassing the spindles.

needle tip remains at the same position during the procedure.

RESULTS

Clinical Studies

This procedure was found to be effective in treating oromandibular (7) and cervical dystonias (8) and spasticity (6), as well as writer's cramp (3,5). Despite the use of ethanol, the clinical benefit of a single injection is still short-lived: it ranges from a few days to a week. Therefore, it is mandatory to repeat the injection every 2 to 3 days or weekly. After 8 to 10 injections, the effect reaches a plateau and lasts more than a few months. This method is labor-intensive, but has the advantages over botulinum toxin injection of being low cost and of being effective in

After targeting the muscle, 80% of the total volume of lidocaine (Fig. 44.3-1) is injected first. Then the tripolar connector is operated to allow injection of 99.5% ethanol (2) in one-tenth of the total volume of lidocaine. This order of injection of lidocaine and ethanol minimizes the pain associated with ethanol injection. Lastly, the rest of lidocaine (20% of the total volume) is injected (3) after operating the connector again. Dividing the injection of lidocaine reduces the discomfort of the subject, because finishing the injection with ethanol would cause an intolerable pain when drawing the needle back. Use of an extension tube is recommended to assure that the

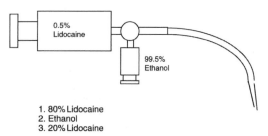

1. 80% Lidocaine
2. Ethanol
3. 20% Lidocaine

FIG. 44.3. Method of muscle afferent block (see text for details).

antibody-positive botulinum toxin-resistant cases (8). Its peak effect was found to be similar to that of injecting botulinum toxin in medium dose (8). In the future, MAB may be found more efficacious in treating occupational cramps than botulinum therapy, which often causes unwanted weakness.

Histologic Studies

Using the rat soleus muscle as a model, we demonstrated that the diameter of bag fibers in the muscle spindles after the injection of lidocaine and lidocaine/ethanol were significantly smaller than those after the injection of saline (8). This bag-fiber atrophy was not explained by direct toxic action of lidocaine or ethanol because there were no findings of muscle destruction and inflammatory cell infiltrates in muscle spindles. Instead, the blockage of gamma fibers innervating these intrafusal muscle fibers was thought responsible for the atrophy. Rosales and colleagues (9) reported similar bag-fiber atrophy in a muscle injected with botulinum toxin. They also noted relative preservation of the extrafusal fibers. The reason for the preferential effect of botulinum toxin upon intrafusal fibers is unclear. The background firing rate is higher for the intrafusal than for the extrafusal fibers, and this increased activity may sensitize the spindle efferent for the action of the toxin.

In the experiment with lidocaine/ethanol injection (8), and in the human study (5), we noted a loss of H reflex with a preserved M wave in injected muscles. This is consonant with the finding of loss of the biceps' jerk reported by Walshe (4), but is difficult to explain by the blockage of gamma efferent fibers alone, because group Ia fibers, but not the spindles, were directly activated in H reflex maneuver (Fig. 44.2). Possibly gamma efferent blockage reduces the excitability of the alpha motoneurons in the spinal cord by abolishing the background activation of the muscle afferents impinging upon alpha motoneurons.

DISCUSSION

MAB is effective in correcting the abnormal muscle activation in Parkinson's disease and dystonia, both of which are thought to be basal ganglia disorders. These findings give us an insight into the physiologic role of the basal ganglia in motor control. The basal ganglia lie between the cerebral cortex and the thalamus, with which they have dense fiber connections forming four to five distinct circuits to allow parallel processing of information. The most studied is the motor loop, which has direct and indirect pathways. The direct pathway disinhibits the powerful inhibition of the internal segment of the globus pallidus/substantia nigra pars reticulata upon thalamic ventrolateral nuclei with a net facilitation on the motor cortex. By contrast, the indirect pathway exerts an inhibitory effect. This dual system provides a center (excitatory)–surround (inhibitory) mechanism to focus its effect on selected cortical neurons. Despite considerable knowledge of the neurotransmitters in these projections, the functional role of the loop in motor control is not precisely understood.

Parkinson's disease primarily affects nigrostriatal dopaminergic neurons and is characterized by bradykinesia (slowness of movement), rigidity of muscles, disturbed postural reflexes and tremor. Hallett and Khoshbin (10) studied the physiologic mechanism of bradykinesia using surface electromyograms (EMGs) in a ballistic elbow flexion movement. They found a fractionated pattern of agonist–antagonist muscle bursts, which were repetitions of the normal triphasic (agonist–antagonist–agonist) muscle activation. The basic abnormality was a smaller-than-normal scaling of movement excursion at each burst, which was compensated for by repeating the normal triphasic pattern. An intriguing feature of Parkinson's disease is the benefit of external sensory cues for initiating and performing movements (kinesia paradoxica). Auditory or visual input can correct the small excursion of movement implying that abnormal scaling of movement is secondary to disturbed use of proprioceptive sensory input. The finding that blockade of muscle afferents with local anesthetic corrected the small excursion of elbow movement in a boy with postencephalitic parkinsonism, as demonstrated by Walshe (4), indicates that blocking muscle afferents rescales the motor excursion.

Dystonia is a sustained involuntary muscle contraction frequently causing twisting or repetitive movements or abnormal postures. It is regarded as a basal ganglia disorder, because focal lesions in the motor loop cause dystonia in the limbs contralateral to the lesion (hemidystonia), and because trihexyphenidyl, an anticholinergic agent frequently used for Parkinson's disease, may be effective in treating the condition. As discussed earlier, the sensory trick suggests sensory-motor mismatch in motor control. MAB seems to abolish this abnormal relationship between sensory input and motor output.

Although the basal ganglia are commonly regarded as a center for motor control, its sensory role has been underemphasized. Animal studies indicate that sensory inputs reaching the basal ganglia significantly differ from those in the lemniscal system in that they show encoding of information that appear to be relevant for motor control (11). Indeed the basal ganglia appear to "gate" sensory inputs at various levels for motor control (12,13).

Lesions of the basal ganglia mostly affect automatic movements that need sensory guidance. It is therefore likely that the basal ganglia control automatic or highly trained movements in relation to relevant sensory inputs (14,15). Tasks impaired in writer's cramp or other occupational cramps could be among these. Indeed the hand representation in the somatosensory cortex (disturbing normal motor sensory integration) was found to be abnormal in writer's cramp (16). Moreover, if extraneous sensory input is fed back for subsequent movement, this would set up a vicious cycle causing further deviation from normal motor control. There are now converging pieces of evidence indicating that this sensory gating for motor control is lost in dystonia (17) and is scaled less than normal in Parkinson's disease (18).

In summary, MAB provides a unique opportunity for investigating sensory-motor integration in dystonia and parkinsonism. It is also expected to broaden the choice of treatment for various movement disorders, enabling the manipulation of the sensory input fed back to control motor output.

ACKNOWLEDGMENTS

This study was supported in part by research grants from Japanese Ministry of Health, Welfare, and Labor, and Ministry of Science, Culture, and Technology.

REFERENCES

1. Gilio F, Curra A, Lorenzano C, et al. Effects of botulinum toxin type A on intracortical inhibition in patients with dystonia. Ann Neurol 2000;48:20–26.
2. Hallett M. How does botulinum toxin work? Ann Neurol 2000;48:7–8.
3. Kaji R, Rothwell JC, Katayama M, et al. Tonic vibration reflex and muscle afferent block in writer's cramp. Ann Neurol 1995;38:155–162.
4. Walshe F. Observations on the nature of the muscular rigidity of paralysis agitans, and its relationship to tremor. Brain 1924;47:159–177.
5. Kaji R, Kohara N, Katayama M, et al. Muscle afferent block by intramuscular injection of lidocaine for the treatment of writer's cramp. Muscle Nerve 1995;18: 234–235.
6. Mezaki T, Kaji R, Hirota N, et al. Treatment of spasticity with muscle afferent block. Neurology 1999;53: 1156–1157.
7. Yoshida K, Kaji R, Kubori T, et al. Muscle afferent block for the treatment of oromandibular dystonia. Mov Disord 1998;13:699–705.
8. Kubori T, Kaji R, Mezaki T, et al. Muscle afferent block for cervical dystonia: a controlled trial with botulinum toxin. Neurology 2000;54:198–199(abstr).
9. Rosales RL, Arimura K, Takenaga S, et al. Extrafusal and intrafusal muscle effects in experimental botulinum toxin-A injection. Muscle Nerve 1996;14:488–496.
10. Hallett M, Khoshbin S. A physiological mechanism of bradykinesia. Brain 1980;103:301–314.
11. Lidsky TI, Manetto C, Schneider JS. A consideration of sensory factors involved in motor functions of the basal ganglia. Brain Res 1985;356:133–146.
12. Schneider JS, Diamond SG, Markham CH. Deficits in orofacial sensorimotor function in Parkinson's disease. Ann Neurol 1986;19:275–282.
13. Tinazzi M, Priori A, Bertolasi L, et al. Abnormal central integration of a dual somatosensory input in dystonia. Evidence for sensory overflow. Brain 2000;123(Pt 1): 42–50.
14. Boecker H, Ceballos-Baumann A, Bartenstein P, et al. Sensory processing in Parkinson's and Huntington's disease: investigations with 3D H(2)(15)O-PET. Brain 1999;122(Pt 9):1651–1665.
15. Passingham RE, Toni I, Schluter N, et al. How do visual instructions influence the motor system? Novartis Found Symp 1998;218:129–141.
16. Bara-Jimenez W, Catalan MJ, Hallett M, et al. Abnormal somatosensory homunculus in dystonia of the hand. Ann Neurol 1998;44:828–831.
17. Murase N, Kaji R, Shimazu H, et al. Abnormal premovement gating of somatosensory input in writer's cramp. Brain 2000;123(Pt 9):1813–1829.
18. Kaji R. The sensory function of basal ganglia. Mov Disord 2002 (in press).

Scientific and Therapeutic Aspects of Botulinum Toxin
edited by M.F. Brin, J. Jankovic, and M. Hallett
Lippincott Williams & Wilkins, Philadelphia, © 2002.

45

Electromyography-Guided Chemodenervation with Phenol in Cervical Dystonia (Spasmodic Torticollis)

Janice M. Massey

Over the last decade, patients with an assortment of movement disorders have benefited from chemodenervation therapy using botulinum toxin injection. The goal of this unique treatment is to weaken muscles that are active in producing the abnormal dystonic movement or posture. Several studies have demonstrated the efficacy of botulinum toxin in cervical dystonia (CD), also referred to as spasmodic torticollis, with improvement of pain or the abnormal movement in 70% to 86% of patients (1–5).

In contrast to conditions such as blepharospasm or hemifacial spasm, chemodenervation in CD typically requires larger doses of botulinum toxin because of the number of muscles involved and their size. With repeated and frequent injections of botulinum toxin, up to 18% of patients develop resistance to this biologic toxin (6). Factors that reduce the likelihood of development of immune resistance include use of the smallest possible dose and an extended interval between injection sessions (7).

BOTULINUM TOXIN RESISTANCE

As the number of patients receiving serial injections has grown, there is an increasing population of individuals treated with botulinum toxin type A who are now resistant (see Chapter 39 for a discussion of immunoresistance). Once immunity develops, no further therapeutic response to botulinum toxin type A occurs and therefore these patients have fewer options for therapy. A small population of patients never has a thera-peutic response to botulinum toxin and could be immune because of prior exposure from food sources or preventive inoculation in some military populations. The frequency of resistance with botulinum toxin type B, recently approved for therapy in CD, is unknown.

PHENOL

Phenol has been used in a number of disease states. It has been used as a topical escharotic agent in dermatologic practice. A number of nonprescription products contain phenol, including several throat and antiitch products. Phenol or alcohol injection into nerve, root, or spinal cord has been used in the treatment of severe spasticity from spinal cord injury for many years. Injection into these structures produces long-standing neural injury. In multiple sclerosis, stroke, and other upper motor neuron diseases, phenol motor point injection, nerve block, or intramuscular neurolysis have successfully treated spasticity (8–13).

Doses up to 1,500 mg per site have been used. Reported side effects include local muscle pain and tenderness and local sensory dysesthesia. No systemic or long-term side effects are known. Industrial toxic exposure may be associated with increased risk of cancer. There is limited experience with the use of intramuscular phenol in the treatment of spasmodic torticollis (14–17).

CHEMODENERVATION WITH PHENOL

Phenol or carboxylic acid produces tissue destruction at the site of application (18). In strong concentrations of 1% to 7%, phenol denatures protein. When injected into nerve or muscle, these structures are denatured. It is a nonbiologic, nonprotein agent and thus no immune resistance develops with chronic usage. Because it is a caustic agent, use of phenol near vital structures raises concern about potential complications.

USE OF ELECTROMYOGRAPHY

In chemodenervation for CD, electromyography (EMG) serves several useful roles. As an extension of the clinical examination, it aids in identifying the presence and degree of abnormal firing patterns in those muscles that are producing the dystonic posture or movement. This information is useful in choosing muscles for injection and their appropriate dosages. In addition, EMG-guided chemodenervation allows for placement of the injected phenol precisely into the muscle. Identification and injection of deeper muscles is possible.

Motor Point Injection versus Intramuscular Injection

Similar to botulinum toxin type A, injection of phenol should ideally be placed at the neuromuscular junctions, which are often clustered together at the motor point of the muscle. The motor point is recognized by determining the point of maximum compound muscle action potential after stimulation of the nerve to that muscle. However, two technical difficulties exist with motor-point injections in neck muscles: (a) In contrast to limb muscles, the motor endplates are not clustered together but are spread across the length of the muscle; (b) In addition, the nerves supplying the muscles are not readily accessible for stimulation, particularly for deep muscles.

Phenol Injection Technique

Table 45.1 outlines the phenol injection technique. Phenol injection can be given intramuscu-

TABLE 45.1. *Summary of phenol injection technique*

- Phenol 1 to 5% solution
- 0.5 to 4 cc injection per muscle based on muscle size
- 20 to 25 cc maximum total dose per session
- Phenol must be spread through the muscle
- Serial injections may be necessary

larly, but this requires EMG guidance to assure that the site of the injection is accurate. With an injectable EMG electrode, motor unit potentials can be localized without a positive deflection and with a maximal rise time. At this site, the electrode is close to the motor endplate. Because of its local anesthetic properties, nearby muscle fibers often rapidly become silent even during injection of phenol.

EMG-guided intramuscular injections allow discrete placement of injected materials and minimize the potential for injection outside of the targeted muscle. Exact placement of the injected bolus is more critical for phenol than with botulinum toxin, which appears to have little deleterious effect on nearby structures other than the neuromuscular junction. There is little local diffusion of an injected bolus of phenol so it must be injected in aliquots throughout the muscle belly.

RESULTS

Fifty-six consecutive patients with cervical dystonia who received EMG-guided intramuscular phenol injection were evaluated by physician and patient assessments of head control, pain, and Toronto Western Spasmodic Torticollis Rating Scale (TWSTR) severity scales (17). There were 22 males and 34 females whose ages ranged from 25 to 83 years. Follow-up was 6 to 46 months. Candidate patients were those considered resistant to botulinum neurotoxin having failed to improve after at least one injection by their referring neurologist and one at our clinic. Patients were considered to have moderate or marked improvement only if all three assessments were in agreement. In no patient were the three assessments all divergent: 45% had moderate to marked improvement; 27% demonstrated mild improvement; and 28% had no improvement. None were worse. The clinical effect was largely reversible, although some patients did sustain improvement. Symptomatic improvement began 2 to 4 weeks after injection. The duration of effect was about 4 to 6 months.

COMPLICATIONS OF PHENOL INJECTION

The most common side effects of phenol injection included lightheadedness during injection, pain at the injection sites, and transitory areas of numbness or dysesthesia over the scalp, neck, or shoulder. Most patients experienced local muscle pain and edema for 1 to 2 weeks. One patient had the sensation of not being able to expand his lungs completely when swimming that resolved after several weeks. Three patients developed paresthesias and mild weakness in the arm or shoulder girdle, presumably from leakage into the brachial plexus or peripheral nerve, all of which resolved by 6 months. One patient had hoarseness and difficulty swallowing immediately after injection with complete resolution in less than 20 minutes. Ice at the injection sites and a nonsteroidal antiinflammatory agent in the first 48 hours decreased local pain.

Several weeks after phenol intramuscular injection, EMG examination showed fibrillations, positive waves, and frequent complex repetitive discharges. Motor unit potentials are very disfigured with marked polyphasia, jiggle, and variable duration from short to occasionally long duration. These findings support a primary muscle effect. Over time, without reinjection, the changes gradually recover although they may persist for years.

COMPARISON WITH BOTULINUM TOXIN

A comparison of 400 units intramuscular botulinum toxin and nerve block using 3 mL of 5% phenol in spasticity showed greater improvement in the group treated with botulinum toxin at weeks 2 and 4, but no differences at weeks 8 and 12 (19). No comparison of phenol and

TABLE 45.2. *Phenol's advantages and disadvantages*

Advantages	Disadvantages
• Alternative for patients with botulinum toxin resistance	• Painful
	• Nearby structures at risk
• No immune resistance	• Labor intensive
• Reinjection as often as tolerated	• Requires EMG guidance
• Inexpensive	

botulinum toxin has been directly performed in cervical dystonia.

Phenol intramuscular injection is painful, labor intensive, and should always be performed under EMG-guidance. Botulinum toxin is less painful and easier to give. The side effect profile of phenol is greater than with botulinum toxin. Immune resistance does not occur with phenol injection. Phenol is inexpensive (Table 45.2).

CONCLUSIONS

With EMG-guided intramuscular injection of phenol, many patients can receive benefit with minimal side effects. Because of the location of vital structures in the neck near the site of injection, the use of phenol chemodenervation is more hazardous than is using botulinum toxins that are specific for the neuromuscular junction. However, because of the level of patient discomfort and potential for side effects, at present, this treatment may most benefit those patients resistant to botulinum toxins.

REFERENCES

1. Tsui J, Eisen A, Stoessel AJ, et al. A double-blind study of botulinum toxin and spasmodic torticollis. *Lancet* 1986;2:245–246.
2. Blackie JD, Lees AJ. Botulinum toxin in the treatment of spasmodic torticollis. *J Neurol Neurosurg Psychiatry* 1990;53:640–643.
3. Green P, Kang U, Fahn S, et al. Double-blind, placebo-controlled trial of botulinum toxin injection for the treatment of spasmodic torticollis. *Neurology* 1990;40:1213–1218.
4. Moore AP, Blumhardt LD. A double-blind trial of botulinum toxin A in torticollis with a one-year follow-up. *J Neurol Neurosurg Psychiatry* 1991;54:813–816.
5. Poewe W, Schelosky L, Kleedorfer B, et al. Treatment of spasmodic torticollis with local injection of botuli-

num toxin. One-year follow-up in 37 patients. *J Neurol* 1992;239:21–25.

6. Brin MF. Botulinum toxin: chemistry, pharmacology, toxicity and immunology. *Muscle Nerve Suppl* 1997;6: S146–S168.

7. Comella CL, Jankovic J, Brin MF. Use of botulinum toxin type A in the treatment of cervical dystonia. *Neurology* 2000;55(Suppl 5):S15–S21.

8. DeLateur BJ. A new technique of intramuscular phenol neurolysis. *Arch Phys Med Rehabil* 1972;53:179–181.

9. Easton JK, Ozel T, Halpern D. Intramuscular neurolysis for spasticity in children. *Arch Phys Med Rehabil* 1979; 60:155–158.

10. Garland DE, Lilling M, Keenan MA. Percutaneous phenol blocks to motor points of spastic forearm muscles in head-injured adults. *Arch Phys Med Rehabil* 1984;65:243–245.

11. Gibson II. Phenol block in the treatment of spasticity. *Gerontology* 1987;33:327–330.

12. Awad EA. Intramuscular neurolysis for stroke. *Minn Med* 1972;55:711–713.

13. Keenan MAE. Management of the spastic upper extrem-

ity in the neurologically impaired adult. *Clin Orthop Rel Res* 1988;233:116–125.

14. Massey JM. Treatment of spasmodic torticollis with intramuscular phenol injection. *J Neurol Neurosurg Psychiatry* 1995;58:258–259.

15. Garcia Ruiz PJ, Sanchez Bernardos V. Intramuscular phenol injection for severe cervical dystonia. *J Neurology* 2000;247:146–147.

16. Massey JM. EMG-guided chemodenervation with phenol in cervical dystonia. *Mov Disord* 2000;15:17.

17. Massey JM. Needle EMG-guided chemodenervation with phenol in cervical dystonia. *American Association of Electrodiagnostic Medicine Course G Syllabus: Chemodenervation* Rochester, MN: American Association of Diagnostic Medicine 2000;21–22.

18. Lack W, Lang S, Brand G. Necrotizing effect of phenol on normal tissues and on tumors. A study on normal tissues and on tumors. *Acta Orthop Scand* 1994;65: 351–354.

19. Kirazli Y, On AY, Kismali B, et al. Comparison of phenol block and botulinus toxin type A in the treatment of spastic foot after stroke: a randomized, double-blind trial. *Am J Phys Med Rehabil* 1998;77:510–515.

Scientific and Therapeutic Aspects of Botulinum Toxin
edited by M.F. Brin, J. Jankovic, and M. Hallett
Lippincott Williams & Wilkins, Philadelphia, © 2002.

46

Immunotoxin

Mark Hallett

Although botulinum toxin (BTX) has been an excellent therapeutic tool, one of its main drawbacks in chronic disease is its relatively short duration of action. The question often arises whether something similar can be done that would provide a longer duration of action. It is known that myectomy can be efficacious in blepharospasm (1–3) and possibly also in spasmodic torticollis (4). If it would be possible to do a chemical myectomy, this might produce a prolonged effect. Other agents are already available that do this, such as phenol and doxorubicin, but these agents are rather toxic and somewhat nonspecific in their action.

Wirtschafter recently reported on his experience injecting doxorubicin in the eyelid of 18 patients with blepharospasm and nine patients with hemifacial spasm (5). Eyelids were repeatedly injected at intervals of 10 or more weeks until the spasms were ameliorated or the patient requested discontinuation. Nine of the patients with blepharospasm completed the full course of treatment and were considered "cured" for more than 1 year. Six of the patients with hemifacial spasm completed treatment, and five were considered "cures," lasting for more than 4.5 to 6 years. The treatment does create considerable local toxicity and particular care is needed to prevent necrosis of the skin overlying the injection site. The toxicity to skin has been circumvented to a large extent by encapsulating the doxorubicin in liposomes (6).

Developing from the large field of immunotoxins (ITX) that are generally used for cancer chemotherapy (7), the idea came to us to develop a "silver bullet" targeting muscle (8). This was made by conjugating a monoclonal antibody directed to the alpha subunit of the nicotinic acetylcholine receptor (MAb 35) to ricin, a toxic protein that inactivates protein synthesis. The idea is that the antibody would selectively attach to muscle allowing the ricin to enter the cell and destroy it. The ITX (Ricin-MAb 35) should not affect any other tissue, and might, therefore, have fewer side effects than drugs such as doxorubicin. Ricin is a polypeptide composed of two subunits joined by a disulfide bond (9). The B chain binds to cell-surface galactose residues and facilitates transport of the A chain into the cytosol. The A chain acts as an *N*-glycosidase inactivating cellular ribosomes. The similarities to the structure and mechanism of botulinum toxin are clear.

The synthesis of our ITX (Ricin-MAb 35) is described in our original article (8). The potency and specificity was examined with several *in vitro* experiments before using it in animals. The cytotoxic effect of ITX and native ricin were tested in tissue culture of cells that do and do not express the acetylcholine receptor. Ricin was equally toxic for both cell types, while ITX was 100-fold more toxic with the receptor-positive cells. Lactose inhibits ricin binding, and it diminished the toxic effect of ricin, but did not influence the effect of the ITX. Hence, the toxicity is indeed specific for cells with an acetylcholine receptor and binding occurs via the antibody and not by ricin's own binding mechanism.

The maximum tolerated dose (MTD) for intraperitoneal injection in mice with 100% survival was 2 μg/kg. Consequently, dosing can be expressed as a fraction of the MTD in order to compare with BTX.

The histologic effects of the toxin were assessed with injections into the gastrocnemius muscle of female Sprague-Dawley rats. At a

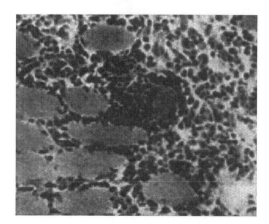

FIG. 46.1. Fresh-frozen transverse section of a muscle biopsy, stained with hematoxylin and eosin (H&E), of the rat gastrocnemius 7 days after injection with 0.01 MTD. Inflammatory cells surround and invade the muscle fibers. (Modified from Hott JS, Dalakas MC, Sung C, et al. Skeletal muscle-specific immunotoxin for the treatment of focal muscle spasm. *Neurology* 1998;50: 485–491, with permission.)

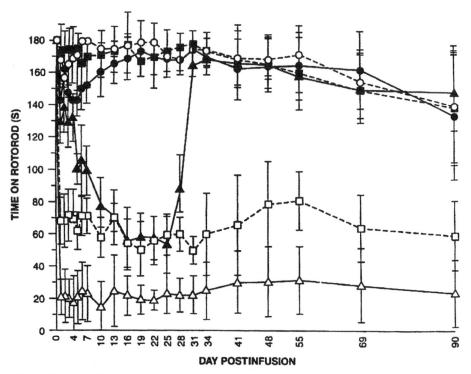

FIG. 46.2. Effects of different doses of BTX and ITX injected into the gastrocnemius muscle of the rat on Rotorod performance. Four rats were in each experimental group. Filled squares are saline; open circles are unconjugated antibody; filled triangles and filled circles are 0.1 and 0.01 LD_{50} of BTX; open triangles and open squares are 0.01 and 0.003 MTD of ITX. (From Hott JS, Dalakas MC, Sung C, et al. Skeletal muscle-specific immunotoxin for the treatment of focal muscle spasm. *Neurology* 1998;50:485–491, with permission.)

dose of 0.01 MTD, at 7 days, changes were seen only at the site of injection and, indeed, only at the endplate region. There was a severe inflammatory response in the endomysial parenchyma and the perimysium. Inflammatory cells invaded muscle fibers similarly to that in primary inflammatory myopathy. Necrosis, phagocytosis, and separation of the muscle fibers were prominent (Fig. 46.1).

In muscle biopsies taken at 30 days, changes were still restricted to the endplate region. There was marked muscle atrophy with increased connective tissue and some residual inflammation in the interstitial tissue. Muscle surrounding the injection site appeared normal.

To assess strength, we used the Rotorod test on female Sprague-Dawley rats injected into a gastrocnemius muscle. The Rotorod test was quantified as the amount of time a rat was able to stay on the rotating rod at 25 or 30 rpm (with a test maximum of 180 sec). Rats were trained to be fully successful for 3 days before any injection. Two different experiments were done. Experiment 1 compared BTX at 0.01 of the LD_{50}, ITX at 0.01 of the MTD, and saline for 100 days. Experiment 2 compared BTX at 0.1 and 0.01 LD_{50}, ITX at 0.01 and 0.003 MTD, unconjugated MAb 35, and saline for 90 days (Fig. 46.2). Results were similar for the same injections. In Experiment 2, virtually no effect was seen for saline, unconjugated antibody, and the low dose of BTX. The higher dose of BTX had a transient effect that was gone in about 30 days. Both doses of ITX had prolonged effects not diminished in the 90 days, and the effect of the 0.01 MTD dose was greater than the 0.003 MTD dose.

The conclusion of these experiments is that ITX appears to be highly selective for muscle, causing focal destruction only in the site of injection and long-lasting weakness at doses with a wide safety margin. We also suggested in the original article that the combined use of ITX and BTX might make sense. BTX would be used first to get the desired effect and to produce an increase in the expression of acetylcholine receptor on the denervated muscle cells. Then ITX could be used; it would attack those denervated muscle cells most effectively, possibly with even a lower dose than is needed for normal muscle.

The effect of this ITX has also been tested in rabbit extraocular muscles (10). Different doses of the toxin were injected into superior rectus muscles of New Zealand White rabbits which were histologically examined at 3, 7, and 14 days. No effect was seen at doses less than 0.01 MTD, and most observations were made with 0.1 MTD. All the rabbits appeared to be healthy and ate normally. Mild conjunctival redness developed at the surgical site in some of the eyes; however, no significant ocular, periocular, or orbital changes were noted in the treated eyes, and no gross changes were visible in the treated muscles at necropsy.

Toxicity of muscle was focal and dose related. At 0.1 MTD, there was substantial inflammatory cell infiltrate by 3 days, which largely disappeared by 7 days. Significant muscle loss was apparent by 7 days (Fig. 46.3). Significantly,

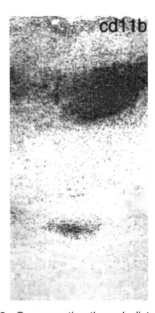

FIG. 46.3. Cross-section through distal superior rectus muscle in the rabbit injected with ITX at 0.1 MTD at 7 days. A large region of the cross-section was almost devoid of myofibers, containing only connective tissue and inflammatory cells. The section is stained for CD 11b-positive inflammatory cells. (Modified from Christiansen SP, Sandnas A, Prill R, et al. Acute effects of the skeletal muscle-specific immunotoxin ricin-MAb 35 on extraocular muscles of rabbits. *Invest Ophthalmol Vis Sci* 2000;41:3402–3409, with permission.)

both the inflammatory reaction and muscle fiber loss were confined to the immediate injection site, and surrounding muscle appeared to be normal. Peripheral nerve and vasculature were also normal. The authors noted specifically the localization of the effect within the muscle epimysium indicating lack of spread as occurs with BTX.

At 14 days after treatment, early signs of muscle regeneration were apparent. However, preliminary evidence from studies at 105 days showed decreased numbers of myofibers and decreased total muscle cross-sectional area. At 1 year, there appears to be a normal number of myofibers, but there is an increase in the heterogeneity of fiber size (Christiansen, Peterson, To, and McLoon, personal communication). In this preparation, there are no data yet on muscle strength.

These studies indicate that ITX is a promising agent for future studies in humans.

REFERENCES

1. Chapman KL, Bartley GB, Waller RR, et al. Follow-up of patients with essential blepharospasm who underwent eyelid protractor myectomy at the Mayo Clinic from 1980 through 1995. *Ophthal Plast Reconstr Surg* 1999; 15:106–110.
2. Anderson RL, Patel BC, Holds JB, et al. Blepharospasm: past, present, and future. *Ophthal Plast Reconstr Surg* 1998;14:305–317.
3. Mauriello JA Jr, Keswani R, Franklin M. Long-term enhancement of botulinum toxin injections by upper-eyelid surgery in 14 patients with facial dyskinesias. *Arch Otolaryngol Head Neck Surg* 1999;125:627–631.
4. Krauss JK, Koller R, Burgunder JM. Partial myotomy/myectomy of the trapezius muscle with an asleep-awake-asleep anesthetic technique for treatment of cervical dystonia. Technical note. *J Neurosurg* 1999;91: 889–891.
5. Wirtschafter JD, McLoon LK. Long-term efficacy of local doxorubicin chemomyectomy in patients with blepharospasm and hemifacial spasm. *Ophthalmology* 1998;105:342–346.
6. McLoon LK, Wirtschafter JD. Direct injection of liposome-encapsulated doxorubicin optimizes chemomyectomy in rabbit eyelid. *Invest Ophthalmol Vis Sci* 1999; 40:2561–2567.
7. Frankel AE, Kreitman RJ, Sausville EA. Targeted toxins. *Clin Cancer Res* 2000;6:326–334.
8. Hott JS, Dalakas MC, Sung C, et al. Skeletal muscle-specific immunotoxin for the treatment of focal muscle spasm. *Neurology* 1998;50:485–491.
9. Sandvig K, van Deurs B. Endocytosis and intracellular transport of ricin: recent discoveries. *FEBS Lett* 1999; 452:67–70.
10. Christiansen SP, Sandnas A, Prill R, et al. Acute effects of the skeletal muscle-specific immunotoxin ricin-MAb 35 on extraocular muscles of rabbits. *Invest Ophthalmol Vis Sci* 2000;41:3402–3409.

NOVEL TOXIN CONSTRUCTS

Scientific and Therapeutic Aspects of Botulinum Toxin
edited by M.F. Brin, J. Jankovic, and M. Hallett
Lippincott Williams & Wilkins, Philadelphia, © 2002.

47

Hybrid and Chimeric Botulinum Toxin Molecules

Eric A. Johnson, Michael C. Goodnough, Carl M. Malizio, William H. Tepp, Sean S. Dineen, and Marite Bradshaw

Botulinum toxin complexes (BTXs) have become important drugs for the treatment of a wide variety of neurologic disorders (1–5). Although strabismus and focal and segmental dystonias were the initial disorders treated, use of botulinum toxin has expanded to include treatment of nondystonic involuntary movements and muscle contractions, spasticity, wrinkles and facial asymmetry, autonomic disorders, pain, and other syndromes (4–6). Potentially, other diseases characterized by hyperactive secretory activity could be treated with clostridial neurotoxins. Furthermore, the binding and channel domains of tetanus and botulinum neurotoxins (TeNT and BoNT) could serve as delivery vehicles for molecules to the nervous system. It is also possible that the catalytic domains of TeNT and BoNT could be genetically altered to recognize other polypeptide substrates associated with disease states, such as proteins in amyloid plaques involved in Alzheimer's disease. However, the development of novel therapeutic agents for these purposes based on BoNT and TeNT will require considerable research and improved understanding of the cellular biology of neurotoxins (NTs), as well as practical methods to manufacture and stabilize novel neurotoxin-derivative molecules.

Despite the successes of BTX as a drug, there are drawbacks to its use, including immunologic resistance in certain patients on repeated injections (7–9) and diffusion of BTX or its constituent neurotoxin component (BoNT) to neighboring muscles, causing undesired effects (8). The paralytic activity of native BTX is not permanent in most human indications, requiring periodic reinjections, often of increasing dosage, which may increase the incidence of side effects. Most of the research efforts on botulinum toxin has been directed toward tissue effects and finding new clinical uses, while relatively little information has been published on improvements of toxin quality, and development of new toxin preparations that could improve the efficacy or decrease the incidence and magnitude of side effects. Our laboratory has been investigating methods to produce and stabilize BTXs, BoNTs, and the light (L) and heavy (H) chains from different serotypes (10–14). These developments should enable the construction of toxin molecule derivatives with improved efficacy and fewer side effects. In this chapter, we discuss early efforts to produce hybrid toxins, consisting of chains/domains of different serotypes, and chimeric botulinum toxins, consisting of botulinum toxin H chain linked to a nonbotulinum toxin that could permanently inactivate exocytosis by killing of the target nerve(s).

Beginning in the 1970s, and continuing until today, various investigators with considerable experience and expertise with clostridial neurotoxins have dissociated the H and L chains of BoNTs and TeNT (15–24). Several of these laboratories have attempted to reconstitute the native NT or hybrid NTs by reformation of disulfide linkage. Generally, the di-chains are formed by specific proteolysis (nicking) of the single-chain toxin molecule, followed by separation of the constituent heavy and light chain in slightly alkaline buffer by treatment with dithiothreitol and urea. Certain laboratories have attempted to improve stability and reconstitution by also including EDTA, sucrose, and other compounds during separation and reconstitution. Dithiothreitol and urea are removed by dialysis to allow disulfide bond formation and other interactions of the protein subunits including hydrogen bonds and ionic and hydrophobic forces.

Careful examination of the reported results in the literature indicates that complete reconstitution of biologic activity by disulfide linkage of the separated chains was generally not achieved (usually ~10% to 35% of toxicity was recovered on reconstitution); furthermore, the protein yields obtained were insufficient for pharmacologic and clinical studies. Several problems have been encountered in reconstitution including low yields of the separated chains from neurotoxin, instabilities of the separated chains, particularly precipitation and fragmentation of the H and L chains. It has been hypothesized that the active conformation of the type A botulinum H chain necessary for binding to its receptor (ecto-acceptor) and for facilitation of membrane permeabilization of the catalytic L chain is lost upon separation from the L chain (25,26). However, our laboratory found preliminary evidence that the H chain alone containing certain ligands can be internalized into cultured neurons (Goodnough MC, Johnson EA, Neale E, Adler M, Oyler G, unpublished results), indicating that further work is necessary to precisely define the regions of BoNTs required for internalization into neurons. These regions required for biologic activity could be defined using systematic genetic deletions of the H and L chains of BoNTs and TeNT. This approach could also be used to define the necessity of an interchain disulfide bond, as has been investigated for ricin (27). The development of a biologically active "H chain," possibly lacking a disulfide, could be used as a building block to construct hybrid and chimeric toxins.

Various laboratories have attempted to construct hybrid BoNTs in which the goal is to biochemically combine constituent L and H chains from different serotypes of toxins. Generally, reconstitution of separated chains from different serotypes results in considerably reduced toxicity compared to the native toxins (24). Further-

more, the hybrid toxin yields are too low to enable detailed biochemical and pharmacologic characterization, as well as clinical testing (Goodnough MC, Tepp WH, Johnson EA, unpublished data). Research is needed to develop methods for construction of stable L and H NT chains for biochemical linkage of toxin components. Genetic strategies are also being explored for generation of hybrids and chimeras involving clostridial neurotoxins (see, for example, reference 28).

Our laboratory has mainly evaluated biochemical approaches for linking chains and domains of toxins. Stability of separated BoNT chains is AHc>BHc>EHc and ALc>BLc>ELc. Separated chains require relatively high sodium chloride concentrations (greater than 100 mmol/L), the presence of a reducing agent such as dithiothreitol, and temperatures below 10°C (50°F) for stability. Additionally, the presence of a mild denaturant such as urea at concentrations up to 2 M has been used to stabilize separated chains.

We have used a series of homobifunctional chemical linkers in efforts to conjugate heterologous heavy and light chains via their free sulfhydryl groups. These linkers have included 1,4-di-[3'-(2'pyridyldithio)propionamido]butane (DPDPB), dithio-bis-maleimidoethane (DTME), and bis-maleimidohexane (BMH). The first two linkers contain reducible disulfide bonds, while BMH is nonreducible. Figure 47.1 shows the structures of these linkers. Figure 47.2 shows the results of one linkage experiment of type A heavy chain and type E light chain.

Figure 47.2 shows a sodium dodecyl sulfate-polyacrylamide gel electrophoresis (SDS-PAGE) photograph showing the reaction products of type A heavy chain and type E light chain using two different concentrations of the linker DTME over time. Lane 1 represents the starting reagents. Lane 2 shows the reaction products after 5 minutes of incubation. The appearance of high-molecular-weight species (150 kDa) indicates that the two heterologous chains are being combined. Lanes 3 and 4 show the same reaction at 15 minutes and 30 minutes of incubation, respectively. The band corresponding to the hybrid toxin at 150 kDa becomes more evident

Reducible

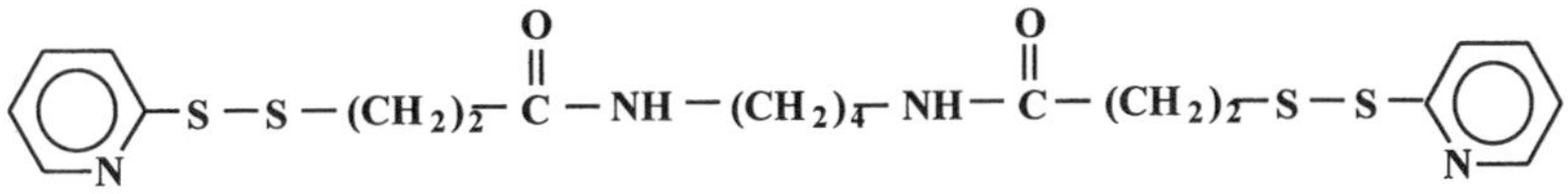

**1,4-di-[(3',2'-pyridyldithio-(propionamido)butane]
spacer arm length 19.9 angstroms
(DPDPB)**

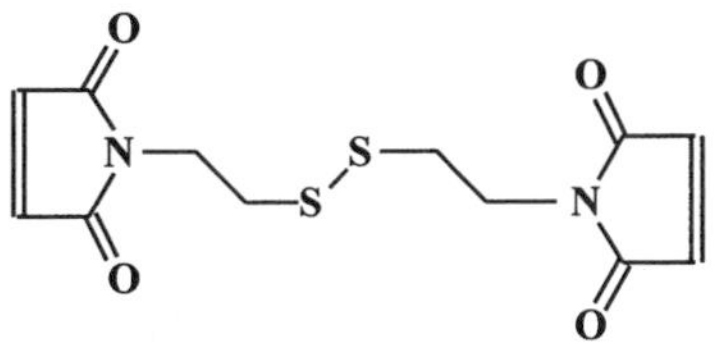

**dithio-bis-maleimidoethane
spacer arm length 13.3 angstroms
(DTME)**

Nonreducible

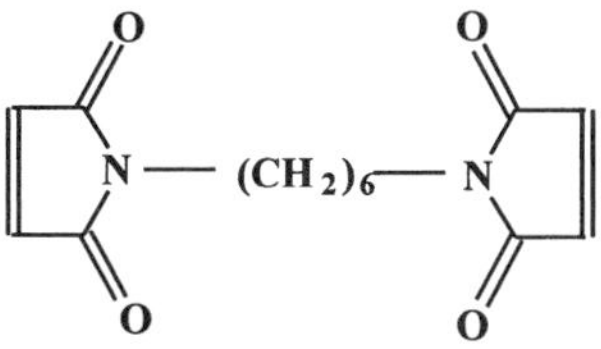

**Bismaleimidohexane
spacer arm length 16.1 angstroms
(BMH)**

FIG. 47.1. Structures of linkers used in synthesis of hybrid botulinum toxins.

as the reaction proceeds. Lanes 5 and 6 represent a parallel reaction using twice the DTME concentration of the reaction shown in lanes 2 to 4. The 150-kDa hybrid toxin band is more evident in this incubation. Additionally, the decreasing concentrations of the starting H and L chains during incubation supports the conclusion that the 150-kDa band is composed of linked BoNT-AHc and BoNT-ELc.

A chimeric neurotoxin was produced biochemically in our laboratory using the heavy chain of type A botulinum neurotoxin and the A chain of ricin (Goodnough MC, Johnson EA, unpublished data). The two components were covalently connected by sulfhydryl linkage using the heterobifunctional linker *N*-succinimidyl-3-(2-pyridyldiothio)-propionate (SPDP). Initial attempts to conjugate the two peptides by their internal sulfhydryl residues did not yield covalent products. The linker SPDP was added to purified ricin A chain at a ratio that yielded approximately one linker per molecule of ricin A chain. Residual linker was removed by size exclusion chromatography and botulinum type A heavy chain that had been freshly reduced added at a two- to threefold molar excess. The excess botulinum heavy chain prevented addition of more than one ricin molecule to the heavy

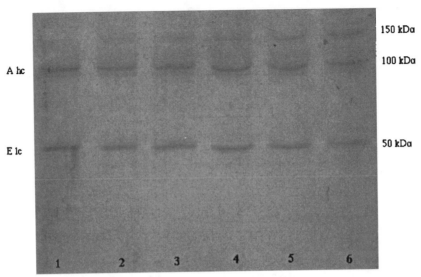

FIG. 47.2. Reaction of purified type E botulinum light chain with type A heavy chain. *Lane 1:* control, no linker; *lane 2:* 0.5 μmol/L DTME, time 5 minutes; *lane 3:* 0.5 μmol/L DTME, time 15 minutes; *lane 4:* 0.5 μmol/L DTME, time 30 minutes; *lane 5:* 1.0 μmol/L DTME, time 5 minutes; *lane 6:* 1.0 μmol/L DTME, time 30 minutes.

chain. Both components of the chimera were low in toxicity to mice (botulinum heavy chain = 1 LD$_{50}$/100 μg; ricin A chain = 1 LD$_{50}$/300 μg), while the resulting construct had a toxicity of approximately 1 LD$_{50}$/50 ng. The construct was immunoreactive to both antisera to type A botulinum neurotoxin and ricin A chain.

By using similar techniques, an SPDP linker was added to purified type B botulinum light chain and purified heavy chain of type A botulinum neurotoxin conjugated to the newly formed sulfhydryl. Both separated chains had toxicities of less than 1,000 LD$_{50}$/mg. The hybrid neurotoxin was immunoreactive to both monovalent antitype A botulinum antiserum as well as type B antiserum. The hybrid neurotoxin had a specific toxicity of approximately 1 LD$_{50}$/ng when tested intraperitoneally in mice.

Many targeted toxins for human therapy are currently produced as genetic fusion protein toxins, generally composed of recombinant antibody fragments (Fv regions) or receptor binding domains genetically fused to the lethal domains of *Pseudomonas* exotoxin A, diphtheria toxin, or various plant toxins such as ricin A chain or saporin (29–34). In addition, new approaches to

targeted cell killing have employed newer killing agents including deoxyribonucleases (35), doxorubicin (36), the fungal toxin clavin (37), agents toxic to mitochondria (38), and agents or treatments inducing apoptosis (39,40).

Botulinum toxin chains and domains can be produced using recombinant DNA expression systems (41–47). Although data is limited, attempts to reconstitute TeNT from rDNA-produced proteins has not enabled full recovery of biologic activity (45,47). Similar reconstitution experiments have not been reported for rDNA botulinum toxin H and L chains. The production of truncated or altered proteins that retain biologic activity could improve the properties of the substrates for construction of chimeric and hybrid toxins including increased solubility, introduction of desired residues for cross-linking, and other desired properties. However, in most laboratories it appears that full-length H chain of BoNT is produced in relatively low quantities in heterologous systems such as *Escherichia coli*, and it may be desirable to use a clostridial host such as a nontoxigenic *Clostridium botulinum* strain developed in our laboratory (48).

Reported research on targeted chimeric toxins

using TeNT or BoNT domains has been extremely limited to date. Francis et al. (28) produced a fusion toxin containing the catalytic and membrane translocation domains of diphtheria toxin linked to the receptor binding domain of TeNT. It was proposed that such constructs could be used to deliver heterologous proteins to neurons, but the efficacy of such a delivery system would appear to be limited in humans because most individuals contain neutralizing antibodies to TeNT. Instead of using the receptor-binding domain of TeNT, it may be possible for delivery to use the receptor domain of BoNT-B, which among the BoNTs has highest homology with TeNT (41,42). Chaddock et al. (49) linked the domains encoding the endopeptidase activity (L chain) and the channel forming region of BoNT-A (LH$_N$/A) chain to wheat germ hemagglutinin lectin (WGA) using a chemical linker [(N-succinimidyl-3-(2-pyridyldithio)-propionate (SPDP)]. Coupling yielded a complex and heterogeneous mixture of products, which on disulfide reduction gave LH$_N$/A as the subunit products identified by electrophoresis. The heterogeneous mixture would not be acceptable as a drug candidate, and additional research is needed to generate a homogenous product with uniform properties. The investigators demonstrated that the construct mixture cleaved the natural substrate, SNAP-25 (synaptosomal-associated protein of 25 kDa), and also inhibited secretory responses in various cell lines. These data indicated that secretory processes in cell types other than those of neuronal origin could be inhibited by cleavage of proteins in the SNARE [soluble NSF (N-ethylmaleimide–sensitive factor) attachment receptor] complex in cells that use the SNARE-mediated secretion mechanism. In an effort to improve the duration of action of muscle paralysis, a skeletal muscle-specific immunotoxin was constructed by chemical linkage of ricin A chain to a monoclonal antibody for the nicotinic acetylcholine receptor (50). The uniformity of the immunotoxin product(s) was not reported. The immunotoxin was cytotoxic to myotubes at a dose 300-fold less than the lethal dose, and caused muscle weakening and paralysis on injection into the gastrocnemius muscles of rats, which was reported to be longer lasting than muscle injected with BTX type A.

CONCLUSIONS AND PERSPECTIVES

New approaches are necessary for production of high yields of uniform H and L chains for biochemical reconstitution of BoNT and TeNT chains with recovery of biologic activity comparable to native toxin. Several approaches are being evaluated in our laboratory. It is possible that nontoxic proteins in the BTX complexes could assist in the refolding, renaturation, and recombination of the H and L TeNT and BoNT subunits. Certain laboratories have reported that nontoxic proteins stabilize the labile NTs in the gut (13,51), and it is conceivable that the nontoxic components could also act as chaperone proteins and assist in the guided folding and recombination of the polypeptide subunits.

Most attempts at reconstituting separated L and H chains of TeNT and BoNT of the same serotype using native sulfhydryl linkage have resulted in low yields and specific toxicities considerably lower than the native toxins. Attempts to form hybrid toxins by reconstitution of L and H chains have been unsuccessful to date in obtaining homogeneous product in good yield and with specific toxicity comparable to native toxins. The highest recovery of BoNT activity has been achieved when chemical linkers have been used to reassociate the H and L chains, but these also have considerably lower specific toxicity than the native toxins. It is apparent that methods are needed to produce subunits or derivative toxins in high yields that can be stabilized with retention of biological activity. Alternatively, if genetic expression of subunits and domains can be achieved with high yields and retention of activity, these could also be used as substrates for chemical linking and construction of novel toxins. Expression systems for clostridial proteins are becoming available (43,48), but methods for solubilizing and reconstituting chimeric proteins as has been accomplished in other systems (34) are needed. Perhaps the most promising technology for production of chimeric toxins containing TeNT or BoNT domains would be to produce fusion toxins, as has been successfully accomplished with other bacterial and plant toxin systems (29–34).

Determination of the three-dimensional structures of BoNT-A (52,53) and BoNT-B (54) has confirmed that these NTs comprised multidomain proteins that have evolved by the assembly of nonhomologous genes. Recently, novel approaches have been used to genetically select for chimeric protein structures with new biologic activities. In one approach (55), functional chimeric proteins containing the N-terminal half of cold shock protein (CspA) linked to various polypeptides encoded by random genomic DNA from *E. coli* was achieved through phage display and genetic selection for resistance to proteolysis. By using this approach, it was shown that functional chimeric proteins were generated by combinatorial segment assembly from nonhomologous proteins, creating novel domains and protein architectures *in vitro*. Other investigators have also used gene-shuffling methodologies to generate proteins with new and novel properties (56,57). Gene shuffling genetic strategies combined with selection for desired properties of TeNT and BoNTs such as resistance to proteolysis, binding to polygangliosides and putative protein receptors, entry into cell cytosol, and proteolytic cleavage of SNARE or other protein substrates could potentially yield chimeric TeNT- or BoNT-based chimeras with novel pharmaceutic potential and ability to overcome current drawbacks of botulinum toxin therapy.

ACKNOWLEDGMENTS

Research in EAJ's laboratory has been supported by the National Institutes of Health, the United States Department of Defense, the United States Department of Agriculture, food industry sponsors, and the University of Wisconsin.

REFERENCES

1. Scott AB. Clostridial toxins as therapeutic agents. In: Simpson LL, ed. *Botulinum neurotoxin and tetanus toxin.* San Diego, CA: Academic Press, 1989:399–412.
2. Jankovic J, Hallett, M. *Therapy with botulinum toxin.* New York: Marcel Dekker, 1994.
3. Moore AP, ed. *Handbook of botulinum toxin treatment.* Oxford: Blackwell Science, 1995.
4. Jankovic J, Brin MF. Botulinum toxin: historical perspective and potential new indications. *Muscle Nerve* 1997;20:(Suppl 6):S129–S137.
5. Dressler D. *Botulinum toxin therapy.* Stuttgart: Thieme-Verlag, 2000.
6. Borodic GE, Acquadro, M, Johnson, EA. Botulinum toxin therapy for pain and inflammatory disorders: mechanisms and therapeutic effects. *Exp Opin Invest Drugs* 2001;10:1531–1544.
7. Jankovic J, Schwartz K. Response and immunoresistance to botulinum toxin injections. *Neurology* 1995;45:1743–1746.
8. Borodic G, Johnson E, Goodnough M, et al. Botulinum toxin therapy, immunologic resistance, and problems with available materials. *Neurology* 1996;46:26–29.
9. Hatheway CL, Dang C. Immunogenicity of the neurotoxins of *Clostridium botulinum.* In: Jankovic J, Hallett M, eds. *Therapy with botulinum toxin.* New York: Marcel Dekker, 1994:93–107.
10. Schantz EJ, Johnson EA. Properties and use of botulinum toxin and other microbial neurotoxins in medicine. *Microbiol Rev* 1992;56:80–99.
11. Goodnough MC, Johnson EA. Stabilization of botulinum toxin during lyophilization. *Appl Environ Microbiol* 1992;58:3426–3428.
12. Johnson EA, Goodnough MC. Preparation and properties of botulinum toxin type A for medical use. In: Tsui JKC, Calne DB, eds. *Handbook of dystonia.* New York: Marcel Dekker, 1995:347–365.
13. Schantz EJ, Johnson EA. Botulinum toxin: the story of its development for the treatment of human disease. *Perspect Biol Med* 1997;40:317–327.
14. Johnson EA. Clostridial toxins as therapeutic agents: benefits of nature's most toxic proteins. *Annu Rev Microbiol* 1999;53:551–575.
15. Matsuda M, Yoneda M. Dissociation of tetanus toxin into two polypeptide fragments. *Biochem Biophys Res Commun* 1974;57:1257–1262.
16. Matsuda M, Yoneda M. Isolation and purification of two antigenically active, "complementary" polypeptide fragments of tetanus neurotoxin. *Infect Immun* 1975;12:1147–1153.
17. Matsuda M, Yoneda M. Reconstitution of tetanus neurotoxin from two antigenically active polypeptide fragments. *Biochem Biophys Res Commun* 1976;68:668–674.
18. Kozaki S, Miyazaki S, Sakaguchi G. Development of antitoxin with each of two complementary fragments of *Clostridium botulinum* type B derivative toxin. *Infect Immun* 1977;18:761–766.
19. Koazki S, Togashi, Sakaguchi G. Separation of *Clostridium botulinum* type A derivative toxin into two fragments. *Jpn J Med Sci Biol* 1981;34:61–68.
20. Syuto B, Kubo S. Separation and characterization of heavy and light chains of *Clostridium botulinum* type C toxin and their reconstitution. *J Biol Chem* 1981;256:3712–3717.
21. Sathyamoorthy V, DasGupta BR. Separation, purification, partial characterization and comparison of heavy and light chains of botulinum neurotoxin types A, B, and E. *J Biol Chem* 1985;260:110461–10466.
22. Maisey EA, Wadsworth JDF, Poulain B, et al. Involvement of constituent chains of botulinum neurotoxins A

and B in the blockade of neurotransmitter release. *Eur J Biochem* 1988;177:683–691.

23. Weller U, Dauzenroth ME, Zu Heringtorf DM, et al. Chains and fragments of tetanus toxin. Separation, reassociation, and pharmacological properties. *Eur J Biochem* 1989;182:640–656.

24. Weller U, Dauzenroth ME, Gansel M, et al. Cooperative action of the light chain of tetanus toxin and the heavy chain of botulinum toxin type A on the transmitter release of mammalian motor endplates. *Neurosci Lett* 1991;122:132–134.

25. Poulain B, Wadsworth JDF, Maisey EA, et al. Inhibition of transmitter release by botulinum neurotoxin A. Contribution of various fragments to the intoxication process. *Eur J Biochem* 1989;185:197–203.

26. de Paiva A, Poulain B, Lawrence GW, et al. A role for the interchain disulfide or its participating thiols in the internalization of botulinum neurotoxin-A revealed by a toxin derivative that binds to ecto-acceptors and inhibits transmitter release intracellularly. *J Biol Chem* 1993; 268:20838–20844.

27. Mohanraj D, Ramakrishman S. Cytotoxic effects of ricin without an interchain disulfide bond: genetic modification and chemical cross-linking studies. *Biochim Biophys Acta* 1995;1243:399–406.

28. Francis JW, Brown RH Jr, Figueiredo D, et al. Enhancement of diphtheria toxin potency by replacement of the receptor binding domain with tetanus toxin C-fragment: a potential vector for delivering heterologous proteins to neurons. *J Neurochem* 2000;74:2528–2536.

29. Kreitman RJ, Pastan I. Immunotoxins for targeted cancer therapy. *Adv Drug Deliv Rev* 1998;31:53–88.

30. Brinkmann U. Recombinant antibody fragments and immunotoxin fusions for cancer therapy. *In Vivo* 2000;14: 21–27.

31. Frankel AE, Kreitman RJ, Sausville EA. Targeted toxins. *Clin Cancer Res* 2000;6:326–334.

32. O'Toole JE, Esseltine D, Lynch TJ, et al. Clinical trials with blocked ricin immunotoxins. *Curr Top Microbiol Immunol* 1998;234:35–56.

33. Winkler U, Barth S, Schell R, et al. The emerging role of immunotoxins in leukemia and lymphoma. *Ann Oncol* 1997;8(Suppl 1):139–146.

34. Speck VD, Murphy JR. Fusion protein toxins based on diphtheria toxin: selective targeting of growth factor receptors of eukaryotic cells. *Meth Enzymol* 2000;327: 239–249.

35. Linardou H, Epenotos AA, Dionarain MP. A recombinant cytotoxic chimera based on mammalian deoxyribonuclease-I. *Int J Cancer* 2000;86:561–569.

36. Remsen LG, Trail PA, Hellstrom I, et al. Enhanced delivery improves the efficacy of a tumor-specific doxorubicin immunoconjugate in a human brain tumor xenograft model. *Neurosurgery* 2000;46:704–709.

37. Dosio F, Arpicco S, Adobati E, et al. Role of cross-linking agents in determining the biochemical and pharmacokinetic properties of Mgr6-clavin immunotoxins. *Bioconjug Chem* 1998;9:372–381.

38. Wallace KB, Starkov AA. Mitochondrial targets of drug toxicity. *Annu Rev Pharmacol Toxicol* 2000;40: 353–388.

39. Kobayashi K, Morita S, Sawada H, et al. Immunotoxin-mediated conditional disruption of specific neurons in transgenic mice. *Proc Natl Acad Sci U S A* 1995;92: 1132–1136.

40. Liu X-H, Castelli JA, Youle RJ. Receptor-mediated up take of an extracellular Bcl-XL fusion protein inhibits apoptosis. *Proc Natl Acad Sci U S A* 1999;96: 9563–9567.

41. Niemann H. Molecular biology of clostridial neurotoxins. In: Alouf JE, Freer JH, eds. *A sourcebook of bacterial protein toxins*. London: Academic Press, 1991: 303–348.

42. Henderson I, Davis T, Elmore M, et al. The genetic basis of toxin production in *Clostridium botulinum* and *Clostridium tetani*. In: Rood JI, McClane BA, Songer JG, et al., eds. *The clostridia. Molecular biology and pathogenesis*. San Diego, CA: Academic Press, 1997: 261–294.

43. Johnson EA, Bradshaw M. *Clostridium botulinum* and its neurotoxins: A metabolic and cellular perspective. *Toxicon* 2001;39:1703–1722.

44. Zdanovsky AG, Zdanoskaia MV. Simple and efficient method for heterologous expression of clostridial proteins. *Appl Environ Microbiol* 2000;66:3166–3173.

45. Li Y, Aoki R, Dolly JO. Expression and characterisation of the heavy chain of tetanus toxin: Reconstitution of the fully recombinant di-chain protein in active form. *J Biochem* 1999;125:1200–1208.

46. Kadkhodyan S, Knapp MS, Schmidt JJ, et al. Cloning, expression, and one-step purification of the minimal essential domain of the light chain of botulinum neurotoxin type A. *Protein Expr Purif* 2000;19:125–130.

47. Tonello F, Pellizzari R, Pasqualato S, et al. Recombinant and truncated tetanus neurotoxin light chain: cloning, expression, purification, and proteolytic activity. *Protein Expr Purif* 1999;15:221–227.

48. Bradshaw M, Goodnough MC, Johnson EA. Conjugative transfer of the *Escherichia coli-Clostridium perfringens* shuttle vector pJIR1457 to *Clostridium botulinum* type A strains. *Plasmid* 1998;40:233–237.

49. Chaddock JA, Purkiss JR, Friis LM, et al. Inhibition of vesicular secretion in both neuronal and nonneuronal cells by a retargeted endopeptidase derivative of *Clostridium botulinum* neurotoxin type A. *Infect Immun* 2000;68:2587–2593.

50. Hott JS, Dalakas MC, Sung C, et al. Skeletal muscle-specific immunotoxin for the treatment of focal muscle spasm. *Neurology* 1998;50:485–491.

51. Oguma K, Fuginaga Y, Inoue K, et al. Mechanisms of pathogenesis and toxin synthesis in *Clostridium botulinum*. In: Cary JW, Linz JE, Bhatnagar D, eds. *Microbial foodborne diseases*. Lancaster, PA: Technomic Publishing Company, 2000:273–293.

52. Lacy DB, Tepp W, Cohen AC, et al. Crystal structure of botulinum neurotoxin type A and implications for toxicity. *Nat Struct Biol* 1998;5:898–902.

53. Lacy DB, Stevens RC. Sequence homology and structural analysis of the clostridial neurotoxins. *J Mol Biol* 1999;291:1091–1104.

54. Swaminathan S, Eswaramoorthy S. Structural analysis of the catalytic and binding sites of *Clostridium botulinum* neurotoxin B. *Nat Struct Biol* 2000;7:693–699.

55. Reichmann L, Winter G. Novel folded protein domains generated by combinatorial shuffling of polypeptide segments. *Proc Natl Acad Sci U S A* 2000;97: 10068–10073.

56. Crameri A, Raillard S-A, Bermudez E, et al. DNA shuffling of a family of genes from diverse species accelerates directed evolution. *Nature* 1998;391:288–291.

57. Ostermeier M, Nixon AE, Shim JH, et al. Combinatorial protein engineering by incremental truncation. *Proc Natl Acad Sci U S A* 1999;96:3562–3567.

Scientific and Therapeutic Aspects of Botulinum Toxin
edited by M.F. Brin, J. Jankovic, and M. Hallett
Lippincott Williams & Wilkins, Philadelphia, © 2002.

48

Novel Toxin Developments: Delivery of Endopeptidase Activity of Botulinum Neurotoxin to New Target Cells

Keith A. Foster

The seven serotypes of the botulinum neurotoxins (BoNTs), A through G, are among the most potent acute lethal toxins known, and are responsible for outbreaks of the lethal food-poisoning disease botulism. Paradoxically, these toxins, particularly serotype A, have, since the pioneering studies of Alan Scott, found increasing use as therapeutic agents (1). The neurotoxins exert their effect by inhibition of synaptic transmission at cholinergic nerve terminals. To do this, the toxins have evolved a highly specialized repertoire of pharmacologic activities, which in recent years have been related to discrete functional domains within the toxin. This highly evolved structure–function relationship is responsible for the potency and selectivity of the neurotoxins, and underlies both their pathologic and therapeutic activities. The understanding of the structure–functional basis of neurotoxin action has enabled component functions of the activity to be dissected out and fragments of the toxin to be employed in the creation of novel agents seeking to employ specific capabilities of the toxins' highly evolved pharmacologic activities in novel therapeutics. This chapter focuses on such studies in relation to the endopeptidase activity of the neurotoxin.

Intoxication of the neuromuscular junction is thought to occur in at least four phases: an initial binding phase, an internalization phase, a translocation phase, and, finally, a neurotransmitter blockade phase (2). The structural basis of these phases resides in three distinct domains within the neurotoxin polypeptide. All BoNTs have a similar structure, consisting of a heavy chain (HC) of approximately 100 kDa, covalently joined, by a single disulphide bond, to a light chain (LC) of approximately 50 kDa (2). Proteolytic cleavage of the H-chain of *Clostridium botulinum* neurotoxin type A (BoNT-A) generates two fragments of approximately 50 kDa each. The C-terminal domain (H_C) is required for target-cell binding, while the N-terminal domain (H_N) is proposed to be involved in intracellular membrane translocation (3). Further support and insight into this structure was recently provided by the x-ray crystallographic resolution of the protein structures of serotypes A and B (4,5). These studies revealed that the neurotoxins adopt a linear arrangement of the three functional domains, with no contact between the catalytic LC and the H_C binding domain. The three domains are spatially distinct with the exception of a loop of the H_N domain, which wraps around the LC, and in BoNT-A occludes the active site, while in BoNT-B it does not completely occlude the active site. The H_C domain consists of two β-strand regions of roughly equal size joined by a single α-helix. The H_N domain of both BoNT-A and BoNT-B contains a coiled-coil cylindrical main body consisting of a pair of antiparallel amphipathic helices twisted around each other with triple helix bundles at each end. While core regions of the long helices show limited homology to the translocation domains of other bacterial proteins, the fold of the BoNT H_N is indicative of a mechanism of pore formation more in keeping with coiled-coil viral proteins having membrane-disruption properties.

BoNTs exhibit a high degree of selectivity for the neuromuscular junction, although they will also bind to and intoxicate other types of neuronal cell. This selectivity is believed to result from specific binding to their target cell by a combination of high-affinity binding events possibly involving more than one component (6). The identities of the cellular receptors for the BoNTs are generally unknown, although it is thought that both gangliosides and membrane glycoproteins may serve as targets for toxin binding in a dual-receptor capacity. Following binding, the BoNTs are internalized, still bound to their receptor, into an acidic endosomal compartment within the synaptic terminal (7), within which it is proposed that the H_N domain undergoes an acid-induced conformational change, leading to the formation of transmembrane pores. The ability of the H_N domain to form channels in liposomes, artificial lipid bilayers, and cell membranes under acidic conditions has been demonstrated (3,7,8). The LC of the BoNT is then believed to gain access to the neuronal cytosol via the H_N-mediated pore. The BoNT LC is a zinc-dependent endopeptidase and once it has gained access to the cytosol, it specifically hydrolyses key components of the soluble NSF (*N*-ethylmaleimide-sensitive factor) attachment receptor (SNARE) complex (9) required for synaptic vesicle docking, fusion, and neurotransmitter release. In nerve terminals, the SNARE proteins are vesicle-associated membrane protein (VAMP, also called synaptobrevin), syntaxin, and a 25-kDa synaptosomal protein (SNAP-25). BoNT-A and BoNT-E cleave SNAP-25, whereas neurotoxin types B, D, F, and G cleave VAMP (10). BoNT-C is unique among the BoNTs in having two identified substrate proteins, both components of the SNARE complex, SNAP-25, and syntaxin (12). Each of the BoNTs hydrolyzes a single, specific peptide bond within its substrate protein, with no BoNT cleaving the same peptide bond as another. Thus, BoNTs are highly specific in terms of both their target cell interaction and their substrate cleavage requirements. Cleavage of SNARE complex proteins by BoNTs destabilizes complex formation such that a failure of the vesicle docking and fusion mechanism occurs, resulting in inhibition of transmitter release from the neuronal cell. This proteolytic activity is the sole reported intracellular activity of the BoNTs.

SNARE proteins are not restricted to neuronal cells. Increasing numbers of isotypes of each of the SNARE protein families are being discovered, and they are considered to be pivotal components of a universal mechanism for vesicle fusion and exocytosis (11). Therefore, the highly specific endopeptidase activities of the BoNTs provide an opportunity for inhibiting SNARE-mediated events, and thereby exocytotic processes including secretion, in a wide variety of cell types.

Unfortunately, the use of native BoNTs is limited by the availability of the requisite toxin receptor(s) on the target cell of interest. Alternative approaches to internalize the active endopeptidase have included techniques such as microinjection, permeabilization or electroporation (12,13). Because of their invasive nature, however, these techniques are less than ideal for the study of complex intracellular processes, and they are entirely inappropriate for the therapeutic use of BoNTs or BoNT derivatives to inhibit secretory events underlying the pathology of disease in nonneuronal cells. To overcome these issues alternative molecules capable of delivering functional endopeptidase to the cytosol of target cells *in vitro* have been investigated.

Under conditions in which the disulfide bond between the L- and H-chains is maintained, trypsin cleavage of BoNT-A results in a 100-kDa species termed LH_N/A (originally described as H_2L in reference 14) representing a catalytically active, non-cell-binding derivative of BoNT-A. By conjugating LH_N/A to alternative targeting ligands, it is proposed to reconstitute the molecule with a cell-binding component while retaining membrane translocation and enzymatic activities. Studies with two alternative targeting ligands, wheat germ agglutinin (WGA) and nerve growth factor (NGF), are reported here. Although generation of LH_N fragments by limited proteolysis has not been reported for all serotypes of BoNT, cloning of the genes for the different serotypes enables recombinant expression of LH_N fragments of all BoNT serotypes and retargeting of their LC activities in a manner akin to that described for LH_N/A.

WGA-LH$_N$/A

WGA, a homodimeric lectin molecule of 36 kDa expressed by the plant species *Triticum vulgaris,* has an affinity for *N*-acetylglucosamine (GlcNAc) and *N*-acetyl sialic acid (NeuNAc) moieties on cell surfaces (15). It has been utilized as a neuronal cell marker, for retrograde transport studies, and for analysis of lectin effects on a variety of cell functions (16). This profile and the degree of characterization make WGA attractive as a novel cell-binding domain for retargeting BoNT LH$_N$ fragments.

WGA-LH$_N$/A conjugate was synthesized by chemically coupling WGA and LH$_N$/A using the heterobifunctional cross-linker *N*-succinimidyl 3-[2-pyridyldithio] propionate (SPDP) as described (17). Conjugation of LH$_N$/A with WGA in this manner generates a heterogenous mixture of high-molecular-weight species; however, when the disulfide bond between LH$_N$/A and WGA was reduced, the heterogenous mixture was shown to consist purely of LH$_N$/A and WGA. It was also established that the catalytic activity of the LH$_N$/A was not compromised by derivatization, with the EC$_{50}$ values (concentration required to achieve 50% substrate cleavage) for BoNT-A, dLH$_N$/A, and LH$_N$/A being 9.0 pM/L, 5.1 pM/L, and 5.9 pM/L, respectively. Therefore, it would be predicted that the enzymic activity of the LH$_N$/A component when introduced into a cell would be similar to that of BoNT-A. Purification of WGA-LH$_N$/A was achieved by a two-step strategy: first, size exclusion chromatography was utilized to remove nonconjugated WGA from the mixture; second, an affinity chromatography step was used to isolate and concentrate species that bound GlcNAc. In this way, the contamination of the construct preparations with nonconjugated WGA and LH$_N$/A components was minimized.

WGA-LH$_N$/A caused concentration-dependent inhibition of secretion from a variety of neuronal and neuroendocrine cells, which correlated closely with cleavage of the substrate protein SNAP-25 in the target cells (17). In all cases, the inhibitory effects of LH$_N$/A alone were extremely low. The ligand-dependent nature of the targeting of the LH$_N$/A was confirmed

by the ability to block both cleavage of SNAP-25 (17) and inhibition of secretion (Fig. 48.1) with excess WGA. These data confirm that both the SNAP-25 cleavage and consequent inhibition of secretion by the conjugate are not a consequence of a WGA effect on cell function.

The effect of WGA-LH$_N$/A on neurotransmitter release was compared with that of BoNT-A in a variety of cell types (Table 48.1). The IC$_{50}$ for inhibition of [^{3}H]-NA release from the established cell lines SH-SY5Y and PC12 cells were determined to be of a similar order for both the WGA-LH$_N$/A conjugate and BoNT-A. In the case of primary neuronal cultures, particularly embryonic spinal cord cultures, however, inhibition of release was significantly reduced in WGA-LH$_N$/A treated cells when compared to the BoNT-A–treated cells (Table 48.1). It is clear, therefore, that the WGA-LH$_N$/A conjugate and BoNT-A do not represent proteins with identical properties of cell binding and intracellular routing.

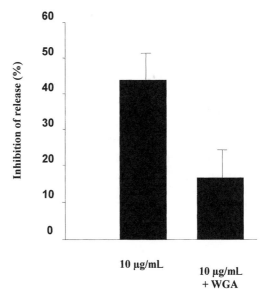

FIG. 48.1. Competition of WGA-LH$_N$/A inhibition of secretion from SH-SY5Y cells by excess WGA. SH-SY5Y cells were exposed to WGA-LH$_N$/A on ice (4°C/39.2°F) for 4 hours in the presence or absence of 100-fold excess WGA, washed and incubated for 16 hours at 37°C (98.6°F) prior to the determination of [^{3}H]-noradrenaline release as described in reference 17.

TABLE 48.1. *Relative efficacy of inhibition of release by WGA-LH$_N$/A as compared to BoNT-A in a variety of cell types*

Cell type	Inhibition of release IC$_{50}$ (mean 6 SEM) following incubation with:	
	WGA-LH$_N$/A	BoNT-A
SH-SY5Y	9.57±0.36 nM/L	5.56±2.37 nM/L
PC12	3.77±0.90 nM/L	4.00±1.30 nM/L
DRG	1.86±0.29 nM/L	0.11±0.03 nM/L
eSC	0.36±0.08 nM/L	0.03±0.01 pM/L

Data are means from a minimum of three independent experiments. SH-SY5Y cells, PC12 cells and eSC neurons were prepared as described in reference 17. DRG neurons were prepared as described in reference 23. All cell types were treated with a range of concentrations of WGA-LH$_N$/A or BoNT-A for 3 days prior to determining stimulated neurotransmitter release. In all cases, the IC$_{50}$ values were calculated from concentration response curves that generated both maximum and minimum inhibitory effects. Stimulated release of [^{3}H]-noradrenaline from SH-SY5Y cells and PC12 cells and stimulated release of [^{3}H]-glycine from eSC neurons was measured as described in reference 17. Stimulated release of substance P from DRG neurons was measured as described in reference 23.

NGF-LH$_N$/A

In addition to demonstrating the ability to retarget the LC of BoNT-A with the lectin WGA, a growth factor has also been used as a ligand to assess the generality of the retargeting concept. NGF, a highly basic 13-kDa protein with three conserved disulfide bridges, is a member of a small group of structurally related growth factors known as neurotrophins. NGF is specific to the peripheral nervous system, where it regulates the survival and development of sympathetic and some sensory neurons (18), and has limited actions on other neuron types (largely central cholinergic neurons of basal forebrain). It has been observed to undergo retrograde transport from the nerve terminal to the cell body in sensory neurons via interaction with a receptor (19). Two receptors for NGF have been identified: TrkA, a high-affinity receptor specific for NGF (20), and p75, a low-affinity, nonspecific neurotrophin receptor. Binding of NGF to TrkA induces receptor internalization, which suggests that NGF could be used as a targeting moiety.

NGF-LH$_N$/A conjugate was synthesized by chemically coupling murine 2.5S NGF and LH$_N$/A using Traut's reagent (N-[4-(p-azidosalicylamido)butyl]-3′-(2′-pyridyldithio)propionamide) as described (21). An important aspect of the conjugation and purification schemes as developed was the maintenance of the biologic activity of the constituent construct components; however, the resulting final yield of purified conjugate was relatively low (approximately 250 μg from 2 mg NGF). The conjugate did retain a capability to stimulate neurite outgrowth in PC12 cells, a property of NGF, with an EC$_{50}$ for the conjugate of 0.12 ± 0.04 nM/L and for control NGF of 0.07 ± 0.02 nM/L. This demonstrates that the majority of the NGF retained its ability to interact with the NGF receptor when coupled to LH$_N$/A. It was also established that the catalytic activity of the LH$_N$/A was not compromised by derivatization, the EC$_{50}$ values for BoNT-A, Trauts-derivatized LH$_N$/A and LH$_N$/A being 8.97 pM/L, 5.1 pM/L, and 5.9 pM/L, respectively. Therefore, as for the WGA-LH$_N$/A, it would be predicted that the enzymic activity of the LH$_N$/A component when introduced into a cell would be similar to BoNT-A.

NGF-LH$_N$/A conjugate displayed a comparable ability to BoNT-A to inhibit depolarization-stimulated release of [^{3}H]-noradrenaline from differentiated PC12 cells following 3 days treatment with an IC$_{50}$ of 1.71 ± 0.39 nM/L as compared to 4.0 ± 1.27 nM/L for BoNT-A (21). By contrast LH$_N$/A had an IC$_{50}$ of 688 nM/L, clearly demonstrating the significant decrease in potency of BoNT-A when the H$_C$ domain is removed. NGF alone was without effect on either the uptake or release of [^{3}H]-noradrenaline. In addition to inhibition of [^{3}H]-noradrenaline release, NGF-LH$_N$/A produced a concentration-dependent SNAP-25 cleavage (21), indicating that the observed inhibition of neurotransmitter release is endopeptidase-mediated. In the presence of competing free NGF, conjugate treatment resulted in significantly less cleavage of SNAP-25, consistent with the entry of the endopeptidase into the cell being dependent upon binding to NGF receptors.

INHIBITION OF INSULIN RELEASE

To demonstrate an ability to retarget neurotoxin endopeptidase activity to cells resistant to

BoNTs because of a lack of the necessary receptor, a cell type is needed that lacks the receptor but has a secretory response dependent on the relevant BoNT substrate. The hamster pancreatic B cell line HIT-T15 is resistant to the effects of BoNT-A, and yet displays SNARE-dependent secretion of insulin when permeabilization of the cell membrane is used to allow the clostridial neurotoxin endopeptidase access to the substrate (13,22). When HIT-T15 cells were incubated with WGA-LH_N/A, and insulin release assessed by radioimmunoassay 16 hours later, a significant dose-dependent inhibition of stimulated insulin release was observed that correlated with increasing cleavage of SNAP-25 (17). At a concentration of 100 $\mu g/mL$ WGA-LH_N/A, inhibition of insulin release was calculated to be $81.6\% \pm 15.7\%$ ($n = 3$), which is in good agreement with previously reported neurotoxin-dependent inhibition of insulin release of approximately 90% (13).

DISCUSSION

LH_N/A can be chemically conjugated to a second protein to form a stable, soluble conjugate able to deliver the neurotoxin endopeptidase activity to a variety of cells *in vitro* by a ligand-dependent process to inhibit secretion via a mechanism involving endopeptidase-dependent cleavage of the natural BoNT-A substrate (17,21). This work represents the first reported replacement of the botulinum neurotoxin cell-binding domain to result in the creation of functional hybrid constructs.

Two different ligands, one a lectin and one a growth factor, have been successfully employed to target the neurotoxin constructs to cells. In both cases, the ligand dependency of the construct activity has been demonstrated by competition with excess free ligand. For the endopeptidase to gain access to its substrate and inhibit secretion via cleavage of SNAP-25, the construct conjugated LH_N/A is required to traverse at least one intracellular membrane. Given the equivalent catalytic activity of the LH_N/A endopeptidase, as assessed in the *in vitro* cleavage assay, the similar overall potencies of the WGA-LHN/A conjugate and BoNT-A in both the PC12

and SH-SY5Y cell lines (17) would indicate that the membrane translocation function of the LH_N/A has not been significantly compromised by conjugation. Indeed, these observations suggest that the H_N domain is fully effective at transporting LC into the cytosol, even though the receptor-mediated mode of entry is different to that employed by native neurotoxin. Thus, it is concluded that the H_N domain has the ability to facilitate translocation of the LC in cell types not associated with the neuromuscular junction.

Furthermore, the effective functioning of the L-chain in the HIT-T15 cytosol, as evidenced by both the cleavage of SNAP-25 and inhibition of insulin secretion, demonstrates that the H_N domain is able to function in a nonneuronal environment enabling translocation of the L-chain. This is the first demonstration of H_N function in a nonneuronal cell. The inhibition of insulin release attained following application of WGA-LH_N/A and internalization of functional endopeptidase into the endocrine cell line HIT-T15 correlated with the cleavage of SNAP-25, and was similar to that previously reported following BoNT-A treatment of permeabilized HIT-T15 cells (13). The ability to inhibit SNARE-dependent release from a cell that is resistant to the actions of surface applied neurotoxin is a significant step forward in the design of a tool for investigation of SNARE-mediated processes.

This study has also indicated differences in potency between the WGA-LH_N/A conjugate and intact BoNT/A. The susceptibility of the established cell lines and primary neuronal cultures, particularly eSC neurons, to BoNT-A-dependent inhibition of transmitter release varies markedly (Table 48.1), with eSC neurons being greater than 10^5-fold more sensitive than PC12 and SH-SY5Y cells. This difference could be a result of the prevalence and/or distribution of the receptor(s) for BoNT-A on the plasma membrane and/or the localized concentration of SNAP-25 near the point of internalization. Therefore, although conjugates of significant potency have been produced, the characteristics of the conjugates in respect of binding, and possibly the intracellular routing, do not simply replicate those of the parental neurotoxin.

Electroporation, permeabilization, or liposome-mediated transfer, are common mechanisms for introducing foreign proteins into cells. Such techniques may, however, compromise cellular functions and are often unsuitable for mixed cell cultures because of the lack of specificity. The ability to target soluble BoNT endopeptidase to the cell of choice is therefore a beneficial alternative to these methodologies. This work demonstrates that a potently active neurotoxin can be detoxified and selectively retargeted with equivalent potency to a variety of cell types *in vitro*. Two very different ligands demonstrate the ability to present the endopeptidase to cells in a form suitable for access to the intracellular substrate and thereby enable cleavage of the substrate. This work establishes that BoNT light chains can be targeted to cells via an alternative route to the native heavy-chain mediated receptor.

The ability to deliver the endopeptidase of BoNT to selected target cells, including ones that are insensitive to native neurotoxin, by replacement of the H_C domain of the neurotoxin with a ligand of choice, opens up the possibility of developing second-generation therapeutics employing the potent pharmacologic properties of the BoNT LC. It will also enable the intracellular routing and kinetics of action of BoNTs in a variety of cell types to be studied in a manner that retains cellular integrity. Although the work described to date is all based upon the LH_N fragment of BoNT-A, the use of recombinant expression systems will enable similar agents employing the LH_N of other serotypes to be produced. Thus, the opportunity now exists to exploit BoNT endopeptidases in the inhibition of secretory disorders for which the native neurotoxins are unsuited. An exciting prospect for novel neurotoxin-based therapeutics is emerging.

ACKNOWLEDGMENTS

The author is grateful to the following for their contribution to the studies described in this chapter: F. Alexander, J. Broadbridge, J. Chaddock, S. Doward, S. Fooks, L. Friis, S. Hiscott, M. Herbert, R. Ling, K. Newton, J. Purkiss, C. Quinn, and C. Shone.

REFERENCES

1. Münchau A, Bhatia KP. Uses of botulinum toxin injection in medicine today. *BMJ* 2000;320:161–165.
2. Simpson LL. The origin, structure and pharmacological activity of botulinum toxin. *Pharmacol Rev* 1981;33:155–188.
3. Shone CC, Hambleton P, Melling J. A 50-kDa fragment from the NH$_2$-terminus of the heavy subunit of *Clostridium botulinum* type A neurotoxin forms channels in lipid membranes. *Eur J Biochem* 1987;167:175–180.
4. Lacy BD, Tepp W, Cohen AC, et al. Crystal structure of botulinum neurotoxin type A and implications for toxicity. *Nat Struct Biol* 1998;5:898–902.
5. Swaminathan S, Eswaramoorthy S. Structural analysis of the catalytic and binding sites of *Clostridium botulinum* neurotoxin B. *Nat Struct Biol* 2000;7:693–699.
6. Halpern JL, Neale EA. Neurospecific binding, internalization and retrograde axonal transport. *Curr Top Microbiol Immunol* 1995;195:221–241.
7. Hoch DH, Romero MM, Ehrlich BE, et al. Channels formed by botulinum, tetanus and diphtheria toxins in planar lipid bilayers: relevance to translocation of proteins across membranes. *Proc Natl Acad Sci U S A* 1985;82:1692–1696.
8. Sheridan RE. Gating and permeability of ion channels produced by botulinum toxin types A and E in PC12 cell membranes. *Toxicon* 2000;36:703–717.
9. Sollner T, Whiteheart SW, Brunner M, et al. SNAP receptors implicated in vesicle targeting and fusion. *Nature* 1993;362:318–324.
10. Montecucco C, Schiavo G. Mechanism of action of tetanus and botulinum neurotoxins. *Mol Microbiol* 1994;13:1–8.
11. Linial M. SNARE proteins—why so many, why so few? *J Neurochem* 1997;69:1781–1792.
12. Foran P, Lawrence GW, Shone CC, et al. Botulinum neurotoxin C1 cleaves both syntaxin and SNAP-25 in intact and permeabilized chromaffin cells: correlation with its blockade of catecholamine release. *Biochemistry* 1996;35:2630–2636.
13. Boyd RS, Duggan MJ, Shone CC, et al. The effect of botulinum neurotoxins on the release of insulin from the insulinoma cell lines HIT-15 and RINm5F. *J Biol Chem* 1995;270:18216–18218.
14. Shone CC, Hambleton P, Melling J. Inactivation of *Clostridium botulinum* type A neurotoxin by trypsin and purification of two tryptic fragments: proteolytic action near the COOH-terminus of the heavy subunit destroys toxin-binding activity. *Eur J Biochem* 1985;151:75–82.
15. Nagata Y, Burger MM. Wheat germ agglutinin: molecular characteristics and specificity for sugar binding. *J Biol Chem* 1974;249:3116–3122.
16. Lis H, Sharon N. Lectins as molecules and as tools. *Annu Rev Biochem* 1986;55:35–67.
17. Chaddock JA, Purkiss JR, Friis LM, et al. Inhibition of vesicular secretion in both neuronal and nonneuronal cells by a retargeted endopeptidase derivative of *Clostridium botulinum* neurotoxin type A. *Infect Immun* 2000;68:2587–2593.
18. Davies AM. Cell death and the trophic requirements of developing sensory neurons. In: Scott SA, ed. *Sensory neurons: diversity, development, and plasticity.* New York: Oxford University Press, 1992:194–214.
19. Stockel K, Schwab M, Thoenen H. Comparison between

the retrograde axonal transport of nerve growth factor and tetanus toxin in motor, sensory and adrenergic neurons. *Brain Res* 1975; 99:1–16.

20. Barbacid M. The Trk family of neurotrophin receptors. *J Neurobiol* 1994;25:1386–1403.

21. Chaddock JA, Purkiss JR, Duggan MD, et al. A conjugate composed of nerve growth factor coupled to a nontoxic derivative of *Clostridium botulinum* neurotoxin type A can inhibit neurotransmitter release in vitro. *Growth Factors* 2000;18:147–155.

22. Sadoul K, Lang J, Montecucco C, et al. SNAP-25 is expressed in islets of Langerhans and is involved in insulin release. *J Cell Biol* 1995;128:1019–1028.

23. Welch MJ, Purkiss JR, Foster KA. Sensitivity of embryonic rat dorsal root ganglia neurons to *Clostridium botulinum* neurotoxins. *Toxicon* 2000;38:245–258.

Scientific and Therapeutic Aspects of Botulinum Toxin
edited by M.F. Brin, J. Jankovic, and M. Hallett
Lippincott Williams & Wilkins, Philadelphia, © 2002.

49

Neuronal Delivery Vectors Derived from Tetanus Toxin

Paul S. Fishman

Tetanus toxin (TTX) enters the central nervous system (CNS) from peripheral tissues with the highest efficiency of any known protein (1). This property has inspired several laboratories, including our own, to attempt to use nontoxic portions of the tetanus toxin molecule as vectors to deliver therapeutic proteins to the CNS. This chapter presents the properties of tetanus toxin, particularly as they relate to binding, transporting, and action of the toxin. The research that has evaluated these aspects for nontoxic tetanus peptides is evaluated, and the use of these peptides to carry potential therapeutics will be assessed.

STRUCTURE AND FUNCTION OF TETANUS TOXIN

Like botulinum neurotoxins, tetanus toxin is a two-chained molecule. Proteolytic cleavage by *Clostridium tetani* of a single-chain protoxin yields a toxin with an approximately 100 kDa heavy chain (HC) linked to a 50-kDa light chain (LC) through a disulfide bridge (2). Three molecular domains have been identified in TTX with similar characteristics to several other bacterial toxins. The carboxyl (C) terminal half of the heavy chain (H_C) mediates neuronal binding and internalization into endocytic vesicles. The amino (N) terminal half of the heavy chain (H_N) forms a pore in the vesicle membrane and mediates the extrusion of the light chain into the cytosol and is referred to as the translocation domain (3,4). The light chain (as is also the case for the botulinum neurotoxins) is a toxic protease that cleaves a membrane protein essential

for synaptic vesicle exocytosis. In the case of TTX the protein substrate is synaptobrevin, also known as vesicle-associated membrane protein (VAMP) (5).

In spite of similarities in structure and function of tetanus and botulinum neurotoxins, they cause dramatically different clinical syndromes (6). Clinical tetanus is characterized by persistent and unremitting contraction of affected muscles (7). The binding and transport properties of tetanus toxin play a major role in dictating the characteristics of this syndrome. Although tetanus toxin can inhibit release at the neuromuscular junction, it is not as potent as botulinum toxin, and this action is usually not clinically significant (8). The action of tetanus toxin is primarily within the CNS.

The source of tetanus toxin in clinical tetanus is usually a wound that provides a suitable anaerobic environment for the bacteria. The toxin diffuses from the wound to local motor neuron terminals and into the general circulation where it has access to all terminals at the neuromuscular junction (NMJ). Although tetanus toxin is too large to cross the blood–brain barrier, it exploits the naked presynaptic terminals of the NMJ to enter the CNS. In a manner similar to botulinum toxin, tetanus toxin undergoes binding and internalization into endocytic vesicles at the presynaptic terminals of the NMJ, but unlike botulinum toxin these vesicles undergo retrograde axonal transport to the motor neuron cell body within the spinal cord or brainstem (9–11). These vesicles then undergo exocytosis from the motor neuron soma and dendrites and the released toxin again undergoes endocytosis by presynaptic terminals in the CNS (12,13). It is at the presynaptic terminals surrounding motor neurons that tetanus toxin shows properties similar to botulinum neurotoxin. The toxin appears to undergo internalization either directly into synaptic vesicles or into endocytic vesicles that are later recycled into synaptic vesicles (14).

In the presence of the normally acid environment of synaptic vesicles, the light chain of TTX dissociates from the heavy chain and is extruded across the vesicle membrane. The catalytic light chain then has free access to cleave synaptobrevin on the cytosolic surface of the vesicle (15,16). The toxin shows a preference to localize and act at inhibitory presynaptic terminals (13,17). This results in preferential inactivation of inhibitory synaptic transmission, leading to a predominance of excitatory neurotransmission onto motor neurons (18,19). The end result is the sustained motor neuron activity and muscular contraction that characterizes clinical tetanus. This occurs initially at muscles close to the infected wound resulting in local tetanus. As the toxin spreads into the circulation it has access to virtually every motor neuron terminal through every NMJ resulting in the widespread involuntary muscle contraction of generalized tetanus. Like botulinum neurotoxin, tetanus neurotoxin has a very long duration of action, with a half-life of approximately 7 days measured by radioisotope methods in the CNS in experimental animals, and a clinical syndrome lasting several weeks in humans (1,7).

NONTOXIC BINDING FRAGMENTS OF TETANUS TOXIN

Studies with nontoxic fragments of TTX have attempted to determine whether they share the properties of TTX that would be useful for a vector for neuronal delivery, including: (a) highly avid and high capacity binding to neurons; (b) neuron-specific binding and internalization; (c) transsynaptic passage between neurons; and (d) prolonged persistence within the CNS. For such a peptide to be a useful vector, all of these properties need to be preserved when linked to another molecule for delivery.

The most well-studied tetanus peptide is the 45- to 50-kDa carboxyl terminus portion of the heavy chain that is now designated as H_C (but also termed B_{IIB}, fragment C, CF, or TTC). This molecule was originally generated by proteolytic cleavage of TTX, but has been expressed in a recombinant form in more recent studies (20–23). This peptide appears to contain the molecular domains responsible for binding and internalization of TTX. The binding properties of TTX, as well as the nature of its receptor, are still controversial.

As with botulinum neurotoxin, the tetanus toxin receptor appears to have both complex ganglioside and protein components (24–27). Unlike the botulinum neurotoxins, however, ganglioside binding may play a more significant role. TTX binding studies reveal two classes of receptors—smaller numbers of high-affinity receptors and larger numbers of low-affinity receptors (28,29). The complex membrane gangliosides GT_{1B} and GT_{1D} probably mediate the lower-affinity, higher-capacity binding (30,31). This form of binding has been the focus of most delivery and transport studies, although its role in the exquisitely high potency of toxicity of TTX is still unclear.

H_C has not only been completely sequenced, but its three-dimensional structure has also been revealed (32,33). The carboxyl terminal portion of H_C contains the ganglioside binding domain and is essential for neuronal binding and transport (34,35). The amino terminus of H_C has structural similarities to the plant lectins and probably binds to carbohydrate moiety of a membrane protein (33,36). This dual binding may be vital to the high potency of the toxin.

Like TTX, H_C shows a high degree of neuronal specificity both *in vivo* and *in vitro* and is widely used to assist in identifying neuronal cells in culture (37,38). Much of its specificity is a result of the unusually high concentration of complex ganglioside in neurons as compared to most other cell types (30). Even many neuronal cell lines do not have sufficient concentrations of GT_{1B} or GT_{1D} to allow them to bind significant quantities of TTX or H_C (20,29). Binding of TTX and H_C is both pH- and salt-sensitive with reduced binding under physiologic conditions (30). H_C is inferior to TTX in both neuronal binding and internalization under physiologic conditions and retrograde transport models (39,40,41). H_C is rapidly internalized after binding in a temperature- and energy-dependent manner (42). H_C does readily undergo retrograde axonal transport (12,20). As with TTX, H_C does not cross the blood–brain barrier. However, the ability to avidly bind motor neuron terminals allows H_C to effectively bypass the blood–brain barrier and enter the CNS via axonal transport.

Presynaptic motor neuron terminals at the neuromuscular junction are one of several neural structures that normally lack a blood–brain barrier. Other sites include peripheral sensory and autonomic nerve endings, hypothalamic secretory nuclei, the vomiting center at the area postrema, and regions surrounding the ventricles. Many exogenous and endogenous proteins that reach the systemic circulation are internalized by neurons with such projections outside the blood–brain barrier (43). TTX exploits these so-called portals to an extent that is unmatched by any other known proteins. Up to 1% of TTX can be detected within the CNS after a single peripheral injection (1). H_C demonstrates similar properties and is internalized by motor neurons from a systemic source at least 300 times more efficiently than a nonspecific protein such as horseradish peroxidase (HRP) (44). H_C does appear to have a preference for motor-neuron terminals as compared to sensory ending in the skin. This may relate to the particularly high concentrations of complex gangliosides at synaptic terminals (and perhaps also to a protein receptor) (45).

H_C also retains TTX's unusual capacity for transsynaptic transfer between neurons (46–48). Many proteins undergo retrograde axonal transport from motor neuron terminals to their cell bodies in the brainstem and spinal cord. Virtually all of these other proteins are retained within vesicular structures of the motor neurons where they are degraded. Some of the plant lectins, such as wheat germ agglutinin, show some transfer to surrounding neurons (49). Both TTX and H_C are predominately transferred from motor neuron cell bodies to surrounding presynaptic terminals. A fraction of tetanus protein

after transfer to these terminals again undergoes retrograde transport to the projecting neuron's cell body. Such retrograde transsynaptic transport has allowed H_C to be successfully used as a tracer to identify neurons that project to motor neurons or autonomic neurons (47,50–52). Such transneuronal transport has also been usually associated not with other proteins, but with neurotropic viruses such as the herpes virus group, which have also been used to map neurons with synaptic connections within the CNS (53).

H_C appears to pass between motor neurons and presynaptic terminals preferentially at regions of synaptic contact (54). The current evidence suggests that endosomes containing TTX or H_C fuse with the motor-neuron somal membrane, releasing their contents into the synaptic cleft. These proteins then bind to presynaptic terminal membranes where they undergo a second round of endocytosis, this time by synaptic vesicles or related vesicles. Once these proteins are internalized into presynaptic vesicles, TTX and H_C have different pathways. H_C lacks the pore-forming and translocation domains of TTX, and remains isolated from the cytosolic compartment of the presynaptic neurons. Evidence from both *in vivo* and *in vitro* studies suggest that H_C remains trapped within the presynaptic vesicle compartment where it may undergo repeated rounds of both exocytosis and reendocytosis (55).

It is well established that the light chains of both TTX and the botulinum neurotoxins must escape from the vesicle and have access to their substrates on the cytosolic surface of synaptic membranes to exert their toxic actions (27,56). Several aspects of this translocation process still remain unclear for the clostridial neurotoxins. It is unknown to what extent residual light or heavy chain is retained within the vesicles (57). It is unclear whether translocation of the light chain across the vesicle membrane results in a truly free molecule within the cytosol or whether it is bound to some extent to the outer membrane surface, with access to its protein substrates. These issues need to be clarified as research attempts to optimize the properties of vectors from clostridial neurotoxins that contain other domains besides H_C.

PROTEIN DELIVERY USING H_C

The potential of H_C as a carrier molecule was demonstrated quickly after its original characterization. Toxicity of TTX in animals could be reestablished by chemically coupling H_C with the other domains of the toxin. Toxicity was correlated with the capacity of this engineered toxin to be transported to the spinal cord (58).

The first potential therapeutic use of H_C to be considered was as an antidote to TTX intoxication. As with clinical botulism, circulating antibody has little impact on the course of clinical tetanus after the disease is established (1). This is likely caused by the inability of circulating anti-tetanus antibody to neutralize toxin after internalization by neurons. Conjugates linking H_C to anti-tetanus antibody directed at the other toxic domains have been created to intercept and neutralize internalized toxin in experimental animals (59).

The development of conjugates of H_C and HRP as a neuronal tracer, emphasized the potential utility of coupling an enzyme to H_C. The first successful use of an H_C-enzyme conjugate as a potential therapeutic involved hexosaminidase (HEX A) (60). The conjugate enhanced the uptake of HEX A by neuronal cells in culture over 15-fold than seen with unmodified enzyme. When neurons genetically deficient in HEX A were exposed to H_C–HEX A conjugates, they demonstrated a marked reduction in stores of its accumulated substrate (GM$_1$ ganglioside). This physiologic effect was correlated with internalization of conjugated protein into cellular vesicles. Similar chemical conjugates of H_C with other enzymes also demonstrate clearly enhanced retrograde axonal transport *in vivo* (both HRP and glucose oxidase) (44,57).

The availability of H_C in a recombinant form stimulated the development of H_C enzyme hybrids. H_C has been expressed as a hybrid protein with the major free radical detoxifying enzyme superoxide dismutase (SOD1). The hybrid enhances the delivery of SOD1 to cultured neurons by approximately 1,000-fold (61). The hybrid also undergoes retrograde and transneuronal transport from an intramuscular injection site *in vivo* (62). Similar results have been obtained after injection of an H_C–beta-galactosidase hybrid, which demonstrates preserved enzyme activity within the CNS (63).

Tests of physiologic and therapeutic efficacy of such H_C–enzyme hybrids have been disappointing thus far. An H_C–SOD1 hybrid has a modest beneficial effect that is not seen with free enzyme in a rodent stroke model (64). The larger hybrid molecule also showed improved pharmacokinetic properties after intravenous injection as compared to rapidly cleared free SOD1. It is unclear whether the beneficial effects seen reflected improved serum SOD1 levels or an H_C specific effect.

Incubation with H_C–SOD1 can substantially raise enzyme levels associated with neuronal cells in culture. These cells, however, were not protected from the cytotoxic effects of starvation, which produces a form of oxidative injury (65). Absolute SOD1 levels did not predict the lack of beneficial effect of H_C–SOD1 in this model. Neuroprotection was observed when enzyme levels were raised to comparable levels (two to three times control) with transfection or transgenic overexpression of SOD1.

These disappointing physiologic tests of H_C–enzyme hybrids are highly illustrative of both the limitations and potential strengths of this form of vector. H_C-linked enzyme has a very different intracellular distribution from enzymes delivered by overexpression of introduced genes. Gene delivery generally leads to a cytosolic distribution of the expressed protein. This cytosolic distribution can be modified if the natural or recombinant gene includes a domain that directs the protein to a specific subcellular target (i.e., mitochondria or secretory vesicles). As discussed earlier, H_C-linked enzymes remain tightly associated with synaptic membranes and vesicles. In the case of SOD1, it is likely that a cytosolic location with intimate contact with important structures such as mitochondria is needed for protection from oxidative injury.

Enzymes linked to H_C can escape into the cytosol if the hybrids also contain an appropriate translocation domain. The entire tetanus toxin molecule can even be functionally reconstituted after expression and purification of recombinant light and heavy chains (66,67). A three-domain hybrid has also been created that contains H_C as its binding domain, as well as the translocation and catalytic domains from diphtheria toxin. Although also a toxic enzyme, the substrate for diphtheria toxin is associated with ribosomes, a more distant cytosolic target than synaptic vesicles. This hybrid protein is extremely neurotoxic *in vitro*, a property not seen with native diphtheria toxin (68). Cellular specificity of this toxin is mediated by its neuronal specific H_C-binding domain, while its cytotoxicity reflects the ability of its diphtheria domain to inhibit cellular protein synthesis. This hybrid toxin has been proposed as a potential means of selectively killing motor neurons driving abnormal contractions when used in a manner similar to long-lasting, but reversible, inactivation of neuromuscular transmission obtained with botulinum toxin.

We are currently developing H_C-hybrid enzymes that are designed to exploit the unique synaptic localization of these proteins. In particular, we have chosen to focus on neurotransmitter modifying enzymes. Because of its importance in the pathogenesis of several neurologic diseases, many therapeutics have been developed that reduce the toxic effects of the excitatory neurotransmitter glutamate. Although extracellular concentrations of glutamate are normally controlled by an energy-dependent transport system, there are several known enzymes with glutamate-degrading capacity. After screening several of these enzymes, we determined that glutamate pyruvate transaminase (GPT, also known as alanine aminotransferase or ALT) has the greatest capacity to rapidly reduce glutamate levels below the neurotoxic range. GPT can protect neurons in culture from both toxic levels of added glutamate, and excessive extracellular glutamate generated by inhibiting cellular reuptake (69). We recently created an H_C-GPT hybrid and are currently testing it in both *in vitro* and *in vivo* models of glutamate excitotoxicity. Our hypothesis predicts that enhanced synaptic uptake and localization will increase both the potency and duration of action of H_C-GPT as compared to free GPT. If this strategy is successful, H_C could be useful in enhancing the action of other enzymes with potential synaptic sites of action. Another candidate

enzyme is glutamate decarboxylase (GAD), which degrades glutamate and synthesizes GABA, a major inhibitory neurotransmitter. The initial success with H_C-HEX A suggests that either HEX A or other enzymes with an intravesicular site of action may also be useful as therapeutics.

H_C has also been evaluated as an adjunct to the therapeutic uses of neurotrophic factors. As with gene therapy (discussed below) the goal of linkage to H_C is to enhance the neuronal specificity of the trophic factor. Although cardiotrophin (CT-1) is neurotrophic for motor neuron, this molecule binds other tissues and shows toxicity for heart and liver. When expressed as a recombinant hybrid, CT1-TTC bound avidly and specifically to motor neurons. This hybrid protein was equally effective in promoting motor neuron survival as unconjugated CT-1 (70).

As mentioned earlier, H_C is inferior to TTX in accumulation in neuronal cells as well as in axonal transport studies. Recently, a full recombinant, but atoxic, form of TTX was created and expressed. This molecule is equipotent to tetanus toxin heavy chain in inhibiting the paralytic and transmitter release effect of TTX *in vitro*. In contrast to its equivalence to heavy chain (and likely H_C as well) *in vitro*, fully recombinant atoxic TTX is 30 times more effective than heavy chain in antagonizing the physiologic effects *in vitro* (71). This degree of superiority is comparable to the superiority of TTX in axonal transport studies. This molecule also possesses translocation properties lacked by heavy chain or H_C, allowing potential passenger proteins linked to the light chain terminus to enter the cytosol.

H_C IN GENE THERAPY

Recent experiments have begun to explore the capacity of H_C as an adjunct to gene therapy. H_C has been linked to the polycationic peptide polylysine in an effort to enhance both the efficiency and neuronal specificity of this nonviral transfection vector (72). H_C coupled polylysine-DNA complexes showed a transfection efficiency several-fold greater than polylysine-DNA alone. H_C-linked polylysine-DNA complexes also showed a high degree of specificity for neuronal cell lines with known TTX receptors. A major limitation of nonviral transfection vectors is their very low efficiency of expression in neurons both *in vitro* and *in vivo*. H_C-linked complexes have not yet been successful in overcoming this limitation.

H_C has also been used to modify viral vectors for gene delivery. H_C has been linked to a fragment of antibody directed to a surface-binding protein of adenovirus. This complex not only masks the normal viral protein responsible for cellular binding, but substitutes the neuron specific H_C-binding domain. This redirected virus shows dramatically enhanced specificity of expression for neuronal cells (73). Such vectors have high potential not only for gene therapy for motor neurons through retrograde transport, but also for enhanced gene delivery within the brain. Although TTX and related proteins do not cross the blood–brain barrier, all neurons in both the peripheral nervous system (PNS) and CNS bind TTX and H_C. Techniques such as direct injection into the brain or cerebral spinal fluid are still commonly employed to deliver genes and proteins to specific CNS regions (74). Vectors modified with H_C would be expected to have enhanced binding to local neurons in this setting.

Gene therapy has also been enhanced by expressing the protein of choice along with H_C. Intramuscular injection of a plasmid for a H_C–beta-galactosidase results in expression of this hybrid protein in muscle. With the transfected muscle acting as a long lasting reservoir, hybrid protein released by muscle is detected in motor neurons, a result not seen with beta-galactosidase alone (75).

OBSTACLES TO DEVELOPMENT OF USEFUL H_C-BASED DELIVERY

As mentioned earlier, neither TTC nor TTX crosses the blood–brain barrier. A growing number of techniques are currently employed to facilitate the entry of large proteins into the CNS. These include methods to disrupt the normal tight endothelial junctions that comprise the blood–brain barrier, or modifying proteins to enhance transcytosis across brain endothelial cells (75–80). None of these methods shows neuronal specificity, so that combining them with a clostridial toxin based vector such as H_C may produce a system with both high brain penetration and neuronal specific delivery.

The most obvious limitation to delivery of H_C-linked proteins, even to their natural target—motor neurons—is the immune system. The vast majority of people in developed nations have been vaccinated against tetanus toxin. H_C is clearly antigenic and was developed as a recombinant protein to facilitate vaccination against tetanus (81). It is also clear that vaccination with either tetanus toxoid or H_C is protective against clinical tetanus (1,23). Passive transfer of antitetanus antibodies has been shown to block the uptake of TTX from the systemic circulation (1,82). The degree to which antitetanus antibodies block uptake of toxin or H_C from an intramuscular injection site is less clear. TTX injected into eye muscles has a paralytic effect similar to botulinum neurotoxin. This clinical effect is a reflection of both well-established blockade of neurotransmitter release at the NMJ (with reduced potency compared to botulinum), and the lack of significant presynaptic inhibition on normal ocular motor neurons leaving only excitatory presynaptic terminals available for inactivation (83).

Even animals vaccinated against tetanus develop local-lid paralysis after intramuscular injection of toxin, although they do not develop symptoms of generalized tetanus (84). This is probably a reflection of the high avidity of TTX for its receptors on presynaptic terminals at the NMJ followed by rapid internalization, and the lack of antibody access to internalized toxin.

We have performed a similar experiment with H_C. When fully vaccinated mice are injected with H_C, there does not appear to be a significant reduction in the amount of H_C transported to local motor neurons. This may also be a reflection of the large difference in quantity of proteins used in retrograde transport experiments (micrograms) compared to physiologic or toxicologic experiments (nanograms). Retrograde transport is a relatively inefficient process in which less than 1% of total protein is typically transported. It is not unexpected that circulating antitetanus antibodies are unable to neutralize an entire large intramuscular reservoir of protein prior to internalization by nerve terminals at the local NMJ.

Other strategies to reduce the immunologic obstacles to H_C-based vectors are also under development. Along with standard immunosuppressive methods, forms of H_C that lack major antitetanus epitopes but conserve molecular domains important for neuronal binding and transport are currently under study (36,85). Similar efforts are also underway involving botulinum neurotoxin-based vectors. Recent studies that combine portions of different clostridial neurotoxins illustrate the potential of such chimeric toxins for both addressing basic science issues of toxin function and as potential therapeutics.

REFERENCES

1. Habermann E, Dimpfel W. Distribution of ^{125}I-tetanus toxin and ^{125}I-toxoid in rats with generalized tetanus, as influenced by antitoxin. *Naunyn Schmiedebergs Arch Pharmacol* 1973;276:327–340.
2. Eisel U, Jarausch W, Goretzki K et al. Tetanus toxin: primary structure, expression in *E. coli,* and homology with botulinum toxins. *EMBO J* 1987;5:2495–2502.
3. Hoch DH, Romero-Mira M, Ehrlich BE et al. Channels formed by botulinum, tetanus and diphtheria toxins in planer lipid bilayers: relevance to translocation of proteins across membranes. *Proc Natl Acad Sci U S A* 1985; 82:1692–1696.
4. Johnstone SR, Morrice LM, van Heningen S. The heavy chain of tetanus toxin can mediate the entry of cytotoxic gelonin into intact cells. *FEBS Lett* 1990;265:101–103.
5. Montecucco C, Schiavo G. Structure and function of tetanus and botulinum neurotoxins. *Q Rev Biophys* 1995;28:423–472.
6. Schiavo G, Benfenati F, Poulain B, et al. Tetanus and botulinum B neurotoxins block neurotransmitter release by proteolytic cleavage of synaptobrevin. *Nature* 1992; 259:832–835.
7. Habermann E. Tetanus. In: Vinken PJ, Bruyn GW, eds. *Handbook of clinical neurology.* Amsterdam: North Holland Publishing Co., 1978;491–547.
8. Habermann E, Dreyer F, Bigalke H. Tetanus toxins blocks neuromuscular transmission in vitro like botulinum A toxin. *Naunyn Schmiedebergs Arch Pharmacol* 1986;311:33–40.
9. Price DL, Griffin J, Young A, et al. Tetanus toxin: direct evidence for retrograde intraaxonal transport. *Science* 1975;183:945–947.
10. Price DL, Griffin JW. Tetanus toxin: retrograde axonal transport of systemically administered toxin. *Neurosci Lett* 1977;4:61–65.
11. Habermann E, Wellhoner HH, Raker KO. Metabolic fate of ^{125}I-tetanus toxin in the spinal cord of rats and cats with early tetanus. *Naunyn Schmiedebergs Arch Pharmacol* 1977;299;187–196.
12. Schwab ME, Suda K, Thoenen H. Selective retrograde transsynaptic transfer of a protein, tetanus toxin, subsequent to its retrograde axonal transport. *J Cell Biol* 1979; 82:798–810.
13. Schwab ME, Thoenen H. Electron microscopic evidence for a transsynaptic migration of tetanus toxin in spinal cord motoneurons: an autoradiographic and morphometric study. *Brain Res* 1976;105:213–237.
14. Matteoli M, Verderio C, Rossetto O, et al. Synaptic vesicle endocytosis mediates the entry of tetanus neurotoxin into hippocampal neurons. *Proc Natl Acad Sci U S A* 1996;93:13310–13315.
15. Katz HJ, Wellhoner HH. Acidification of the cytosol inhibits the uptake of tetanus toxin in NG108–15 and NBr-10A neurohybridoma cells. *Naunyn Schmiedebergs Arch Pharmacol* 1996;353:606–609.
16. Williamson LC, Neale EA. Bafilomycin A1 inhibits the action of tetanus toxin in spinal cord neurons in cell culture. *J Neurochem* 1994;63:2342–2345.
17. Ligorio MA, Akmentin W, Gallery F, et al. Ultrastructural localization of the binding fragment of tetanus toxin in putative gamma-aminobutyric acidergic terminals in the intermediolateral cell column: a potential basis for sympathetic dysfunction in generalized tetanus. *J Comp Neurol* 2000;419:471–484.
18. Curtis DR, deGroat WC. Tetanus toxin and spinal inhibition. *Brain Res* 1968;10:208–212.
19. Curtis DR, Felix D, Game CJA, et al. Tetanus toxin and the synaptic release of GABA. *Brain Res* 1973;51: 358–362.
20. Bizzini B, Stoeckel K, Schwab M. An antigenic polypeptide fragment isolated from tetanus toxin: chemical characterization, binding to gangliosides and retrograde axonal transport in various neuron systems. *J Neurochem* 1977;28:539–542.
21. Helting TB, Zwisler O. Structure of tetanus toxin. I. Breakdown of the toxin molecule and discrimination between polypeptide fragments. *J Biol Chem* 1977;252: 187–193.
22. Makoff AJ, Ballantine SP, Smallwood AE, et al. Expression of tetanus toxin fragment C in *E. coli*: its purification and potential use as a vaccine. *Biotechnology* 1989; 7:1043–1046.
23. Halpern JL, Habig WH, Neale EA, et al. Cloning and expression of functional fragment C of tetanus toxin. *Infect Immun* 1990;58:1004–1009.
24. Pierce EJ, Davison MD, Parton RG, et al. Characterization of tetanus toxin binding to rat brain membranes. Evidence for a high-affinity proteinase-sensitive receptor. *Biochem J* 1986;263:845–852.
25. Schengrund C-L, Ringler NJ, DasGupta BR. Adherence of botulinum and tetanus neurotoxins to synaptosomal proteins. *Brain Res Bull* 1992;29:917–924.
26. Marxen P, Fuhrmann U, Bigalke H. Gangliosides mediate inhibitory effects of tetanus and botulinum A neurotoxins on exocytosis in chromaffin cells. *Toxicon* 1989;27:849–859.
27. Williamson LC, Bateman KE, Clifford J CM, et al. Neuronal sensitivity to tetanus toxin requires gangliosides. *Biol Chem* 1999;274:25173–25180.
28. Rogers TB, Snyder SH. High-affinity binding of tetanus toxin to mammalian brain membranes. *J Biol Chem* 1981;256:2402–2407.

29. Staub GC, Walton KM, Schnaar RL, et al. Characterization of the binding and internalization of tetanus toxin
in a neuroblastoma hybrid cell line. *J Neurosci* 1986;6:
1443–1451.

30. Goldberg RL, Costa T, Habig WH, et al. Characterization of fragment C and tetanus toxin binding to rat brain
membranes. *Mol Pharmacol* 1981;20:565–570.

31. Walton KM, Sandberg K, Rogers BT, et al. Complex
ganglioside expression and tetanus toxin binding by
PC12 pheochromocytoma cells. *Biol Chem* 1988;263:
2055–2063.

32. Umland TC, Wingert LM, Swaminathan S, et al. Structure of the receptor binding fragment H_C of tetanus neurotoxin. *Nat Struct Biol* 1997;4:788–792.

33. Emsley P, Fotinou C, Black I, et al. The structures of
the H(C) fragment of tetanus toxin with carbohydrate
subunit complexes provide insight into ganglioside
binding. *J Biol Chem* 2000;24:8889–8894.

34. Shapiro RE, Specht CD, Collins BE, et al. Identification
of a ganglioside recognition domain of tetanus toxin
using a novel ganglioside photo-affinity ligand. *J Biol
Chem* 1997;272:30380–30386.

35. Herreros J, Lalli G, Montecucco C, et al. Tetanus toxin
fragment C binds to a protein present in neuronal cell
lines and motoneurons. *J Neurochem* 2000;74:
1941–1950.

36. Sinha K, Box M, Lalli G, et al. Analysis of mutants
of tetanus toxin H_C fragment: ganglioside binding, cell
binding and retrograde axonal transport properties. *Mol
Microbiol* 2000;37:1041–1051.

37. Dimfel W, Habermann E.[125]I-labeled tetanus as a neuronal marker in tissue cultures derived from embryonic
CNS. *Naunyn Schmiedebergs Arch Pharmacol* 1977;
290:329–333.

38. Mirsky R, Wendon LMB, Black P, et al. Tetanus toxin:
a cell surface marker for neurones in culture. *Brain Res*
1978;148:251–259.

39. Bakry N, Kamata Y, Sorensen R, et al. Tetanus toxin
and neuronal membranes: the relationship between
binding and toxicity. *J Pharmacol Exp Ther* 1991;258:
613–619.

40. Weller U, Taylor CF, Habermann E. Quantitative comparison between tetanus toxin, some fragments and toxoid for binding and axonal transport in the rat. *Toxicon*
1986;24:1055–1063.

41. Fishman PS, Parks DA, Patwardhan AJ, et al. Neuronal
binding of tetanus toxin compared to its ganglioside
binding fragment (Hc). *Nat Toxins* 1999;9:15–16.

42. Halpern JL, Loftus A. Characterization of the receptor-
binding domain of tetanus toxin. *J Biol Chem* 1993;268:
11188–11192.

43. Fishman PS, Savitt JM, Farrand DA. Enhanced CNS
uptake of systemically administered proteins through
conjugation with tetanus C-fragment. *J Neurol Sci* 1990;
98:311–325.

44. Broadwell RD, Brightman MW. Chemistry of undam-
aged neurons transporting exogenous protein in vivo. *J
Comp Neurol* 1979;185:31–74.

45. Fishman PS, Carrigan DR. Motoneuron uptake from the
circulation of the binding fragment of tetanus toxin.
Arch Neurol 1988;45:558–561.

46. Buttner-Ennever JA, Grob P, Akert K, et al. Transsynaptic retrograde labeling in the oculomotor system of the
monkey with [125]-tetanus toxin BII$_b$ fragment. *Neurosci Lett* 1981;26:233–238.

47. Evinger C, Erichsen JT. Transsynaptic retrograde transport of fragment C of tetanus toxin demonstrated by
immunohistochemical localization. *Brain Res* 1986;
380:383–388.

48. Fishman PS, Carrigan DR. Retrograde transneuronal
transfer of the C-fragment of tetanus toxin. *Brain Res*
1987;406:275–279.

49. Jankowska E. Further indications for enhancement of
retrograde transneuronal transport of WGA-HRP by
synaptic activity. *Brain Res* 1985;341:403–408.

50. Horn AKE, Buttner-Ennever JA. The time course of
retrograde transsynaptic transport of tetanus toxin fragment C in the oculomotor system of the rabbit after
injection into extraocular eye muscles. *Exp Brain Res*
1990;81:353–362.

51. Manning KA, Erichsen JT, Evinger C. Retrograde transneuronal transport properties of fragment C of tetanus
toxin. *Neuroscience* 1990;34:251–263.

52. Cabot JB, Mennone A, Bogan N, et al. Retrograde,
transsynaptic and transneuronal transport of fragment C
of tetanus toxin by sympathetic preganglionic neurons.
Neuroscience 1991;40:805–823.

53. Sams JM, Jansen AS, Mettenleiter TC, et al. Pseudora-
bies virus mutants as transneuronal markers. *Brain Res*
1995;687:182–190.

54. Fishman PS, Savitt JM. Transsynaptic transfer of retrogradely transported tetanus protein-peroxidase conjugates. *Exp Neurol* 1989;106:197–203.

55. Figueiredo DM, Matthews CC, Parks DA, et al. Interaction of tetanus toxin derived hybrid proteins with neuronal cells. *J Nat Toxins* 2000;3:963–979.

56. Mochida S, Poulain B, Weller U, et al. Light chain of
tetanus toxin intracellularly inhibits acetylcholine release at neuro-neuronal synapses, and its internalization
is mediated by heavy chain. *FEBS Lett* 1989;253:47–51.

57. Beaude P, Delacour A, Bizzini B, et al. Retrograde axonal transport of an exogenous enzyme covalently linked
to B-II$_b$ fragment of tetanus toxin. *Biochem J* 1990;271:
87–91.

58. Bizzini B, Grob P, Glicksman MA, et al. Use of the B-
II$_b$ tetanus toxin derived fragment as a specific neuro-
pharmacological transport agent. *Brain Res* 1980;193:
221–227.

59. Habig WH, Kenimer JG, Hardegree MC. Retrograde
axonal transport of tetanus toxin: toxin mediated antibody transport. In: Liu TY, et al., eds. *Frontiers in biochemical and biophysical studies of proteins and membranes.* New York: Elsevier, 1983:463–473.

60. Dobrenis K, Joseph A, Rattazi MC. Neuronal lysosomal
enzyme replacement using fragment C of tetanus toxin.
Proc Natl Acad Sci U S A 1992;89:2297–2301.

61. Francis JW, Hosler BA, Brown RH Jr, et al. CuZn superoxide dismutase (SOD-1) tetanus toxin fragment C hybrid protein for targeted delivery of SOD-1 to neuronal
cells. *J Biol Chem* 1995;270:15434–15442.

62. Figueiredo DM, Hallewell RA, Chen LL, et al. Delivery
of recombinant tetanus-superoxide dismutase proteins
to central nervous system neurons by retrograde axonal
transport. *Exp Neurol* 1997;145:546–554.

63. Coen L, Osta R, Maury M, et al. Construction of hybrid
proteins that migrate retrogradely and transsynaptically
into the central nervous system. *Proc Natl Acad Sci U
S A* 1997;94:9400–9405.

64. Francis JW, Ren JM, Warren L, et al. Postischemic infusion of Cu/Zn superoxide dismutase or SOD:Tet451 re-

duces cerebral infarction following focal ischemia/reperfusion in rats. *Exp Neurol* 1997;146:435–443.

65. Matthews CC, Figueiredo DM, Wollack JB, et al. Protective effect of supplemental superoxide dismutase on survival of neuronal cells during starvation. Requirement for cytosolic distribution. *Mol Neurosci* 2000;14: 155–166.

66. Li Y, Aoki R, Dolly JO. Expression and characterisation of the heavy chain of tetanus toxin: reconstitution of the fully recombinant di-chain protein in active form. *J Biochem (Tokyo)* 1999;125:1200–1208.

67. Li Y, Foran P, Fairweather NF, et al. A single mutation in the recombinant light chain of tetanus toxin abolishes its proteolytic activity and removes the toxicity seen after reconstitution with native heavy chain. *Biochemistry* 1997;33:7014–7020.

68. Francis JW, Brown RH Jr, Figueiredo D, et al. Enhancement of diphtheria toxin potency by replacement of the receptor binding domain with tetanus toxin C-fragment: a potential vector for delivering heterologous proteins to neurons. *J Neurochem* 2000;74:2528–2536.

69. Matthews CC, Zielke HR, Wollack JB, et al. Enzymatic degradation protects neurons from glutamate excitotoxicity. *J Neurochem* 2000;75:1045–1052.

70. Bordet T, Castelnau-Ptakhine L, Fauchereau F, et al. Neuronal targeting of cardiotrophin-1 by coupling with tetanus toxin C fragment. *Mol Cell Neurosci* 2001;17: 842–854.

71. Li Y, Foran P, Lawrence G, et al. Recombinant forms of tetanus toxin engineered for examining and exploiting neuronal trafficking pathways. *J Biol Chem* 2001;276: 31394–31401.

72. Knight A, Carvajal J, Schneider H, et al. Nonviral neuronal gene delivery mediated by the H_C fragment of tetanus toxin. *Eur J Biochem* 1999;259:762–769.

73. Schneider H, Groves M, Muhle C, et al. Retargeting of adenoviral vectors to neurons using the Hc fragment of tetanus toxin. *Gene Ther* 2000;7:1584–1592.

74. During MJ, Naegele JR, O'Malley KL, et al. Long-term behavioral recovery in parkinsonian rats by an HSV vector expressing tyrosine hydroxylase. *Science* 1994;266: 1399–1403.

75. Coen L, Kissa K, le Mevel S, et al. A somatic gene transfer approach using recombinant fusion proteins to map muscle-motoneuron projections in Xenopus spinal cord. *Int J Devl Biol* 1999;43:823–830.

76. Bartus RT, Elliott PJ, Dean RL, et al. Controlled modulation of BBB permeability using the bradykinin agonist, RMP-7. *Exp Neurol* 1996;142:14–28.

77. Poduslo JF, Curran GL. Increase permeability of superoxide dismutase at the blood–nerve and blood–brain barriers with retained enzymatic activity after covalent modification with the naturally occurring polyamine putrescine. *J Neurochem* 1996;6:734–741.

78. Elliott G, O'Hare P. Intercellular trafficking and protein delivery by a herpesvirus structural protein. *Cell* 1997; 88:223–233.

79. Schwarzce SR, Ho A, Vocero-Akbani A, et al. *In vivo* protein transduction: delivery of a biologically active protein into the mouse. *Science* 1999;285:1569–1572.

80. Friden PM, Walus LR, Musso GF, et al. Antitransferrin receptor antibody and antibody–drug conjugates cross the blood–brain barrier. *Proc Natl Acad Sci U S A* 1991; 88:4771–4775.

81. Fairweather NF, Lyness VA, Maskell DJ. Immunization of mice against tetanus with fragments of tetanus toxin synthesized in *Escherichia coli*. *Infect Immun* 1987;55: 2541–2545.

82. Habermann E, Erdmann G. Pharmacokinetic and histoautoradiographic evidence for the intraaxonal movement of toxin in the pathogenesis of tetanus. *Toxicon* 1978;16:611–623.

83. Dastur FD, Shahani MT, Dastoor DH, et al. Cephalic tetanus: demonstration of a dual lesion. *J Neurol Neurosurg Psychiatry* 1977;40:782–786.

84. Fezza JP, Howard, Wiley R, et al. The effects of tetanus toxin on the orbicularis oculi muscle. *Ophthal Plast Reconstr Surg* 2000;10:1–13.

85. Figueiredo D, Turcotte C, Frankel G, et al. Characterization of recombinant tetanus toxin derivatives suitable for vaccine development. *Infect Immun* 1995;63: 3218–3221.

Subject Index

A

Abducens (VI) nerve paralysis, botulinum toxin in management of, 190–192

Accommodative esotropia, botulinum toxin in management of, 193–194

Acetylcholine (ACh) release, botulinum neurotoxin-A inhibiting, 171

ACh. *See* Acetylcholine (ACh)

Achalasia, botulinum toxin-A in management of, 295–299
  after failure of myotomy or pneumatic dilatation, 299
  cost-effectiveness of, 298
  diagnostic use of, 299
  for high-risk patients, 298–299
  in pediatric population, 299
  pneumatic dilatation compared with, 298
  side effects of, 295–296
  studies of, 297–298

Adductor spasmodic dysphonia (ADSD)
  botulinum neurotoxin-A injections for, 179–180
    BOTOX titration in, 208
    with breathing spasms, 211–212
    dosing strategies for, 210–211
    functional changes following, 180–184
    injection in, 208–211
    injection technique for, 208–209
    lidocaine in, 207–208

ADSD. *See* Adductor spasmodic dysphonia (ADSD)

Anal fissure, chronic, 274–279
  pathophysiology of, 274–275
  treatment of
    botulinum toxin in, 277–279, 300
    calcium channel antagonists in, 277
    conservative, 275–276
    muscarinic agonists in, 277
    with nitric oxide donors, 276–277
    surgical, 276
    sympathetic neuromodulators in, 277

Anal sphincters
  anatomy and physiology of, 269–272
  internal, disorders of, botulinum toxin-A in management of, 300

Anismus, botulinum toxin-A in management of, 300

Antibody(ies) (Ab)
  anti-BoNT-A
    H_C regions recognized by, 386–390
    regions recognized by, with H_C used as immunogen, 392–393
  anti-H_C, regions recognized by, 395–396
  to botulinum neurotoxin, 103–104
    clinical implications of, 409–414
    depletion or inactivation of, 423
    detection of, 417–418
    frequency of, 413
    overcoming of
      by increased botulinum toxin doses, 422–423
      by using different botulinum toxin preparations, 423
      by using different botulinum toxin serotypes, 423
    prevention of, 413–414
    prevention of formation of, 424
    protein load and, 104–105
    spontaneous disappearance of, 421–422
    titers of, interpretation of, 418–421

Arm spasticity, botulinum toxin-A in management of, 225–226, 228

Arytenoid rebalancing, botulinum toxin-A in management of, 214

Axillary hyperhidrosis, botulinum toxin-A in management of, 304–305, 307

B

Baclofen, in tetanus management, 159

Basal ganglia, in motor control, 457–458

Belt region, of botulinum neurotoxin-B, 21, 34
  role of, 35–36

Benzodiazepines, in tetanus management, 159

Bethanecol, in chronic anal fissure management, 277

Binding domain, of botulinum neurotoxin-B, 30, 32–33

Blepharoplasty, botulinum toxin-A as adjunct to, 292

Blepharospasm
  alternative treatments of, 202
  botulinum toxin-A in management of, 173

Blepharospasm (*contd.*)
    duration of action of BTX-A in, 201
    follow-up evaluation and treatment in, 198
    initial eyelid treatment in, 198
    initial ophthalmologic examination in, 198
    pharmacologic adjuvant therapy combined
        with, 197–198
    side effects of, 201–202
    spontaneous resolution of blepharospasm
        after injection in, 202
    treatment of residual eyelid and eyebrow
        spasms in, 199–200
    treatment of residual facial spasms in, 200
    treatment of subsequent residual eyelid and
        facial spasms in, 200–201
    treatment outcomes in, 197
BoNT. *See* Botulinum neurotoxin(s) (BoNT)
BOTOX. *See* Botulinum neurotoxin (BoNT),
        serotype A, therapeutic (BOTOX,
        DYSPORT)
Botulinum neurotoxin(s) (BoNT). *See also*
        Clostridial neurotoxins (CNTs)
  action of
    cysteines role in, 79–80
    disulfide bond role in, 79–80
  antibodies to, 103–104 (*See also* Antibody(ies)
    (Ab) to botulinum neurotoxin)
  antigenicity of, clinical implications of,
    409–414
  binding of, to presynaptic membrane of
    neuromuscular junction, 49
  chimeric, 471–473
  cortical motor area excitability and, 174–176
  domains of, roles of, 80
  effects of, at neuromuscular junction, 167–170
  efficacy of, weakness and, 167–168
  endopeptidase activity of
    correlation between quaternary structure and,
        83–84
    delivery of, to new target cells, 477–482
    factors stimulating, 78
    molecular basis of, 75–86
    NAP-enhancement of, 82
    structural basis of, 76, 78
  exocytosis blockade by, durations of, 95–98
  genomic organization of, 81–82
  hybrid, 469–-471, 472–473
  immune recognition of, 385–404
  immunology of, 383–437
  immunoresistance to
    clinical implications of, 409–414
    frequency of, 413
    prevention of, 413–414

  intracellular substrates of L chains of, 75
  laryngeal physiology and, 179–185
  metalloprotease activity of, 3–9
  modes of action of, 41, 75
  nicking-mediated activation of, 82–83
  pharmacology of, 89–141
  physiologic mechanism of action of, 455–458
  proteolytic mechanism of, 24–25
  recombinant vaccines against, 431
  serotype A
    antibodies to, H_C regions recognized by,
        386–390
    binding domain of, 17–19
    botulinum neurotoxin-B compared with, 35
    central nervous system function and,
        171–176
    chemodenervation at motor nerve terminals
        by, features of, 98–100
    immunologic considerations on, 103–105
    L chain of, active site of, mutagenesis of,
        7–9
    light-scattering studies of, 15–17
    molecular weight of, determination of, 13
    neuroparalysis by, extended duration of,
        91–100 (*See also* Neuromuscular
        paralysis by BoNT-A)
    on projection density map, 12–13, 14
    structural forms of, enzymatic activity
        difference between, 84, 85
    structure of, 12, 15, 17
    synaptic vesicle trafficking and, 61–72
    therapeutic (BOTOX, DYSPORT), 103
      for achalasia, 295–299
      for adductor spasmodic dysphonia,
        179–184
      analgesic effects of, initial observations
        on, 233–234
      for anterior rectocele, 280–282
      for arytenoid rebalancing, 214
      for blepharospasm, 197–202 (*See also*
        Blepharospasm, botulinum toxin-A in
        management of)
      for bruxism, 234–236, 347–348
      in cerebral palsy, 217–221 (*See also*
        Cerebral palsy (CP), botulinum toxin-A
        in management of)
      for chronic anal fissure, 277–279, 300
      for chronic constipation from pelvic floor
        dysfunction, 279–280
      commercially available preparations of,
        comparison of, 136–137
      for cosmetic disorders, 287–292
      for cranial dystonia, 197–202 (*See also*

Cranial dystonia, botulinum toxin-A in
management of)
for delayed gastric emptying, 282
for detrusor hyperreflexia, 355
for detrusor-sphincter dyssynergia,
353–355
discussion of, 138–140
electrical stimulation and, 169
for essential voice tremor, 213
exercise and, 169–170
extralaryngeal uses of, in laryngopharynx,
214–215
for focal hyperhidrosis, 303–308 (*See also*
Hyperhidrosis, focal)
for gastrointestinal disorders, 269–283
glycogen depletion assay of, 136
for headache, 238–245 (*See also*
Headache)
for hemifacial spasm, 197–201, 202–204
for infantile hypertrophic pyloric stenosis,
282
injections of, measurement of, 135–140
for myofascial pain syndrome, 236–238,
312–319
for obesity, 282
patient resistant to, botulinum toxin type F
for, 451–453
physiologic effects of, laryngeal
physiologic changes from, 185
potency of, 106
in prevention of posterior glottic stenosis,
214
for puberophonia, 214
resistance to, chemodenervation with
phenol in, 459–461
for spasticity, 223–231 (*See also*
Spasticity, botulinum toxin-A in
management of)
for sphincter of Oddi dysfunction,
282–283
"spread" effects of, compared with
BoNT-B, 127–129
spread of paralysis from, 123–131
for strabismus, 189–195 (*See also*
Strabismus)
for stuttering, 212–213
for temporomandibular disorder, 234–236
for tics, 338–340
for tremors, 323–334 (*See also* Tremors)
for ventricular dysphonia, 213–214
for vocal tics, 213
serotype B
belt region of, 21, 34
role of, 35–36

binding domain of, 30, 32–33
botulinum neurotoxin-A compared with, 35
catalytic domain of, 30, 32, 33–35
crystal structure of, 29–38
enhanced catalytic activity of, 36
ganglioside binding of, evidence for, 36–37
reduced form of, 36
structure of, 17
description of, 30–35
therapeutic (MYOBLOC), 115–122
for cervical dystonia, 371–380 (*See also*
Cervical dystonia (CD), botulinum
toxin-B in management of)
characterization of, 115–116
complex integrity of, 119
potency of, 106
production of, 116–118
purity of, 118–119
quality of, 118–120
specific activity of, 119–120
"spread" effects of, compared with
BoNT-A, 127–129
spread of paralysis from, 123–131
stability of, 120–121
translocation domain of, 30, 33
tyrosine phosphorylation of, 36
serotype C, therapeutic, clinical trials with,
441–449
serotype E
administration of, neuroparalysis duration
from BoNT-A and, 94
therapeutic, clinical trials with, 441–449
serotype F, therapeutic, for botulinum toxin-A
resistant patients, 451–453
serotypes of
cross-reactions of, therapeutic applications
and, 396–400
serum cross-reactivity between, antigenicity
of BTX and, 413
therapeutic
activation levels of, comparison of,
105–106
antibodies of, neutralizing versus
nonneutralizing, 103–104
antigenic potential of, comparison of,
105–111
applications of, consequences of cross-
reactions to, 396–400
clinical uses of, 123
cross-reactivity of, 109–110
duration of action of, 108–109
potencies of, comparison of, 106–108
properties of, 103–112

Botulinum neurotoxin(s) (BoNT) (*contd.*)
  safety of, 110–111
  spread of paralysis from, study of,
    123–131 (*See also* Paralysis from
    botulinum neurotoxins, spread of, study
    of)
  uses of, 149–150
  structural features of, 78–79
  structural view of, in numerous functional
    states, 11–26
  synaptic vesicle recycling and, 67–71
  toxicity of, three-step model of, 11, 13
Botulinum toxin (BTX). *See* Botulinum
  neurotoxin(s) (BoNT)
Botulism
  classes of, toxin production sites in, 427
  clinical, 145–150
    clinical manifestations of, 146–148
    management of, 147–148
    pathogenesis of, 145–146
    prevention of, 148–149
  vaccines for, 427–435
Brow lift
  botulinum toxin-A in management of, 290–291
  surgical, botulinum toxin-A as adjunct to,
    291–292
Bruxism
  botulinum toxin-A in management of,
    234–236, 347–348
  temporomandibular disorders and, 261
BTX. *See* Botulinum neurotoxin(s) (BoNT)

C

Calcium, dependence of synaptic vesicle exo- and
  endocytosis on, 69, 71
Calcium channel antagonists, in chronic anal
  fissure management, 277
Casting, as adjunct to BTX-A for cerebral palsy,
  221
Catalytic activity of botulinum neurotoxin-B,
  enhanced, 36
Catalytic domain
  of botulinum neurotoxin-A, endopeptidase
    activity and, 76, 78
  of botulinum neurotoxin-B, 30, 32, 33–35, 78
Cataracts, strabismus after surgery for, botulinum
  toxin in management of, 192
CD. *See* Cervical dystonia (CD)
Central nervous system (CNS), function of,
  botulinum neurotoxin-A effects on,
  171–176

animal experiments on, *in vitro* and *in vivo,*
  171–172
human studies on, 172–173
Cephalic tetanus, 155
Cerebral cortex, motor areas of
  effects of botulinum neurotoxin-A on, 173
  excitability of, botulinum toxin and, 174–176
Cerebral palsy (CP)
  botulinum toxin-A in management of, 217–221
    adjunctive treatments in, 220–221
    dose in, 218–219
    duration of effect of, 219
    indications for, 218
    side effects of, 219–220
  botulinum toxin in management of, 194
Cervical dystonia (CD)
  botulinum toxin-A in management of, 359–369
    adverse effects of, 362
    with BOTOX, clinical trials on, 359–363
    cost effectiveness of, 362–363
    with DYSPORT, clinical trials on, 360,
      361–362, 365–369
      dose equivalence of, versus BOTOX,
        367–368
      dose-response relationships in, 366–367
      immunogenicity in, 368–369
      long-term outcome in, 368
      secondary nonresponsiveness in, 368–369
      short-term, 365–366
    electromyography guidance for, 361–362
    immunogenicity of BTX-A in, 361
  botulinum toxin-B in management of, clinical
    efficacy studies of, 371–380
    demographics of, 374, 375
    design of, 372–374
    efficacy assessments in, 374–377
    results of, 374–379
    safety in, 377–379
  EMG-guided chemodenervation with phenol in,
    459–461
Cervicogenic headache, botulinum toxin-A in
  management of, 238–239
Chimeric botulinum neurotoxins, 471–473
Chin, trembling, hereditary, botulinum toxin-A in
  management of, 333
Clathrin, endocytosis mediated by, synaptic
  vesicle recycling and, 67, 69, 72
Clostridial neurotoxins (CNTs). *See also*
    Botulinum neurotoxin(s) (BoNT);
    Tetanus neurotoxin(s) (TeNT)
  binding of, double receptor model of, 52–53
  genetics of, 3–5
  internalization of, 53–54

intracellular zinc-endopeptidase activity of, 55
metalloprotease activity of, 6–7
modes of action of, 41
neuronal intoxication by, 5–6
neuronal recognition of, 17–20
presynaptic receptors of, 5–6
receptor-binding domains of, 41–47
  study of
    methods of, 43–44
    results of, 44–47
  structure of, 4–5
  substrate binding of, 21–24
  substrate specificity of, 21–24
  toxin translocation in, 20–21, 22
  translocation of, into neuronal cytosol, 54–55
Cluster headache, botulinum toxin-A in
        management of, 240–241
CNS. *See* Central nervous system (CNS)
Constipation, chronic, from pelvic floor
        dysfunction, botulinum toxin for,
        279–280
Cosmetic disorders, botulinum toxin-A in
        management of, 287–292
  adjunctive use of, 291–292
  common uses of, 288–291
  dilution and handling for, 288
  injection technique in, 288
CP. *See* Cerebral palsy (CP)
Cranial dystonia
  alternative treatments of, 202
  botulinum toxin-A in management of, 197–202
    follow-up evaluation and treatment in, 198
    initial eyelid treatment in, 198
    initial ophthalmologic examination in, 198
    pharmacologic adjuvant therapy combined
        with, 197–198
    treatment of residual eyelid and eyebrow
        spasms in, 199–200
    treatment outcomes in, 197
Crow's-feet, botulinum toxin-A in management
        of, 289–290
Crystal structure, of *Clostridium botulinum*
        neurotoxin serotype B, 29–38
Cysteines, in botulinum neurotoxin action, 79–80
Cytosol, neuronal, translocation of tetanus
        neurotoxins into, 54–55

D

Débridement, wound, in tetanus management, 159
Detrusor hyperreflexia, 351–353
  botulinum toxin-A in management of, 355

Detrusor-sphincter dyssynergia (DSD), 353–355
Diazepam, in tetanus management, 159
Disulfide bond, in botulinum neurotoxin action,
        79–80
Disulfide bond reduction, botulinum neurotoxin-A
        endopeptidase activity mediated by, 76,
        78
Dopamine antagonists, dystonic reactions to,
        tetanus differentiated from, 156, 157
Dot blot assay, in BTX antibody detection, 412
Double receptor model of clostridial neurotoxin
        binding, 52–53
Dry eye, complicating BTX-A treatment of
        blepharospasm, 201
Dysphagia, from botulinum neurotoxin therapies,
        111
Dysphonia
  spasmodic (*See* Spasmodic dysphonia)
  ventricular, botulinum toxin-A in management
        of, 213–214
Dysphonia plicae ventricularis, botulinum toxin-A
        in management of, 213–214
DYSPORT. *See* Botulinum neurotoxin, serotype
        A, therapeutic (BOTOX, DYSPORT)
Dyssynergia, detrusor-sphincter, 353–355
Dystonia(s)
  cervical, botulinum toxin-A in management of,
        359–369 (*See also* Cervical dystonia
        (CD), botulinum toxin-A in
        management of)
  cranial, botulinum toxin-A in management of,
        197–202 (*See also* Cranial dystonia)
  focal hand, 251–257 (*See also* Focal hand
        dystonia)
  laryngeal, 179–180
  muscle afferent block for, 455–458
  occupational, 251–257 (*See also* Focal hand
        dystonia)
  oromandibular
    botulinum toxin-A in management of,
        343–347
      muscle selection for, 344–345
      results of trials of, 345–347
    temporomandibular disorders and, 261
  tongue protrusion, botulinum toxin-A in
        management of, 347
  upper limb, botulinum neurotoxin-A injections
        for, 172–173
Dystonic reactions to dopamine antagonists,
        tetanus differentiated from, 156, 157

E

EDB-test. *See* Extensor digitorum brevis test
        (EDB-test)

Electromyography (EMG)
  in botulinum toxin-A treatment of focal hand
      dystonia, 253
  chemodenervation guided by, with phenol in
      cervical dystonia, 459–461
  in guidance of BTX treatment of cervical
      dystonia, 361–362
ELISA. *See* Enzyme-linked immunosorbent
      assays (ELISA)
Endocytosis, in internalization of botulinum
      neurotoxins, 75
Endopeptidase activity of botulinum neurotoxin
  conditions stimulating, 78
  correlation between quaternary structure and,
      83–84
  delivery of, to new target cells, 477–482
  molecular basis of, 75–86
  NAP-enhancement of, 82
  structural basis of, 76, 78
ENS. *See* Enteric nervous system (ENS)
Enteric nervous system (ENS), functional
      organization of, 272–273
Enzyme-linked immunosorbent assays (ELISA)
  in BoNT vaccine efficacy studies, 434–435
  in BTX antibody detection, 418
Equinovarus, spastic, botulinum toxin-A in
      management of, 226
Esophageal sphincter, upper, dysfunction of,
      botulinum toxin-A in management of,
      299–300
Esophagus, spasms of, diffuse, botulinum toxin-A
      in management of, 299
Esotropia
  accommodative, botulinum toxin in
      management of, 193–194
  infantile, botulinum toxin in management of,
      193
Exocytosis blockade
  by botulinum neurotoxin-A, time courses of,
      neuroparalysis duration and, 92–94
  by botulinum neurotoxin serotypes, durations
      of, 95–98
  by clostridial neurotoxins, 29, 67–72
Exotropia, intermittent, botulinum toxin in
      management of, 194
Extensor digitorum brevis test (EDB-test), in
      BTX antibody detection, 418
Extraocular muscles, disorders of, botulinum toxin
      in management of, 193
Eye, dry, complicating BTX-A treatment of
      blepharospasm, 201
Eyebrow spasms, residual, after BTX-A
      treatment, management of, 199–200

Eyelid spasms
  botulinum toxin-A in management of
      initial, 198
      subsequent residual after, treatment of,
          200–201
  residual, after BTX-A treatment, management
      of, 199–200

F

F-TAT. *See* Frontalis type A test (F-TAT)
Face
  asymmetry of, botulinum toxin-A in
      management of, 291
  wounds of, repair of, botulinum toxin-A in, 292
Facial lines, hyperfunctional, botulinum toxin-A
      in management of, 287–292
Facial spasms, residual, after BTX-A treatment
      management of, 200
      subsequent, treatment of, 200–201
Facial (VII) nerve, aberrant regeneration of,
      botulinum toxin-A in management of,
      203–204
Fibromyalgia, myofascial pain syndrome
      distinguished from, 310
FM-labeling, in synaptic activity demonstration,
      66–72
Focal hand dystonia
  botulinum toxin-A in management of, 253–257
      efficacy of, 256–257
      muscles injected for, 254
  differential diagnosis of, 252
  epidemiology of, 251–252
  history of, 251
  physiology of, 251–252
  signs and symptoms of, 252
Focal hyperhidrosis, botulinum toxin-A in
      management of, 303–308
Foodborne botulism
  clinical manifestations of, 146
  prevention of, 148
  toxin production in, 427
Forehead lines, horizontal, botulinum toxin-A in
      management of, 290
Frey's syndrome, botulinum toxin-A in
      management of, 307
Frontalis type A test (F-TAT), in detection of
      immunoresistance to BTX, 410
Frown lines, glabellar, botulinum toxin-A in
      management of, 288–289

G

Gangliosides in binding, 41–42
  of botulinum neurotoxin-B, evidence for,
      36–37

results of, 47

study methods for, 44

Gastric emptying, delayed, botulinum toxin-A in
    management of, 282

Gastrointestinal tract (GIT)

    pelvic floor anatomy and physiology and,
      269–274

    smooth muscle of, disorders of, 295–301 (*See
      also* Achalasia)

    smooth muscles of

      contraction of, 273–274

      neuromyogenic properties of, 272

Genes, synthetic BoNT(H$_C$), design of, 431–432

GIT. *See* Gastrointestinal tract (GIT)

Glabellar frown lines, botulinum toxin-A in
    management of, 288–289

Glottic stenosis, posterior, botulinum toxin-A in
    management of, 214

Glycogen-depletion assay, in BTX-A activity
    quantitation, 136–137

Granuloma, vocal fold, botulinum toxin-A in
    management of, 214

Gustatory sweating, 303

    botulinum toxin-A in management of, 307

H

H$_C$, of antibodies, reaction with, after
      immunization with peptides, 400–404

H$_C$ domain, of tetanus toxin, 51, 486–487

    in binding process, 52–53

    in gene therapy, 489–490

    protein delivery using, 488–489

      useful, obstacles to development of, 490–491

H$_C$ gene, for tetanus neurotoxin

    binding domain of, identification of key
      residues within, 44, 46–47

    functional domains of, analysis of, 44, 45

    mutants of, cloning and expression of, 43

H$_C$ region(s), of botulinum toxin-A

    recognized by anti-BoNT-A antibodies, from
      three outbred host species, 386–389

    recognized by anti-H$_C$ T cells, 393–395

    recognized by mouse anti-BoNT-A antibodies,
      389–390

H$_{CC}$ region, of tetanus neurotoxin, binding and,
    42–43

Head tremors, botulinum toxin-A in management
    of, 323–327

Headache

    botulinum toxin-A in management of, 238–245

    cervicogenic, botulinum toxin-A in
      management of, 238–239

cluster, botulinum toxin-A in management of,
    240–241

migraine, botulinum toxin-A in management of,
    241–245

    double-blind, placebo-controlled study of,
      244–245

    open-label, prospective study of, 243–244

tension

    botulinum toxin-A in management of,
      239–240, 241

    temporomandibular disorders and, 261

Heavy chain(s) (HC)

    disulfide-linked, botulinum neurotoxicity and,
      79–80

    in hybrid botulinum toxin production, 469–473

    N-terminal part of, in clostridial neurotoxins,
      functions of, 51

    of neurotoxins, role of, 80

    of tetanus neurotoxin, 51

Heavy chain (HC) domain(s), of clostridial
    neurotoxins, 41

Hemifacial spasm

    alternative treatments of, 202

    botulinum toxin-A in management of,
      202––203

Hemimasticatory spasm, 348

Hereditary trembling chin, botulinum toxin-A in
    management of, 333

Hirschsprung's disease, botulinum toxin-A in
    management of, 300

Holotoxin

    hydrodynamic radius of, 15–17

    structure of, 17

HTIC. *See* Human tetanus immunoglobulin
    (HTIG)

Human tetanus immunoglobulin (HTIG), in
    tetanus management, 159

Hybrid botulinum neurotoxins, 469–471,
    472–473

Hyperhidrosis

    axillary, botulinum toxin-A in management of,
      304–305, 307

    focal, botulinum toxin-A in management of,
      303–308

    palmar, botulinum toxin-A in management of,
      304, 306–307

Hypocalcemic tetany, tetanus differentiated from,
    156, 157

I

Immunization

    with peptides, reaction with H$_C$ of antibodies
      and T cells obtained after, 400–404

    tetanus, 160–161

Immunoglobulin, human tetanus, in tetanus
    management, 159
Immunologic considerations on botulinum
    neurotoxin therapies, 103–105
Immunoprecipitation assay (IPA), in
    immunoresistance assessment, 411
Immunoresistance, to BTX
  clinical implications of, 409–414
  frequency of, 413
  prevention of, 413–414
Immunotoxin (ITX), 463–466
Indoramin, in chronic anal fissure management,
    277
Infant botulism
  clinical manifestations of, 146–147
  prevention of, 148
  toxin production in, 427
Infantile esotropia, botulinum toxin in
    management of, 193
Infantile hypertrophic pyloric stenosis, botulinum
    toxin-A in management of, 282
Insulin release, inhibition of, botulinum
    neurotoxin-dependent, 480–481
Intoxication, neuronal
  by botulinum neurotoxins, mechanism of,
    427–428
  by clostridial neurotoxins, 5–6
IPA. See Immunoprecipitation assay (IPA)
ITX. See Immunotoxin (ITX)

L

Laryngopharynx, extralaryngeal uses of botulinum
    toxin in, 214–215
Larynx
  disorders of, botulinum toxin-A in management
    of, 212–215
  functional changes in, following BTX-A
    injection, 180–184
  hyperfunctional, botulinum toxin-A in
    management of, 207–215
  physiology of, botulinum toxin and, 179–185
Leg spasticity, botulinum toxin-A in management
    of, 226, 228–229
Light chain(s) (LC)
  of botulinum neurotoxins, loops in, 78–79
  of clostridial neurotoxins, functions of, 51–52
  disulfide-linked, botulinum neurotoxicity and,
    79–80
  in hybrid botulinum toxin production, 469–473
  of neurotoxins, role of, 80
Light chain (LC) domains of clostridial
    neurotoxins, 41

Limb tremor, botulinum toxin-A in management
    of, 327–330
Linkers, in hybrid botulinum toxin production,
    470–472
Lorazepam, in tetanus management, 159

M

MAB. See Muscle afferent block (MAB)
Meige's syndrome, 343
    botulinum toxin-A in management of, 197–202
      (See also Cranial dystonia)
Melolabial folds, botulinum toxin-A in
    management of, 291
Meningitis, tetanus differentiated from, 156, 157
Metalloprotease activity, of clostridial
    neurotoxins, 6–7
Methylprednisolone, for myofascial pain
    syndrome, botulinum toxin-A versus,
    237–238
Micturition, anatomy and physiology of, 351–353
Migraine, botulinum toxin-A in management of,
    241–245
  double-blind, placebo-controlled study of,
    244–245
  open-label, prospective study of, 243–244
Monkey hand model of muscle paralysis from
    botulinum toxins, 124–129
Mouse diaphragm assay (MDA), in BTX antibody
    detection, 412, 419–420
Mouse protection assay (MPA), in BTX antibody
    detection, 409–411, 419–420
Mouth, dry, from botulinum neurotoxin therapies,
    111
MPA. See Mouse protection assay (MPA)
MPS. See Myofascial pain syndrome (MPS)
Muscarinic agonists, in chronic anal fissure
    management, 277
Muscle(s)
  extraocular, disorders of, botulinum toxin in
    management of, 193
  smooth, of gastrointestinal tract
    contraction of, 273–274
    disorders of, 295–301 (See also Achalasia)
    neuromyogenic properties of, 272
Muscle afferent block (MAB), for dystonia,
    455–458
Myectomy, limited, botulinum toxin-A combined
    with, for aberrant regeneration of facial
    nerve, 203–204
MYOBLOC. See Botulinum neurotoxin (BoNT),
    serotype B, therapeutic (MYOBLOC)

Myofascial pain syndrome (MPS)
  botulinum toxin-A in management of,
      236–238, 312–319
    antinociceptive mechanisms in, 316
    clinical developments in, 312–315
    diluent in, 318–319
    dosing guidelines for, 317–318
    injection technique for, 317
    patient selection for, 316–317
    technical considerations on, 316–319
  central sensitization model of, 311
  dysfunctional muscle spindle model of,
      310–311
  energy crisis model of, 310
  fibromyalgia distinguished from, 310
  irritable motor endplate model of, 310–311
  peripheral sensitization model of, 311
  therapeutic approaches to, 311–312
Myotomy, for achalasia, failure of, botulinum
      toxin-A after, 299

N
NAPs. *See* Neurotoxin-associated proteins (NAPs)
Neck
  lines in, botulinum toxin-A in management of,
      291
  spasticity in, botulinum toxin-A in management
      of, 229
Neonatal tetanus, 155–156
  prevention of, 160
Nerve growth factor (NGF), delivery of
      endopeptidase activity of botulinum
      neurotoxin and, 480
Nervous system
  central (*See* Central nervous system (CNS))
  enteric, functional organization of, 272–273
Neuromodulators, sympathetic, in chronic anal
      fissure management, 277
Neuromuscular junction (NMJ)
  active, botulinum toxin and, 168–169
  blockade of, in tetanus, 153
  effects of botulinum toxin at, 167–170
    phases of, 477
  presynaptic membrane of, binding of clostridial
      neurotoxins to, 49, 50
Neuromuscular paralysis, by BoNT-A
  duration of, BoNT-E administration and, 94
  extended duration of, 91–100
  time courses of exocytosis blockade and,
      92–94
Neuronal intoxication, by clostridial neurotoxins,
      5–6

Neuronal recognition, of clostridial toxins, 17–20
Neurons, cultures of, in synaptic transmission
      studies, 62–66
Neurotoxin-associated proteins (NAPs)
  biologic activity of, 80–81
  botulinum neurotoxin and toxicity and, 80–82
  botulinum neurotoxin endopeptidase activity
      enhanced by, 82
  in botulism, 75
  genomic organization of, 81–82
  types of, 80–81
Neurotoxin complex protein, antigenicity of BTX
      and, 412
Neurotoxins
  botulinum (*See* Botulinum neurotoxin(s)
      (BoNT))
  clostridial (*See also* Clostridial neurotoxins
      (CNTs))
  tetanus (*See* Tetanus neurotoxin(s) (TeNT))
NGF. *See* Nerve growth factor (NGF)
Nicking-mediated activation of botulinum
      neurotoxin, 82–83
  comparison of serotypes, 105–106
Nifedipine, in chronic anal fissure management,
      277
Nitric oxide (NO) donors, treatment of anal
      fissures with, 276–277
NMJ. *See* Neuromuscular junction (NMJ)
NO. *See* Nitric oxide (NO)
Nystagmus, botulinum toxin in management of,
      193

O
Obesity, botulinum toxin-A in management of,
      282
Occupational dystonia, 251–257. *See also* Focal
      hand dystonia
Oculomotor (III) nerve paresis, botulinum toxin in
      management of, 192
OMD. *See* Oromandibular dystonia (OMD)
Ophthalmopathy, thyroid, botulinum toxin in
      management of, 192
Oromandibular dystonia (OMD)
  botulinum toxin-A in management of, 343–347
    muscle selection for, 344–345
    results of trials of, 345–347
  temporomandibular disorders and, 261
Orthoses, as adjuncts to BTX-A for cerebral
      palsy, 220

P
Pain, botulinum toxin-A in management of,
      233–238
  in bruxism, 234–236

Pain (*contd.*)
    in headache, 238–245 (*See also* Headache)
    initial observations on, 233–234
    in myofascial pain syndrome, 236–238
    specificity of, 234
    in temporomandibular disorder, 234–236
Palatal myoclonus, botulinum toxin-A in
        management of, 333–334
Palatal tremor, botulinum toxin-A in management
        of, 333–334
Palmar hyperhidrosis, botulinum toxin-A in
        management of, 304, 306–307
Pancuronium bromide, in tetanus management,
        159
Paralysis
    from botulinum neurotoxins, spread of, study of
        comparison of "spread" effects for BoNT-A
            and BoNT-B, 127–129
        discussion of, 129–131
        factors influencing spread in, 130–131
        materials and methods of, 124–126
        minimum effective dose determination in,
            126–127
        results of, 126–129
        safety of spread in, 129–130
    neuromuscular, by BoNT-A, extended duration
        of, 91–100 (*See also* Neuromuscular
        paralysis by BoNT-A)
Parkinson's disease, muscle afferent block for,
        457-458
Pediatric patient, achalasia in, botulinum toxin-A
        in management of, 299
Pelvic floor
    anatomy and physiology of, 269–274
    dysfunction of, constipation from, botulinum
        toxin for, 279–280
Peptides, immunization with, reaction with H$_C$ of
        antibodies and T cells obtained after,
        400–404
Phenol, EMG-guided chemodenervation with, in
        cervical dystonia, 459–461
Physical therapy, as adjuncts to BTX-A for
        cerebral palsy, 220
Pichia pastoris, design of synthetic BoNT(H$_C$)
        genes and production in, 431–432
PKC. *See* Protein kinase C (PKC)
Pneumatic dilatation, for achalasia
    botulinum toxin-A compared with, 298
    failure of, botulinum toxin-A after, 299
Polysialogangliosides, in clostridial neurotoxin
        binding, 52
Protein(s)
    in clostridial neurotoxin binding, 52

neurotoxin-associated, in botulism, 75
vesicle-associated membrane, in botulinum
        neurotoxin serotypes, 75
Protein kinase C (PKC) in tetanus neurotoxin
        neurotoxicity, 53
Proteolytic mechanism of botulinum neurotoxins,
        24–25
Pseudotetanus, tetanus differentiated from, 157
Ptosis, transient, complicating - treatment of
        blepharospasm, 201
Puberphonia, botulinum toxin-A in management
        of, 214
Pyloric stenosis, infantile hypertrophic, botulinum
        toxin-A in management of, 282

R
Recombinant DNA expression systems, in hybrid
        botulinum toxin production, 472–473
Rectocele, anterior, botulinum toxin-A in
        management of, 280–282
Retinal detachment, strabismus after, botulinum
        toxin in management of, 192
Risus sardonicus in tetanus, 154
Ross syndrome, 303

S
Safety, of botulinum neurotoxin therapies,
        110–111
Salbutamol, in chronic anal fissure management,
        277
SCM-test. *See* Sternocleidomastoid test (SCM-
        test)
Seizures, generalized tonic-clonic, tetanus
        differentiated form, 156–157
SNAP-25. *See* Synaptosomal-associated protein of
        25 kDA (SNAP-25)
SNARE complex formation, synaptic vesicle
        membrane fusion mediated by, 11, 14
Spasm(s)
    eyebrow, residual, after BTX-A treatment,
        management, 199–200
    eyelid, botulinum toxin-A in management of
        initial, 198
        subsequent residual after, treatment of,
            200–201
    hemifacial
        alternative treatments of, 202
        botulinum toxin-A in management of,
            202–203
    supraglottic, botulinum toxin-A in management
        of, 213–214
    in tetanus, 154

Spasmodic dysphonia, botulinum toxin-A in
        management of, 207–215, 330–333
    for abductor dysphonia
        dosing strategies for, 211
        injection technique for, 209–210
    adductor, 179–180
    for adductor dysphonia
        dosing strategies for, 210–211
        functional changes following, 180–184
        injection technique for, 208–209
    in adductor laryngeal breathing dystonia,
        211–212
    in anterior commissure release failures, 211
    BOTOX titration in, 208
    injection in, 208–211
        other methods of, 212
    lidocaine in, 207–208
    in nerve-section failure patients, 211
    positioning for, 208
Spasmodic torticollis, 359. *See also* Cervical
        dystonia (CD)
Spasm(s)
    esophageal, diffuse, botulinum toxin-A in
        management of, 299
    hemimasticatory, 348
Spasticity
    botulinum toxin-A in management of
        advantages/disadvantages of, 231
        in arm spasticity, 225–226, 228
        clinical use of, principles of, 228
        doses for, 230–231
        follow up of, 231
        functional electrical stimulation in, 227
        indications for, 227
        injection technique for, 230
        in leg spasticity, 226, 228–229
        literature on, problems interpreting, 227–228
        mechanism of, 225
        in neck spasticity, 229
        ''neuroprotective'' effect of, 225
        other studies on, 226–227
        patient selection for, 228
        phenol versus, 227
        role of, 224–225
        situations to avoid in, 229–230
        trial evidence on, 225, 226
    definition of, 223
    importance of, 224
    pathophysiology of, 223–224
Speech, vocal fold vibration for, 179
Sphincter(s)
    anal, anatomy and physiology of, 269–272
    upper esophageal, dysfunction of, botulinum
        toxin-A in management of, 299–300

Sphincter of Oddi dysfunction, botulinum toxin-A
        in management of, 282–283, 300–301
Spinal cord
    function of, botulinum neurotoxin-A and
        animal studies on, 171
        human studies on, 172
    tetanus neurotoxin activity in, 49–50, 71
SSV. *See* Synaptic vesicles, small (SSV)
Sternocleidomastoid test (SCM-test), in BTX
        antibody detection, 418, 419
''Stiff-person syndrome,'' tetanus differentiated
        from, 157
Strabismus
    adult, botulinum toxin in management of,
        192–193
    botulinum toxin-A in management of, 189–195
        clinical results of, 189–190
        dosage for, 191
        indications for, 189–190
        injection technique for, 194
        technical complications and difficulties with,
            194–195
    childhood, botulinum toxin in management of,
        193–194
    paralytic, botulinum toxin in management of,
        190–192
    postcataract, botulinum toxin in management
        of, 192
    postretinal detachment, botulinum toxin in
        management of, 192
Strychnine poisoning, tetanus differentiated from,
        156, 157
Stuttering, botulinum toxin-A in management of,
        212–213
Styryl dye, in synaptic activity demonstration,
        66–72
Supraglottic spasm, botulinum toxin-A in
        management of, 213–214
Sweating, gustatory, 303
    botulinum toxin-A in management of, 307
Sympathetic neuromodulators, in chronic anal
        fissure management, 277
Synaptic transmission, studies of, 62–72
    neuronal cultures in, 62–66
Synaptic vesicles
    recycling of, 61–62
        botulinum neurotoxin exposure and, 67–71
        tetanus neurotoxin exposure and, 67–71
    small (SSV)
        increase in, in tetanus neurotoxin
            intoxication, 50
        in tetanus neurotoxin internalization, 53–54

Synaptobrevin. *See also* Vesicle-associated
        membrane protein (VAMP)
    in botulinum neurotoxin serotypes, 75
Synaptosomal-associated protein of 25 kDa
        (SNAP-25)
    BoNT-A–truncated, persistence of, 94–95, 96
    in botulinum neurotoxin serotypes, 75

T

T cells
    anti-H_C, regions recognized by, 393–395
    reaction of H_C with, after immunization with
        peptides, 400–404
    recognition profiles of, mapping of, 390–392
    regions recognized by, with H_C used as
        immunogen, 392–393
Temporomandibular disorders (TMDs)
    botulinum toxin-A in management of,
        234–236, 348
        evolution of, 262–265
        feasibility study on, 262–263
        final thoughts on, 265–266
        long-term follow-up of, 265
        pilot study on, 264
        preliminary study on, 263–264
    classification of, 260–261
    definition of, 259, 260
    interdisciplinary manifestations of, 261
    pathophysiology of, 261
    treatment of, 261–262
Tension headache
    botulinum toxin-A in management of,
        239–240, 241
    temporomandibular disorders and, 261
TeNT. *See* Tetanus neurotoxin(s) (TeNT)
Tetanospasmin, action of, 152–153
Tetanus
    cephalic, 155
    clinical aspects of, 151–161
    clinical manifestations of, 153–156
    complications of, 155
    diagnosis of, 156–157
    differential diagnosis of, 156–157
    epidemiology of, 151–152
    generalized
        clinical manifestations of, 154–155
        management protocol for, 158
    localized, 155
    neonatal, 155–156
        prevention of, 160
    neuroanatomic basis of, 49–50
    pathogenesis of, 152–153

    pathophysiology of, 49–50
    treatment of, 157–160
Tetanus neurotoxin(s) (TeNT). *See also*
        Clostridial neurotoxins (CNTs)
    binding domain of, structure of, 17–20
    binding of
        double receptor model of, 52–53
        neurospecific, 52–53
        to presynaptic membrane of neuromuscular
            junction, 49, 50
    cellular mechanism of action of, 52
    competition binding assays for, with rat brain
        synaptosomes, 44
    function of, 485–486
    H_C domain of, 51 (*See also* H_C domain of
        tetanus toxin)
    H_C gene for
        binding domain of, identification of key
            residues within, 44, 46–47
        functional domains of, analysis of, 44, 45
        mutants of, cloning and expression of, 43
    H_{CC} region of, binding and, 42–43
    internalization of, 53–54
    intoxication with, synaptic vesicle fusion and,
        64–66
    intracellular zinc-endopeptidase activity of, 55
    L chain of, 51–52
    metalloprotease activity of, 3–9
    modes of action of, 41
    N-terminal part of H chain in, 51
    neuronal delivery vectors derived from,
        485–491
    neurospecificity of, 52–53
    nontoxic binding fragments of, 486–487
    pathophysiology of, 49–50
    radioiodination of, 43–44
    structure-function relationships of, 50–52
    structure of, 485–486
    synaptic vesicle recycling and, 67–71
    targeting of, 52–53
    translocation of, into neuronal cytosol, 54–55
    transsynaptic migration of, 49, 50
Tetany, hypocalcemic, tetanus differentiated from,
        156, 157
Thyroid ophthalmopathy, botulinum toxin in
        management of, 192
Tics
    botulinum toxin-A in management of, 338–340
    clinical phenomenology of, 337
    pathophysiology of, 337–338
    vocal, botulinum toxin-A in management of,
        213
TMDs. *See* Temporomandibular disorders
        (TMDs)

Tongue protrusion dystonia (TPD), botulinum
        toxin-A in management of, 347
Tonic-clonic seizures, generalized, tetanus
        differentiated from, 156–157
Torticollis, spasmodic, 259. *See also* Cervical
        dystonia (CD)
Tourette syndrome, pathophysiology of, 337–338
Toxin complex
    serotype A
        antibody mapping studies of, 13–14, 16
        hydrodynamic radius of, 16, 17
        stability of, 11–17
        structure of, 11–17
Toxin translocation in clostridial neurotoxins,
        20–21, 22
Toxoid vaccines, botulinum, 428–431
TPD. *See* Tongue protrusion dystonia (TPD)
Translocation domain, of botulinum neurotoxin-B,
        30, 33
Tremor(s)
    botulinum toxin-A in management of, 323–334
        mechanisms of action for, 334
    head, botulinum toxin-A in management of],
        323–327
    limb, botulinum toxin-A in management of,
        327–330
    palatal, botulinum toxin-A in management of,
        333–334
    voice, botulinum toxin-A in management of,
        330–333
    voice, essential, botulinum toxin-A in
        management of, 213
Trigeminopathy, definition of, 266–267
Trisialoganglioside, binding of botulinum
        neurotoxin to, 75
Trismus in tetanus, 154
Trochlear (IV) nerve paresis, botulinum toxin in
        management of, 192
Tyrosine phosphorylation of botulinum
        neurotoxin-B, 36

U

UBI test. *See* Unilateral brow injection (UBI) test
Unilateral brow injection (UBI) test, in detection
        of immunoresistance to BTX, 410, 411
Urologic disorders, 351–355
    anatomy and physiology of micturition and,
        351–353

V

Vaccination, tetanus, 160–161
Vaccines, for botulism, 427–435
    botulinum toxoid, 428–431
    efficacy of, 432–435
        ELISA in study of, 434–435
    potency of, 432, 433
    recombinant, 431
    regulatory issues and requirements for, 435
VAMP. *See* Vesicle-associated membrane protein
        (VAMP)
Vecuronium, in tetanus management, 159
Ventricular dysphonia, botulinum toxin-A in
        management of, 213–214
Vesicle-associated membrane protein (VAMP), in
        botulinum neurotoxin serotypes, 75
Vocal fold, granuloma of, botulinum toxin-A in
        management of, 214
Vocal fold vibration for speech, 179
Vocal tics, botulinum toxin-A in management of,
        213
Voice tremor
    botulinum toxin-A in management of, 330–333
    essential, botulinum toxin-A in management of,
        213

W

WBA. *See* Western blot assay (WBA)
Weakness, botulinum toxin efficacy and, 167–168
Western blot assay (WBA), in BTX antibody
        detection, 410
WGA. *See* Wheat germ agglutinin (WGA)
Wheat germ agglutinin (WGA), delivery of
        endopeptidase activity of botulinum
        neurotoxin and, 479–480
Wound botulism, toxin production in, 427
Wound débridement, in tetanus management, 159
Wounds, facial, repair of, botulinum toxin-A in,
        292
Writer's cramp, 251–257. *See also* Focal hand
        dystonia

Z

Zinc-endopeptidases, clostridial neurotoxins as,
        29, 55